AF688313

Discovering Life: Homeopathic Portraits

Discovering Life: Homeopathic Portraits

An In-Depth Modern Clinical Materia Medica

Luc De Schepper
M.D., Lic. Ac.

Full of Life Publishing ♦ Santa Fe, NM

DISCLAIMER

The information in this book is presented for informational purposes only. All therapies, treatments, or energetic interventions of any nature should be undertaken only under the direct guidance and care of a properly trained and legally qualified healthcare professional specializing in the service rendered. Nothing described in this book should be construed by any reader or any other person to be a diagnosis or treatment for any disease or condition. Neither the author nor the publisher can accept any responsibility for any ill effects resulting from the use or misuse of the information contained herein. Any uses or misuses of the information presented here for educational purposes are the responsibility of the reader. The names and other identifying characteristics of the persons included in this book have been changed.

CONTACTING THE AUTHOR

The author welcomes feedback from the readers mailed to the publisher's address below. To order other books by Dr. Luc, please visit his website at drluc.com

© 2013 by Luc De Schepper. All rights reserved.
Printed in the United States of America
Full of Life Publishing
P.O. Box 31025
Santa Fe, NM 87594

ISBN-10: 0942501195

ISBN-13: 978-0-942501-19-3

Editing: Amari Barash
Art direction: Yolanda De Schepper

Back cover photo: Dr. Luc in his opening speech at the European Congress of Homeopathy in Riga, Latvia, 2010

DEDICATION

To the Healing of Mankind

Contents

Introduction xi

Part One: The Modern Materia Medica

The Blueprint of the Modern Materia Medica 3
Notes to the Reader 17
Glossary 21

Part Two: Homeopathic Portraits

Aconitum napellus 35
Agaricus muscarius 43
Agnus castus 49
Alumina 55
Ambra grisea 67
Anacardium orientale 73
Argentum nitricum 83
Arsenicum album 91

Aurum foliatum 105
Baryta carbonica 121
Calcarea carbonica 135
Causticum 155
China 167
Cocculus indicus 177
Conium maculatum 189
Cuprum metallicum 197
Fluoricum acidum 203
Gelsemium 211
Graphites 217
Helleborus niger 223
Hyoscyamus 233
Ignatia 247
Kali bromatum 255
Kali carbonicum 263
Lac caninum 277
Lachesis muta 285
Lycopodium clavatum 313
Lyssinum 339
Magnesia carbonica 351
Medorrhinum 357

Mercurius solubilis ... 371
Natrum carbonicum ... 381
Natrum muriaticum ... 391
Nitricum acidum ... 419
Nux vomica ... 429
Petroleum ... 443
Phosphoricum acidum ... 451
Phosphorus ... 459
Platina ... 473
Plumbum metallicum ... 487
Pulsatilla ... 497
Sepia ... 511
Silicea ... 527
Staphysagria ... 543
Stramonium ... 559
Sulphur ... 571
Tarentula hispanica ... 589
Thuja occidentalis ... 603
Veratrum album ... 617

References ... 625

Introduction

As it was at the beginning of the twentieth century, homeopathy is at a crossroads. Students and practitioners of homeopathy are dealing simultaneously with allopathically biased studies and ever-increasing exposure to new approaches in homeopathy that are not always based on sound homeopathic laws and principles. Divergent opinions can and should exist for the sake of progress. However, a truly objective person takes account of objections to his opinions and decides how he proposes to meet them; he discusses rival views and shows why he cannot accept them. Hahnemann was such a person. Unfortunately, people like Hahnemann are often regarded as egotistic, threatening and dogmatic. In homeopathic circles these days, it is much more comfortable to live and let live without criticism. There are always new techniques being espoused in homeopathy with neo-gurus promising an easier way to the simillimum—and yet not only do most of their contributions not add anything, but they increase the noise that drowns out the music and insight of classical homeopathy, impeding its true progress. Too many homeopaths fall into the process of transference, hearing what they want to hear and failing to respond critically. Such neo-gurus make deliberate and conscious use of the very real human tendency toward transference, and they achieve great success by doing so.

Erudition is extensive knowledge acquired chiefly from books. Scholarship involves intellectual self-discipline, which consists of the scrupulous consideration of objections and alternatives. Both are needed in any scientific exploration. But dogmatism is always a threat to such exploration: it blocks the objections and alternatives to any new theory! A truth that has been merely learned adheres at most like transplanted skin, but a truth won by independent thinking can truly be owned. It is my goal, in this materia medica, to make a scholar out of the reader as well as a critical thinker—one who constructs his opinion by collecting the opinions of others, employing in-depth analysis, and laboriously thinking for himself. To develop the skill needed to succeed in today's challenging circumstances, the ideal practitioner should be cautious yet courageous and inquisitive: a born adventurer and discoverer. By discovering life as proposed in this book, practitioners can learn to see patients in a light that will enable them to assist others in living their lives to the fullest. In doing so, they will also come to live their own lives more fully.

Why Portraits?

The descriptions of remedies in this book are akin to artistic portraits: in a portrait, the painter seeks to communicate the psychological and spiritual as well as the physical essence of the subject. This process is analog to finding a remedy by what is described in homeopathic literature as using the totality of symptoms combined with the patient's peculiar and unusual symptoms to find the simillimum. A painted portrait is not the same as a photograph of a person; no photograph can possess the emotional depth of a well-rendered painting. While a snapshot is considered a realistic image, it does not necessarily convey important truths about its subject; furthermore, despite its realism, it might at times even be misleading. A photograph, posed or not, mechanically records an individual's appearance at a particular moment in time. Unlike a snapshot, a portrait is not at war with time; it takes no account of time's succession, because it captures the sitter's multifaceted inner reality. And just as the classically trained homeopath carefully observes his patient, a painter observes his subject for hours in his studio so that during the sitting a range of traits, emotions, and expressions are translated to the canvas—producing a fuller and deeper understanding of the human being, both physically and psychologically. A variety of life's milestones can be described, some imposed by fate, others through individual choice, but all form the intricate story of layers of human life. From a homeopathic perspective, the most important reason to paint a portrait rather than take a snapshot (that is to say, to prescribe based on the essence and totality of the picture) is that a portrait alone seeks to describe a soul. The portraits of homeopathic remedies in this book describe not just what Jung refers to as the *persona*; they also describe the sitter's Self.

During the time a homeopath spends with his patient, noting details gathered over many hours of observation, he can come to know things not apparent on the surface—the way the person expresses himself, the manner of his behavior towards others, the tendency to exaggerate facts or minimize them, bringing what is underneath to the surface. Spending time with patients allows them to unfold. The portraits in this book are based upon countless hours spent with a variety of patients presenting many aspects and facets of each particular remedy. I try to thoughtfully and completely present the intricacies of each remedy portrait, based on reliable provings of the Masters but also expanded with descriptions of the psychological and philosophical aspects of the person who visits the homeopath in a particular remedy state.

Most people are unable either to penetrate the unconscious aspects of the human mind or understand the enigmatic message of dreams; for the majority, then, the unconscious remains forbidden and dangerous terrain. Generally speaking, much of the ego's conscious content is therefore relegated to the shadow side in an effort to protect the integrity of the ego—because the suppressed content is too hurtful and shameful to bear. Hopefully, the soul-penetrating portraits in this work will provide a basis for revealing this hidden territory: a start on the road to Self-realization.

The Role of Free Will

Free will is an individual's ability to make choices between good and evil; thinkers have written many volumes that question the extent to which life is an exercise of choice. Some allopathic scientists, including the well-respected author and physician Oliver Sachs (a front-runner in the field of neurology), think that every choice we make is predetermined by the neurophysiology of the brain. In contrast, the eminent psychologist Viktor Frankl, the father of logotherapy, who spent years in concentration camps during World War II, thought that he and his fellow inmates—despite their dire constraints—had a choice between trying to survive and purposely running to their deaths into the electrical barbed wire fences. Frankl thought the prisoner spiritually responsible for what was happening to him psychically regardless of his circumstances. So how does homeopathic science differ from the allopathic determinism postulated by Sachs or from the psychological constructs described by Frankl in explaining the behaviors of individual prisoners?

If we were to examine the family background of each of the camp inmates homeopathically, it would become apparent that each individual's predominantly activated miasmatic state influenced some to show life-affirming behaviors and others to do the opposite. This scientific approach applies when any powerfully negative event takes place, shaking a person's status quo and providing circumstances for positive change—or for ruin. For some, catastrophe leads to a life of depression and despairing drunkenness (syphilitic miasm); others choose to live a life of thrill-seeking and reckless behavior (sycosis); still others choose to become better people by looking for help or by becoming helpers themselves (psoric miasm). The willingness and ability to take on the challenge of constructive change as a new reality in life is one of the major differences between those who grow through adversity (psoric miasm) and those who are destroyed by it (sycotic and syphilitic miasms). Carl Jung expressed this concept by stating that, in the case of constitution and temperament, the patient cannot elect his response to a specific situation, especially in reaction to a strongly loaded emotional event (or in a *highly feeling-toned complex*); Jung described such reactions as predetermined hereditary fixed response patterns. Individuals who do not undergo therapeutic genetic (miasmatic) intervention remain under the powerful influence of their unique miasmatic backgrounds.

Generally speaking, our society instructs its members from a young age about moral questions and the difference between right and wrong; how, then, can we explain increasingly violent behavior in our culture, especially among young children and teenagers? The incidence of heinous acts being committed by youth, including mass murder, has escalated at an alarming rate in the last decade. With each devastating occurrence, the same questions in the media pop up: How can this happen? How can we prevent it from happening again? Then, purported experts in human behavior and science start beating the same old drum of examining genetic testing, environmental factors, and the perpetrator's upbringing. It is akin to examining a cadaver in search of a soul. Allopathic science can offer no true insights into why such acts are occurring, and the solutions proposed run the usual gamut of banning weapons and identifying potential offenders early by means of better psychiatric diagnosis, ubiquitous labeling, and early treatment with a stupefying cornucopia of prescription drugs. Yet, even if properly identified, what would the solution be within a system that offers only suppression in the sense of legal and medical intervention? Society's failure to curtail the spread of the violence epidemic is not only reflective of a lack of understanding of free will; it also provides evidence of the failure of allopathic medical treatments to rectify or even assuage the abnormal moral code (syphilitic miasmatic predominance) apparently followed by those who perpetrate horrible events. By contrast, a homeopath knowledgeable in miasmatic management possesses the tools to restore the patient's native soil to health and to remove the blockage produced by his genetic background, allowing the indicated remedy to work in a timely and effective manner.

Awakening Consciousness

The scientific mainstream acknowledges that even animals and plants share part of the universal consciousness on a rudimentary level. Modern science is making strides in demonstrating that animals and plants have some degree of feelings and awareness, verified by the fact that animals such as dogs, dolphins, cats, and others demonstrate certain levels of emotion and intelligence. However, the consciousness of most human beings is still dormant or, rather, partially unused, as man relegates about half of his consciousness (awareness of shameful, sad, and truly shocking events—things we are afraid of) to the unconscious. Consequently, he is unable to develop his full potential as a spiritual being unless he can integrate the dark elements of the unconscious into his consciousness; this is a process that is met by formidable resistance in most. Although the spark of consciousness is latent in every human psyche, most of mankind, unaware of it, walks the world in a state of somnambulism, mesmerized by the mechanical external manifestation of our own subconscious creations.

Although the brilliant Carl Jung mapped the psyche and sought to understand the individual in his totality in order to release him from the bondage of the Cyber delusion (CD), Jung's psychoanalytic tools were limited. This fact resulted in significant losses of time in removing obstructions from patients' psyches. And five millennia before Jung, Traditional Chinese Medicine (TCM), through its energetic intervention as an empirical science, recognized different blockages and could remove them through an array of therapies (acupuncture, moxibustion, and herbology). But TCM, although it shares many principles with homeopathy such as the emphasis on individuality and the approach to the direction of the cure, differs from homeopathy in that it cannot address the genetic (miasmatic) background; it also lacks the specificity required to address the subtle differences among emotions. For instance, an emotion such as fear is addressed in TCM with a correction of the Kidney imbalance, but no differentiation in treatment is made for different kinds of fear: fear of crowds, the future, disease, the dark, lightning, failure in business, etc. Homeopathy is capable of matching more than one remedy to each kind of fear, with every remedy, again, showing a subtle difference from the others; in this way, homeopathy accomplishes the identification of the remedy closest to the clinical picture of the patient (the simillimum). It was Hahnemann, in 1816, through erudition as well as the attainment of clinical success with miasmatic theory, who pinpointed the deviation from the normal moral code, or the lack of guilt, in unwell individuals and started the road to explaining and preventing the horrible events that seem to proliferate in humankind today. Hahnemann's theory remains unknown to allopathy.

The Role of Psychotherapy

An important question often arises in our quest to help patients along their path of individuation and health: in addition to homeopathic treatment, should the patient be referred to an experienced (non-homeopathic) psychotherapist? In examining this important question, we must first determine what the term "experienced" means. Too often, this word is used simply to refer to the length of time spent in the profession; such usage assumes (often wrongly) that experience equates to proficiency. While length of experience might be an important criterion when searching for a car mechanic, barber, trial lawyer, or restaurant chef, experience alone does not qualify the psychotherapist, physician, or homeopath to whom you are considering entrusting your mind and body. Many health care providers have been dogmatically instructed in schools that fail to focus on critical thinking; these providers have passed through a system that awards credentials based on rote and conformity and, unfortunately, have learned little about curing their patients either in their schooling or in their subsequent practices. As Jung asserted: "The study of medicine consists on the one hand in storing up in the mind an enormous number of facts, which are simply memorized without any real knowledge of their foundations, and on the other hand in learning practical skills, which have to be acquired on the principle 'Don't think, act!' Thus it is that, of all the professionals, the medical man has the least opportunity of developing the function of *thinking*."[1]

The *Diagnostic and Statistical Manual of Mental Disorders* (*DSM*) has spawned a culture of simplistic diagnosis. It is a rather crude approach and concludes that the seat of psychiatric illness is the brain (which encourages the performance of numerous specialized brain tests). Unfortunately, to the detriment of millions, this approach ignores the crucial aspect of the development of consciousness, which contributes to the incapacity of allopathy to differentiate between justified sadness as a result of losses, deception, betrayal, and other noble misfortunes (as Traditional Chinese Medicine [TCM] calls them) and clinical depression without any apparent basis. Allopathic treatments turn the patient's mind into a commodity for the pharmacological and health insurance world. Gone is any real connection to the patient. The lumping of individual patients into categories and the ignoring of their individual expressions remain the biggest tragedies perpetrated by allopathy; these errors are committed in the interest of consolidating manifold issues under a common name with a prefabricated

1. Carl G. Jung, *Dreams*, trans. R.F.C. Hull (Princeton University Press, 1974), 63.

diagnosis and standard of care, thus violating the sacred principle of individuality. Suppression of the patient's symptomatic disease expressions through heavily toxic medication kills the soul. Loving attentiveness to stricken souls (physically and especially psychically) would be far more effective, and the gentle homeopathic remedies that treat disease roots should replace the mind-numbing poisons of allopathic medications.

While it is tempting to want to believe that the mental health community knows how to assist a patient once a (possibly elusive) diagnosis is assigned, this is unfortunately usually not the case; furthermore, psychiatric diagnostic labeling is often the beginning of additional difficulties and suffering, creating a far deeper layer of both psychic and physical harm and yet another obstacle to overcome for an already weakened patient. Rarely does anyone practicing Western medicine address the issue of the impact of assigning diagnostic labels to a suffering individual; it remains certain that allopathic medicine has not been able to indicate how a label helps the patient.

DSM-II (The *Diagnostic and Statistical Manual*, appearing in 1968) contained 297 categories, and *DSM-V* (appearing in 2013) contains 374. Logically speaking, the increase in the number of categories and the amount research entailed in arriving at such revelations over the last 45 years should connote a commensurate increase in successful cures and treatments. Alas, this is most certainly not the case. Why should so much new knowledge yield so little fruit? One must consider the possibility that the inherent fundamentals undergirding the "Bible" of mental health diagnosis are wrong, and that no amount of legitimate fact-gathering or categorizing laid upon a faulty foundation can produce a cure. But what is wrong with the theoretical foundation upon which the *DSM* rests? It follows the same allopathic model that relies upon suppressive medication. Such so-called treatment suppresses or extinguishes symptoms while not only missing but often deepening the root of the disease in the process. This reflects a reliance on a linear Newtonian approach when, in fact, the living human organism is more correctly treated with the quantum approach taken by the medical sciences of both homeopathy and Traditional Chinese Medicine.

When the National Institute of Mental Health, a seat of power driving world mental health policy, decided to break from the *DSM-V*, its director declared that the brain is the "alleged seat and cause of psychiatric suffering" and announced the decision to put NIMH's research dollars into a new classification system—the Research Domain Criteria (RDoC)—with the intention of incorporating genetics, imaging, and cognitive science and focusing more on neurological systems rather than just constellations of symptoms. RDoC would classify psychopathology based on observable behavior and neurobiological measures. With this materia medica, I hope to strengthen the ability of the homeopath to hold true to the laws and principles of homeopathy—even in the face of our modern epidemics—by framing the remedy portraits within the modern context and by means of using a model of consciousness, with an emphasis on exploring the **mind** of the patient.

Presently, the majority of physicians habitually and reflexively dole out prescriptions based upon what is called, in medical jargon, standard of care. So it is with psychotherapists. Certain fixed diagnoses (name-giving) are treated with such-and-such approach, learned according to this-and-that theory, according to the book that represents the guideline of a particular school of thought (hence the *DSM*). Clinging to authoritarian theories and techniques that cannot move a patient forward hinders the development of independent and critical thought. Most practitioners refuse—which is to say, are afraid—to step away from dogmatic beliefs, and to the detriment of themselves and their patients, they never veer from one-sided, sectarian exclusiveness of thought. The temperament, constitution, and life story of a psychotherapist (and of a practitioner in any other medical field) influences her treatment of patients if she has not looked at and treated herself holistically—in other words, as one entity consisting of mind, body, and spirit. I have observed that psychotherapists often enter their profession as a result of youthful experiences and traumas; these must be resolved before commencing clinical practice, else such events continue to roam in the unconscious, inadvertently putting patients in danger of projection or transference from the therapist.

As in any context, the good and the not-so-good exist side by side in the medical profession; just as there are more Volkswagens than Rolls-Royces, the truly excellent and thorough practitioner is a rarity. I believe that a practitioner deserves to be called excellent when he has developed knowledge, sympathy or empathy, energy, objectivity, discipline, immersion in the profession, patience, and, above all, a love of people. For the excellent practitioner, every patient is an individual, a new puzzle—new and different at each step of that person's ongoing treatment. Concentration is also a necessary condition for the mastery of an art, one that is a rare commodity in our culture. A good practitioner shows respect for the individual and for the very principles of respect; as such, she restrains from interfering with a patient's domain of choice and wholeheartedly assists a person even if he should later choose a different mode of treatment. This is yet another component of the ethics that a healer should follow: responsiveness (*respondere*, from the Latin *pons*, or bridge, and *ponder*, or weighty: constructing a weighty bridge to the patient). Responsiveness is answering by making a weighty bridge, one that can withstand the weights of prejudice, self-interest, and boredom in order to attend to another's need and reality. There is also the ethics of caring for all people (and for all living things), the Golden Rule of Humanity as announced by Confucius (6th century B.C.): do no harm, and do unto others as you would do unto those you love.

Unfortunately, human values are too often undermined by economic rules and needs, and the medical profession has not been immune to these: like others, physicians routinely concern themselves with overhead and stock performance as well as their desires to buy new homes and other material items; our culture creates economic incentives for the practitioner, and these often pose the greatest obstacle to excellent treatment. For example, a psychotherapist has the clock in front of him, and at the end of the hour, the journey has just begun—often with no end in sight. The patient is now further bound to his past: grievances, traumas, and other misfortunes have become part of the luggage on his back, and as such, he continues to be controlled and influenced by the contents of that baggage. The real question should be and remain: How do we get rid of the baggage? How do we integrate unconscious contents into consciousness?

According to Aphorism 2 of the *Organon*, this integration should be done rapidly, gently, and permanently. Does psychotherapy fulfill these criteria? The criterion of gentleness is the most likely to be met; there are wonderful therapists who, in many instances having experienced trauma themselves, will carefully handle the tragic issues of the wounded patient. The other two criteria (rapidity and permanence) of Aphorism 2, though, pose a grave problem in the context of the practice of psychotherapy. Due to the limits of the medical tool chest available to him, even Carl Jung, whom I consider to be one of the greatest geniuses of all time, routinely followed schizophrenic and psychotic patients for many years. And although he often understood them well, some of these patients descended further into the hell of their delusions with no rescue in sight. Don't think for a moment that Jung would have approved of the use of mind-numbing allopathic drugs; he often expressed how much he valued the individuality of his patients. Clearly, the psychotherapeutic process takes substantial time, commitment, and money! Many obstacles remain in this process. The true roots of problems remain undiscovered or unrecognized in allopathic medicine while the suppression of symptoms substitutes for treatment—and this is one of the lesser obstacles in the path of true treatment.

Another challenge is that the patient's own point of view is always somewhat distorted and incomplete, and the psychotherapist's suggestions can lead to the danger of incorporating and transferring those intimations. In turn, this can result in the fabrication of a story, maybe even a myth with little truth, which both parties can ponder for years to come as the story fails to integrate the dark elements from the unconscious into consciousness. Does one need to understand every piece of the past story in order to move on, to make peace with the past? I don't think that hours and hours talking about the past encourages a healthy focus on the present. Certainly, dreams understood can reveal a patient's progress on his individuation path, and they may suggest various possibilities as to how a patient might endeavor to become more complete, but dreams almost never reveal a single, clearly indicated correct solution. Another potential obstacle is that many therapists are either *Nat-mur* or *Calc-carb* personalities, and when studying these portraits, the reader will become aware that persons in these states often have a propensity for mulling things over. Such an approach encourages patients to haunt the past, sniffing it like a bloodhound and tracking it relentlessly. In such circumstances, a patient originally injured in the soul and haunted by an event can experience stagnation (*stagnation of thoughts* [Nat-m]), as indicated by the rubric *sad thoughts persistent* and *haunted by unpleasant thoughts of* (Nat-m); now, *he talks about nothing but murder, fire and rats* (Calc-c). It is the task of every healer involved with a patient in such a state to move her forward in accordance with the principles set forth in Aphorism 2, to move them away from this dark fantasyland and break the chains that bind them to their demons while focusing on living in the present and organizing the future. Homeopathic remedies and the suggestion of new meaning in life will help the patient to reach these goals more quickly. A good therapist does not befriend the patient through commiseration; rather, he is eager to move the patient forward with whatever good techniques he possesses. Hopefully, he also refers the patient to a good homeopath so that the healing process can evolve according to Aphorism 2 of the *Organon* without descending into unhealthy rumination about the past. The good therapist puts the central focus on objectivity, alertness, and openness, allowing him to do transforming work so that patients can make their own decisions about moving on with life rather than feeling that they need permission to do so.

The Study of Disease in This Materia Medica

Our patients drive us to ask questions that require answers. The construction of the portraits in this book can illuminate answers in a clear manner based on the real provings of the Masters. Though every homeopathic remedy portrait has a story with a beginning, a middle, and an end, the patient's story will have a distortion. As a practitioner, according to a basic tenet, you will see that the pattern in that distortion most resembles a particular portrait. The power of the Cyber delusion often holds a person in its chains and captures him in a vicious cycle until the Cyber delusion is broken by the judicious dosing and intake of the individually indicated remedy. As practitioners of allopathic medicine, we learn the conception of disease together with the idea that diseases follow a course from their onset to their climax or crisis, followed either by a happy or a fatal resolution; however, allopathic case histories tell us nothing about an individual or about that individual's true prognosis. Allopathic collections of data often reveal nothing of the experience of the person struggling to survive his disease, nor do they take into account the actions of the Vital Force in its attempts to reorganize the chaos produced by fixed ideas. Modern science approaches human beings with a *soulless medicine and a bodiless psychology*, and because of this, a comprehensive understanding of disease is absent. What cannot be not accommodated in the conventional framework of medicine disappears mysteriously and is forgotten, else it is entirely replaced with a new name. The old disease gives birth to a radical new disease: allopathic medications have the potential, for example, to carry the patient from stupor to the other end of the spectrum with tics and frenzy, resulting in the need to name a new disease.

To get to the crux of a patient's suffering, we must deepen our approach to each case with a narrative that reflects three elements: the motor and drive, or libido, behind his thoughts and actions (expressed by the CD); the causality that allowed the CD to prosper in the first place; and the ways in which the individual deals with his suffering (his compensations). The study of disease and identity/individuality cannot be disjoined. As Hahnemann asserted, there are no diseases—there are just patients with diseases! Sir William Osler, the famed early-twentieth-century allopathic doctor and professor, echoed the same principle: "The good physician treats the disease. The great physician treats the patient who has the disease." The study of the onset of disease also demands the study of the inner world that a patient creates spurred of the deregulation of her Vital Force. We don't just examine the outside of the patient by observing her behavior; the homeopath must also try to get inside. The portraits in this book, based on the true provings of each remedy included, reveal not only the physical, mental, and emotional foundations of the persona, but also the mysterious tale of the shadow side as presented in the clinic. Every sickness is a musical decomposition, and every cure is a musical composition. The experience of recovery is not unlike a coming out, a process in which the patient—with judiciously applied doses of the simillimum—begins to peek out from an enclosed world and reach a place of clarity where he is suddenly freed from the fixed ideas of the Cyber delusion. These portraits are individuals, each of whom inhabits a world of his own. In order to understand more of the disease-provoking potential of the CD, in the next chapter, "Blueprint of the Modern Materia Medica," we will study the birth and dissolution of the CD.

What is New in This Materia Medica?

What makes this materia medica different from others? Why a new materia medica among the glut of existing ones? One of the most confounding aspects of homeopathy, which I have noticed while teaching throughout the world, is the difficulty that both students and experienced practitioners have in translating the language of the patient into the language of the materia medica. This book addresses that need. This is done partly through sharing observations with creative in-depth applications, avoiding a sterile accumulation of statistical facts that would add nothing to the truths and knowledge of health and disease in the human body. A pure citation of the proving symptoms without in-depth analysis would, likewise, offer too little explanation to apply in the daily practice. In addition to providing practical information that is both accurate and rich in detail, this book also addresses a major issue of the old materia medica: the use of cryptic language which does not always resonate with our present idiom. For instance, in *Hering's Guiding Symptoms*, we can read in the provings for the same remedy both "taciturn" and "loquacious"—on the same page. What can the student of homeopathy do with this information? How does one deal with this apparent inconsistency? The addressing of the dominant miasmatic state of the patient when he presents in the clinic leads to ready understanding of such an apparent contradiction; these expressions refer to behaviors that take place in two different miasmatic states (syphilitic and sycotic).

Some modern materia medicas, in their attempts to offer something new, take the road of the esoteric and speculative, disconnecting entirely from the old provings—a mortal sin in clinical homeopathic application. Others simply take on most of the Masters' cryptic and archaic language without adding anything to it but a few small nuggets from their own clinical findings. The result is that such materia medicas remain, at best, obscure for the modern practitioner; at worst, they may be dangerously misleading. In other words, remedies need to be able to reveal their stories through illumination with additional languages—those of philosophy, psychology, and TCM—while confirming the real provings of the Masters. In such a manner, using accessible vocabulary and describing situations directly applicable in a contemporary clinic, this book tells a fuller, more accurate, and more individual story for each remedy.

This book offers a solution to the difficulties the homeopath encounters in the practice through the application of in-depth, modern psychology and philosophy to the Masters' proving symptoms. By learning how to translate the patient's common language into the language of this materia medica, the practitioner will greatly facilitate her work in the clinical setting. This book is the first materia medica to present modern, cohesive stories about remedies: it is as if the patient were present on consult. The rubrics in the *Essential Synthesis*, as well as Hering's and T.F. Allen's proving symptoms, are used as references. Provings are primarily from Hering's *The Guiding Symptoms of the Materia Medica,* with some exceptions: T.F. Allen is indicated, Kent's *Lectures on Materia Medica*, other rubrics can be found in *The Essential Synthesis , Edited by F. Schroyens, Homeopathic Book Publishers and Archibel S.A., 2007* (indicated by their intensity).

I have added live cases from the clinic in some remedy portraits in order to make the descriptions even more accurate and vivid; rubrics corresponding to patients' statements are added in the text in italics. (Intimate details about these cases are omitted to protect patient privacy.) The connection with the enigmatic language and symbols of dreams is also broached in this materia medica; it provides a homeopath's introduction to seeing dreams, in an accurate context, for what they are: messengers from the unconscious presenting a view that enlarges, completes, or compensates the conscious attitude. It is beyond the scope of this book to elaborate on dream interpretation (which will be the subject of a future book). But the reader will become aware that dreams are indeed an unconscious reaction to a conscious, individual situation, confirming individuality as a sacred homeopathic principle.

Throughout the portraits, differential diagnoses with common complementary remedies are analyzed, again facilitating the homeopath's work in the clinic by encouraging an understanding of the fine nuances of remedies in the same rubric. Delusions, rather than possessing obscure meanings, are explained and often grouped in a central theme so that their enigmatic message truly becomes the beginning of the remedy's story. Initially, in my student years, I buried myself in thousands of the Masters' papers that were stored in the belly of the medical library at the University of Michigan in Ann Arbor—the place where Kent once taught homeopathy. I then put the information together for my own use in a manuscript I called *Gems and Pearls*; this manuscript was available to some of my students, but I never published it officially. These wonderful tips from the practices of the Masters deal mainly with the physical aspects of disease (without neglecting the emotional and the picture as a whole) as homeopathy at that time was (as it still is) far ahead of allopathy when it came to conquering common daily illnesses as well as epidemics of measles, scarlatina, pertussis, typhoid fever, dysentery, malaria, cholera, and others. For the first time, this information is now added and expanded to each portrait to enhance the full picture and to present characteristic, clinically proven physical indications for both acute and chronic conditions of the remedy in question. You will find them under the heading "Golden Tips from the Masters" at the end of each portrait. It must be said, as a reminder, that these clinical tips in no way indicate specific remedies for specific diseases: as always, the totality of the symptoms must be taken into account before prescribing the simillimum. The Golden Tips, though, often serve as a key to unlock the creaky gate to a true treasure.

Why I wrote This Book

My life as a physician, for four decades now, has been dedicated to helping people who are misunderstood, abandoned, and often even tossed aside. Children have always had a special place in my heart. I started medical school in Belgium in 1964. Seven years later, I was one of 36 left of the 770 we started with in the first year. Medical school indeed allows the survival of only the fittest; it is a breeding ground of high competition, disregarding empathy and fellowship in pursuit of one of the few final places. It is indeed an ironic training for people who are supposed to become compassionate healers. Upon graduating and after being wined and dined by the pharmaceutical companies in France and Belgium, I started private practice. Having been programmed by scientific medical dogma for seven years, and believing wholeheartedly that allopathic medicine was the only medicine that merited any consideration, I was jolted into reality on my very first day of practice. Shortly thereafter, I was forced to recognize what little difference I was making in my patients' lives and was deeply disillusioned. I remember my first cases as if they were yesterday. My first real patient (not counting the case of my dog, who loved food and would swallow anything I presented) was a 15-year-old girl with a complaint of chronic headaches. Her headaches were triggered by weather changes, which was unfortunate as the weather in Belgium changes about four times a day throughout the year. She thought, after having tried all the existing medications, that this new young gun (me!) fresh out of medical school would have the latest answers and solutions. Of course I had none.

The next patient was a lady in her forties whose face is still etched in my memory. She had suddenly lost her speech after witnessing the death of her best friend. Countless therapies had failed before she came to me, and for the grace of God, I had no idea why she came to me as I had no answer either. Now, I believe that this was an important message for me: these cases exposed me from the beginning to the fact that conventional medicine had great limitations, even with regard to understanding patients. Unconsciously, I understood that the Newtonian physics on which conventional medicine is built was too linear. The patient is approached like a sum of auto parts, a physical machine being put together, and whenever there is one part malfunctioning, only that part needs to be fixed. Such a reductionist, linear approach cannot give us an accurate understanding of disease and health. I realized that I had to start thinking out of the box, and from my readings in quantum physics, I thought it more logical to assume that there is always an interaction between all body parts: when one part is sick, other parts are "derailed" also. This is the only truly *holistic view*.

The combination of caring, boredom, restlessness, and wanting to be able to understand those mystery cases threw me forcefully in another direction, as if I had been picked up by a sudden twister. I wanted to free myself of the blinders of modern civilization's dogmatic beliefs and was about to challenge the sacred foundations of Western medicine. On the spur of the moment, I entered two three-year schools of Traditional Chinese Medicine (TCM) in Amsterdam and Paris at the same time. By academic standards, I became a radical, a medical heretic, leaving the ivory tower of science in which I had dwelled for seven years. Some of my friends openly questioned if I had suffered a head trauma. Had a coconut fallen on my head before I had even set foot in Africa? Some suggested that I move to the United States (which I eventually did), because I sounded to them like the rattlesnake oil salesmen from the Old West. But I was determined to put the spiritual wisdom of ancient modalities into the equation to improve my patients' mental and physical health. It was in Holland and in France that I was exposed to the possibilities of homeopathy, a science that caught my attention because of its simplicity, efficacy, and cost effectiveness: a combination that would make it possible for me to fulfill my dream of providing health care to the poorest around the world, even as a single individual.

Finally, in my fifties, when my children left the nest, I was able to begin teaching and helping the poor in S. Africa and Kenya, India, China, and Sri Lanka among other places. It was in those simple worlds that I learned the most about sharing, love and respect for Nature, and the hardships that women and children confront on a daily basis. To this day I have not regretted the change of my life's course. On the contrary, I feel that I have earned far more appreciation from my patients and derived far more satisfaction than I ever could have dreamed of if I had remained an allopathic physician. Nature and its Laws have been and will remain my teachers. I know that I received the greatest reward on earth: that of a life based on service to others. I will always remember the immortal words of Dr. Samuel Hahnemann, the founder of homeopathy: "I did not live in vain." This is the only legacy that I, too, wish to leave.

The catastrophe of the sick individual should move us all. It should move us in both senses of the word: touching our feelings and impelling us to action because something amazing can be achieved. This awareness must refer to the human being as a whole, not to her isolated and fractured features. It is not enough to be aware of the effects of toxic elements in our environment (internal and external), of the weakening of humans in the last decades, and of the abnormal findings or biomarkers that result from in-depth investigations. It is necessary to become aware that all these features are part of an individual's system—a system that must inevitably express itself. We must thoroughly understand that nothing is achieved if one fights isolated symptoms and suppresses them; rather, one must change the background, the metaphorical soil in which those symptoms are rooted. The understanding of one part of man entails an understanding of each other part, which requires great flexibility of thinking. We have to become aware that we must return to Nature, be guided by its infallible laws, and liberate ourselves from technologies that promise to dissect and reduce the human being to the smallest possible particle but that neglect to look at the human being as a totality that is actually very different from a mere summation of all its components.

Dissecting the patient to his smallest fibers is nothing but dehumanizing him: real changes can only be achieved through the integration of all his parts: physical, emotional, mental, and spiritual. Awareness should lead to alternatives. If only the false statement that there *are* no real alternatives is made, there can be no rational and adequate action to change the status quo. The field of medicine must still learn to follow the examples set by physics and biology, to embrace the quantum paradigm! I hope that this book will awaken people to the fact that there do exist true alternatives—real possibilities of improving the lives of countless individuals in our generation and in those to come! The alternative is a true revolution in science and medicine, a revolution that paradoxically confirms the veracity of the old proven sciences of homeopathy and TCM as effective models of healing. The alternative suggested here is that of radical changes in science and medicine to be achieved by converting a large segment of present and future physicians. We must put an end to the present situation in which a healthy pharmaceutical economy is possible only at the cost of unhealthy human beings. Every homeopath has the opportunity, without doing harm to himself, to conduct a short proving of remedies upon himself, or at the least to take the remedy indicated for his imperfections—because there is nothing like trying it on your own body if you want to grasp what a given remedy can do!

I hope that this book will be a tool for the homeopath to remain composed and inquisitive in the face of many mystery illnesses, and that it will help with whatever difficulty he may face: be it a despairing, out of balance, or angry patient, or trying to make sense of a complicated clinical case. This book is meant to help the homeopath to remain the Sherlock Holmes he has to be without falling into emotional traps; only in this way can he retain and hone his power and his reasoning abilities.

Part One:
The Modern Materia Medica

Blueprint of the Modern Materia Medica

In the homeopathic practice, we are confronted daily with the need to make a differential diagnosis between two or more remedies. To do so, we require a more structured and narrative picture of those remedies—still and only based upon the reliable provings of the Masters. In addition to the Golden Tips from the Masters, the other three parts of the structure of the portraits—the Cyber delusion, causalities and compensations—are explained in this section.

The Cyber Delusion

Definition

Cyber delusion (CD) comes from the Greek *cybernetes*, meaning "the helmsman": he who steers the ship and constantly adjusts the tiller of the ship in response to the information obtained from the environment. The helmsman is the Cyber delusion or fixed idea that steers the ship, the sum of the personal unconscious and conscious. Most people are only partially aware of the conscious part of their life and completely unaware of their unconscious forces, so the CD, hidden and roaming in the vast unconscious darkness, steers and dictates the ego, master of the conscious (the tiller). It is in the unconscious, in other words, that the CD hides in the shadow side, the dark and neglected side of each person that in reality steers man's consciousness! This is quite a frightening thought, considering that this CD is repressed or unacknowledged by most and therefore remains primitive and archaic. So a rather primitive and unsophisticated entity is the orchestrator and conductor of man's life. The perfect road to individuation, to becoming a psychologically balanced individual, would (of course) go in a straight line; this, however, is never possible, even for those few who have the introspection and the courage to investigate their shadow sides. Even individuals who are truly spiritual will often fall off the proverbial wagon when circumstances force them to operate in their inferior conscious function (see further).

So this forceful entity, the CD, dictates everything you think (mental), everything you feel (emotional), and everything your body feels (physical); in other words, the CD is the director of your holistic mind-body entity. The Cyber delusion is the impetus of the individual's every thought and action and becomes part of the shadow, an archetype hidden in the unconscious of the individual that contains everything that is too painful, shameful, or negative for her to deal with.

One can also be dominated by a false or negative Cyber delusion. Many people cling to dreams that they lack the talent to achieve and waste their entire lives chasing them. Many people, in the grips of their CD, get goose bumps all over when they announce their big plans to become the next famous actor, author, athlete, or singer. They are convinced that they have extraordinary talents that they don't see in other people but that others will surely recognize in them. When this is not the case, it is the task of the good homeopath to help such a person fall softly—but not far—and land—but not hard—on the comforting, carpeted floor called the truth. It is homeopathy's goal to make clear to the patient his own hidden contents (his shadow) to be integrated into consciousness, rather than putting the shining light solely on the part visible to others: the mask, or persona, which is only one half and often even less than that of a person's real existence!

Birth of the CD

Every emotional state produces an alteration of consciousness. That is to say, a certain decrease of consciousness is produced as well as a corresponding strengthening of the unconscious. Jung's work on dementia praecox, as published in *The Psychogenesis of Mental Disease,* presents a useful definition of delusion as well as a further approach to its understanding. As René Masselon, a contemporary of Carl Jung, pointed out in *Psychology of Dementia Praecox,* we can clearly see that "certain memories, once intimately connected with important events of the patient's life [such as heartbreak, great fear, and strong incidences of indignation like that caused by rape, etc.], tend to reproduce themselves and occupy the patient's conscious mind continually. [...] By continually reproducing themselves, **such thoughts tend to coagulate** and there is the formation of emotional impoverishment."[1] In Jungian terms, this is the perfect

1. C.G. Jung, *Psychology of Dementia Praecox*, trans. R.F.C. Hull (Princeton University Press, 1960), 12. Emphasis added.

definition of delusions, stereotyped ideas, or *idées fixes*. One extreme situation is the schizophrenic person's coagulation of his mental life with the passive registration of events in his immediate environment: an *abaissement du niveau mental* (literally, a "lowering of the mental level," a term coined by Pierre Janet in 1889 in *L'Automatisme psychologique*), or what Jung called a consciousness disintegration.

Any one of us might have the feeling at some point in our lives that we are all alone in this world and that no one cares about us (isolation through betrayal by a spouse or best friend, the loneliness of an immigrant, or the differences and frustrations that accompany a physical handicap, to name a few examples), but most often this is a fleeting moment: not a delusion, but an illusion. A delusion is an illusion in an advanced state. In our homeopathic repertory, we often find the same remedies under both rubrics (delusion and illusion), and it is really a matter of intensity. If, months or even years after the fact, a psychological trauma still evokes the sentiment that I am all alone in the world and no one cares about me, and if all of my actions and thoughts are ruled by this notion, then it can be defined as a delusion. Such a fixed idea dominates the life of the patient; everything he thinks, does, and plans is fueled by that delusion. It is this state of distracted attention that creates a sort of consciousness vacuum in which certain ideas, especially fixed ones, can penetrate more easily than in periods of full attention when many stimuli are stored in the conscious. This creates a vicious cycle for the patient who is already submerged in his Cyber delusion. The patient's psychic activity tends to turn inwards, driving an unending elaboration of the same thought, thus building up the force of the Cyber delusion. This process takes place in very much the same fashion that a tropical storm gains strength blowing over the sea (a relative fixed symbol that equates to unconscious life) and attains the status of a class five hurricane unless it downgrades when landfall occurs (equating to the return of consciousness, when the ferocity of the psychic thought process decreases).

The strong delusion of being unloved, for example, hinders concentration; the patient is unable to tear himself away from it and to funnel his activity and interest into other, more positive and productive channels. Once there is consciousness lowering and disintegration, delusions are created and then freed from all restraint; they are, therefore, able to occupy the ego-consciousness. As the delusional ideas obstruct the patient's rational thoughts, he becomes unable to exert control over his ideas; thus, the delusions can no longer be eliminated from the conscious process. They remain fully operative and prevent further personality development as well as keeping the patient from fully understanding and enjoying life. This process shows how the patient becomes a prisoner of his delusional thoughts, especially the Cyber delusion, over and over again.

These fixed thoughts, which are often morbid, overcome the patient and have powers of their own that are hard to control. One will observe that most delusions or fixed ideas come from fixed emotions. Recurrent or long-lasting unresolved emotions are apt to create patterns in our brains, memories that will be triggered by the slightest, even innocent, insinuation. Eventually, we maintain these particular emotions—anger that flares up easily, involuntary weeping, a sense of anguish and foreboding, obsessive-compulsive behavior, etc.—because we have become addicted to them and they have become part of our personality (in the language of our repertory, *thoughts, persistent*)!

The psychological trauma that can create, amongst other conditions, OCD, autism, and a host of other behavioral disturbances such as violence, intolerance to contradiction, dictatorial behavior, and so on, often originates at a very young age. The extent to which the word "young" is used here should not be underestimated as it can include intrauterine emotional events. Allopathy has still not linked the emotions of the pregnant mother to the unborn fetus, even though we see the results of unfortunate intrauterine trauma in many of our young patients. As a result, for many diseases, such as OCD or violent (even murderous) behavior in children, the homeopath can answer the two most important questions that allopathy always fails to address: "What is the cause of this behavior?" and "Is there an effective therapy for my child?" These questions also hold true for many adults with similar conditions.

One must keep in mind that, in order to preserve human health, a small quantity of sorrow, fear, anger, or want is required at all times—just as a ship needs a ballast to maintain stability. This is well known in Traditional Chinese Medicine (TCM), but it is now confirmed even by allopathic studies that encounters with tiny portions of emotions erect a set of primitive defensive mechanisms starting in utero and teach the fetus about cause and effect. And suppressed emotions in adults always cause more damage to our defense systems than honestly expressed emotions. Repressed emotions fester, creating painful fixed ideas.

Importance of the CD

Like a good homeopath, Jung recognized that *abaissement du niveau mental* (consciousness disintegration) may be caused by various triggers like fatigue, fever, intoxication, anemia, religious fanaticism, intense affects, or shocks like hearing bad news. It may also be caused by constitutional and hereditary factors. Recognizing this reveals both the danger and the necessity of homeopathic and psychotherapeutic intervention in any neurosis or homeopathic delusional state in order to prevent its progression into a full-blown psychosis. The neurotic and (homeopathically speaking) delusional patient is approaching a dangerous divide: as long as he can hold out on the neurotic side, he remains somewhat in control. As cancer can be a sign of one's true feelings and could, therefore, be considered a true friend who is trying to warn the cancer patient to change his lifestyle and protect his boundaries, so should one accept neurosis as one's truest and most precious counselor. Instead of attempting to eliminate the neurosis through suppression with allopathic drugs, one should find out what the neurosis is trying to tell us about ourselves. In this way, we don't cure the neurosis, but the neurosis heals us!

Unfortunately, many neurotic patients, under the continual strain of an unresolved, persistent, and intensified delusion, cross over the danger line. They are no longer considered neurotic and must now be identified as psychotic. Many psychotic patients have struggled as unrecognized neurotics before finally succumbing and drowning in the overwhelming tsunami of schizophrenia! Several of the same negative forces (delusions, neuroses) can be found in the unconscious of normal people, appearing in countless dreams where the neuroses have found a safe haven. People often remain blissfully ignorant of these forces until a trigger induces a dangerous deepening of the problem, leading to a psychotic break. In the clinic we often see that people on the eve of a psychotic outburst are upset by things they have never minded before; now these matters have become stumbling blocks and obsessions. Here again, without knowing it, Jung touches on the homeopathic miasmatic theory, in which a trigger is seen to produce a flare-up of the dominant miasm's numerous expressions.

In treating most psychosomatic diseases, one should concentrate more than anything on the psychological traumas that have led to the fixed ideas or delusions of the patient. But why do homeopaths give so much importance to delusions? In general, in the homeopathic practice, delusion rubrics are scarcely used and frequently misunderstood. When homeopaths attempt to find the simillimum, we must take into account the rubrics of Aphorism 153: "rare, strange, and peculiar symptoms," and there is no doubt that delusions belong in this category. Let's not forget that there is a second important requirement for selecting the simillimum: symptoms must have remained permanent over some time! Since a delusion is a fixed idea, it is by definition permanent. Therefore, a delusion should be considered to be among the most valuable symptoms for the determination of the simillimum since it clearly belongs to the A153 rubrics. The delusion, in the homeopathic sense—and even according to Jung—always contains some grain of truth, but the quality of life of the individual and of the people around her is affected by the patient's inability to let go of this fixed idea.

The feeling-tone (intensity/character) of delusional thoughts (especially the CD) is so strong that no matter what the emotional excitation or trigger, only the delusional thought is re-lived over and over again. Take, for example, the psoric phase of *Aurum's delusion, neglected his duty*. No matter how much praise and acknowledgment he receives from others, all incoming positive thoughts are consumed by the negative thought "I did not do enough" (*imagines he is neglectful and deserves reproach in consequence*, Hering). The well-selected remedy, possibly *Aurum* in such a case, will be able to release this person from his delusional fetters, allowing him to take up the task of finding some sort of existential meaning that will enable him to continue living, some sense of self-worth that can replace his resignation and mournful retrospection. Being imprisoned by a delusion destroys a person's capacity to feel joy and compassion and leads to the patient's emotional isolation, as expressed in *Aurum's* delusional proving symptoms: *He imagines he cannot succeed in anything; he does everything wrong; he is in disunion with himself; he thinks he is not fit for this world and longs for death; he sees obstacles everywhere; he imagines he lost his friends' affection*, Hering). Eventually, in *Aurum's* syphilitic phase, the emotional alienation parallels the intellectual estrangement (*mental dullness, feels stupid; loss of memory*, Hering) and, when physical pathology sets in, heart troubles and hypertension commence.

Measuring the Strength of the CD

Is the presence of this CD a new phenomenon? Not at all! It is certainly as old as humankind, but as civilization took root, the prevalence of the CD increased dramatically—and the higher the civilization, the more delusions emerge. When it comes to rational science, entities like Vital Force, Qi, and the CD are in the realm of the immeasurable (although they can be described and therefore do come under the umbrella of the empirical sciences). Because measurement is the foundation of modern science, though, science will not concede the existence of anything unless we can measure it. But entities like the CD and the nothings hiding away in the subconscious are always measured by the discomfort and suffering they cause and the diseases they will eventually yield. In that aspect, every day of human existence is a measurement of the incredible power of the CD, the invisible rudder which, in spite of one's conscious belief and objections, is the master of life's ship.

Indeed, how could we measure the depth at which we have released the demon (the CD), the beast in the cage (Shadow side)? We only know how much of the pain, the grief, or the jealousy is left in the subconscious when we stumble on a trigger that points to the old high feeling-toned complex (Never Well Since or Ailments from). All of a sudden, the complex that we thought had been exorcized and removed from the cage, or at least domesticated, comes to consciousness with a viciousness and biting growl that wounds us again and again and makes us doubt our progress on the journey of our individuation. It is again the raw emotion we feel, and the self-assuredness of our persona is shattered like a mirror into a thousand pieces. We might react with the most incredibly primitive emotions, emotions we might have denied ever existed in us. Of course, it is always easier to deny the existence of evil rather than to accept the necessity of reckoning with it.

How to find the CD

In the Materia Medica

I will restate here in brief some of the criteria I used in order to determine a delusion to be the Cyber delusion of a particular remedy.[2]

1. For me, the first obvious criterion was that, among the many different delusions of a remedy, the CD should be either black type (3) or italics (2). In other words, the fixed idea was present among most of the provers of the remedy. One example is the delusion of *Aconite*: *he is about to die. Aconite* is a well-known remedy for women in labor with their first child who may be paralyzed by fear of the impending delivery. Among all its

2. For details, please refer to my book *Advanced Guide for the Professional Homeopath*, Chapter 6.

delusions, *Aconite* has only this delusion in bold type. Additionally, *Aconite* is the only bold type remedy in this rubric, and no other remedy has the same intention or meaning as other remedies in this rubric!

2. If all delusions of a particular remedy are graded "1," that is, are listed in plain type, we can try to determine a delusion in which only this remedy is found. For example, in the *Silica* proving we find the delusion *left half does not belong to the right one,* which expresses the dual nature of *Silica*—who is timid in public and, often, a tyrant at home. Only *Silica* is found in the repertory under this rubric.
3. Often, the essence of the CD is also expressed by other delusions found in the provings of the same remedy. For example, *Lac caninum* has the CD *he is dirty,* which is also expressed in the delusions *he is small, he is looked down upon, he is despised, he is short,* and *he is insulted.* When many delusions express the same theme, that theme points clearly to the CD.
4. The CD gives birth to secondary delusions. The CD of *Lachesis* is *he is about to be injured by his surroundings* and he *is wronged,* which leads to further suspicious behavior and secondary delusions such as *he will be sent to the asylum* and *the medicine is poison.*
5. Last but not least, a person needing a remedy with a particular CD will always return to his CD after executing a series of defensive compensations and displacements. In other words, the remedy story begins and ends with the CD. For instance, no matter how many positive or negative compensations *Aurum* executes, he always will come back to his CD, *I neglected my duty,* unless the homeopathic remedy frees this victim from his chains.

In the Clinical Setting

A Cyber delusion is the expression of the dominant, ruling emotion. It is the driving force behind the actions, thoughts, and plans of the patient, and it will create secondary delusions along the way. Therefore, all compensations and secondary delusions have their origin in the Cyber delusion. It is imperative for everyone (as we all have a Cyber delusion) to execute compensations, which can be regarded as defense mechanisms that enable us to flee from the Cyber delusion (when it is negative) or to reinforce it when it is positive. The patient will try hard to compensate, to stay away from his inevitable fate, but he will have to face this Cyber delusion at some point in his life. The patient's good delusion, obviously, is also bad for him as it impedes his self-growth. If we don't ask enough about the motivations behind the psychological behavior of the patient, she will express compensations far away from the Cyber delusion, therefore leading the homeopath to prescribe for the mask rather than the shadow side, a mask that is formed by all these compensations. The mask represents the simile (compensations), but the shadow side is the simillimum (the Cyber delusion)! An ancient Chinese proverb expresses the same: Confucius says that to return to the root is to find the meaning, but to pursue appearance is to miss the source! When I find the Cyber delusion, the light bulb goes on: I see the essence of my patient. All his mental/emotional and physical compensations are determined and guided by this primary delusion.

Another hint is that, during the case taking, the patient often betrays his CD when a very painful issue is touched upon, by even as so much as a small hint, reference, or thought. At this point, the patient may react with telltale indicators such as silence, anger, irritability, crying, hesitation, or stuttering. When this happens, the homeopath must realize that his words or gestures have evoked the memory of a painful Never Well Since (NWS) event in the patient's homeopathic history. Be sure to record such a reaction during the consult, along with the source of the reaction, so you can know how the CD was touched upon.

Compensations

As a physician, I have observed that the number one regret dying people have is that they lacked the courage to live life true to themselves—not according to what others expected of them (social and professional persona). By investigating the shadow side and integrating its contents into consciousness, people can live unbound by fear of failure or disapproval. Rather, they can become individuals ready to accept setbacks; with courage they continue to go forward, to try a little more. These are people who adopt the attitude "I will" rather than thinking "I should have..." Unfortunately, most people continually resort to compensations rather than taking the opportunity to become more complete individuals.

In the blessings as well as in the calamities of life, less depends upon what befalls us than upon the way in which it is met: how do we react to and compensate for pleasures and misfortunes in life? Compensations are an attempt to reorganize the chaos inflicted by the CD, a process of continuous rehabilitation on an unstable basis, an attempt to reach homeostasis and to regain and preserve identity. The portraits in this materia medica are to be studied as phenomena of health and disease placed in the endless forms of individual adaptations by which human organisms (individuals) adapt and reconstruct themselves when faced with the challenges and vicissitudes of life. Depending on the judiciously administered remedy, for some, such reorganization transforms the dark and negative side of the CD into the plus of positive compensation. For others, caught in a vicious cycle, the attempt might only lead to more disorganization until they are finally liberated by the homeopathic remedy that is their simillimum. We must remember that it is not the existence of the problem itself (the NWS), but the patient's attitude toward it (compensation), that gives it the power for good and evil. Out of grief may come determination and undaunted courage or degradation, meanness, and spiritual apathy. Out of riches and power may come selfishness, self-gratification, and materialism (as with *Nux-v*) or the understanding that it is important to be, not to have, presenting us with the opportunity to serve and to practice the art of giving—like a balanced *Aurum*!

Persona Malformations as Compensations

For many in this world, compensations will lead to a malformation of the persona, or the formation of a pseudo-ego. As a defense—and depending on her constitution, dominant miasmatic background, and individual experience—the person constructs a thick, multicolored mask (excessive persona) that is hard to penetrate and effective at hiding the skeletons in the closet. These skeletons are usually personal characteristics exactly opposite of those that she shows. People with an excessive persona will do anything—lie, boast, act cynical and dictatorial, retreat when not on familiar ground, manifest narcissistic behavior, rejoice in the misfortune of others, steal, deceive, or resort to the most vile and primitive instincts of humankind such as violent jealousy, malicious behavior, and even killing. But in spite of the fearful and ferocious front a person puts forth, the individual with an excessive persona battles the demons of inadequacy, cowardice, and lack of self-confidence throughout his life. These demons sap his Vital Force, often leading to many physical illnesses and maladjustments in his relationships, especially at home. *Lycopodium* and *Silicea* are two known examples of this frequently encountered persona. In dreams, such a person always has too many clothes on; he might take a jacket off and find that another one appears! He might be overly decorated in gaudy uniforms, armor, or dresses, but he will never be able to reach the necessary nakedness of selfhood! When reading their portraits in this book, the reader will get a sense of how *Lycopodium* and *Silicea* have come to be in such a thwarted and uncomfortable situation, to be suffocated in their heavy armor, unable to change their attitudes or self-image.

The inadequate persona is the opposite of the excessive one. One does well to distinguish between the *hereditary* formations of such a mask, of which *Bar-c* is the prime example (*Bufo* is another one), and the *acquired* inadequate persona formation. The latter is a result of *ailments from domination,* of which *Alumina, Anacardium, Staphysagria, Stramonium,* and *Nit-ac* are examples as well as remedies not described in this book such as *Viola-tricolor, Hura Braziliensis* and *Carcinosin.* While the individual with an inherited inadequate persona needs and welcomes someone else's guidance and control, the other form of domination is imposed on the individual: either out of jealousy, maliciousness, and cruelty, or to help (read "dominate") the person on his individuation path out of "love and concern" while unconsciously making an emotional amputee of the person—until he is rescued by the indicated homeopathic remedy. As his life is entirely guided by someone else, the dominated person has dreams of appearing naked, unprotected, and vulnerable, or of sitting in a car that is being driven by someone else, which symbolizes the fact that someone else is in control of his life. In contrast to the meaning of appearing naked in a dream for someone with an inadequate persona, appearing naked in a dream can also have a positive connotation when it occurs in a person who, thanks to the homeopathic remedy and his own courageous introspection, is able to appear naked voluntarily—to be himself without feeling the need to put up a mask. He can let his hair down, so to speak.

A third form of malformation is the identification with the persona, thus forming a pseudo-ego. Unbeknownst to the person, he entirely misses the aim of living a full life unless balanced through therapy. Such a person, regardless of circumstances, is and always plays the role portrayed by the persona: he is the CEO at all times, the captain of the ship who acts like he is always ordering everyone on his ship in case of emergency, the physician who talks comfortably about his profession but is ill at ease in any other conversation, and the mother who suffers from empty-nest syndrome. Such a mask is very rigid and glued onto the patient's face. It is a one-sided mask with only one color, not a multi-faceted one like that of the excessive personality; the individual who identifies with his mask is married to his persona, to his profession. This person is a rather boring type who zealously keeps his mask on and dominates conversation at all costs. If one tries to steer the conversation away from this lopsided personality, he will quickly interject with topics in which he is competent: this is the shield and dress that makes him feel important and admired. Of course, he is mistaken! Others, excepting simple souls, don't see him as a strong, well-adjusted social being; rather, they know that he is like a mere child who has little explored his psyche and, consequently, has an underdeveloped personality. Unbeknownst to himself, he is nothing but the role he plays, identifying himself solely as belonging to a certain category of people (lawyers, physicians, judges, etc.); he is always dressed in the appropriate uniform—the only set of clothes he possesses—and he therefore belongs to the class of people who can hardly make the first step toward becoming truly human. In dreams, his clothes may be glued to his skin, prohibiting the skin from breathing; he might also appear with diseased skin, another symbol of identification with the persona. When he loses his position, retires, or is struck by a disease, his single set of clothes is taken away and he is left with nothing but an empty shell. *Arsenicum, Platina, Veratrum-a,* and *Nux-v* are examples of this identification with the persona.

To correct these malformations, we must become aware of ourselves as individuals separate from the external demands made of us. We have to acquire a sense of responsibility and a capacity for judgment, and we have to use our personae to facilitate social interactions. The persona of a physician facilitates the examination of the patient, while the patient contributes to the examination by adopting the persona of the patient. But this should only happen in the physician's office or in the hospital! When it is appropriate, the physician can change out of his representational clothes and into something more comfortable; he can also be naked sometimes (let his guard down). If our clothes stick to us or seem to replace our skin, we are likely to become ill! We must use our social and professional masks in the right circumstances so as to form an adequate ego and an adequate mask to meet the outer demands of the world we live in. One should never mistake the role for the man.

A further goal of this materia medica is to help homeopaths aid their patients in attaining the highest form of completeness: by uncovering what is hidden and unknown in the individual's shadow side, integrating the dark unconscious elements into consciousness, and accepting the soul mates of anima and animus. A great block to personal individuation and the achievement of Self-realization is removed when, with the help of the simillimum, a person finds the courage to investigate his unconscious. Once a patient becomes more complete through the acceptance and acknowledgment of the skeletons in their closet, and desires to change and integrate the darkness into her consciousness, that person can become a soloist. He can do what so few among us can: achieve ego loss, in the sense of indifference to the opinions of those who are driven by envy, competition, and ignorance. He enjoys life regardless. Such an individual does not say "I enjoy Rome": rather, he says "I enjoy myself in Rome." We should remember that wealth and beauty do not last; character and individuation do! Through the investigation of the unconscious, aided by the simillimum, the homeopath helps the patient to remove the obstruction blocking his power; then, the patient can make the most advantageous possible use of the personal qualities he possesses. The freed individual goes on to live a life full of meaning and rich in thought.

Notes to the Reader

Patient confidentiality: Patients' names and circumstantial details of their lives have been changed to protect their anonymity. All quotes are word-for-word from patients, and the actual details of their conditions, remedies, and case development are all accurate.

Names of remedies: Remedy names are indicated in *regular Italic font* and given as they would be used in conversation, with common sense prevailing: *Arsenicum* is of course *Arsenicum album*, *Aurum* is *Aurum metallicum*, *Calcarea* is *Calcarea carbonica*, and so forth, with the most common and frequently used remedy assumed. Long remedy names are abbreviated as they would be in conversation, such as *Nat-mur*, and *Kali-bich*. Remedy names appearing in the same font as the font of the original proving: for example (<> *Platina*) indicates that the remedy was included as part of the original proving and is not a separate addition of the author of this book. Remedy names appearing next to italicized proving symptoms as with this example: withdrawn (*great sorrowfulness with constant inclination to sit in a corner buried in thought—sits still, wrapped in deep sad thoughts and notices nothing* (Puls!). *Puls!* indicates the author has linked another often indicated remedy with the proving that was not part of the original proving (In this example, "*Puls!*" is the author's addition).

Common homeopathic abbreviations in the text:

CC = Chief complaint
DD = Differential diagnosis

Gender of pronouns: To avoid the awkward "he or she" or "s/he," the pronoun referring to a practitioner is sometimes male and sometimes female.

Quotations from the *Organon*: The word "Aphorism" or use of the "A" with a number always refers to the *Organon*.

Provings: The provings from the homeopathic materia medica are original and all words are unaltered from the original texts. The original provings are woven into the language of this book but offset in italics. Similar provings have been grouped together, but when they are not from a single proving the reader will understand as such by the manner of the punctuation used, and the punctuation will differ from that used in the original provings. The original language and punctuation of provings is indicated by the use of the different italicized font setting as such.

Example 1. The Cyber delusion of a remedy is noted by a proving emphasized in ***bold italics:***

> The all-consuming Cyber delusion of *Aconitum*, ***he is about to die,*** reflects an immense fear of dying and points to a particular event and time in the future **when** this will happen.

Example 2. Original provings are copied verbatim from the sources and are set within the text of the author of this book by using italics contained within the flow of regular text. To demonstrate this, the following is a short excerpt from the text of this book in which there are seven separate provings from the homeopathic materia medica woven into a portrait in this book:

> Such a woman will need more support than ever (*desire to be magnetized*) to guide her through this period of terror and fright, because she will be overcome by irrational and hysterical behavior (*hysterical fainting; hysteria in plethoric subjects; laughing alternating with rage and spasmodic frenzy*). Her usual intelligence and common sense go out the door (*diminished intellectual power, cannot perform even light mental work*). One can easily see how such a woman, when no understanding is forthcoming from husband and family and when she is not supported by *Aconite*, can become delirious and frantic (*delirium with talk about death; delirium especially at night, raves and springs out of bed with excessive sweat in the morning*).

The seven provings/rubrics excerpted from a portrait in this book in the above example:

1. *desire to be magnetized*
2. *hysterical fainting*
3. *hysteria in plethoric subjects*

4. *laughing alternating with rage and spasmodic frenzy*
5. *diminished intellectual power, cannot perform even light mental work*
6. *delirium with talk about death*
7. *delirium especially at night, raves and springs out of bed with excessive sweat in the morning*

Example 3. The regular font and non-italic punctuation joins different provings together, and such uses throughout the portraits should signal to a homeopath that they reflect the same idea. The following example contains nine different provings symptoms:

> This appears as *chorea* and *twitches and jerking everywhere* (*eyelids, left side of the face, blinking of the eyes*; *trigeminal neuralgia with a feeling like a frostbite*; *trembling of the mouth*; *twitching of the abdominal muscles*; *jerking of extremity muscles on falling asleep*; *tingling and burning on the spine with cold spots along the spine* and *jerking or twitching ceasing on falling asleep, as if electric*).

The nine proving symptoms from the above text excerpted from a portrait in this book:

1. *Chorea*
2. *twitches and jerking everywhere*
3. *eyelids, left side of the face, blinking of the eyes*
4. *trigeminal neuralgia with a feeling like a frostbite*
5. *trembling of the mouth*
6. *twitching of the abdominal muscles*
7. *jerking of extremity muscles on falling asleep*
8. *tingling and burning on the spine with cold spots along the spine*
9. *jerking or twitching ceasing on falling asleep, as if electric*

References: Are placed in footnotes throughout the portraits, although if unobtrusive they are included in the text. A bibliography is provided at the end of the book. Bracketed comments interpolated into quotes or text in regular type [thus] are by the author of this book.

Glossary

Anima: An archetype that represents a man's unconscious, eternal, feminine other, the male's recessive female or Yin aspect. The anima, corresponding to the maternal eros, and therefore naturally abundant in women, is the personification of all feminine psychological tendencies in a man's psyche, such as: his vague feelings and moods; fears, anxieties, depressions, reactions, prophetic hunches, and impulses; capacity for love, emotions and relationships; spontaneity, sensitivity, receptivity, adaptability, warmth, empathy; love for nature and animals; and especially his possible connection to, and interest in, the unconscious as well as to everything that is spontaneous in psychic life. The first picture of the anima comes from the man's mother and then from the grandmothers, stepmother, mother-in-law, sisters, lovers, wife, and any woman with whom he has a relationship. The anima is also shaped by the father's ideas about women.

Animus: Corresponds to the man's anima; represents the woman's recessive maleness or Yang aspect: her urge for action, her capacity for judgment and discrimination. The animus has both positive and negative aspects, as does the anima. The animus enters unconsciously and automatically into any situation that requires initiative, action, determination, authority, rationality, and understanding (logos). A negative animus in a woman can be a voice in the unconscious that says: "You are hopeless. Why even try? There is no point in doing anything. Life will never change for the better." The animus, if in balance, gives the woman capacity for reflection, deliberation, courage, objectivity, and self-knowledge. The first model of animus for the woman is formed by the father, followed by grandfathers, stepfather, father-in-law, brothers, lovers, and any men with whom a relationship exists. The animus is also shaped by the mother's idea about men.

Archaic (undifferentiated, primitive) Ego: The primitive or undifferentiated ego that starts growing around age two. A child's ego is called the prenatal ego, a primitive ego and its make-up is primarily from the mystical participation to the parents. Up until age five the child is close to the collective unconscious. From age five on, there is a transition from the prenatal psyche into ego consciousness, as a psychological separation takes place when the child goes to school, venturing out of the shelter of the house and parents. Therefore age five is a crucial age for either sex as any psychological or physical trauma occurring around this time will hinder further development of the child.

Archetypes: Manifest both on a personal level (through complexes) and collectively (as characteristics of whole cultures). Archetypes make up the collective unconscious. Archetypes are responsible for the striking similarity in theme and imagery shared among myths, folk tales, and fairy tales worldwide as well as for the parallels found among the dreams of individuals. Archetypes offer compelling evidence that there is a stratum of shared unconscious resemblances in all human beings. Jung called those resemblances archetypes of the collective unconscious; they are the psychic structural components of the collective unconscious, and they appear as figures, structures (temples, pyramids, craters of the moon), and situations (menarche, menopause, etc). For many, the drama of failed idealism and spiritual longing is an archetypal experience of the modern world. Some examples of archetypes, in addition to the shadow, the anima, and the animus, are the hero (based on overcoming obstacles and achieving certain goals), the Divine Child (innocence), the Divine Mother (nourishment and protection), and the Old Wise Man (image of meaning and wisdom). Archetypes have both positive and negative facets. For instance, the old wise man can appear as a shaman (positive) or as an evil wizard (negative).

Attitude functions of introversion and of extraversion: Extraversion is the psychological orientation that orients the libido toward the outer world. Introversion is the psychological orientation that orients the libido toward the inner world and personal unconscious. Both attitudes are present in everyone, but one always dominates. A healthy person accesses and exercises both as appropriate.

Autism Spectrum Disorders/Autism (ASD): A state in which an individual is trapped in the personal unconscious and even remaining close to or trapped in the collective unconscious. The person with ASD has not separated psychologically from his parents or started on the necessary road to ego consciousness. Remaining close to the collective unconscious means being trapped in childish fairy-tale language with an obstructed desire to acquire external stimuli; as a result, a longing for protection, safety, and nourishment drives a wish to stay in the womb. The external world seems an untenably dangerous and frightening place, encouraging the individual to withdraw deep into the unconscious and create a fantasy world with imaginary companions.

Alzheimer disease: We are in the midst of a brain failure epidemic. By 2040, it is estimated that more than 100 million people will suffer from some form of dementia. For homeopaths, ALZ is one of the expressions of an active syphilitic miasm, affecting first the short-term memory and later the long-term memory. Aging is a transition to the syphilitic miasm, and the speed at which this process takes place depends upon three factors: the individual's lifestyle, her inherited traits, and any suppressive allopathic treatments that she may have undergone (accelerating the process from psora to sycosis and finally to the syphilitic miasm).

Attention deficit hyperactivity disorder (ADHD) and Attention deficit disorder (ADD): Two conditions whose symptoms, allopathically speaking, include a very short attention span, restlessness, and behavioral disturbances (including violence). Homeopathically, both conditions are expressions of the sycotic miasm, in which all symptoms carry an excessive tone. Mind, body, and emotions are captured by a whirlwind, leaving the victim in a state of nervous debility with extreme mood swings and a physical body capable of adapting to neither atmospheric changes nor food absorption.

Collective unconscious: The shared mind of our ancestors; their ways of thinking and feeling; their ways of experiencing life, the world, good, and evil. The collective unconscious stands for all the psychological contents that belong not just to one individual, but to many of the human or animal species. These are collective miasmatic traits and can be found in any culture. The collective unconscious contains a number of patterns, or archetypes, common to the whole of humanity. Examples include events such as puberty and menopause, as these are universal to every people and culture, even those with no historical or cultural connection. Even in animals, we see the collective unconscious at work in the nesting instincts of birds; the migrations of whales, butterflies, birds, and caribou; and in the swimming of salmon upstream at same time each year. One illustration of a collective reaction is the urge of the beaver to build dams, which comes from an instinctual reaction to the sound of running water.

Conscious functions: In his *Analytical Psychology: Its Theory and Practice*, Jung discusses four different functions that can be distinguished in each individual's consciousness: sensation, thinking, feeling, and intuition[3]. The four functions square off in pairs and are diametrically opposed to each other. The first pair consists of the thinking and feeling functions, which are rational functions. Both necessitate judgment and evaluation. The other functional pair, sensation and intuition, is the irrational pair. In the latter function of each pair (feeling and intuition), everything is based upon the absolute intensity of mere perception. Each of the two non-diametrically opposed functions is of secondary importance: it is an auxiliary or complementary function that changes the nature of the person. Each is useful only insofar as it serves the dominant function without claiming superiority. In other words, the secondary function has a different nature from, but is not antagonistic to, the primary or superior function. The so-called inferior function is unconscious and, for that reason, projected upon a non-ego. For instance, the thinking type can have either sensation or intuition as a secondary/auxiliary function. This means that an individual can be a thinking-sensation type but rarely will be a feeling type at the same time. The fourth archaic and primitive function (feeling in this case) is, as a rule, entirely beyond the control of a person's will and therefore makes its appearance on inopportune moments when a highly feeling-toned complex is touched upon, surprising the patient and everyone around them. Further differentiating and elaborating the auxiliary functions (in this case, sensation and intuition) creates a more balanced person. But for the thinking type, feeling will always remain the Achilles heel. Thinking is an objective judgment. It tells you what a thing is. Thinking names things. Feeling tells you what a thing is worth to you and has to do with the expression of the personal or subjective value which we give to that which we perceive. For instance, when we say, "I don't like this dress" or "I do like it," we have placed a personal value on what we have perceived: agreeable or disagreeable, good or bad, etc. Sensation is concrete perception of objects and individuals by means of our five senses, the primary source of information. Our senses tell us *that* something is, not *what* it is (for that we need the thinking function). Sensations perceive things as they are and not otherwise. Reality comes to us through the five senses! Intuition is a sort of guess about the possibilities of the reality we perceive. Your senses tell you that there is something; your thinking tells you what it is; and feeling tells you whether or not you like it, whether you accept it or reject it: a subjective judgment. Intuition tells you what *may* be

3. C.G. Jung, *Analytical Psychology: Its Theory and Practice: The Tavistock Lectures*, trans. R.F.C. Hull (Princeton, 1960), 16-20.

("I have a hunch!"). Sensation and feeling should not be confused; the difference between them is well expressed in the French language (*sensation* and *sentiment*).

Corrective and reductive dreams: Examples of compensatory dreams in which the conscious attitude of the dreamer is so one-sided that it fails to recognize the optimal possibilities of life. Corrective and reductive dreams are vivid and comprise a contrasting but purposefully compensating content as an expression of the self-regulation of the psyche, establishing a psychological balance. A perfect example of reductive dreaming is the sort that takes place in the lopsided *Lycopodium* (with his self-confident, boasting, power-seeking attitude), who has dreams in which his boat founders, he fails exams, or in which he is unable to reach his destination.

Cyber delusion: A fixation on one person or sensation/thought at the exclusion of all other incoming stimuli that creates a vacuum in the ego of the person through a lowering of the mental level. The ego becomes occupied by one fixed idea—the Cyber delusion—so that no other thoughts or interests can penetrate the ego. The Cyber delusion, a masked figure of the unconscious, now becomes the driving force behind each thought, each plan, and each action of the person possessed by it. It is the dominant force and ruling emotion that rules his unconscious; it becomes part of the patient and, unless resolved by effective therapy, continues to grow and dominate, leading the patient ever closer to a state of psychosis. The Cyber delusion is at the center of the disease process of the individual. All of her mental, emotional, and physical compensations are propelled, determined, and guided by this primary delusion. The Cyber delusion always gives birth to secondary delusions when it is not resolved through adequate therapy.

Delusion: Most of the homeopathically defined delusions have the potential to create pathology on the physical, mental, and emotional planes. All delusions, in the homeopathic sense, contain a germ of meaning, a kernel of truth; they therefore encompass a much wider range of meaning than they do in allopathic medical terms. In allopathy, delusions are linked to grave psychological illness such as schizophrenia. Behind a delusion lies a personality, a constitution, a temperament, a life story, and a pattern of hopes and desires. However, these pathologies are still called neuroses because their intensities are not (yet) sufficient to push the individual beyond the danger line to psychosis.

Delusions of grandeur: The confusion of ambitions, hopes, dreams, and desires with actual accomplishments and realities. Jung would call such delusions an inflation of the anima.

Delusions of reference: The gross misjudgment of any small acute circumstance, small gesture or word, or perceived situation. When someone with delusions of reference meets with a mishap, he immediately jumps to the conclusion that he has been deliberately injured, insulted, or treated maliciously.

Depersonalization: The process by which person who hovers around the danger line between neurosis and psychosis may, at any time, with the slightest additional stress, succumb to a psychosis.

Dissociation: The danger of the rupture of the ego, master of consciousness, when unconscious contents overwhelm the conscious, fracturing the ego and leading to schizophrenia (a moderately severe or severe psychotic state in which the sufferer flees into a world of fancy illusions).

Ego: Master of consciousness, center of the psyche, mainly reflecting the dominant conscious function. The ego makes up the persona (but is not identical to it) as we acquire a sense of responsibility, morality, and capacity of judgment.

Eros: From the Greek word for sensual love. Eros reflects the function of human relationships (sexual and others).

Essence: In Traditional Chinese Medicine (TCM), represents a specific kind of energy which plays a very important role in human physiology. Stored in the kidneys (according to TCM) but circulating throughout the body, Kidney essence determines growth, reproduction, development, sexual maturation, conception, and pregnancy. Essence is mostly derived from the parents. Some of it is lost with each illness, and it is difficult to replenish.

Highly feeling-toned complex: A psychological picture of a traumatic event contained in the unconscious. A highly feeling-toned complex constitutes the distressing personal and painful private side of psychic life; it is, therefore, often suppressed or repressed. In homeopathy, it is analogue to the Never Well Since (NWS), Ailments from (A/F), or causality.

Ignoble misfortune: A misfortune befalling someone because of his own wrongdoing or as a result of his overestimation of his own capacities (see *Delusions of grandeur*).

Individuation: The process through which a person becomes psychologically an individual, standing apart from the masses, and learns to be indifferent to vile opinions and strict conformism as well as to peer pressure. Individuation allows a person to find meaning in life, to find his voice, and to attempt to follow the path to Self-realization—a goal achieved by few.

Libido: Psychic energy without whose power nothing moves. This is much more than Freud's more specific definition of libido as sexual drive or sexual energy; it is the energy of the psyche responsible for powering all of man's drives. It is of paramount importance, along with the Vital Force (VF) or Qi.

Logos: The principle of logic and structure. Logos is traditionally associated with spirit, the paternal and male world, and the God-image.

Multiple sclerosis (MS): In allopathy, a demyelinization throughout the CNS; in homeopathy, an expression of the syphilitic miasmatic state.

Mystical participation: The transference to the unborn fetus of emotions attached to events suffered by the pregnant mother through the psychogenic umbilical cord. Jung called this process *participation mystique*, or mystical participation, a term coined by the French anthropologist Lévy-Bruhl to refer to the child's perception of the conflicts between parents and his beginning to suffer from those conflicts as if they were his own.[4]

Neurosis: "A neurosis is a dissociation of personality due to the existence of complexes [the homeopathic NWS]. It is normal to have complexes but if these complexes are incompatible to the patient, the part of the personality which is too contrary to the conscious one becomes split off. If the split reaches the organic structure, the dissociation is then called a psychosis, a schizophrenic condition, as the term denotes."[5] "The mildest forms of neurosis are the lapses of consciousness, for example, slips of the tongue, suddenly forgetting names and dates, inadvertent clumsiness leading to injuries, misunderstandings of memory, as when thought to have said something or done something that they have not, etc." [6]

---

4. C.G. Jung, *The Development of Personality*, ed. and trans. Gerhard Adler and R.F.C. Hull (Princeton University Press, 1981), 124.

5. Jung, *Analytical Psychology*, 188.

6. C.G. Jung, *The Practice of Psychotherapy*, trans. R.F.C. Hull (Princeton University Press, 1933), 57.

Noble misfortune: A misfortune that befalls a person because of unfortunate circumstances or fate rather than as a result of his own wrongdoing. This noble misfortune can include naivety, and misjudgment.

Obstructed personality: A lack of individuation; a psychic arrest stemming from any of a number of childhood psychic traumas creating a situation in which the individual is incapable of moving forward. The individual with an obstructed personality is ill-equipped to deal with the challenges of life because he performs with a wrong persona (an excessive or inadequate one, or one with which the individual has identified). One can be born with an obstructed personality through mystical participation. In allopathy different disease names are attributed to the obstructed personality for either a child or adult: from ASD to selective autism, to ADD, adult ADD to timidity and aggressiveness

Parallel dreams: Dreams whose content derives from a recent event witnessed by the patient. They do not have a compensatory or self-regulating message or effect, and they recur as long as the stimulus continues to occur or as long as it is kept in the memory of the patient.

Persona: The persona, or mask, is oriented toward society or, more precisely, toward the expectation that society has of the individual. This persona is not part of the unconscious, as it is created by the ego; rather, it resembles the ancient actor's mask that was worn in early plays, just as our multiple personae (socially, professionally) represent the roles we play on the world stage. Persona indicates something of what the person is like, just as the mask suggests the role or emotions of the actor. According to Schopenhauer, persona is "that which somebody represents in contradiction to what he actually is." Schopenhauer also mentions the notion in his *Essays and Aphorisms*: "Persona really means an actor's mask, and it is true that no one reveals himself as he is; we all wear a mask and play a role."[7]

Personal unconscious: The private life of the psyche, chiefly containing the so-called feeling-toned complexes; the painful ailments from (A/F), homeopathically speaking. The personal unconscious encompasses the archetypes, shadow, anima, animus, and the fourth archaic

7. Arthur Schopenhauer, *Essays and Aphorisms*, trans. R.J. Hollingdale (Middlesex, England: Penguin, 1976), 168.

undifferentiated conscious function as well as the Cyber delusion; it is distinct from the collective unconscious.

Projection: Feelings that are not accepted as one's own and are therefore dealt with by being attributed to others. Our shadow side is often projected onto others, for example when we discover many qualities in others that are in fact unconsciously present in ourselves. To find out what the patient is projecting, ask him the following: "Describe the personality type that you find most despicable, most unbearable, and most impossible to get along with? What do you hate most in a person? What characteristics make you angry in others?" Most likely (not always, of course) the patient will produce a description of his own repressed characteristics—those of which he is utterly unconscious. Such qualities are so unacceptable precisely because they represent his own repressed side. This is psychological projection, and when we exercise it, we often pronounce moral judgments with the deepest conviction. What we don't understand is that what we combat in our neighbor is usually our own inferior side.

Relatively fixed symbol: The symbols that appear in dreams. In order to gain far-reaching insight into dreams, the homeopath must be experienced in the matter of relatively fixed symbols. These constitute something like an enigmatic language and can be more fully understood when studying dream analysis. The insights that result have great diagnostic and prognostic values. We refer to the symbols as relative, not absolute, because we cannot know for certain that their occurrences in dreams signal no other meaning. The meaning of any particular dream symbol may differ among people—or even for the same person at different stages of his life.

Repression: Deeper than suppression. Sad, cruel, shameful, and embarrassing events can be so powerfully relegated to the unconscious that the patient is left with no recollection of them. Usually, such a patient consults for physical events but is unable to connect her ailments with any previous misfortunes. Often, dreams bring the necessary message from the unconscious, helping to expand upon and elaborate the patient's consciousness. When repressed emotions are uncovered and processed, it can bring the patient to wholeness and independence.

Self: Includes the totality of the psyche (sum of consciousness and unconscious) that manifests itself in an individual. The Self is the center of this totality, whereas the ego is the center only of the conscious. The Self is what you really are, not what you want to be or imagine you ought to be. It is the archetype of wholeness and the regulating center of the psyche, a transpersonal power that transcends the ego.

Self-realization: The highest level one can reach, personified by the number seven. Few people reach this level and one can say that it is reaching the God within each of us. It is the ultimate goal of the individuation path, which requires much introspection and examination of the personal unconscious.

Shadow side: An archetype hidden in the unconscious of the individual that contains everything about her that is too painful, shameful, or negative to be dealt with consciously. The term "shadow" refers to that part of the personality which has been repressed for the sake of the ego preservation so that it will not be fractured. It is the darker side of our personality, the one that we do not consciously display in public. It is that part of us which we do not allow ourselves to express—at least not voluntarily—but it very often finds its expression through projection upon someone else or in uncontrolled and socially unacceptable behavior that is triggered accidentally. The Jungian counterpart to the homeopathic NWS is the complex, which can be traced to some experience in the life of the patient which made a deep and shocking impression: one so painful that it could not be endured for long in consciousness and has therefore been repressed. Our dark sides—or shadow sides—remains unknown, though they are the most important parts of us; they are riddles for speculation, masses of suppressed and unexplored facts. Everyone has a shadow, and in dreams the shadow appears as an inferior human being of the same gender as the dreamer (that is, an alter ego). The shadow is not wholly bad. While most shadow sides possess all the traits that individuals want to hide and suppress, there are also people who, in conscious life, live below their potentials. Their positive qualities—those insufficiently developed functions—are cast away into the shadow side rather than being employed and cultivated. This kind of personal darkness contains the rejected *positive* contents of a human psyche; whether intentionally or not, these aspects are inadequately exercised in the conscious life of an individual. Thus, the undeveloped qualities remain in an archaic form, causing the individual to miss his true vocation—and the meaning of life itself!

Suppression: The disappearance of symptoms that have not been healed but have been sent to deeper levels, from the physical to the emotional and mental plane. A clear example in allopathy: suppressed eczema transforming into asthma and then into seizures, an expression on the deepest physical level (central nervous system [CNS]).

Symbol: The best possible expression for something unknown. The image or word implies something more than its obvious and immediate meaning. From the Greek *sym*, meaning "together," and *bolo*, meaning "to throw," combining to mean "that which has been thrown together."

Transference: "When two chemical substances combine, both are transformed. This is what precisely happens in transference. It is inevitable that the doctor should be influenced to a certain extent and even that his nervous health should suffer. He quite literally takes over the sufferings of his patient and shares them with him."[8] The homeopath is no exception to this transference process; much more so than the regular physician, she is involved in the recovery of her patient's well-being because she spends far more time with the patient than does an allopathic physician (except, of course, for a psychiatrist). Depending on the miasmatic state of the physician, unconscious contents shared with the patient may be activated in him which would otherwise remain latent. A homeopath should realize that, in her profession, and with the great empathy and patience she shows to her patients, the transference process is always lurking around the corner; it is, in fact, concomitant to the homeopath's work and career. Through knowledge of the miasmatic states and with the help of the homeopathic remedies, the process is processed in the right way when it occurs, especially if the homeopath is knowledgeable in dream analysis.

8. C.G. Jung, *Psychology of the Transference*, trans. R.F.C. Hull (Princeton University Press, 1966), 7-8.

Part Two: Homeopathic Portraits

Aconitum napellus (Aconite, Acon). Monkshood

The Cyber Delusion

The all-consuming Cyber delusion of *Aconitum*, ***he is about to die***, reflects an immense fear of dying and points to a particular event and time in the future **when** this will happen (*prophesying, predicts the time of death, and bids friends goodbye*). This situation typically arises in the primigravida when she anticipates possible dangers of, and has irrational fears of, the unknown delivery process (*fear of death during labor and during pregnancy*; *delirium with talk of death*). In a society in which every little pain is annihilated with painkillers, the reality of severe pains linked to the delivery inundates the mind of the excitable woman and can take on enormous dimensions even before the pains are experienced (*insanity, from intolerable pain*). This should not come as a surprise; James Kent called the primigravida "a nervous race horse," and there is no better remedy than *Aconitum* to avoid miscarriage later in the pregnancy (seventh or eighth month) when the delivery process comes nearer (*gen, fem, abortion, with fear of death*; *abortion, last months*). Other delusions confirm this message of gloom and doom (*delusion, she has an incurable disease* and *delusion, of being doomed*). Notice the despair of this person ahead of the event that seems to be looming as an ever-increasing threat to her well-being and that of her fetus (*despair of recovery* and *doubtful of recovery*). Continuous physical confusion and unrest (*gestures, confused, involuntary motions of hands* and *hurry in movements*) are warning signs of impending loss of control.

Disconnection with reality sets in as the person in an *Aconite* state is overcome with the intensity and duration of this emotional excitement (nervous excitement): *delusion, floating in the air* and *delusion, she will become insane*. Her sense of security is also affected: *delusion, she is away from home*—home being a relatively fixed symbol for security and protection, especially during pregnancy. When someone wants to return to the womb (return home), it means also returning to the unconscious, even the collective unconscious, to be near to the archetype of the Divine Mother (symbol of love, nourishment, and security). It is not uncommon in these circumstances that the primigravida—although previously often a very independent woman—becomes now more dependent on partner, family, and friends, who serve as a security blanket during these frightening times in anticipation of the unknown (*frightened easily; fear of impending death; long-lasting fear; ideas haunt her, cannot get rid of them*). Such a strong neurosis always risks developing into a psychosis, depending also on the patient's constitution (with their tendency toward a multitude of fears, *Phosphorus* and *Calcarea* are especially at risk).

Such a woman will need more support than ever (*desire to be magnetized*) to guide her through this period of terror and fright, because she will be overcome by irrational and hysterical behavior (*hysterical fainting; hysteria in plethoric subjects; laughing alternating with rage and spasmodic frenzy*). Her usual intelligence and common sense go out the door (*diminished intellectual power, cannot perform even light mental work*). One can easily see how such a woman, when no understanding is forthcoming from husband and family and when she is not supported by *Aconite*, can become delirious and frantic (*delirium with talk about death; delirium especially at night, raves and springs out of bed with excessive sweat in the morning*). This last proving is understandable given that, during sleep, a person loses all inhibitory capacities and reasoning powers to control her fright; her unconscious and suppressed fears now have free reign to disturb her sleep and create nightmares (*at night anxious dreams, several times waking with a start; awakened by nightmare* and *vivid dreams of day's occurrences* [which are parallel dreams related to events from previous day]; *restlessness with continual tossing*).

Causalities

Fright

Being in a very nervous state and prone to falling into an imbalance even in response to everyday common events (*ailments from emotional excitement*) as well as events that would disturb and shock a person in a healthy state, the pregnant mother's fear will now take on huge dimensions (*fear of suffocation*), especially in a woman with a sensitive constitution such as *Phosphorus* or *Arsenicum*. For instance, witnessing an accident and being suddenly confronted with death (*ailments from fright, from the sight of an accident*) will release the vast arsenal of suppressed material from her unconscious; this material will crash with tsunami-like force on her fragile ego, testing the solidity and integrity of her ego consciousness. I remember a case in which my patient witnessed the death of her best friend; the incident rendered her completely "speechless" (diagnosed allopathically as "hysterical aphasia"). But *Aconite* has in its provings *stupid, eyes closed, facial muscles twitch, mouth compressed with no power of speech* and can be indicated for such a response to witnessing an accident; it can also be indicated for those who have narrowly escaped death or danger, which can leave an indelible impression on the psyche (for example, when one has almost died from a heart attack, almost drowned, or come close to dying in a car accident, earthquake, tsunami, etc.). The thought that death has knocked on the door, and that it may do so again at any time, can often lead to a continuous and recurrent recall of this trauma through certain events or words pointing to this suppressed painful highly feeling-toned complex; now, the remedy *Aconite*, needed acutely before but not administered, will lead to a chronic state in which *the fear of the fright remains,* also expressed as *fear because of a previous fright* and in which *Opium* will now be indicated. Indeed, a strong negative emotion is often dealt with by depositing it into the subconscious in order to move on in life. Unfortunately, depositing this frightful emotion elsewhere is not equivalent to curing it, just as beheading someone is not the solution to a headache. Failing to work toward integrating this painful highly feeling-toned complex into consciousness results in the emotion retaining its archaic or primitive character; the holder will be surprised by the strength of this emotion when it is suddenly released at some inopportune moment in which an event, a gesture, or simply a word brings it up.

Anger

Fright also takes another form as the supersensitive expectant mother needs more reassurance and support from her immediate family. This pregnant woman is a volcano about to erupt, and when assistance is not forthcoming, there is *anger with fright* and *anger with silent grief,* a withdrawal into the unconscious (*delusion of fancy illusions*), and another precarious emotional state that becomes a brewing storm in the unconscious, capable of being set loose at any time when an innocent word or gesture points to the Cyber delusion. This sensitive person views such perceived (not necessarily real) lack of support as an *ailment from mortification*: "Why are you not here when I need you the most?" Fear (often) and fright (always) will be displaced by anger: fear is an emotion that threatens the integrity of the ego more than anger, and fear always cultivates the defense mechanism of anger. With any angry person, one always needs to ask first: "What are you afraid of?"

Excessive Joy

Traditional Chinese medicine (TCM) recognized long ago the danger of *ailments from excessive joy* leading to instability of the Fire Element (Heart, Pericardium, circulation) with emotional instability, insomnia, hysteria, and the risk of cardiovascular disease (stroke, heart attack). This emotional factor (joy often coupled with anticipation anxiety) naturally increases when the woman is pregnant for the first time, especially in the case of many trials with in vitro fertilization (IVF) or in the case of having suffered many miscarriages. Such a high-anxiety woman is naturally overcome by the fear of death of the fetus, the unborn being an intimate physical and psychological extension of her own self. There is probably no more high-anxiety situation (*she is beside herself*) in life, as this pregnant woman is hypervigilant at every milestone in the pregnancy process and fearful of every result from every test during pregnancy; she lives from week to week, as she is often overcome by her Cyber delusion that she (or her fetus) will die (*anxiety in paroxysms*). In this day and age, with the autism epidemic, such fear has extended not only to death of the child but also to the fear of having a child with special needs, which can be translated into ailments from *death of a child* or *ailments from death of loved ones* (it is not the normally developing child that was expected).

Compensations

Oversensitivity

Aconite is suitable to the sanguine temperament, a fire that often needs only a small trigger to consume the person in an enormous flame, even to the point of immediate combustion; this excessive reaction is easily seen on the mental, emotional, and physical planes. On the mental level, there is *confusion of the mind with difficulty of concentration* and *weakness of memory for what he has just done*, but the vulnerability seen in the *Aconite* state exists especially on the emotional plane with *violent anger* (created and fueled by fright), *being besides herself, inconsolable*, and *sensitive to noise* (where the slightest noise is unbearable), *light and children* as well as emotions related to *oversensitivity to the pain*: *insanity from intolerable pains*; *despair with the pain*; *restlessness during pain*; *unbearable pains and shrieking with the pain*. One recognizes *Aconite*'s value as a first-class remedy in a sudden heart attack or angina pectoris as well as a remedy for the contractions of the birthing process. On the physical plane, this restless *patient tosses in bed, with anxious moaning and groaning* and shows *convulsive and confused gestures with involuntary hand movements*.

Social Indifference

One would think that a person needing the attention and care of others would be very affectionate, almost clinging to others. Nothing is further from the truth in the case of *Aconite*, with the exception of her behavior with her most immediate support such as husband or family. She *has aversion to people,* and *has no affection for anybody during pregnancy; answers laconically yes or no.* There is almost a total indifference towards her friends. One can see the immense power of *Aconite's* Cyber delusion, which has created a huge vacuum in the ego consciousness: this vacuum is occupied entirely by that fixed idea that she (and her fetus) will die, so no other thoughts or emotions can penetrate the ego consciousness. There is simply no place for them, even to the point of *indifference to loved ones*! And when her ego is filtering the outside information to determine what can come into the consciousness of this overly preoccupied person, only that which pertains to her CD is absorbed. Despite her actual situation (*she cannot banish anxious apprehensive thoughts even in gay company; intolerant to contradiction* and *contrary and obstinate*), the CD has become a fixed idea that can resist even the most eloquent and rational argument and blow her fears up to immense proportions. At the same time, she has a *chaotic and confused and alternating behavior* as there are moments that she *wants to be carried* (supported) and *desires to be caressed and magnetized*: after all, she needs an audience to express the contents of this frightening Cyber delusion. Otherwise, she remains very *suspicious,* a precaution to avoid any harm that may come to her; even innocent comments or well-meaning advice are met with much resistance (*easily offended*). Trying to lighten up her mood with humor or music has the opposite effect: she *takes every joke in bad part* and *music is unbearable and makes her quite sad.*

Fear of the Unconscious

It is clear that the person in an *Aconite* state, consumed by the idea that she will die, wants to remain hypervigilant. At night, when sleep should set in, all these inhibitory processes fall away; now, an *Aconite* patient is at the mercy of all the suppressed emotions that have been hiding in her unconscious. Control becomes impossible, and she is now overwhelmed by fearful ideas that make her delirious: *delirium, at night, springs suddenly from bed and escapes; delirium, talks about death and looks fixed on one point, staring.* One can see a kind of paralytic fear overwhelming her in her sleep, and for this reason, the person *has aversion to bed and shuns bed.* The power of the suppressed and controlled emotions is far too frightening to lose control over it (*desire for light* or consciousness and *fear of the dark,* which is one of the relatively fixed symbols for the unconscious), as this mighty destructive force—the unconscious bursting with frightful elements—is able to attack the ego integrity of the person (*anxiety on going to sleep*).

Aggravation from Music

Many positive compensations available to other remedy characters seem to be out of reach for *Aconite*. Music is one example. Any kind of music aggravates her situation; she has a *strong aversion to music as it causes her headaches,* and there is even *sadness from music.* It is interesting to note that religion, so often a rescue route to the relief of any kind of emotional and physical suffering, also fails to deliver *Aconite* from her anguish as the patient is overcome by *despair of recovery. Industriousness* is not an available compensation either. Rather, it is a kind of frenzied "being busy," an unproductive activity (*undertakes many things, perseveres in nothing; hurry in occupation*), while *mental work fatigues.* Unproductiveness is caused by *excessive disagreeable restlessness, as he is in the greatest haste and every obstacle that delays his rapid pace is excessively annoying.*

Golden Tips from the Masters

- Indicated as one of the three von Boenninghausen croup remedies *Aconite—Hepar-s—Spongia,* to be taken two hours apart in this sequence (in a 200C or 1M potency in water) and repeated if necessary if the attack is not completely over. Seldom does the patient have to repeat it!
- In the case of poisonous bites and stings, it is a first choice together with *Ledum*
- In an angina pectoris attack, it will still the anguish of the stinging, stabbing pain: *screams with the pain*
- Acute inflammatory processes: first stage with watery discharges (storms that blow over quickly) anywhere in the body presenting as the **4 Fs**: **F**ast, **F**ever, **F**right, and **F**ulminant (explosive), from sudden violent changes and from being exposed with deficient clothing
- Sudden onset of cold with high fever or Bell's palsy after exposure to dry, cold, windy weather around midnight or from the intensely hot weather of summer (diarrhea and/or vomiting)
- Threatening miscarriage late in the pregnancy (last trimester) due to increasing fear of the delivery
- Faintness after frightful event
- Fear of walking across a busy street
- One of the main remedies in agoraphobia
- Acute onset of trigeminus neuralgia caused by cold exposure
- Injuries to the eyes with a foreign object
- Retention of urine in newborns
- Blue babies and cyanosis of extremities and nails (*Laur, Carbo veg*)
- Remedy for panic attacks: it is considered the homeopathic Valium
- Music makes her so sad it is unbearable
- Heart disease with fear and restlessness
- Angina pectoris, pericarditis, and simple hypertrophy
- One cheek red, the other one pale, with anxiety and chilliness, always indicates *Aconite*

- In insomnia from anxiety, restlessness, anguish, and fear. When there is tossing and turning and despair of ever being able to fall asleep, *Aconite* is simply scientific magic.
- In pneumonia followed by pleurisy, one dose of *Aconite* followed by a dose of *Sulphur* (its chronic) will give relief and will prevent return of a similar attack
- For severe menstrual and labor pains when the patient screams aloud at the slightest touch, cannot bear light, and changes position continuously
- #1 remedy for urinary retention of the newborn (*Causticum* for the mother!)

Agaricus muscarius (Agar). Fly Agaric

The Cyber Delusion

The fixed idea determining all of the actions and thoughts of *Agaricus* is expressed by the Cyber delusion ***her legs don't belong to her***. This is also conveyed in the delusion, *her arms do not belong to her*. In other words, her extremities (legs and arms), the human being's instruments and muscles to achieve, to act, and to take initiative and responsibility for things, seem to be under the power of someone else (*delusion, he is under superhuman control*). An *Agaricus* patient wishes to be responsible for his actions but feels that, in reality, he only follows the commands of others. The person in an *Agaricus* state senses that he is being controlled and made dependent. Such an internal battle is always followed by an Adlerian masculine protest, by a quest for power, a striving for a place in the sun, even if it is just in his mind. As a result, his sense of perception is greatly disturbed, leading to two opposing character presentations. One of these is the presence of delusions of grandeur (*delusion, he is a great person and he is an officer*), common in a personality that at all costs tries to maintain his own (albeit blown-up) mask of power and muscle. The other presentation is that of being smaller (*delusion, his whole body is diminished* and *delusion, of being smaller*), which reveals the other side of the coin: his shadow side, that of a weak-willed individual who seeks the guidance of a stronger personality, perhaps a guru for life (*irresolution*) on whom he bestows excessive love and praise (*embraces his companions; kisses the hands of his companions; dependent on others*).

This dependence is easily seen in an interview when even an adult person continually looks at his companion, wringing the hands (*gestures, involuntary motions of the hand*) while waiting for an answer from her. A parent or spouse in an *Agaricus* state will always ask: "When are you coming home? When are you going to sleep? What are we going to do?" and constantly calls on the person on whom he is dependent (*childish behavior*). The delusions of being smaller evoke further fixed ideas of a disturbed sense of perception, as everything now seems bigger than it is in reality: *delusion, distances are enlarged* and *delusion, a small hole appears like a frightful chasm.* Such a dichotomy in the personality is apt to create a fearful, insecure person, one that may even be arrested in his development *(development of children arrested)* and who needs to hide these shadow feelings behind an excessive mask of grandiosity (*egotism, reciting his exploits*). The world is full of more or less mediocre people who think they are great and who have a great need for others to think of them as great. As usual, an excessive persona (which is part of *Agaricus*—a reaction to his true persona, the inadequate one as seen further) will at all costs avoid having his mask ripped off during a conversation, avoid being exposed: he might be *loquacious but answers no questions*! This is sometimes partly due to his stuttering: *mind, speech, incoherent; mouth, speech stammering; mouth, speech difficult; mouth, speech difficult, from spasms of the tongue; mouth, speech stammering, from excitement.*

Causalities

Ailments from Fright and Emotional Excitement

Agaricus has an inadequate persona, which always leads to a struggle in life to deal with the everyday obstructions and cobblestones that life can throw at him. Life is never a smooth road, but *Agaricus*' archaic ego does not know how to distinguish small things from big ones, as some of his delusions indicate: *delusion, a small hole appears like a frightful chasm.* Therefore, any bad news, even trifles, is blown up and easily becomes part of *Agaricus*' makeup. When he reads about a person dying from cancer, he is immediately gripped with intense *fear of impending disease,* and especially a *fear for cancer.* These delusions are particularly exacerbated when a loved one or a family member dies. *Agaricus* weeps when telling his symptoms (*thinking of complaints aggravate; pities himself*). The vulnerability and lack of ego defense show clearly as his shock goes immediately to the deepest level of the physical plane: the central nervous system. This appears as *chorea* and *twitches and jerking everywhere* (*eyelids, left side of the face, blinking of the eyes; trigeminal neuralgia with a feeling like a frostbite; trembling of the mouth; twitching of the abdominal muscles; jerking of extremity muscles on falling asleep; tingling and burning on the spine with cold spots along the spine* and *jerking or twitching ceasing on falling asleep, as if electric*). *Agaricus* can be incapacitated by multiple tics of extreme violence coming in volleys every few seconds. It is important to notice that these chorea movements **disappear when sleeping** and when occupied (*generalities, chorea, sleep, during, ameliorate* and *occupation ameliorate*). When the person swims, sings, or works evenly and rhythmically and finds a place which is tension-free, he is tic-free!

Under the eruptive, comical, even foolish surface, *Agaricus* is a deeply serious person—and a man in deep despair. Fear of death is typically found in people who have forgotten to live and have never been able to find a meaning in life. Certainly, the dependent *Agaricus* is such a person. The thought of cancer is seen as destructive evil for this person to such an extent that he even has *fear of losing his reason* as he is incapable of withstanding the rush of such a fateful conception. This is especially true upon going to bed, when his inhibitory conscious mechanisms are not operating (*thoughts, rush, flow of, in the evening in bed* and *shrieking during sleep*). An interesting and paradoxical aspect of *Agaricus* is that, even with so many fears, the *Agaricus* child is not afraid of going on roller coasters; he *runs about in most dangerous places.*

Ailments from Sexual Excesses

An archaic ego often looks to compensate through increased sexual activity. However, increased sexual activity and masturbation lead to a loss of precious fluids. As is well known in homeopathy and Traditional Chinese Medicine (TCM), such loss leads not only to physical exhaustion and general debility of the CNS but also to frequent damage to the soul: *sadness after coition, sadness after masturbation* and *from sexual excesses.* This will remove that person even further from reality in life as the loss of precious Vital Force or Qi will also lead to short-term memory weakness (*memory, weakness of for what he has just done; for expressing oneself,* and *for what he has just thought*), more *irresolution* and *indecision,* and *anxiety about health,* all well-known characteristics of a loss of Kidney Qi, as it is known in TCM.

Ailments from Reproaches

This trigger is especially important in children who may be slightly developmentally delayed (*retarded development with twitches*) and have learning difficulties leading to nervous tics, convulsions, and noticeable trembling and chorea when being reproached by parents, teachers, or coaches (*offended easily, takes everything in bad part*). Because of their archaic egos, these children will exhibit alternating silly, foolish and depressed behavior (*chaotic confused behavior; dancing grotesque; foolish delirium* and *cheerful alternating with sadness*). They are also uncoordinated in their movements (*awkward, drops things; gestures, involuntary motions*) as a result of a mental defect, and therefore are often delayed in walking and talking" (combining the features of two remedies, the "*late learning to talk*" of Natrum Muriaticum and the "*late learning to walk*" of Calcarea carbonicum due to bone weakness); even at a later age they still speak in fragments: *speech, by jerks while making many mistakes.*

Compensations

Hiding

Fueled by his delusions of grandeur and at the same time tormented by the opposite fixed idea of being small and vulnerable, *Agaricus* will do anything to keep his excessive and inadequate mask from being ripped off; the true person can and shall not be discovered: *aversion to answer; refuses to answer; loquacious but does not answer; loquacious* and *changing quickly from one subject to another* and *laughing loudly.* All these are overcompensations for his profound sense of insecurity at every turn and for his basic sense of inferiority. His emotional vulnerability and instability are also expressed by *attempts to escape* and *aversion to being touched* as well as *avoiding company* and *desiring solitude,* remarkable for such a dependent person. This is mainly due to his *childish character,* as he is disappointed when friends are not available to be with him when he wants it (they are working, in school, or occupied with their own families). In this *Agaricus* joins other characters like *Silica, Nat-mur, Kali-c, Lachesis,* and *Tarentula,* who tightly guard the skeletons deposited in their cupboards (in the unconscious) as they fear that an in-depth questioning will expose their real motivations: feelings of vulnerability, suspicion, high anxiety, and insecurity. But by keeping his secrets under tight control, *Agaricus* runs the risk of having that growing primitive beast of the unconscious, residing in the shadow side, come crashing down into his consciousness, leading to a sense of instability (*fear of insanity, of losing his reason*). Anyone who needs to keep tight control over his shadow side spends a lot of energy trying to keep his mask on day-to-day. The person who concentrates mainly on the ego consciousness (delusions of grandeur) and pays little attention to his shadow side is bound to lose control over his tightly controlled world, which is nothing but a house of cards that will tip over with the least touch. And his main compensation then becomes aggression and rage, leaving no place for understanding and love (*rage, constant*).

The Blaming Game

When not looking into his shadow side, and trying to discover what he has hidden there, *Agaricus* retorts to the natural human reaction: one of projection. It is always the other person's fault. "**You** have this problem; **I** don't!" The ego, in this instance, plays the role of a clown in the circus (reflective of the twiching character of *Agaricus*) whose gestures (*violent gestures; grasping at things; involuntary motions of the hands* and *strange attitudes and positions of the head*) are intended to persuade the audience that all the changes on the stage are brought about by the faults of others. It is simply covering up his unconscious motives—those of letting others always decide what he should do when he is confronted with difficulties in life so that when something goes wrong, he can blame them. Such rationalization borders on *cowardice*, something that will be denied with great vehemence (*delirium, raving and raging* and *obstinate; violent*). *Agaricus* is somebody who thinks he is always on top of things; in reality, though, he does not know how to put order in his own house because he never reaches down below the surface into the unconscious. This explains why he would show *despair bordering on rage*! What becomes apparent in *Agaricus*' character is a large amount of confusion (*mistakes in speaking, using wrong words; confusion of the mind as if intoxicated* and *concentration difficult with difficulty learning things*).

Aggression and Rage

Through his daily efforts to maintain his inadequate mask, *Agaricus* exists in an almost permanent state of aggression on the outside; inwardly, this stems from a partly conscious and partly irrational attitude toward the tasks which life imposes. This reflects a *childish behavior* and *resembles a child with arrested development*, as normally a child from age five on learns to take responsibility and to discriminate between good and bad. Not so in the *Agaricus* state! It is almost as though the person for whom *Agaricus* is indicated is convinced that every individual really exists in **his** egotistic and irresponsible state. This aggressiveness (*constant rage*) might not always be obvious but boils up when such a person resorts to *alcoholism* to numb his feelings of inadequacy: *rage during drunkenness*, in which he now shows all his muscle, an untapped source for such a long time and therefore released in immense strength (*rage, strength increased*). But even when trying to hide this rage, it is shown in his face as *twitching of the face* is seen by everyone (*generalities, chorea, accompanied by, muscles, twitching of*). He is a person who is always at war, on a constant path of aggression (*battles, war, talks of*). The purpose is to ward off these inadequacies that he has so tightly stored in his subconscious.

Golden Tips from the Masters

- Tic douloureux
- Trigeminal neuralgia
- Chorea (quivering and twitching everywhere, now in one part, then in another): <before thunderstorm, >during sleep, >during occupation
- Main remedy for frostbite or NWS
- Bechterew's disease
- Headache as if a nail is being pounded into the skull
- Delirium tremens (the DTs) in alcoholics
- #1 remedy for chilblains, worse during menses
- Raynaud's syndrome
- Headaches in spinal patients as if from cold needles
- *Agaricus* belongs to the tubercular diathesis

Agnus castus (Agn). Chaste tree

The Cyber Delusion

Once someone is in an *Agnus* state, the overwhelming fixed thought is found in the delusion ***he doubts if anything had existence.*** In other words, there is definitely dissociation with reality, but it is not so much because of a psychotic break as can be observed occurring in the schizophrenic states applicable to *Lachesis* or *Anacardium* (*two wills*). It is also not the case that the separation from reality is drug-induced as it is in *Anhalonium* (with the Cyber delusion *he is separated from the world*). Rather, in *Agnus'* case, it is mainly due to a depletion of the Vital Force or Qi; a general debility and depression of the Vital Force are marked on all planes: on the mental plane *forgetful of purchases, goes off and leaves them,* on the emotional plane with *indifference to external things,* and on the physical plane with *great debility and impotence.* As a consequence, the world is now viewed as in a haze; nothing seems very real anymore. Such a separation from reality can only occur if the Qi or Vital Force has been lost; this force is causally and intimately connected with the foundation of all energies in the body—the Yin and Yang energies—and the organ that houses this foundation: the Kidney.

One of the functions of the Kidney in Traditional Chinese Medicine (TCM) is to house the *Essence*, which is a precious substance determining the basic constitution, strength, and vitality of the individual. Essence is inherited mainly from the parents and is partly replenished by the Qi extracted from food. The Kidneys are also the source of fire in the body, which is called "Fire of the gate of Vitality;" this provides an idea of what happens when the Kidney Qi is depleted, as can be seen in this *Agnus* portrait. The Essence is also the basis of sexual life and the material foundation for the manufacture of sperm in men and ova in women (important when we consider the source of depletion of this Essence as in the person in the *Agnus castus* state); furthermore, it controls the onset of the various stages in life, i.e. birth, puberty, menopause, and death! Aging itself is due to the physiological diminishment of a person's Essence during life. When the Essence is weak, there will be lack of vitality and infertility or sexual weakness, all cardinal expressions of a person in an *Agnus* state. As usual, when one is so inadequate in various ways, the only way of surviving such scenario is to put up an excessive mask or persona, showing the opposite of one's shadow side: *Agnus* hides besides a well-constructed persona of *delusions, of wealth*. He might think he is still wealthy (especially in the domain of sexual prowess) but, unfortunately, that is a thing of the past; through his persona and delusional thinking, though, he can vehemently deny such a decline (*exaltation of fancies*).

Causalities

Ailments from Sexual Excesses

With the introduction of the internet and the increased sycotic tendencies in the population (fueled by vaccinations, antibiotics, cortisone, etc.), *Agnus* is a remedy that will be needed more and more in the future and, increasingly, by a younger population. TCM knew the dangers of sexual excesses centuries ago (described in the Chinese essential text of health and healing, *The Yellow Emperor's Classic of Medicine* [*YECM*]); TCM called these excesses "unregulated affairs of the bedroom" or "excessive labors of the bedroom." *YECM* describes numerous sexual techniques and provides advice and guidelines on healthy frequency of intercourse, adjusted according to one's age and according to the seasons (increasing in spring and decreasing in winter).[9] Sexual intercourse—the Way of Tao—was deemed by the Chinese to be healthy; intercourse is also mentioned in Aphorism 77 and in Aphorism 5, in which Hahnemann discusses lifestyle and habits and their role in maintaining health. Allopathy can learn something from TCM and homeopathy regarding regular sex and health benefits; allopathy touts sex as a wonder drug (reducing stress, risk of cancer, high blood pressure, and heart disease among other things, but no one has worked out the best dosage—the amount needed for maximum benefit or an optimal orgasm count. TCM and homeopathy see it differently and more accurately. Excessive sexual activity does not allow the body to recuperate and restore Kidney Essence (in contrast to sexual activities not culminating in orgasm, which are not thought to be depleting the Kidney Essence); references to "excessive sexual activity"

9. Ni Maoshing, *The Yellow Emperor's Classic of Medicine: A New Translation of the Neijing Suwen with Commentary* (Boston and London: Shambhala, 1995).

denote activities leading to actual ejaculation for men and orgasm for women. *Agnus castus* is definitely an example of the aberrant psychosexual development and immaturity that Hahnemann and TCM connected with disturbances of the Kidney Essence such as those mentioned above.

Just like *Lycopodium*, *Agnus* is an individual who has only reached the most superficial level of love in his life; this is called a *sexual attitude*. In other words, there is a sexual attraction towards the other person but nothing more. Flirting is second nature to such people (*lascivious*) and belongs to their social persona. In other words, this is the kind of person (like those needing *Lycopodium*, *Medorrhinum* and *Fluoricum-acidum*) who deliberately ignores the uniqueness of the other person and only looks for the immediately satisfying sexual act. If the partner leaves *Agnus* unsatisfied, that partner is immediately erased from the social agenda. These characters lack the quality of happiness in love and, therefore, must compensate for it in the number of sexual encounters and trophies they can assemble. The hunt for women (or men) often is a quest for substitute gratifications and typically fails to provide the expected satisfaction. But the disappointed and dissatisfied hunter often fails to get the point and seeks more conquests, as if quantity might make the difference. As this approach to "love" is purely physical and never integrates the physical attraction with the psychic structure of the partner (which would be infatuation or an *erotic attitude*), these excessive labors of the bedroom inevitably lead to a loss of precious fluids, always bringing with it a state of exhaustion on every plane as well as causing specific symptoms such as blurred vision, night sweats, lower backaches, sensitivity to cold, weak knees, ringing in the ears, and frequent urination, all symptoms of a Kidney weakness and all belonging to the *Agnus* homeopathic picture.

TCM also considers the circumstances in which sexual activity takes place. For example, having sexual intercourse in a state of drunkenness or while on street drugs or as the result of a rape is considered extremely harmful to any resulting fetus, causing delayed development on many planes. Although TCM is mainly concerned with excessive sexual activity as a cause of a disease state, an unhappy sexual life lacking in warmth and affection is also an important and frequent cause of disease. As mentioned before, *Agnus* has no quality of happiness in his love life, so deep down there is great unhappiness and anxiety; these become causes of disease in themselves.

Repeated Attacks of Gonorrhea

A debauched lifestyle and a history of promiscuity leading to recurrent gonorrhea most often create the basis of the *Agnus* state (*impotence with gleet, especially with those who have frequently had gonorrhea*). It does not come as a surprise that, for immature characters like *Agnus*-c and *Lycopodium*, a monogamous attitude is impossible as physical desire is never conjoined with a desire for psycho-spiritual union. These are characters who have built up their personae partially on their sexual prowess, leading to a problem as repeated orgasms and loss of seminal fluid weakens the Kidney energy: sexual energy is a manifestation of the Kidney Essence, and each orgasm quite simply depletes some of this Kidney Essence. The cause of disharmony in *Agnus* is simply to be found in the person's habits and lifestyle, creating a *false chronic disease* (see Aphorisms 277 and 5). Balance is a key to health: balance between rest and exercise, balance in diet, but also balance in sexual activity, something which is sorely lacking in the *Agnus* person. Identifying the causality of the disharmony is necessary in order to advise specific changes to restore harmony: it is not enough to just administer the remedy! In Chinese medicine we have a saying: "Examine the pattern to seek the cause!"

Compensations and Consequences

A False Persona

Initially, to keep up the past glory of the hunter and his delusions of grandeur, he puts up a false social mask. He remains *amative and amorous* as this was always part of his makeup, even in his successful *lascivious* days, but at this time he has **become** his mask (identification with the persona): this is a formation of pseudo-ego that is very rigid, defensive, brittle, and fragile. This pseudo-ego is subject to constant pressure from within to uphold that image (*hysteria, lascivious*): "I am still a very attractive and virile man, able to continue my sexual excesses." In reality, as much as he looks strong on the outside, he is fragile and weak on the inside! He still tries to express himself through *eccentricity*: yes, the saying is that the clothes make the man, but unfortunately, this man has become the clothes! Underneath, there is nothing left but a ghost of the past with no substance or strength: *mental work is impossible* and there is brain fag; but worse, his sexual prowess has received a terrible blow (sexual neurasthenia): *there is often a complete loss of sexual desire and sexual erections; his penis is so relaxed that even voluptuous fancies excite no erections; the testes are cold, swollen, hard and painful and there is a small flaccid penis.* In company, he exhibits *loquacity* and can talk as if he still has sex every day (like *Selenium*, but *Selenium* still has sexual desire). The mind is still *obscene and lewd*, but his body is prematurely aged by masturbation and previous debauchery. *Agnus* is therefore also indicated when an older man marries a younger woman and becomes impotent, but also in a young man with a history of sexual excesses and secret vice who now finds himself newly married and impotent and whose young, beautiful wife excites no more erections.

Anxiety and Weariness of Life

When a person observes a steep decline in his health on every plane and realizes that his whole constitution is undermined, he thinks that his end is obviously near and that he must be suffering from a terrible disease (*anxiety about health*; *hypochondriasis*). Of course, such a person is always astonished and incredulous to hear that his sexual activity might have something to do with his problems. What he does not realize is that many sexual problems, such as *impotence* or *premature ejaculation*, often require first of all a decrease in sexual activity if there is to be any chance of successful treatment through the remedy. It is ironic, of course, that this "chaste tree" or shrub (a mixture of ripe berries, leaves, and flowers) was used originally to kill the sexual drive of medieval monks so that they would stay away from the sins of sex (**of course what it can kill it can also restore!**). As his sexual conduct always served as *Agnus*' flagship in life, and now this ship has capsized, *Agnus* is now overcome with a *weariness of life* similar to that of the *Phosphoricum-acidum* patient, who also has ailments from loss of fluids. Observing his debilitated condition, the resulting depressive state is so deep that *Agnus*' Cyber delusion becomes reality: *he doubts if anything has an existence*. Worse, he *has a presentiment of death and believes that soon he will die and that he cannot be helped*. He is now *doubtful about his recovery and discouraged with onset of indifference to external things* (which always were so important in his life). Kent states that these "pale sickly and sad mortals, heart-broken over their early life, lament over their misspent life."[10] Such a person is often diagnosed with neurasthenia or chronic fatigue, but what he needs is *Agnus castus*! Then this person will rise from the depths of his depression (*incapacity for business*; *discouraged*; *fear he will die soon* and *loathing of life*) and realize that, as long as he can work productively, he is not finished with life. This possibility can add a few lines to his life story—lines that may set his whole personal picture in a new perspective.

---

10. J.T. Kent, *Lectures on Homeopathic Materia Medica* (New Delhi: Aggarwal Book Centre, 1990), 35.

Golden Tips from the Masters

- Nonspecific urethritis (NSU) with impotence
- *Milk disappearing in nursing women after sadness and despondency*
- Chronic effects of sprains
- Biggest keynote: feeling of coldness at testes. He keeps looking to see if his fly is unzipped
- Often used when an older man marries a younger woman and then becomes impotent without sexual desire

Alumina (Alum). Aluminium oxide

The Cyber Delusion

Alumina's Cyber delusion is ***her consciousness belongs to another***. In other words, the ego, master of consciousness, is a pseudo-ego; someone else is molding the ego of this person, whether child or adult. The process of individuation is entirely guided by someone else who will make all the choices for the person involved—causing children trapped in this state, to grow up to be pseudo-adults. Some will call it domination and others will call it well-meant "guidance," but the result is the same: the victim loses his identity and is lost on his road to becoming a true individual. In the typical family of such a child, there is little genuine affection; in place of love, there is constant pressure to be bright and cheerful, to conform, and, above all, to do one's best and stand out. The aim is for the child to achieve what the parents could not, implying, therefore, that one should be grateful to have the chance to become a doctor, attorney, teacher, famous pianist, athlete ... anything, but most likely in order to fulfill the unlived life of the parent. One is expected to always put up a good face, no matter how one feels. The *Alumina* child, therefore, learns to hide her feelings, as expressions of individual needs and choices are taboo. No one in her family is allowed to show anger, and sadness is not permitted as everything is done for the "benefit" of the victim. Other delusions or fixed ideas confirm the idea of being dominated and loss of identity: *his head belongs to another. Delusion, errors of personal identity; delusion, of being double* and *delusion everything is unreal.* Furthermore, some fixed ideas leave no doubt that the person's identity has been hijacked by another person: *delusion, someone outside of his body saw or spoke*; *delusion, when he says something, it seems to him as though somebody else has said it*; *delusion, when he speaks, someone else is talking* and when he sees something it seems as though he saw it through somebody else's eyes, *delusion, seeing, cannot see, transfer himself into another, and only then he could see* (only *Alum*). Healthy relationships depend upon the tricky balance between love and dependency on one hand

and individual separation on the other. *Alumina* cannot find this healthy balance, as shown in her behavior: *timidity alternating with assurance,* and *vivacious alternating with absentmindedness.*

There is only one theme in *Alumina's* delusions: the formation of a confused person who has a sense of duality, who is not in control of himself, and who has lost his identity. Everything points to the formation of an inadequate persona. After the formation of an *Alumina* state in a child, the child is unlikely to be allowed to make any decision; the parents make them all for her. Such inflexibility is destructive when incorporated into the structure of parent-child interactions so that the parent is the sole authority on the legitimacy of the child's experiences. Whatever the child wants, in his actions, choices of friends or clothing, the parents say "no." It is always "let-me-tell-you-what–to-do and whom-to-be-with," an intrusiveness that silences its victim. It does not matter how minor a decision the *Alumina* child is making or how knowledgeable he is about it, the meddling parent will correct it. Unfortunately, such a parent has a responsibility and compassion system in overdrive, often personifying the overbearingly caring personality with an outsize feeling of duty for her child, seeing and creating problems where there are none. The parent wants to mend the nonexistent hole in the child's life and feels a keen sense of guilt if he does not try. "Let me tell you what to do. I don't want you to make the same mistakes I did" is the battle cry! Parents force the *Alumina* person to break off a passionate early love affair because there is "no future in it." *Alumina's* identity is erased: she has no name and no voice!

To accommodate her parents' inflexibility, the *Alumina* child suppresses her real thoughts, real feelings, and even her own sense of self as a person with independent desires and needs (*delusion, of being double; delusion, her head belongs to another*). Choices are irrelevant, because acting on her own preferences threatens the parental relationship. The idea can be clearly seen in these delusions: whatever the child is saying or seeing is really said by someone else or seen by someone else (*mistakes in speaking, using wrong words, what he does not intend*); there is another "body" taking over for her body *(outside of his body someone else saw or spoke)*. In *Alumina's* pathology, there is a progressive loss of voice and paralytic weakness of the larynx, which is symbolic for having lost her voice at home and in society. She is always double in the sense that she feels she is one person split in two: one part weaker and more insecure, belonging to her, and the other foreign and more dominated, belonging to someone else. *Alumina* looks in the mirror and does not precisely know who she is. She does not view herself as ugly and short like *Lac caninum*, the Cinderella of the materia medica, but at the same time, she realizes that she is not capable of voicing opinions. Even when she tries, there is always someone who advises her, who tells her what to do instead, leading to total *confusion, indecisiveness* and *pent-up anger*. In other words, there is total domination of her as an individual, often under the disguise of a well-meant active guidance, which is mainly overactive and excessive. It can lead to secondary fixed ideas in the victim: "Did I do something wrong?" (*delusion, he had committed a crime* and *delusion, he is a criminal*) or "Why is everything so unreal?" (*delusion, everything seems unreal*). Emotional turmoil can be so overwhelming that the victim has the feeling of becoming insane (*delusion, she will become insane*). "How can I survive this?" (*delusion, threatened by a fatal accident*). Can you imagine being such a person, kept in the shackles of domination? He does not know what to do anymore, or who he is, or what he wants. Domination can take many forms in the development and formation of the individual and is a theme that must be carefully investigated to reverse the *Alumina* state of a patient. Being kept in the shackles of another individual, one should not be surprised that one possible theme in dreams found in *Alumina* is that of flying. Following the Law of Compensation, such a dream is symbolic of a longing for freedom and joy, a wish to be liberated and get rid of the shackles and traditional taboos stemming from her negative childhood experiences. Such a dream of flying refers also to ascending to the sky, an age-old symbol for God or transcendence; so flying, in this case, refers to coming closer to the authentic self or true self and meaning of life. This is, of course, just one of many possible dream motifs of an *Alumina* state. Other dream motifs always refer to the person not being in control of his life (like sitting in the back seat of a car) or having wings on, as a winged figure represents a part of the dreamer beckoning him to a higher, more spiritual, more detached perspective, a higher level of consciousness or liberation from the oppressive situation represented by *Alumina's* conscious life. Another possible *Alumina* dream theme is being in a barber shop. A barber, cutting hair, is symbolic of someone who can change your persona, the way you look—especially when hair symbolically represents power (the lion's mane, Samson's hair) and beauty. So this can be an anxious dream for *Alumina* as the dreamer is in someone else's hands or influence.

Causalities

Ailments from Domination

Alumina's main causality is domination. Domination can take different forms. The most frequently occurring one is not even malicious; it is done in the name of love. It does not involve direct physical abuse of the person, but is more an emotional abuse in which the child is enslaved by the opinions and directions of an authority—a guru, teacher, leader, coach, or, more frequently, the parent. What the authoritarian figure often forgets is that true love preserves the condition of one's individuality instead of squashing it, and that true love permits the person to be himself. But this parent's idea of love is more one of receiving than giving. "Let me tell you what you should do, because I know what is best for you," says the figure of authority. What the domineering person really has in mind is what is best for **him**, not for the child. This supposed selfless devotion is nothing but a cloak under which the interests of the parents hide. Contrary to appearances to the outside world, not one grain of real love is ever given to the child who is in such a situation! It is often the case that the parents themselves suffered from suppression (political suppression, poverty, or being the victim of a crime, for instance) and therefore draw unwarranted conclusions about the evil in the world; hence, they want to make sure that their children are "better off" than they were. ("I give you the opportunity to go to this school, and you'd better make something of it; I never had that chance.")

Many parents have announced to me their laudable intention of sparing their children the experiences they had to go through in their own childhoods. The truth is that the *Alumina* child is a normal child making common mistakes; the parent mistakenly infers that he needs extra guidance when the truth is that most children commit the same "misdeeds." Such a negative first relationship can doom this child to become trapped over and over again in self-destructive behavior (*upon seeing blood, or knives, horrible thoughts throng her mind; she feels for instance, as though she would commit suicide, although she has the greatest aversion to it; T.F. Allen*). But when questioned as to whether they themselves have overcome these misfortunes, parents are firmly convinced that the damage from their own suffering has absolutely been corrected. Actually, this is rarely the truth. If, as children, they have been brought up too severely, then they spoil their own children with a tolerance that borders on insanity; if, in childhood, certain facts of life were concealed from them, those facts are then thrown open to their children by methods of enlightenment that are just as painful. "I never got any guidance from my parents, so I will guide you because you are too young to know what you are doing. I want to make sure you don't commit my mistakes; that's how I ended up being pregnant with you!" The father figure might be in the military and is often a person who is used to taking and dishing out orders. In other words, he lives in a structured world in which everything seems simple, because everything in his life is dogmatic, subjected to military rule and a code of conduct. As a good soldier, he is used to obeying orders, even to killing others; he is, after all, the property of the military. He does as he is told without asking why, and he expects the same from those under his authority. When the child asks "Why?" the answer is "Because I said so."

As I have seen often in practice, the child has to make up for the deficiencies of the parent, for all the failed ambitions and hopes that parent ever had: now the parent wants to give the child the opportunity he never had. But such a parent is behaving with no concern for the life and the growth of his child, so there is really no love! These are parents who were unable to fulfill their own ambitions, and they therefore embody them in a gifted child whom they either pamper or whip up into a showpiece, always to the detriment of the future adult (as is evident from the lives of many infant prodigies). Thrusting the "very best" they can do for their child down his throat is nothing but pressuring him to achieve what they themselves so miserably failed to do. Parents basically tend to fall to the other extreme of the old sin. "I never got any guidance from my parents, so I will guide you forcefully because you are too young to know what you are doing!" Everyone has to commit his own errors in order to become an individual, as this offers him or her the occasion to see how he or she deals with adversity in life. *Alum* and *Anac* both have *weak wills*. If this disharmony between the self-conscious and the ego persists, it can evolve into a neurosis (*hysteria*; *hypochondriasis*) or even a psychosis in which the conscious is now overwhelmed by unconscious contents (schizophrenia). True personality is a gem that can develop only by slow stages in and through life, and children need to be able to make their own mistakes; otherwise, we rob them of their childhood. Such a child simply becomes a pseudo-adult, and society has created many such handicapped people.

Critical Father, Overprotective Mother: Ailments from Anticipation and Anger

A real danger for a child with developmental problems (Autism Spectrum Disorder [ASD], for instance) is the critical father who is in denial of the shortcomings of his child. When such a father's primary mode of giving attention is to show disapproval and admonishment, praising and displaying love only when he is pleased with his child's conduct, the mother's love will most often shift into an overprotective mode. Then, often unknowingly, the growing child is kept on the infant level, and the mother compensates by eagerly fulfilling all his infantile wishes and helping him in unnecessary ways. The mother of one of my patients was in total denial of her daughter's innate low IQ, and she absolutely believed her daughter was going to be the next Marilyn Monroe because the daughter was genuinely warm with lots of kinky blond hair. Although this child was visibly disturbed as well as with the presence of some degree of retardation, the mother was convinced of the girl's talent, saying to me, "Believe me, I know talent when I see it." That, too, is domination, and in a form sometimes more insidious than active domination. Such acts of "unselfishness" on which people often pride themselves, "living only for their children," do not create happiness and closeness in relationships with their children; rather, these children remain stuck in an infantile attachment to the mother, whose aim is to be loved but not to love. The mother enslaves the child in the name of love and duty, but in reality, she does not allow the victim to breathe unless it is through her. This negative or dark side of the Mother archetypal figure takes life instead of giving life, presenting herself as morally impeachable; this creates *ailments from anticipation* and *anger*, two additional emotional states that will imprison the person needing *Alumina*. For the person in *Alumina* state, who has no effective sense of herself as an individual nor any apparent meaning in her life, the emerging threat of destruction from dangerously pent-up violence becomes very real (*fear of his own impulse*; *fear of losing his reason, of inanity*; *suicidal disposition, with a knife or razor*).

Ailments from Humiliation

The thinking of parents of an *Alumina*-created child is: "Children should be seen but not heard." And woe to the child that is heard! A child that is rambunctious, impulsive, volatile and seeking his own identity (*Sulphur* and *Phosphorus* come to mind)! *Alumina* is over-protected and mercilessly guided by the family. In other words, the family forces the child to be something other than what she naturally is. It leads to the *Alumina* state, resulting in errors of identity: the child does not know who she is and what to do (*irresolution*; *undertakes many things, perseveres in nothing*); the parent shapes the child into something she is NOT. It is like looking in the mirror and asking, "Is this really me? Was it really me who did this?" (*delusion, everything seems unreal*; *confusion as to his identity*). And if this child resists being what others want her to be, only humiliation and scorn come her way (*ailments from mortification and being scorned*).

Compensations

The Formation of a Wounded Animus

Both situations—cruel domination and benevolent exertion of over control by parents—occur. But in both cases, parents will chain the child by damaging the animus, which is the domineering archetype in the male but also the necessary recessive maleness in the female. Animus is the decision-making power; it stands for adventure, spontaneity in action, and the acting power to change things. For both sexes, animus represents the urge for action and the capacity for judgment and discrimination. The animus enters unconsciously and automatically into any situation that requires initiative, action, determination, authority, rationality, and understanding (Logos). For a man, the formation of a handicapped and deficient animus has consequences for the rest of his life, handicapping him in his traditional role of the "acting" man. It often results from having an overprotective mother or one with many rules and regulations (like a *Kali-c* mother). He has a longing for life in the world; as a handicapped adult, he will make fitful starts in a world that he encounters as very challenging because it is nothing like the one that was offered by his mother. When aggression is repressed (for instance, because one has learned not to reveal one's anger or because everything was made too easy for one as a child), the result is often a frustrating impotence and boredom (*time passes too slowly*; *intolerable ennui*; *trifling things seem insurmountable*). The lack of necessity to achieve anything through one's own efforts (because everything is taken care of) brings about a sense of hopelessness stagnation (*no desire to do anything, especially anything serious*) and a dangerous buildup of unexpressed and non-personalized violence, including self-destructive urges (*mania to kill himself with a sharp weapon*). Challenges make demands on the conscious side, the masculinity of a man, on his courage and resolution. But unknowingly, the saint-like, dutiful *Kali-c* mother has forcefully injured her son's animus in order to still her own anxiety.

The young girl growing up in these circumstances does not fare much better! A woman cannot become a fulfilled being without consciously integrating a minimal amount of aggressiveness, assertiveness, and independent reasoning. A woman must also be hard (animus) in the sense that she should be enduring, independent, have judgment and determination. Lack of animus in a woman will lead to weakness and incompetence, a woman who is too soft (*quiet disposition*) and fearful of any new situation requiring judgment and action; this makes her the potential victim of other domineering people who may appear in her life.

Anger Directed Inward

Anger about the domination is common and to be expected, but as a child still searching for a dominant conscious function and independence, the *Alumina* victim often directs anger at herself, expressing it in a syphilitic or destructive way. As the intensity of authoritarian control rises, particularly in the case of a person with sensitive constitution, there might come a tremendous sense of despair expressed through suicidal tendencies, especially upon seeing sharp instruments: *impulse to cut herself even though she abhors the idea* or *suicidal disposition, on seeing blood or a knife, she has horrid thoughts of killing herself, though she abhors the idea; morbid impulses to shoot himself; suicidal with a razor, suicidal with a knife; suicidal, to be run over* and *suicidal from sadness* all reflect the destructive miasm and the self-destructive tendency of the *Alumina* state:

> One of my patients was an intelligent young lady, 25 years old, who as a child had been forced to spend hours every day practicing the piano—even during her vacations, while her peers would play outside and have fun. This had enraged her so much that by the time she consulted me, she had often attacks of fierce anger upon which she retired to her room and cut her arms "with the finest surgical knife" she could find. And her scars were explained to her parent, with whom she still lived, as cat scratches. Her parents had no idea that their daughter's only relief was found in seeing her blood streaming out of her body. It makes one think of "the blood boiling over," a severe expression of anger. If ever there was a manual for breeding psychological distress, it is this required perfectionism that seeps into the psyche and keeps its victim from ever discovering what she really likes or creating her own identity. It is like presenting a report card at the end of each day, a critical self-evaluation: "Where did I fail, where did I succeed?" I also remember the sad eight-year-old girl that was standing in the midst of a road with heavy traffic. To the question "Why?" she responded that she "wanted to be killed (*suicidal, to be run over*)."

To elude her emotions, *Alumina*, as seen before, resorts to self-injury/cutting. Such self-sabotaging behavior is deployed to short-circuit the emotional cascade, in the hope that the physical sensations from the destructive behavior—the pain from self-injury—will distract her from her upsetting thoughts. Stopping the emotional cascade and reducing her emotional pain feels good in the moment and is the "helper" that is needed like a false friend; the negative consequences of the behavior, though, persist, and *Alumina* is harmed, especially when this behavior is repeated. It is especially women who resort to self-treachery like self-injury or comfort eating, while men are more likely to develop problems with physical aggression and drug and alcohol use (*Nux-v* being the prototype of such behavior). *Alumina* will be needed more and more in this society as forms of self-defeating behavior are on the rise—especially self-injury/cutting in adolescents. Ailments from domination lead to sadness, dissatisfaction and depression and often lead the victim to withdraw from others and stop engaging in activities they enjoy (*indifference to pleasure; indifference, joyless; discontentment*). By withholding such healthy compensations from herself, she only increases the depression; self-injury then feels "right" because it helps her escape momentarily intense and overwhelming negative emotions (*fears to be left alone lest he should injure himself*).

Anger Directed Outward

Alumina can also have the tendency to kill someone else when they see a knife (*desires to kill at sight of a knife or a gun*). In the case of *Alumina*, there is chaotic thinking even about committing violence: *he wants to cut himself although he abhors the idea of seeing blood.* This confusion is also expressed by *cobweb sensation in the face* reflecting a senseless going back and forth, a highly unstable irresolute state which can boil over any time. It is clear that the central idea in *Alumina* is a fight over control between the parent and the child, a struggle to avoid total submissiveness. As a result, the child develops *contradictory states* because she fights to regain control: a destructive person fights back, but there is also the psoric aspect of looking for support, a natural first instinct. We see this duality in: *timidity alternating with assurance; obstinate, resists the wishes of others* and *defiant; anxiety with fits of paroxysms* and *anxiety as if guilty of a crime* and *cowardice* as well as *courageous alternating with fear*. Such a child is at times submissive, and at other times will show rebellion (*barking, growling like a dog; contrary; disposition to contradict*). Together with *Mercury* and *Syphilinum*, *Alumina* is one of the strongest syphilitic hereditary remedies, so destructive expressions on every plane are predominant. Strong physical expressions of this remedy are *paralysis, constipation* and an Alzheimer's-like lack of memory; all of these are related to a person who is frozen, can't go forward, and does not dare to move without the consent of the parent or authority figure.

Such a strongly present conscious situation is always compensated with dreams carrying the opposite theme in the unconscious. These dreams are also a compensation to stop the unfortunate victim from falling into an abyss of despair and destruction by alerting him to the danger. The theme of the dream is often one in which the dreamer finds himself in a car driven by someone else or in which the dreamer is seated in the back of the car. In dreams, a car is the relatively fixed symbol for the urge or libido, not only sexual libido but also libido in general: the urge to get somewhere, the drive for independence, freedom, personal choice, and decision-making. Whoever is in the driver's seat in your dreams is influencing your life, either with your permission or, as in *Alumina's* case, through dominance. *Alumina* wakes up from the dream and, unfortunately, does not usually realize how meaningful it is: the dream is a severe warning to which he must listen if he wishes to change his life for the better. As Rainer Maria Rilke wrote: "[...] Here there is no place / that does not see you. You must change your life."[11]

Fighting for More Independence

Alumina's self-worth depends on conditions beyond his control: if he is "successful," he is valuable for the family and will be loved for being what his parents want him to be. If he is not successful, he is worthless in terms of maintaining or resurrecting the family's honor, and he will therefore not be loved. It leads to an immense degree of insecurity and confusion which can hardly be overestimated (*delusion, he is worthless, Anac, Thuj*). If respect and love for a person depend only on success in a competitive world, that person's self-esteem and self-confidence are bound to be shaky as any failure or setback inevitably leads to insecurity, helplessness, and a deep sense of inferiority and self-loathing. These are emotions which the *Alumina* person will constantly fight. Instead of being able to proclaim: "I am what I do," *Alumina* must say: "I am what you want me to do or desire me to be." *Alumina* has no genuine identity: he is only known to others as a substitute person of someone else—someone who manipulates the strings of his life story as if in a puppet theater. *Alumina* finds himself in a relationship in which he fights for more independence, since he needs to sacrifice too much in order to please other people. She always does what others want of her; she is not

11. Rainer Maria Rilke, "Archaic Torso of Apollo," *The Selected Poetry of Rainer Maria Rilke*, trans. Stephen Mitchell (New York: Vintage, 1989), 61.

allowed to take her own space in this world as remaining obedient is the only way to secure the love and support of the people she depends on. She is active in her own squashing, not just acquiescent. I had a patient who, while traveling, would say, "Oh, let's go to this place, we are so close, to see this or that." And her husband would always reply, "You really don't want to see that, right?" and she would say, "Of course not," because she knew **he** did not want to.

Taking away a person's individuality may create an *Alumina* state, especially if there is a destructive background in the family (mental disease, neurological destructive diseases, alcoholism, or autoimmune disorders). It will stir up the victim's feelings of hopelessness and despair as well as emotions of feeling small and dependent on someone else. *Alumina* is so controlled that impulses come on suddenly and take him by surprise, as when he grabs somebody's hand or acts violently and impulsively. The theme in *Alumina* is trying to **regain control**; this means control of the body (the child and the adult suffer from severe constipation and an Alzheimer's-like memory loss), control of the limbs (weakness is present), control of the impulses (sudden violent anger attacks alternating with timidity), and control of the emotions (*indifference to pleasurable things*; *injure himself, fears to be left alone, lest he should*). *Alumina* has a great fear of losing control. Since her mental will has been undermined, the will from the muscles is also taken away, leading to *great exhaustion of strength, especially after walking in open air*. Therefore, the patient cannot be hurried (*hurry, awkward from*). This mind/body **disconnect** is seen through the person's inability to move properly, having no balance despite wanting to be in control of the situation. *Alumina* also shows *aversion to the color red.* As a relatively fixed symbol, the color red stands for love, emotions, blood, passion, and life. Certainly, as discussed before, all this is absent in *Alumina*'s life, leading to an unconscious aversion to something that represents what is so lacking in her life.

Golden Tips from the Masters

- Dryness is the central idea (sweating is rare even during exertion), except in the vagina (leucorrhea): constipation with weakness of the rectum, with slight or no urge; dryness of the skin, wrinkled and cobweb sensation because of premature aging of the skin. Grayish look.
- Desires indigestibles (*Calc*)
- Alzheimer remedy (brain is "dried up")
- Multiple sclerosis remedy (*Con, Gels, Nat-m, Caust*): starts as a semi-paralysis, for a long time merely an inactivity before evolving into a complete paralytic state (paralysis of flexors and extensors)
- Strong catarrhal tendency wherever mucous membranes exist
- Remedy for broken-down voice in singers through overexertion with a peculiar tickling (*Arg-met*)
- Remedy for myelitis with spasmodic condition of the back and band sensation about the body and limbs, a sensation of a tight cord around the body
- #1 remedy for lead poisoning
- #1 remedy for constipation in young infants/newborns when nothing else is found

Ambra grisea (Ambra). Morbid secretion of the sperm whale

The Cyber Delusion

The Cyber delusion is ***sees diabolical, ugly and hideous faces crowded upon him, especially on waking***. This person is overcome by visual hallucinations (*delusion, sees specters, ghosts, devils, frightful images*) and is often a markedly nervous, sensitive, and self-conscious person. Although also a remedy for children, *Ambra* is mainly a **geriatric** remedy (*old age premature*; *he is unable to reflect in old age, feels stupid*). It is upon awaking, when one opens his eyes and is confronted with light (*shuns light*), the relatively fixed symbol of consciousness, that these ugly visions occur (*frightened upon awaking*). Reality indeed is often a shock, too much for *Ambra's* markedly fragile ego to bear. As *Ambra* has also *delusions, of fancy illusions,* one can understand that this is a person who tends to flee into the unconscious and create his own special, safe world where he is confronted only by creations of his own imagination. This is a person who needs his own space and privacy, away from others who now crowd upon him like ugly diabolical faces; he is easily overcome when the slightest demands are placed upon him. This creates a fear of *others approaching him* and general *misanthropy*. The causality will explain such behavior: Has everything becomes too much, too demanding for him, so that reality has become a hell from which he wants to escape? Indeed, the CD reflects strong causalities that have exhausted the Vital Force of the *Ambra* person: a diagnosis of mental and physical neurasthenia (*mental work impossible in old age*) is correctly applied to him, and anyone in such a fragile condition is at risk of falling into the *delusion, of becoming insane.*

Causality

Ambra's greatest ailment from (A/F) is *ailments from* ***business failure*** (*ailments from reversal of fortune*), a failure which is a *mental shock to him*. Because of his sensitive nature, this creates easy embarrassment (*ailments from embarrassment,* second only to *Sulphur*). *Ambra* is not only a *sensitive* person but also a very serious one who can be *full of cares and worries* and is *greatly affected by daily cares.* He takes his problems to bed (*anxiety in bed; she is haunted by unpleasant thoughts*); this creates *much sleeplessness after going to bed,* preventing him from falling asleep as his mind is full of his business (*sleeplessness, from cares, of business; from activity of thoughts about business*); *ailments from reversal of fortune* are always on his mind. There is nothing that drains someone's energy more than loss of sleep, and *Ambra* is no exception. Part of it is that this person is very attached to his family, for which he feels very responsible, but in *company he is rather embarrassed.* Another part is that he has *fear for poverty,* so business is always on his mind. This leaves little place for pleasurable things as they rather distract from what he wants to achieve: *fear from music* with a very special keynote that his *cough is aggravated with trembling by music or when playing the piano* (DD *Nat-c*). This cough is also aggravated *at the sight of strangers; <when persons are present.* Being an introvert, *Ambra* does not relate to music well; this is an individual who does not know how to deal with the emotions evoked by music. Nothing should distract him, so he appears rather *indifferent to joy and suffering,* and *even agreeable things* as he maintains the focus and seriousness of the disciplined businessperson; this will eventually lead to *ailments from mental work.* It is above all this failure in business that causes him *grief and bereavement. Ambra* is so single-minded, so oriented toward one aspect of life, that he neglects the lighter side and falls into *despair.*

Nature always punishes us with a disease when we suppress our feelings. In *Ambra's* case, the affliction usually remains psoric, or functional in nature, with *vertigo upon least exertion* (a non-descriptive dizziness as he must wait a while when getting out of bed) and *impaired hearing* as well as *functional metrorrhagia*—all symptoms that, in Traditional Chinese Medicine (TCM), indicate a deficient Kidney Qi. This is understandable as mental fatigue drains the precious Kidney Qi much more than does physical exertion. All this leads to the development of a person who becomes old-looking at an early age and who starts questioning the "meaning of his life," descending into a state of melancholy when business crumbles and when friends and family members die around him; there seems not enough spirit left in his body to be able to put up a good fight.

Compensations

Search for Privacy: Withdrawal

Concerned about his professional persona, this single-minded person definitely has an *aversion to the presence of strangers* and even *aversion to smiling faces* as he is overcome with anxieties, embarrassment, and worries over which he broods but about which he does not want to talk—at least not with an unknown person (*fear of others approaching him* and *fear of being looked at*). This is an added difficulty for the homeopath, who will have to probe gently; *Ambra* will not be forthcoming in admitting embarrassment suffered in business. It is not that he has an excessive persona in which he will hide lack of confidence, but rather that he shows identification with his persona. The only thing that is important is his business; it is the sole topic of his mind and conversations, all day long and, alas, also on going to bed, as we have seen before. So he looks rather like an asocial introvert who has an *aversion to answering* if it is not in the interest of his business and who gets *irritable from conversation* as it is a distraction from his goals in life. He surrounds himself with "barbed wire and hockey gear" in order to avoid any embarrassment. Few people will gain his trust or penetrate the elaborate defense mechanisms he has built up, so communication with the homeopath can be difficult as even the therapist can fall under the definition of his Cyber delusion. He takes his search for privacy to a different level, as he seems to be embarrassed about anything that he considers private: he avoids going to the bathroom when not at home (*company aversion to, the presence of strangers during stool and during urination*), is painfully aware of his own body odor, and is very discreet even when simply blowing his nose. *Ambra* is truly the opposite of so many people who are always searching for pleasure, parties, and free time and then don't know what to do with their leisure time. The austerity of *Ambra's* character combined with the over-intensity of his behavior makes him look humorless around the campfire or the barbecue. This is an introvert who always mulls things over (*absorbed, buried in thoughts*), who observes, hesitates, and ponders, a person who does not like to improvise. This is a person who looks for refuge in his home and workplace (his other home); the more crowded he thinks a place may be, the more reluctant he is to visit it (*anxiety in a crowd*; *fear of narrow places*). *Ambra* is really a cautious, anxious, and rather timid person (*timidity appearing in public*; *bashful in company*) with a nervous temperament; he expects and often sees obstacles where none exist and is guarded when performing any task, which often leads to a lack of lust for life (*weary of life*; *loathing at life*).

The Destruction of Consciousness

Consciousness is only increased by being exposed to stimuli from the environment and making split-second decisions, to accept or reject, acting like a filter. Increased consciousness is also augmented by the release of repressed unconscious contents that are made conscious. What happens to the *Ambra* person? He deliberately turns away from any incoming inner source while also withdrawing from society. Depleted energy is seen on every level in his consciousness. Mentally, he *has a weakness of memory for what he has read* and has a level of forgetfulness that is typical of a much older person (*forgetfulness of old people; he has to read everything three or four times and then does not understand it; unable to reflect in an old age*), even resembling *imbecility*. His speech is not an asset as he rather *rambles and changes quickly from one subject to another, continuously speaking in questions*. Emotionally, any contact with people outside of the immediate family is rejected (*conversation aggravates; indisposed to talk* and *indifference to loathing of life* and *sits weeping, wrapped in deep sad thoughts with indolence to work, especially in the morning*). He is so strongly indifferent that he does not even wonder why he is not excited over these wonderful things that would move the heart of a well-balanced person. Physically, he struggles with many functional problems due to exhaustion. Because of the lack of exterior stimuli coming to *Ambra's* ego, this strange Cyber delusion has a great opportunity to fill the vacuum created in the conscious, and it therefore separates this person more and more from the real world, bringing him closer to the abyss of psychosis. Everything is *as in a dream* while *time passes too slowly and appears longer*. The pressure to always exert himself to obtain success in his business easily reaches a breaking point when he is confronted with failure—to the point that he will lose his mind (*delusion, is about to get insane*). His dissociation from reality is expressed by his way of talking. As Kent mentions, "...there is a fleeting inquisitiveness, jumping from one subject to another, asking one question and then another without waiting for an answer"[12] which makes one think of *Lachesis*, another character who can descend into the abyss of insanity, in that case because of his fiery and often unbalanced character. *Ambra* seems present but is not; he remains somewhere between consciousness and unconsciousness in his dreamy, absent state.

12. Kent, *Lectures*, 67.

Golden Tips from the Masters

- Indicated in stage fright (*Gels, Arg-n, Lycopodium*)
- Nondescript vertigo in the elderly on the least exertion
- Impaired hearing in the elderly without any organic defect of the ear
- Analogue to *Nat-m* with dwelling on disagreeable things

Anacardium orientale (Anac). Marking-nut Tree

The Cyber Delusion

Anacardium's Cyber delusion brings much insight to this important remedy: ***a devil is speaking in one ear, an angel in the other, prompts him to do murder or acts of benevolence***. Certainly this is a person suffering from a Dr. Jekyll and Mr. Hyde complex, from an inner conflict (*contradiction between reason and will*). Here is a split personality (*feels and thought he had two wills, one commanding to do what the other forbids; thinks he is double; duality, sense of*) who seems to be able to demonstrate totally opposite behavior unexpectedly, without any apparent reason, from acts of goodness to the most evil acts known to humankind. Worse, *Anacardium* has no control over who will win this battle: the devil or the angel, the bad or the good. He suffers from a mental schism: there are moments in which he enjoys doing harm, yet he is then overcome with guilt. *Anacardium* causes a situation of "disinhibition." These are thoughts that all of us can have in passing but that normally are inhibited. With *Anacardium*, these thoughts persevere in the back of the mind, and the struggle starts between control and loss of control when some of these thoughts are released without his consent or intention at the most inopportune moments. He is overcome by rage and panic, leading to sudden *violent rage so violent he could have stabbed someone*, a raging storm which is an expression of *Anacardium's* dark side. The more he loses the battle between good and evil, the more his heart hardens, which is symbolic of his name: *Anacardium* is derived from the Greek *an* ("without" or "not") and the Latin *cor* or "heart," combining to mean "without a heart." And at some stage, following one moral defeat after another, *Anacardium* may reach a point of no return unless liberated by homeopathic doses of *Anacardium*.

Anacardium is possessed by his Cyber delusion and is scarcely able to achieve real identity amid the tremendous pressure and chaos it creates. There is a constant fight between an "It" and "I." Sometimes the "I" vanquishes and reigns over the "It," and at other times the

"It" overwhelms the "I." Part of this is because *Anacardium* has the delusion that *he is under super human control.* Don't think that such a delusion only appears at the end of severe pathology; sometimes such a Cyber delusion is expressed at a young age. I had a beautiful eight-year-old girl as a patient who was extremely cruel and unfeeling towards her mother but fearful of, and obedient to, her alcoholic father. When I asked her why she behaved this way, she answered: "I can't help it, **someone makes me do it**," expressing the delusion of being under the influence of a powerful being, a sort of possession by primitive impulses and urges (*delusion, being possessed*). So *Anacardium* can resort to unacceptable acts of cruelty.

The *Anacardium* patient seems to be a victim, at least as far as the kind of etiology is concerned (see Causalities below). But he certainly doesn't act like a victim. He has *want of moral feeling*; he often *curses* and does physical violence without any remorse. Our materia medica says that the devil speaks in one ear and the angel in the other, but when the devil wins, the patient feels no remorse and performs the requested deed with no scruples. When the good voice (the angel) regains ground in her mind, the patient feels terrible afterwards. The continuous and horrific battle expressed by this Cyber delusion is also expressed by the delusions, *thinks he is demoniacal*; *the devil whispers blasphemous words*; *delusion of being double*; *delusion, someone is in bed with him*; *a devil sits in her neck and tells him most offensive things*; *delusion, strange figures accompanying him, one on his right, the other on his left*; *being possessed*; *he is three persons*; *he is possessed of two wills.* Clearly, many of the proven delusions of *Anacardium* are additional expressions and confirmations of our Cyber delusion, revealing a lack of control and much confusion in the patient's behavior as well as a fixed idea of *separation from the world* because of the battle between two wills. This will lead to an obstructed personality, a lack of ego growth or individuation, or what we could call a psychic arrest. Even a partial loss of contact with reality engenders a profound sense of insecurity, irresolution, and abandonment closely resembling the atmosphere of a nightmare. In conventional medicine, such a child may receive many diagnoses ranging from ASD, ADHD, or Selective Autism to Tourette's syndrome and, especially, Infantile Bipolar Disease (IBD):

> One of my patients with autism strongly exhibited this battle between bad and good by creating an alter ego. His alter ego was Draco (a character from the YouTube BabyTV Channel), a goofy, happy, and cute dragon that plays with a ball (a game of self-exploration), and he always spoke using this dragon character's

voice. He would say "Draco will hit you" or "Draco loves Mommy" or "Draco bumped Mommy's head." And when his mom said "Yes, Draco bumped my head but I am OK," he cried so much that he had to be restrained because he wanted to strike himself. One sees the great battle between good and evil and the confusion it creates. Draco makes him assume the role of the ruler, the one in command of his darker side, on which all the responsibility of this child is placed. Draco gave my patient the chance of living on the side of power. There was even a time that my patient announced to his mom: "Draco will bump Mommy." When his mom replied, "Does Draco want to bump Mommy?" he said yes but then proceeded to hug her. The mom told me, "This seems very schizophrenic to me, a dual personality of sorts." Jung referred to such behavior as that of a child suffering from a "moral inferiority."[13]

Causalities

Ailments from Parental Domination

Parental domination is one of the most common triggers of an *Anacardium* state. Parental domination refers not only to that of natural parents, but also to any authority figure, including other family members, teachers, priests, gurus, coaches, etc. As expressed by the Cyber delusion, it is often only one of the parents who plays the role of the "devil": for instance, an alcoholic father, a mother who is a prostitute, or an overly strict military father with a lack of feelings and flexibility. The "superhuman being" can also be a coach, teacher, and guru who plays the father or model role who begins to impose his own set of distorted rules and regulations. With each step on the wrong path, it becomes more difficult to return to the fork in the road where a wrong decision was made. *Anacardium's* relative hardness delays the ultimate pathology for *Anacardium*, which will be a late-onset psychotic break with the appearance of a schizophrenic state, when the ego is overwhelmed by the contents of the unconscious. Indeed, in the case of *Anacardium*, there is hardness and cruelty harbored deep down in the shadow side as a compensation for the conscious, one-sided low self-confidence, as well as a *disposition to malice as even the slightest offence makes him excessively angry.*

13. Jung, *Development of Personality*, 150.

The term "superhuman being" can be relative. For a very weak, chaotic, confused person, or anyone in a vulnerable position, everyone out there looks like a superhuman or giant. For a naïve child with an undeveloped ego, a parent or any adult with authority seems to be of enormous proportions. For a mesmerized follower, a guru seems to attain gigantic dimensions, and for the beginning homeopath, a master homeopath seems to have godlike qualities. These relationships can be called dysfunctional. In a balanced family, no one enjoys dogmatic authority, but only that authority to which he is entitled by reason of his labors and abilities. Alas, in *Anacardium's* case, we often have a *pater familias* who will assert absolute, even cruel and unjust dogmatism and authority, unchallenged by anyone.

Any child growing up in such a household will exhibit an inadequate persona. It is a form of an obstructed personality in a person, a malformation of the persona or the formation of a pseudo-ego in child or adult alike. It can take three forms: an inadequate persona (*Anac, Bar-c*), an excessive persona in which a thick mask is formed to hide inadequacies (*Lyc, Sil*), or identification with the persona (*Ars, Sulphur, Verat-a*) in which the person has become the persona, a lack of expanding one's interests, to form a one-sided, one-colored mask. But for the inadequate persona, as is the case with *Anacardium*, the individual feels that he possesses no conscious, freely chosen, well-serving guidelines about his self-growth and direction in life. His ego is emptied of libidinal energy, the very source of life. He is convinced that no one believes anything he says is worth listening to as it is always somebody else who makes decisions for him. In other words, the "face" or persona that is presented to the outside world is in reality a face imposed and molded by others: it is the other person's face, not his (DD with *Alumina*)! The inadequate personality is he who looks in the mirror and poses the questions: "Who am I? What is my name?"

The persona is the opposite of the shadow. The symbols of the persona appear in dreams as images of clothes, hats, dress, uniforms, armor, and masks. They also may be expressed in awards, diplomas, the characteristics of a profession or trade, or a variety of status symbols (stethoscope, wig, etc.). When one appears in his pajamas, it means he has no persona, since he is in the garment suited to the unconscious! But persons with an inadequate persona like *Anacardium* often have dreams of appearing naked, of feeling unprotected and vulnerable. Being naked in a dream can also have a positive side. It is when the person, through either psychoanalysis or homeopathic remedies, makes progress in his individuation process and now lets his guard down, so to speak, able to look at himself as he really is.

An inadequate or false ego formation can also be the result of hereditary weakness or idiocy (as in *Bar-c* and *Bufo*) as well as the formation of an inadequate persona through neglect of the individual (as is the case in *Hura braziliensis*, *Lac-c* and *Lyssin*). No matter what the etiology of this foreign mask is, it will always lead to the formation of individuals who are morbidly sensitive to criticism (*offended easily*) and demonstrate low self-worth, leading to a life of great dependency on others. In general, we can say that an *Anacardium* state can be brought about mainly by abuse, sexual abuse, contradiction, domination in children, rudeness of others, and violence.

Ailments from Anticipation Anxiety

The maintenance of such an *Anacardium* state and the deepening of the Cyber delusion are supported by subsequent *secondary ailments from*. If someone in a child's life, for instance, always decides what she should do, how she should dress, what friends to choose, what books to read, who to socialize with, etc. (I refer here even to the parent who means well), the child will be nothing more than a slave without a voice. All decisions are taken without heart and purely according to the intellectual thinking *(logos)* function of the conscious. One of the first consequences in the child will be a high degree of *anticipation anxiety*: *There is always anguish and apprehension as of imminent misfortune. He troubled himself about every trifle, as if it would cause great injury, with solicitude about the future.* Indeed, paying attention to every trifle is crucial (*conscientious about trifles*)! Approval or disapproval is totally dependent on how well behaved this child can be—that is, the one her parents want her to be, regardless of who she really is.

Ailments from Contradiction

This child is contradicted in everything she wants, does, or expresses as it does not conform to the master plan of the ruler of the house, so the child clashes constantly with the *modus operandi* of the parent(s). *Ailments from contradiction*, therefore, figure prominently in *Anacardium's* picture. All too often, an intellectual, *logos*-oriented parent (especially one in a thinking profession such as a scientist, lawyer, or doctor) can impose his preferences on his child who, for instance, may be naturally more inclined to the arts as she is the feeling type (Eros) and not the thinking type. Forcing someone to function in his archaic conscious function (that is, the weakest conscious function) leads to many neuroses and future failures in life! This person may never find the meaning of his life.

These causalities stemming from childhood will carry over into adulthood if there has been no appropriate therapy (counseling, homeopathic remedies) and resolution. More often, a situation has been created in which the individual is incapable of moving forward, and the childhood crime, often delegated to the unconscious, translates now in adulthood into many compensations resulting from that one Cyber delusion, which is mostly unknown to its possessor. The childhood crime has now created a dysfunctional adult, who is in a worse condition than a defective child, an adult who always needs support from his immediate family, especially the mother: this person is unable to attempt to understand and develop the innate potentialities of his or her psyche. Somewhere along the road, such a person gets stuck, even unbeknownst to himself.

These ailments from contradiction also take a somewhat different form. I refer here to conflicts between the parents in the presence of the child. One of the children in my practice became "autistic" because the father threatened to kill his wife in front of the child (*abusive husband insulting wife before children*). Such a child, caught in the crossfire and frightened to death, becomes confused as she loves both parents; she now becomes a split personality, choosing one parent one moment, then the other the next. Even less traumatic events have led to infantile schizophrenia. An example is the story of five-year-old "Renee," whose father had a mistress and who heard her mother say, "I will kill myself if he leaves me." This frightened Renee so much that, from that moment on (just at an age at which the child tries to become separate from the parental ego and become more independent), the growth of her ego was harmed for several years with frightened momentary experiences of dissociation. This only worsened around puberty, with flaring up of the syphilitic miasm and a deep descent into schizophrenia from which she recovered only years later.[14] A similar situation can arise when the parents of a young child divorce. I remember the case of a fifteen-year-old boy whose parents had divorced when he was six. He was living with his mother. The breakup

14. Marguerite Sechehaye, *Autobiography of a Schizophrenic Girl: The True Story of "Renee"* (New York: Penguin, 1994), 22.

of his family at this young age had created such confusion and guilt in him that he went from excessive coprolalia (*swearing, obscene and lewd*) to extreme violence and rage, smashing holes in the wall.

Compensations

Lack of Self-Confidence

The *Anacardium* child, because of lack of control and disorientation, will easily and unexpectedly change from positive to negative compensations (unlike most suffering children, who resort first to positive compensation steps). One of the first victims of such a situation is *Anacardium's* confidence: she will suffer greatly from *lack of self-confidence* under the constant control of the parent. The lack of self-confidence is always a very deep pathology in *Anacardium*. (*Bar-c* and *Anac* are the most outspoken in this rubric.) With *Bar-c*, an undeveloped *Calc-c*, there is dwarfishness of the mind from birth on (hereditary, miasmatic influence). *Anacardium*, on the other hand, suffers from the domination from others or is overcome from too much mental effort by trying to prove himself to his parents in order to gain their love. *Anacardium* can have periods of the same shyness and lack of self-worth as *Bar-c* as she walks on the street, thinking that people are criticizing her. At first, the *Anacardium* child will try to overcome this through hard work, knowing that he is capable of succeeding, trying to prove the parent wrong, and, above all, trying to receive approval from the parent. The continuous great demands put on her by others and herself (as she tries to eradicate her inadequacy and prove to others that he is worthy of receiving love and approbation through increased hard work) will eventually lead to an opposite, undesirable state: *aversion to mental work* and *ailments from mental exertion*. This is a child who will flee her homework and who has great anticipation anxiety before tests. *She cannot be persuaded of doing anything; she has no pleasure in anything.* There is *indifference to everything; indifference to irritating disagreeable things; to joy and suffering of others; to his religion and to pleasure. She is disinclined to talk and there is estrangement from individuals and society, with fear of the future. There are bad effects from mental exertion, as it brings on a tearing pressing headache to forehead, temples and occiput.* You can see what a wonderful remedy *Anac* can be for students who are preparing for exams and suffering from great anticipation anxiety with mental neurasthenia.

Paranoia and Timidity

Anacardium's ego is assaulted step by step, enslaved to the ego of that "superior" being (the dominating person), so timidity and being stuck and obstructed are always on *Anacardium's* path: *timorous in all his actions; he views everything, more anxiously and timidly; he always thinks of being surrounded by enemies and has deep thoughts, meditating over his present and his future destiny. The future seems to him very dangerous as if nothing were imminent but misfortune and danger; he has distrust in his own power and suffers from despondency.* This becomes a very vicious cycle for the *Anacardium* child: he wants to prove himself to others and himself, but *he has so little confidence in himself that he despairs of being able to accomplish what is demanded of him.* No wonder such a child is easily left behind in the classroom.

Intolerance of Contradiction

A strong feeling of inferiority is obviously at the bottom of *Anacardium's* neurosis, a clear case of Adlerian psychology in which the inferiority gives rise to a power complex. For Adler, and as seen in *Anacardium's* case, the delusional system is a "masculine protest," a striving for power to safeguard his threatened individuation (*abusive; violent anger; blasphemy*). When one feels submerged in feelings of inferiority, one must have some compensatory reaction of superiority in which to take refuge. Unfortunately, this interplay between inferiority and superiority never results in a normal adaptation to life, since either one state or the other must prevail. If a child fails to adapt to a new situation, he may be seized with rage to try to compensate for his sense of defeat. Pushed by an extremely painful conflict (his sense of inadequacy and incompetence and his will to succeed in spite of it) *the child takes everything in an ill manner* and *becomes violent, passionate* and *contrary at a slight offense. He is very intolerant of contradiction.* The rage emerges like a tsunami and just has to run its course. But then, a few hours later, *Anacardium* feels terrible about herself, guilty and despicable (*anxiety, conscience, as if guilty of a crime; reproaching himself; delusion, he is demoniacal*). And then she can't even bear to look at herself in the mirror: nothing is right, everything is wrong, and *Anacardium* is crying inside.

His behavior can also look more and more foolish: *extreme merriment and laughing when he should be serious* (*laughing about serious matters*), an indication of the sadness behind the mask. *Anacardium* can resort to *continuous talking of senseless things and use of profane language with swearing and thinking himself to be a demon.* In this use of *profanity,* we can recognize the unfortunate victim of Tourette's syndrome, irresolvable in allopathy. Loss of control in this child is easily observed. *A slight offense makes him extremely angry, as he takes everything in bad part and becomes violent.* It goes even to the point of *want of moral feeling with depravity, inhumanity, wicked, cruel* and *hardness of heart,* the latter proving reflecting its own remedy name. This is seen in cruelty to animals and people (*joy at misfortune of others*).

Mental Exertion

The *mental exertion* also takes its toll on *Anacardium* as his memory completely fails, something he was dreading all along: *her forgetfulness troubles her so much that she loses her appetite; he remembers with difficulty; he retains nothing in his memory; he is deficient in ideas and he soon loses his subject without being aware of it; his great forgetfulness makes him very morose. His memory is better in the afternoon than in the morning. Anac* is a great remedy for the student who feels a lot of pressure to succeed because of earlier unfounded criticism (when parents or teachers haven't acknowledged his worthiness, often comparing him to a successful sibling). Towards the end of the preparatory period, even before the actual examination, the *Anacardium* person forgets everything he studied from sheer exhaustion and extensive effort: *his thoughts leave him and everything intellectual is hard for him. Exertion of the mind brings also on a tearing pressing headache in forehead, temples and occiput. He becomes very indifferent and unfeeling. There is obtuseness of the senses as he hardly notices what passes around him.* One recognizes easily the picture of some ASD children. I often have seen that the child, aware of what this mental effort in school does to him, starts feigning strong headaches in order to avoid going to school.

At the end, because of failure of memory, his contradictory moods, a profound inferiority complex, a constant guessing about a course of action, and failure of accomplishments due to constant disappointments and criticism, the fixed idea *everything appears as in a dream* (showing the disconnection and loss of control of the ego) is created; he feels as if his spirit were separated from his body, contributing to continued confusion and a return to his Cyber delusion, the mental schism from which he suffers.

Golden Tips from the Masters

- *Anacardium* is a combination of *Lycopodium* and *Nux vomica* intensified
- Etiology is humiliation and suppression, much like *Staphysagria*: they are put down by society and want revenge
- Religious fanaticism like *Verat-a*
- #1 for Tourette's syndrome with swearing
- Multiple personality syndrome
- Paranoid schizophrenia
- Feels better when eating: indicated in some cases of stomach ulcer
- Mass murderers with auditory hallucinations

Argentum nitricum (Arg-n). Silver nitrate

The Cyber Delusion

The central fixed idea of *Argentum* is that ***he is despised and forsaken*** (***abandoned***). The main idea is that he is forsaken, and thus a person in an *Arg-n* state immediately thinks that it must be because he is despised (*delusion, he is repudiated by his relatives*), not appreciated and loved. Most of the time it has nothing to do with reality, yet this fixed idea occurs frequently to the child or the pregnant mother because of increased anxiety and fear. In the case of a pregnant woman, especially a primigravida, her state may cause an increase of anxiety. This may create a state of oversensitivity to small events which normally would not bother her, such as her partner working many hours or making a business trip to another state. One can see immediately the kind of hopelessness and despair that takes the person in its firm grip, leading to great restlessness in everything she does and contributing to a situation in which she is always on the verge of a nervous breakdown or fears a heart attack (*delusion, die, he was about to die; while walking, he thinks he will have a fit which makes him walk faster*). It is even more than a forsaken feeling, as his frail nerves imagine all kinds of disasters: *delusion, he has an incurable disease; delusion everything fails* and *delusion, he cannot succeed and does everything wrong,* while irrational thoughts about danger loom everywhere around him, leading to ritualistic and superstitious behavior (*impulse to do strange things*): *delusion, while walking in the street corners of the house project so that he fears he will run against them* and *houses on each side of the street and would approach and crush him.* One can see his *fear of being enclosed in narrow spaces and a sense of isolation* (*agoraphobia,* which imprisons him in his home), which creates a very needy and fearful person who always wants a trusted person close to him. When that person cannot always be there for her, she is convinced that *she is neglected* and not loved. The delusion (an internal barometer with constantly falling self-esteem) that everything will fail and that she cannot succeed makes *Arg-n* a difficult person in work environments, reinforcing his

Cyber delusion, as he tends to be an obstructionist stirring up doubts in others and eroding confidence in novel ideas and projects. Without any doubt, *Arg-n* can be called a remedy for the neurotic person for whom every small task becomes a hopeless difficult enterprise and every minor discomfort a fatal disease. *Arg-n* is the most fearful and worrisome remedy in our materia medica, and nothing, even the most rational reasoning, can convince such person that she is OK (*obstinate, headstrong; she had the queerest objection against whatever was proposed*). To any reasonable argument, she always will retort, "Yes, but WHAT IF..." What if this or that happens? No reasonable argument can convince this person; another "what if" can always be found intellectually (archaic thinking function). The person in an *Arg-n* state has a hard time grasping how others could feel safe in the same situation; her fixed response overrides the primitive thinking function and is unable to quell the tsunami of her dominant feeling function until the indicated doses of *Arg-n* frees the patient from this black hole resulting from the "what ifs." *Arg-n* will always find the cloud in any silver lining, discouraging anyone from taking a bold initiative or step forward in life.

Not surprisingly, this forsaken feeling creates a kind of depression and confusion as expressed by another delusion: *she is enveloped by heavy black thick clouds,* taking away her reasoning capacity (*delusion, has softening of the brain*) as such a person even believes that *she is lost to the world beyond hope.* No one is there and willing to help her, and for a child this fixed idea of being forsaken can appear anytime that mom is not nearby or when the child enters school and is now left behind in a new environment for the first time. Everything around her looks unfamiliar and looms larger than normal, adding to the overwhelming sense of danger (*delusion, objects and distances are enlarged,* and *delusion, everything is changed* and *familiar things seem strange*).

Causalities

Anticipation Anxiety

The main causality is anticipation anxiety and stress (*emotional excitement*) related to certain events: first-time pregnancy, anxiety about a new job, entrance exams for a new career, testing by a psychologist or school tests, waiting for the results of a medical test, or anything that creates high anxiety about an *upcoming event as well as mental work.* Let's take the example of a pregnant woman whom I saw in my practice. She was expecting her first child, and it was very much wanted. Suddenly she experienced uterine pains in the beginning of the pregnancy. She was examined but nothing could be found. She thought little of it, but the pains persisted. When there was any small problem, she became terrified that something was really wrong, that something was going to happen. She felt in physical danger. Additionally, she stated, "I thought I might have an extra uterine pregnancy." She even went to a university clinic for further testing, but nothing was found. Yet she did not believe the reassurances, which is additionally reflective of *Argentum nitricum's* fixed ideas that *she is lost beyond all hope to the world; and she was about to die.* At this very moment, her husband had to travel overseas. She pleaded with him not to go: "I wanted my husband to stay just in case something happened to me"—reflecting *fears of impending disease,* and *fear something will happen.* In spite of her pleading, her husband left, reassured by the words of the doctors; this created, in the pregnant mother, the fixed idea that he did not care (*delusion, she is despised; forsaken; and repudiated by relatives;* the fixed idea, *that she is neglected*). "I felt that I could not count on him, and I told him when he called that he did not have to come back. It took a long time to repair, much longer than the pregnancy," she reported (*hatred, unforgiving to those that have offended*). "I called close friends to let them know what was going on with me, just in case I needed their assistance during the night, and I went to sleep worrying again," she stated (*fear something will happen*). Like *Aconite,* the *Arg-n* person is convinced that harm will come her way (*prophesying and predicting time of death*). Her husband leaving town at the moment of her insecurity and her feeling of impending danger made her very nervous. "What if something should happen while he is gone?" she asked (*A/F emotional excitement; persistent tormenting thoughts*). This "what if" emotion (expressing fear) was transferred to the fetus through mystical participation, through the psychological umbilical cord, creating a child with the same strong emotions that the mother had experienced during and after the pregnancy.

Fear, Fright and Emotional Excitement (Stress)

Without any doubt, *Arg-n* is the greatest phobia remedy of our materia medica. Anything that can create a sensation of *isolation* and not belonging to this world (*forsaken, sensation of isolation*), real or perceived, creates *fear and fright*! Fright also includes stressful situations such as anxiety and shock upon hearing bad news, seeing a dead body, witnessing an accident, or fright after an airplane crash. It also includes insecurity about a job, a relationship, or health; fear of poverty; and *fear of failure* and *stage fright* occurring days before the event. In children this fear will be manifested with *enuresis nocturna,* or bedwetting. In fact, this is very often caused in the child through a family situation of anxiety or insecurity. There is no other emotion that is more inappropriately channeled than fear. Fear and fright throughout life are always threatening to destroy the integrity and control of a person's life. Rather than facing and dealing with such overwhelming emotions, people give in to anger as it provides a way to avoid dealing with the more menacing feeling of fear. Often, for children in an *Arg-n* state, fear is translated into anger or temper tantrums. We can even see it in animals: when dogs feel fear, do they not react with anger and barking? Adults fare no better: *disappointment leads to loss of ambition* and *easy angry outbursts.* Because their nerves are getting the best of them, any *mental exertion aggravates* with *difficulties of thinking and comprehending* as they always seem to be in a fog. The slightest stress, like leaving the home, where they feel secure, overcomes them with a feeling of dread (*fear when ready to go to church or opera*); this phobia of perceived danger and *helplessness* can go so far that, even in their own home, they will withdraw to one room and resort to *weeping from hopelessness* and *loss of will from melancholia.*

Compensations

Need for Protection and Purposeless Activity

The Cyber delusion creates in child and adult alike an intense fear of his surroundings (*fear to walk past certain corners; fear in a crowd* and *public places* or *agoraphobia*) and fear for his health (*fear of impending disease; delusion, he has an incurable disease* or *his heart will stop beating while sitting*) as well as insecurity in his capabilities (*delusion, everything will fail* and *he cannot succeed as he is doing everything wrong*). In order to keep control over these situations, the *Arg-n* person can become *busy fruitless.* Even the smallest task (he makes a mountain out of a molehill), like cleaning up his room or balancing a checkbook, becomes a severe test, and *Arg-n* will not start this task if he thinks he cannot do it perfectly (*he undertakes nothing lest he fail*). The *Arg-n* state produces an unbalanced, often irrational and impulsive person with weakening mental faculties (*he feels very much affected bodily and mentally; he does not undertake anything lest he should not succeed, but he suffers from mental work*). Often, strange and crazy ideas float in his mind, such as: I should jump from a bridge, or I should touch this person suddenly and make him jump; often the impulses are so strong that *Arg-n* needs to muster all his mental strength not to do such foolish things. Purposeless activity is driven by an internal compulsion, as the person is driven by anxiety. *Busy fruitless* is no activity but mere *busyness.* The person is acted upon by this internal force which leads to Obsessive Compulsive Disorder (OCD), which means that he is forced to do something against his own will by an inner force that he is unaware of, such as avoiding certain corners of the streets, counting steps (*superstitious*), or the flapping and spinning of the child in an autistic state. This is also a person who indulges his urge to triple-check and to organize. This non-productive activity refers to its quality, as purposeful behavior results in useful personal changes and growth of the ego, which is not the case in *Arg-n*. Remedies such as *Veratrum* as well as *Bar-c* have excessive amounts of this fruitless activity or passivity. But when the anticipation anxiety rules (hesitation), *anxiety about any upcoming event* occurs, and he is overcome by *despair in hypochondriasis,* the *Arg-n* person eventually refuses to leave his home and prefers to stay in bed (*desire to remain in bed*); he becomes a prisoner in his own home. This stage follows the *Arg-n* state of strong *desire for company,* as this person always feels a need to talk about his anxieties (*desire to talk to someone; talks anxious about his condition with wife and children; talks of nothing but one subject – his fears*). However, in the end, unable to find people to listen to his continuous *lamenting and wailing about his sickness,* this person becomes isolated from society.

Morbid Need for Affection

Arg-n has a morbidly intense need for affection and attention. Remedies such as *Pulsatilla* and *Hyoscyamus* can also come to mind, but in the case of an *Arg-n* person there is neither violent nor sexual behavior, nor lewd talk, nor even jealousy present. Contrary to *Pulsatilla* and *Hyoscyamus,* who consider the younger sibling as competition for attention, the *Arg-n* child can have a younger sibling and, if anything, would be very concerned for her safety, always looking after her. He is very protective of his younger sibling, a trait reflecting the state of the expectant mom while pregnant with him, when she was overly protective of her unborn fetus and going from one physician to another (or having many tests done just to make sure that "nothing can happen and everything is OK"). The *Arg-n* child is not jealous of his sibling, but he experiences so much anxiety about whether his mother loves him (he needs the protection!) that he constantly asks his mom, "Do you really love me?" We see the child's clinginess and constant need to be reassured of his mother's affection. He asks for hugs all the time, but he wonders: "Can I trust her when she says she loves me?" It does not come as a surprise, therefore, that he is *sensitive to admonition,* which rips his soul apart. A child like this is often excessively sensitive to a small insignificant snub or offense (*melancholy since an undeserved slight with the fixed idea that he was neglected and despised by his family*). Hence his morbid sensitivity to admonition! The *Arg-n* person, often with *a weakness for what she is about to say,* can have a feeling (fixed idea) of being despised: "I am dumb; I deserve to be punished," which may very well feed this delusion.

Anger

As mental work aggravates him and causes *difficulty of thinking and comprehending,* an *Arg-n* child can become *excitable and contrary.* Sure that he will fail, he *desires to remain in bed* as the mental work fatigues him greatly. He can become antagonistic toward himself, exhibiting low self-esteem ("I am dumb") even to the point of asking for punishment and abuse. He speaks eloquently, though with a *rambling loquacity* (such children with autism usually belong to the high-functioning group), and cries easily (*weeping from hopelessness*). Anger expresses itself symbolically on the physical plane: the *Arg-n* child is always a colicky baby from birth on, keeping the parents awake at night. Moreover, *Arg-n* is one of the best remedies for colicky babies. This was often seen when physicians or nurses used to put silver nitrate drops in the eyes of newborns to avoid transference of gonorrhea (Ophthalmia neonatorum). Many past incidences of colic were caused by these prophylactic drops.

Anger can turn into aggressivity when someone invades *Argentum nitricum's* space (*fear of narrow places such as elevators, tunnels, and dentist; fear in crowds, agoraphobia*). Such a person always needs an exit: if the *Arg-n* child sleeps with other children in a big room, he will never sleep in the middle of the room but will always stay near the exit so as to know that, in case something happens (the "what if something happens"), he will be ready to escape. *Arg-n* has an extreme fear of the dentist as he is locked in a narrow space without an exit—and at the mercy of the "one with the drill!" Although the child *desires company,* and *has aversion to solitude,* he is quite content to play by himself at home and school, the latter becoming a safe second home. He shows the same *fear something will happen* except when he is in a safe environment, surrounded by people he knows: home or the familiar school. Otherwise, outside of these two safe environments, the *Arg-n* person feels neglected when expected attention is not forthcoming: especially attention desired from his parents or from people who play the role of parents/relatives. These may include the homeopath, teacher, guru, or, in the case of an adult, the spouse. Someone trusted must stand by him at every moment of his life, especially to shoulder the burdens of life and deal with the dangers in life: *he looked around as if expecting someone to help him out.* He needs this support to still his anxieties!

Restlessness

The physical body is always in tune with the restless mind. Unless he has become a prisoner of his home, reluctant to step out into the world, hurry is always a part of driven *Arg-n*. *He is always in a hurry when walking; always in a hurry to arrive for the appointed time.* If he has to meet someone, he has anticipation anxiety, breaks out in a sweat, and may experience urgency to make a stool. Whoever is with him at that time has to hurry too (*everybody must hurry*). Such a person will always be extra early for appointments (*fear of being late*) and has a difficult time waiting in your waiting room. This restlessness is also reflected in the gastrointestinal tract: *diarrhea when excited* and *diarrhea as before going to the theater.* The latter proving is easily seen in the *Arg-n* person. Anytime he goes to a movie theater, a restaurant, or a speaking engagement (which seems worse than approaching death), or even to work, he will have a tendency toward diarrhea and will need to know where the toilet is. I had a patient who needed to travel one hour to work on a busy freeway, but he never succeeded in reaching his destination without stopping as, in the middle of his trip, he always had to park his car on the side to hurry to have a bowel movement. *Arg-n* cured him. **There is also no better remedy for stage fright and fear** before an examination when diarrhea sets in **days before** the event takes place.

Golden Tips from the Masters

- It is the left-sided *Lycopodium*: *Lyc* is the closest remedy to *Arg-n*
- Best remedy for sweet and salt cravings at the same time (patients overdose on sweets, resulting in diarrhea and eructations with general feeling of being sick)
- Fear of one's own thoughts and losing control
- Remedy for claustrophobia and agoraphobia
- Major diabetes and hypoglycemia remedy (*Phos*, *Sygizium*)
- Major stomach ulcer remedy (*Kali-carb*)
- Fear of narrow bridges and high places causing vertigo
- "Speaker's" throat: feeling of having a thorn in the throat making him constantly clear his throat (*Arum triphyllum*)
- Conjunctivitis with yellow-green discharge, the inside of the eye looks like raw meat and eyelids stick together. #1 remedy for conjunctivitis in children
- Sensation of expansion in the head from studying too much
- Hot-blooded people >from fresh air
- #1 remedy for eructations and flatulence
- Brings relief to some beginning cases of Alzheimer (*weakness for expressing oneself, for what he is about to say*)
- *Gelsemium* is the exhausted state of *Arg-n*: overexertion leads to this exhausted state
- In dull headaches of business and literary men (Richard Hughes)
- A nursing infant with green diarrhea because the mother ate candy (Kent)
- It has a complementary action to *Lachesis* concerning diseased blood vessels with atheromatous degeneration and varicose veins
- A complementary action is also seen with *Pulsatilla*: he wants cold air, cold drinks, cold things like ice and ice cream, and suffocates in a warm room
- Often indicated in Colitis ulcerosa patients with great anxieties and phobias as ulceration is found everywhere in this remedy: it heals the ulcers
- Cannot lie on right side as it causes palpitations: outspoken symptom
- Feeling of something sticking in the throat (*Hepar*, *Nit-ac*)
- #1 Remedy for colicky babies

Arsenicum album (Ars). White arsenic

The Cyber Delusion

Arsenicum is one of those people who ought to come with an instruction kit. *Arsenicum's* Cyber delusion is ***he is sick***. From in the beginning of his existence, he feels very sick (at least in his mind), which is also expressed by the delusions *his time has come to die*; *he is being doomed*, and *he is about to receive an injury*. In *Arsenicum's* mind, there are always the gloomy forebodings and thoughts of death because of the "incurability" of his symptoms. This irrational fear of death is outspoken in *Ars* and results from the failure to live, an expression of a guilty conscience for wasting one's life and missing the opportunity to do something productive with one's talents. To die with the thought that life was in vain, to die without having lived, is unbearable—yet it is *Arsenicum's* fate because of his sterile approach to life. *Arsenicum* has never found true pleasure, had serenity of mind, or experienced the absence of fear. *Arsenicum* lives under the illusion that destiny can be controlled and life and health mastered by the right actions; he believes that misery and disease are but malfunctions which may be righted by giving more effort and adopting the proper approach. *Arsenicum* cannot keep his composure and realism and look straight into the abyss that life can be.

There is no doubt that his health issue is primordial, so his Cyber delusion has everything to do with the **preservation of health and survival**, the most basic human instinct (*when alone he falls to thinking about disease and other things, which he can scarcely keep out of his mind*). This will lead him to be very fearful and anxious about almost everything. *Arsenicum* always seeks scientific revolutions which provide the ultimate consolation: the promise to delay aging, overcome any illness, free him of unavoidable suffering, and, one day, even cheat death itself. The quest for longevity! Of course for *Arsenicum*, nothing but a dissatisfying state comes from such thoughts and cares. He always suffers from a neurosis, namely, an obsession with being sick and especially with having cancer. He has already consulted all available specialists, who in turn have performed all possible X-rays and tests. They have all assured him that he has no cancer. But *Arsenicum* will tell the homeopath: "I know that I have no cancer, but I still could have one" (*thoughts of incurability of his complaint*). Who or what is responsible for this imaginary yet persistent idea? It is his Cyber delusion!

This survival instinct brings on paranoia as *Arsenicum* has other fixed ideas: *he is being watched; he has done wrong; he is about to be arrested; there are conspiracies against him; he had murdered someone* and *he has offended people*. One can sense his overwhelming feeling that his life and safety are at stake, as in his mind, *he has done wrong* and *he has committed a crime against others* who will now try to harm him and who are watching him closely. This creates a tremendous state of hypervigilance so as not to make any mistakes. One needs other people in order to survive, but at the same time, *Arsenicum* is a high-strung person who is not easily influenced by other people's opinions. Overwhelmed by fears (especially *fear for cancer*), *Arsenicum* has the feeling that it is "my life and I must take care of it. I must make sure I am happy. I must sure that my family and I will not die from starvation" (*fixed idea that he and his family will die from starvation*). As *Arsenicum* strives for an unobtainable perfection, he is also sure that no physician yet has discovered his elusive illness (*thoughts of death and the incurability of his complaint*).

Causalities

Ailments from Anger and Anticipation Anxiety

The greatest ailments from, or triggers, are *ailments from anticipation* and *ailments from anger with anxiety*. In a child, such emotions can invade by means of mystical participation as the fetus is tied not only to the physical but also to the psychological umbilical cord of the mother. Through mystical participation, because of the close psychological bond existing between child and mother from the day of conception until at least age five, the newborn *Arsenicum*'s prenatal ego will have absorbed much of what roams in the unconscious of the mother, especially the fixed ideas mentioned before. It will create a child who is restless, irritable, and excessively anxious (especially at night) from day one—a child who can only be quieted when carried around. At the same time, such a child will eat greedily and more than he needs, and he will often exhibit colicky pains and acid reflux after eating. And incidences of anticipation and anxiety are common for the pregnant mother, especially if she has had miscarriages or failed IVF (in vitro fertilization) attempts in the past, which can increase her anxiety level even further. Being more sensitive than normal, the pregnant mom reacts more strongly to triggers that normally not would be a problem; she is disturbed if her partner travels, worries about what to do in case of bleeding, feels more anxious at night, and needs company. There is also fear for the delivery, fear for miscarriage, fear for having an abnormal child in this age of the Autism Spectrum Disorder (ASD) epidemic, fear her own health will be affected, fear she will not be a good mother, *fear of being left alone*, fear *for being alone in bed at night, lest he die* (*Arsenicum* in high potency is a great remedy to bring comfort and peace to the dying patient). This constant *fear for evil* befalling the woman during pregnancy can be so intense and last so long that the fetus can hardly escape taking on these emotions. Hence, this is a child, and later an adult, that will be very *anxious at night in bed, driving him out of bed or tossing about in bed*. The anxiety can already start around *twilight*. The anxiety can be so strong that it leads to *anguish with palpitations with a feeling of constriction in the chest*. The child is *full of cares even about trifles* and *can be beside himself*, as fixed ideas of doom and gloom can take over. What *Arsenicum* needs to learn is that everyone needs a certain amount of worry, anxiety, pain, or trouble, just as a ship requires ballast in order to proceed on a straight and steady course. This is what is called real life.

Pecuniary Loss and Financial Debacle

Another trigger that will create an *Arsenicum* state is pecuniary loss or a financial debacle: this can be money lost in the stock market, a job or home lost by the pregnant mother (or her partner), or having unexpected taxes to pay as money was mismanaged; these can lead to a severe and long-lasting emotional state infecting the unborn fetus with the same feeling, which will influence the child as he grows up:

> I remember the case of a young professional who took money out of her IRA without realizing she had to pay taxes on that amount. When her accountant told her so, she went into a great, despairing *Arsenicum* state, becoming irrational and claiming that she reacted to every remedy given, even in the smallest amount. She ended up fearful that she would harm herself and therefore was putting the remedy in 13 successive cups from each of which she took one drop; she asked a friend to carry the remedy when she accompanied her to another doctor

to test her sensitivity for it. She was convinced that she was poisoned beyond relief from her remedy (*despair of recovery; doubtful, medicine is useless*). Appropriate doses of *Arsenicum* were able to dissolve the irrational despairing state.

Compensations

Looking for Company

A person who is overcome by anxiety and anticipation has as a first compensation and defense mechanism a *desire for **company***, a source of protection. That strong desire for self-preservation is fundamental, and people in despair need to count on someone whom they can trust, someone of whom they are 100% sure. A child with an archaic ego will always seek the company of the mother or father and go from one to the other. An adult will look for the spouse, a best friend, and yes, his physician, who will have to notify Mr. *Arsenicum* when and where he plans to take a little vacation, giving the patient the means (telephone, email) to reach the physician while he is away. There is great fear of losing needed support, so when the mom or dad is sick, or someone he knows in the family dies, this great fear of death is translated into *fears something may happen to his relatives*, a projection of his own fears. Fear of disease can also extend to his friend's sicknesses: first of all, these will be contagious to his spirit so he will have *gloomy forebodings while lying in bed*, creating a very restless sleep. No wonder, as his mind is *thinking about disease and other scary things which he can scarcely keep out of his mind leading to fear of being left alone*. In fact, this person, like the *Calcarea* person, fears suffering and disease almost more than death. Such a child wants to be in the parents' bed; a little light in his room is not sufficient. But the child *often talks in his sleep, revealing his deepest secrets*, usually his *extensive fears* and *despair of recovery*.

The child overcome by fears is usually a very *serious child, who almost never laughs*. Unfortunately for this child, seriousness is usually met with seriousness, while laughter and openness from adults come from similar emotions in children. Such a child, therefore, has few friends in school; obviously, the *Arsenicum* adult or child, afraid he is going to lose his sole support, becomes too dependent on his friend. The resulting clinginess usually does indeed lead to losing that friend, so his greatest fear comes true. He will face the hardship in life alone, and he is convinced that others have conspired against him to bring him to this precarious position (*delusion, there are conspiracies against him*). If his mom is also an *Arsenicum* person, then looking for company takes on a different meaning: her unfortunate child will be the object of numerous visits to a variety of physicians, undergoing a multitude of tests and treatments. As one can see, that will only increase the anguish in this child, as he will think that something must be deadly wrong with him as the topic of such an intensive investigation. Conversely, the child can also become the adult! I remember such a case in my practice: the 11-year-old daughter was playing the mother to her own mother, who was seized by the inner drive to have her child undergo checkups in response to any innocent trifle. Her mom always brought me baked goodies, of course always made with the healthiest organic ingredients, but what was more interesting to me was how this poor girl talked to her mom like an adult, trying to reassure her mom that she was OK. Ailments from early responsibility and anticipation anxiety are two unfortunate triggers for future cancer development.

Unfortunately, the *Arsenicum* person *despairs and weeps and imagines no one can help him; he is convinced that he must die*, and *there is excessive anguish with oppression of the chest driving him from one place to another for relief* (which means from one physician's consult to another). To further compensate for his *delusion, he is sick and dying*, the *Arsenicum* person talks a lot about her health and the newest discoveries of the benefit of vitamins and natural products to everyone who will listen: *great loquacity while awake and asleep* (that means that the child will keep up the parent to be reassured all the time). The adult *Arsenicum wakes up children and wife to talk to them. He wept and whined and whimpered. It is pitiful complaining with great anxiety and restlessness, often leading to lamentations and despair of life*. Of course *Arsenicum* talks always about his "health problems" and his fear of death and suffering. Restlessness is seen everywhere in these children: as they go from one place to another, from mother to father, or to another family member, they become suddenly overtired and then *want to be carried fast* from one room to another.

Fear of death is an essential characteristic of *Arsenicum*. Fear of death, in a healthy person, should result in a desire to live life meaningfully to the last breath. Alas! This is not the case for the *Arsenicum* person. For mankind, the terrifying certainty of death necessarily appeared with the faculty of reason. But this certainty of death can only terrify those who have a guilty conscience towards life. Only those who have betrayed their own souls (*Carcinosin, Staph* and *Lachesis*, to name a few cursed with the penalty of the unlived life) are frightened by this inevitable event. It is also the *Arsenicum* person who cannot let go, exhibiting on his deathbed the mental and physical restlessness for which this remedy is so effective and well known. *Arsenicum* has never reached his goal—perfection—and therefore cannot exit from his unfulfilled life. The hypochondriacs, like *Arsenicum, Calc-c, Cann-i* and *Nit-ac,* have so much anxiety about catching a disease that they pursue the *delusion, they can never die.* It is a foolish quest for longevity or even immortality! Their emotional states lead to a multitude of allopathically attributed disease names, of which the best known is OCD, as a means to control their anxiety and paranoia (the simplest forms of schizophrenia). A full-blown picture of schizophrenia and *insanity* is possible, caused by *fright, grief* and *persecution mania.*

Hypochondriasis

Anyone can experience a sudden brush with hypochondriasis. We feel pain in the thorax, the cough does not disappear, and we think for a moment: "Is this lung cancer?" But then it disappears the next hour. We might have a mole appear on the neck and not even think of it until a concerned and well-meaning friend tells us: "If I were you I would let a dermatologist look at it." (Of course, the dermatologist is never content to just look at it: he wants to biopsy it and cut it out, just in case.) And a touch of deep-seated fear, of our powerful survival instinct momentarily arises. What if it is cancer? I don't mean to say that one should never consult a physician, but the *Arsenicum* person takes hypochondriasis to new heights. The Greeks invented the term to describe ailments caused by the movement of the upper region of the abdomen—from *hypo* (below) and *chondros,* or "breast bone cartilage." By the late 19th century, hypochondriasis had come to mean something entirely different. Hypochondriasis is the fixed idea that one suffers from an incurable disease or that no physician has yet discovered the disease from which he is suffering. It is a life based upon the raw, carnal fear of forthcoming disease and death. In any given year, Mr. *Arsenicum* may be convinced that he is dying of (in no particular order): brain cancer, stomach cancer, bowel cancer, pancreatic cancer, skin cancer, MS, and Lyme disease (*fear of death; anxiety about salvation*). When one ailment is dismissed by his physician, he inevitably rushes to Google to find out why his doctor is wrong. "What! I don't have pancreatic cancer? Then it must be..." Of course, when *Arsenicum* googles "blurred vision and tumor," a whopping 200,000 results come back, many of which confirm his worst nightmares. One also has to tiptoe around Mr. *Arsenicum,* fearful of brushing against him and drawing his ire for exposing him to "viruses and bacteria" (*delusion he is about to receive an injury*). He is the germophobe by excellence and leads a personal crusade against the bacteria, viruses, fungi, other still-to-be-found microorganisms, and dirt that exist everywhere. He dreads ATMs, computer keyboards, babies, handrails, shopping carts, door knobs—you name it. This terror can manifest itself in obsessive hand-washing (*washing, hands, always washing the hands; cleanness, mania for*) or an aversion to others' touch, all syphilitic traits for the dominant psoric *Arsenicum* person. Outside of the operation room, as we know, scientists debate whether there is really any reason to fear germs so much, but marketers of hand sanitizers do a good business nonetheless. It is no surprise that *Arsenicum* evinces an extraordinary affection for the ultimate groomer among animals, the cat (*animals, love for cats*). *Arsenicum* is also convinced that trifling imperfections are a matter of life and death (*conscientious about trifles*). And as long as these trifles are not corrected, he is convinced that his health is at great risk. The hypochondriac talks in exaggerated, hysterical tones about a multitude of ailments; these are frequently such trifles as: "Why is this nail not growing as fast as my others?" "What does this white spot on my skin mean?" etc. The patient's painful expression and his hurried loquacity confirm that he views these "imperfections" as life-threatening and direct expressions of ill health. It is more than fear—it is anguish, a syphilitic expression leading to pessimism, irresolution, anguish, irritability, and even hostility if not taken seriously (*disposition to contradict; contemptuous; cursing*). "Doctor, I know I have already had this stool test several times," he says, "but I want you to retake it in a different lab. I think the others missed something." "I know I am dying because, well, I just know. I am certain of it. I can feel it. These other physicians are wrong. I know they are wrong. I wish I could believe them." The hypochondriac is dreaded by the physician as he constantly besieges the physician with messages and faxes regarding his imminent death. Usually, though, he outlives his physicians and tortures them with exaggerated or non-existent disease states. Even if he improves 90% with your remedy, he will focus on the remaining uncured 10% and declare that he has not improved at all. He is driven by the quest for perfection, the fear of suffering, the despair of possible recovery (*despair of recovery, during convalescence*), and the always-present threat of imminent death (*anxious about salvation*).

One example of typical *Arsenicum* communication came from an obsessively anxious patient who sent me a fax after leaving five telephone messages during my busy workday asking for reassurance. I could not describe *Arsenicum's* mind better than he did, as the following in fact expresses many of his delusions:

"I don't think I will make it through the day, my heart is pounding so much."

"I have waves of weakness in my arms and I am extremely nervous."

"I feel like I have to pace and walk all the time."

"I have feelings of fear of I don't know what."

"I think I am going to die." (He said this four times that day.)

"My hands tremble and I have gas in my abdomen. I think there is something seriously wrong."

"I know I can't get through this day! I feel shortness of breath on exertion or lying down."

"If this is of any value to you [he is not sure!], we can discuss it the next time we talk."

Well, to be sure it was of great value, and there was no need to see him or to talk further: he needed *Arsenicum*!

Hoarding

Why is it that some people feel such a strong urge to hold onto things, while others shred, dump, and recycle with ease? According to allopathy, the behaviors of packrats may have some genetic basis. Homeopathy knows that it is caused by a psoric miasmatic predisposition. The *Arsenicum* person's security is based upon hoarding and saving, while spending, even if necessary, is felt to be a threat. Spending must be tightly controlled to provide for future catastrophes, "just in case something happens." He lives in his castle, and has surrounded himself, as it were, by a protective wall, and his main aim is to bring as much as possible into this fortified position and to let as little as possible out of it. *Arsenicum's* belongings pile higher and higher over time in unwieldy stacks, choking off access to closet shelves. Tackling the mountain of stuff is impossible due to *Arsenicum's* cherished attachment to items, which makes it painful to dispose of them. *Arsenicum* tends to develop emotionally fraught relationships with the things she owns. Emptying her shelves directly into a dumpster would certainly evoke a heart attack in *Arsenicum* (also *Sulphur*). His miserliness encompasses money, food, and material things (toys for children); it extends, also, to feelings and thoughts. Love is a possession; he does not give love but tries to get it by possessing the beloved. He knows everything but is sterile and incapable of productive thinking. He shows a tight-lipped mouth and an enormous desire for possession (*greed*) about anything that is around him (greedy and protective of what he has): "This is mine: my family, my toys, my books..." He does not want to share and, in fact, keeps what he does not need; he even resorts to *kleptomania*. When a five-year-old child has books that he read when two years old, but he wants to hang on to them and refuses to give them to his younger sibling, it is an expression of the homeopathic proving of *Arsenicum*: *his desires are greater than his needs; he eats and drinks more than is good for him*. This leads easily to avarice with secondary delusions; now, he is afraid that others will take his belongings (*suspicious, mistrustful*): *Delusion, someone is under the bed; delusions, he is about to receive an injury; sees rats; sees thieves;* and *thieves are in the space under his bed. He imagines that he sees burglars in his room, and listens under the bed; he is bathed in cold sweat;* and *runs about the house, looking for thieves*. Understandably, he loves to have money to stay afloat in life and is afraid to lose it or spend it: this is the child who willingly puts every small amount of money he receives in a bank account to accrue interest. When the adult or child loses money, it leads to deep grief (*ailments from financial loss; melancholy after financial loss, cannot be consoled; thinks he will have to die with his family from starvation*). If you shortchange him even by a penny, he can become very angry. The *Arsenicum* person saves everything and gives nothing away (no garage sales!). And he is convinced that everyone is overcharging him for the smallest task they perform: he constantly thinks that people rob him. Unfortunately, the *Arsenicum* tightwad amplifies the importance of the future instead of enjoying himself in the present, a phenomenon called hyperopia. This medical term denotes problems associated with farsightedness. Too often, the beautiful moments of life can be drowned out by a cacophony of self-consciousness and unending anxiety. Life unfolds in the present, but *Arsenicum* often lets the present slip away, allowing time to rush past unobserved, squandering the precious seconds of his life as he worries about the future and ruminates about the past. The key for *Arsenicum* should be thinking about what he will regret in the long term, but alas—that is never on *Arsenicum*'s mind!

Sterile Orderliness: Obsessive-Compulsive Behavior

The expressions of obsessional neurosis are multiple, but all carry great intensity: extreme meticulousness, a great eye for detail, exaggerated love for order and symmetry, fanatical cleanliness, and pronounced germ phobia are a few, all of which can be found in the *Arsenicum* person. This obsessional neurosis stems from excessive consciousness and conscientiousness. It is the result of striving for one hundred percent, for absolute perfection, and is therefore doomed not only to fail but also to create a pattern of repetition the moment one starts any process. It is an exhaustive (and exhausting) search for unobtainable perfection! As the person knows that he cannot achieve a hundred percent in **everything**, he thinks that maybe he can achieve perfection in one specific area of his life. He becomes a "hot spot" observer, demanding extremely high standards of neatness and order in a very particular area. In *Arsenicum's* case, the person seeks success in excessive, ritualistic hand-washing, cleaning his house or his desk, planning every action of the day on paper, itemizing schedules, stocking his refrigerator with bottles of Evian water, all with labels facing outwards (or there will be hell to pay!), bringing his own plastic silverware to the one restaurant he patronizes, organizing of all the items in her household in name-tagged boxes, stocking food for at least a hundred days (Dooms day is always looming), and writing twenty-six pages of complaints to his homeopath; *Arsenicum* is capable of all of this. It is all based upon *Arsenicum's* desire for absolute **security**, something he can fall back on in case of disaster. The process of cleaning does make *Arsenicum* feel that he has achieved some small thing in an unmanageable world. It gives the illusion of order. These obsessions, however, can also impair one's ability to function. I had a patient, a motivational speaker, who felt the urge to spend hours scrubbing his hands in the bathroom before a scheduled speech. He was convinced that if he went onstage without doing so, he would inflict a mysterious disease on his audience (*delusion, contaminated, everything one is touching is,* only *Arsenicum*). The sad thing is that such behavior imposes the laws of his personality on others (especially close family), which is not only sick but also suffocating and selfish behavior. But *Arsenicum* can become a high achiever because of this so-called pathology—not in spite of it. For accountants, lawyers, editors and engineers, *Arsenicum* is a good fit.

One of the most common characteristics of the *Arsenicum* person (adult and child) is a pedantic and sterile orderliness. There are certain rules to be followed. He cannot endure things that are out of order and will automatically rearrange things (*conscientious about trifles; he cannot rest when things are not in proper place*). In the child's case, you see this in the way he lines up his toys or arranges his books and gets very upset if anyone upsets the harmony of his world or fails to return an object to its proper place. *Arsenicum* wipes her shoes vigorously on the doormat even though she is planning to remove them. This is symbolic for *Arsenicum* as he tries to master the outside world by avoiding its intrusion. Compulsive cleanliness is an expression of his need to cut off contact with the outside world. Things beyond his own frontiers are felt to be dangerous and unclean, and he annuls menacing contact by *compulsive hand washing,* similar to the religious washing rituals prescribed after contact with unclean things or people. Things have to be put in their proper place but also in their proper place in time, leading to obsessive punctuality. Order and security are the driving forces, but all this is sterile, as life starts to resemble death. From there comes *Arsenicum's* great fear of death and preparation for it! However, we must remember that exposure to infectious agents is essential for the growth and development of the immune system. So in fact *Arsenicum* shoots himself in the foot by not challenging his immune system; only exposure allows the body to create specific antibodies to be are stored and summoned to defensive duty when a similar bug poses a threat.

Obviously, perfection (so much desired by the *Arsenicum* person) is unobtainable (*delusion, he will never be happy in his own house*), and therefore the *Arsenicum* person always thinks he has not put in enough effort (*delusion, he neglects his duty*). *He is dissatisfied and angry with himself all day and thinks he has not accomplished enough and reproaches himself bitterly.* For the pre-verbal child with ASD, this will lead to a lot of frustration and temper tantrums: *very cross, irritable and whining.* This is a child that does not like his clothes to be soiled by food or drinks as he is very *fastidious.*

Ars is a person who feels compelled to examine all the options before him before making a decision, which leads to *irresolution.* As a result he is frequently beset with regret and self-blame (*reproaching himself*) about the road not taken. In doing so he incurs a hefty psychological cost: *despair of life,* guilt (*anxiety of conscience as if guilty of a crime*), and an existence *full of worries.* Always displeased with the option he chooses, he is *full of worries about trifles* and unhappy with the one he chooses as there are so many others that appear to be better on further contemplation (*delusion, he has done wrong*). Rather than yielding better results, this leads to procrastination (*postpones everything till the next day*). Procrastination is arational, without reason—because the real issue is emotional. In *Arsenicum's* case, the issue is the fear of doing something wrong and not finding the perfect solution.

Depression/Anger

When no form of support is found, anguish can overwhelm the *Arsenicum* person and a deep form of depression can set in: he *feels uncomfortable and takes pleasure in nothing; the least thing troubles her as she has a hypersensitive delicate mood. The least trifle fills her with solicitude and care. Her mind is depressed and sad and great despondency and indifference follows.* What does not help him is that when *ideas crowd upon him, he is too weak to repel them in order to dwell upon* ***one*** *idea only*! Such extraordinary mental activity leads suddenly to a lack of focus and a sudden exhaustion and weariness that seems out of proportion to the effort that the *Arsenicum* person has put forth.

At this point, when negativity dominates, the *Arsenicum* person can show his dark side: he *can be cruel and malicious, and loves to make people and animals suffer. He becomes angry at himself when he makes mistakes* and often it is about nothing (*anger about trifles*); in addition, though, *he reproaches others* for his misfortunes. He can demonstrate excessive *censorious behavior*, especially if friends or family members disturb the order of his world. Being malicious and manipulating people comes in many forms, but the M.O. is always to provoke and then make the other person feel that they have no reason to react—and that it is all the other person's fault to begin with! *Arsenicum shows envy at the qualities of others.* Arsenicum gets *confused but washing the face with cold water ameliorates.* At this point, such a *child does not bear to be looked at as it aggravates his mental symptoms.* No matter what you do or say, *Arsenicum will take everything in bad part and shows a peevish and morose character. He is convinced people are plotting against him and becomes extremely suspicious.* His withdrawal from the outside world is expressed in *frequent spells of unconsciousness and absences* and withdrawal into a dream world (*delusion, of fancy illusions*).

Golden Tips from the Masters

- *Arsenicum* is the acute of *Nat-s* and *Thuja*. Excellent for the acute asthma attack, but a complete cure will require anti-sycotic remedies such as *Med, Nit-ac, Thuja* and *Nat-s*.
- Refuses to take the medicine as he feels he is incurable: "There is no use in having the doctor come; I am going to die."
- Fear of incurable disease (cancer, AIDS) dominates (*Nit-ac, Lach*)
- #1 remedy for the dying patient to die peacefully (1M potency)
- Whereas *Aconite* reflects a big storm soon over, *Arsenicum* is enduring and recurrent torment
- #1 for food poisoning from bad water (compare with *China*: from bad meat)
- An extra pillow under the head relieves the asthma attack with *Arsenicum*.
- Everything aggravates by cold except cold applications for headaches; body pains >warmth. Relief of all the complaints of the body from warmth in general when he is easily chilled
- #1 for hypersensitive people (DD *Phos*)
- Big keynote: sneezing without relief
- At any stage in a cancer patient's treatment, *Arsenicum* can be needed to combat fatigue, anguish, and shortness of breath. It is the best remedy for palliation of a cancer patient where burning, stinging pains have entirely disappeared as in uterine and breast cancer
- Keynote: weakness of the patient out of proportion
- *Arsenicum*, the famous remedy for cancer, works brilliantly when a dose of *Carcinosin* is given first (Richard Hughes)
- *Ars* drinks little and often. *Bryonia* drinks much at a time and seldom. *Ars* eats much at a time. *Bryonia* eats often and little (J.H. Clarke). *Ars* is thirstless in **chronic** conditions
- *Ars* has proven to be curative in epithelial cancer of the lips, face, and tongue (Hughes and Kent)
- *Ars* has no rival for severe forms of aphtae
- *Ars* is a classic remedy for bleeding cancer and has an equally great reputation for the cure of lupus

- Use the Morgan bowel nosode in cases of asthma in children where *Ars* and *Nat-s* have failed
- #1 remedy for gangrenous lesions (*Lachesis*)
- Swelling of the lower eyelid (*Kali-c* has swelling of upper eyelid)
- Periodicity (every week or two weeks) in malaria attacks
- With *Ferrum*, #1 remedy for anemia

Aurum foliatum (Aur). Aurum metallicum or gold

The Cyber Delusion

Aurum foliatum has the Cyber delusion ***he has neglected his duty and deserves reproach.*** The essence of this remedy is to be the first, to be the best. The *Aurum* patient (child or adult) always thinks he does not do enough for other people or for himself (*delusion, he has done wrong*) to achieve the highest ambition he fosters; *he always thinks that he is neglecting something for which he will be reproached; he seems to carry with him this internal restlessness, and it took from him all perseverance and energy.* A person of great capacity, such as someone matching the *Aurum* profile, is likely to have a great task ahead of him but also, assuredly, a more difficult life. One's crown is also one's cross. The *Aurum* person is very serious, studies and works hard and systematically (*industrious*), and feels the burden of preparing for future performances; people expect much from him, compounding the pressure he puts on himself. For *Aurum*, who does not merely think how to spend his time but tries to *use* it to achieve, the important thing is his personality: his moral character, intelligence, and *industriousness*. Gold is the symbol of perfection, of freedom and immortality, and a person instilled with such a character always strives for the purest ideas and goals, even if it leads to great personal sacrifice. But it can also lead to the highest goal: achieving true happiness, as the happiness we receive from ourselves is definitely superior to that which we can receive from our surroundings. *Aurum* is a person who is firing on all cylinders in order to rise to a challenge. He feels a sense of personal mastery over the goal he has set, and the activity is so intrinsically rewarding that, although the task can be difficult, action feels effortless.

Conscientiousness is one of *Aurum's* natural inborn qualities and fundamental personality traits. He exemplifies what he holds important; his values infuse his life. Conscientiousness is equal parts *industriousness,* impulse control and organization. Conscientiousness is also called responsibility. Responsibility and responding have the same root, being derived from the Latin *respondere*, "to answer." To be responsible, for *Aurum*, means to be ready to respond when and where he is needed. *Aurum* is very invested in his own family, in community, and in the world at large. These investments call for people to be more responsible, and *Aurum* responds to that call. This is at the root of *Aurum's* life and, ultimately, his suffering. *Aurum* fills his life to the very brim with goal-oriented deeds for mankind, just as one might fill a cup to the very brim with wine. It is a remedy suited to a child or adult who seems to have the fundamental conviction that he is destined to achieve a superior position in life and extraordinary feats, that it is his birthright. He knows he has great qualities and convictions, and he believes in his own ideals (destined to help people, to become a CEO, great filmmaker, great writer, great healer, etc.). *Aurum* possesses a productive obsession: it is rooted in love, interest, and desire to better our shared circumstances here in this world. *Aurum* always thinks big! He learns to banish distractions so that he can concentrate on his ultimate goal. *Aurum* is hardly a person who looks at himself in the mirror and sees a person who might have done this but didn't, or who loves that but, for some odd reason, took no active interest in it. Without hesitation, he ups the ante and gets obsessed. He prefers grand pursuits to ordinary ones and stands in solidarity with other members of his species who have opted for big thinking and big doing. He cultivates this productive obsession to the point of exhaustion, walking a long arduous journey with dips and peaks. His mantra is: "I am doing this and I will succeed." He is a vessel of light, and in his presence we are reminded of our own neglected heights; we are embarrassed to be less than we could be. Socrates, Gandhi, Buddha, Mother Theresa, and Nelson Mandela come to mind. *Aurum* always has a strong sense of purpose. He radiates righteousness and force of will, and his single-minded focus on the larger significance of what he is doing becomes obvious.

Some humans have the rare tendency among the world's creatures to give to those to whom they are not genetically related. Among those, one recognizes *Aurum* people who are particularly prone to benevolence and philanthropy, marked by their kindness, focus, intensity, and great inner strength. Even when the sacrifice is so great that they risk their very lives, they believe the rewards of giving outweigh its consequences, staking their lives upon their values. Ordinary riches can be stolen from a man, but the real riches in the treasure house of *Aurum's* soul cannot be taken from him. *Aurum* is living proof of one of the paradoxes of happiness: man needs more than pleasure to live the best possible life. The broader definition of good living blends deep satisfaction and a profound connection to others through empathy and unconditional service, a rich, full, and meaningful joy. Compassion, altruism, wisdom, insight—sometimes only the trials of adversity can foster these qualities, as is the case for *Aurum*. These ideals often lead to isolation and even mockery by his contemporaries; he is often more appreciated much later, even after his death. But for *Aurum* it does not matter, as long as he realizes the nobility of the soul that is within him. A well-balanced *Aurum* person is in general very productive and animates whatever he touches (the proverbial meaning of "everything he touches turns to gold"). He is a person who carries out the responsibilities he himself has taken on: he is a person free of fear, even in the face of death threats or imprisonment. He might use his wealth to undertake philanthropic enterprises, contributing to the general good of his fellow men.

The person in an *Aurum* state is generally closed (introvert), refined, and highly disciplined and ambitious. Because of their serious-mindedness and ambition (*serious, earnest*), such people can lose their sense of lightness about life; it is as if a constant background of sad music has been playing in accompaniment to the events in their life. *Aurum* children are usually more adult than their friends and choose their friends very carefully. In fact, usually they have few friends, and are often busy by themselves, wanting to be left alone but bullied in school. The *Aurum* child is very intellectual, precocious, and too serious for his own good. The reaction of the outside world to a joyous child is joyous; the reaction to a serious child is serious, and *Aurum* does perceive the difference; this doesn't protect him, though, as he, driven by his CD, cannot change his character. He has a strong belief in his own ego, but his only fear is of failure (*delusion, everything will fail*; *delusion*; *he cannot succeed and does everything wrong*), this can lead to a fixed idea of *not being appreciated* and a *forsaken feeling*, a sense of loneliness (*delusion, he has lost the affection of his friends* and *the delusion, that his friends have lost all confidence in him*). Especially in American culture, sports stars are much more valued in school than academic stars, who are often dismissed as "nerds." This can cause self-condemnation (*reproaches himself*), *a constant looking into self*, and a deep depression in the *Aurum* personality, who goes so far as to think that no one out in the world understands him or wants to connect to him (*delusion, he is unfit for this world*). *Aurum* can victimize himself by telling himself that he has not achieved enough, that he has not put out enough effort, and that he has let down his friends. *Aurum* has at the end of his road a negative inflation, which is a state of feeling too bad rather than too good. He feels that he is in no way good enough for this world, that he is always at fault or always wrong. He is, therefore, oversensitive to criticism, both real and imagined. He *sits still, wrapped in deep, sad thoughts and notices nothing* and broods about whether people appreciate him, which of course only intensifies the fixed idea. *Aurum's* perfectionism and conscientiousness create a harsh internal environment as they fail to teach *Aurum* how to accept his inevitable limitations. He is always on the defensive and constantly feels attacked. Any statement or fact is interpreted as criticism; any obstacle, any difficulty, any relationship problem proves that he is no good, that he is a failure: *delusion, everything will fail; delusion, she is lost; delusion, does nothing right*. There is a constant threat that eventually all roads lead to depression, melancholy, tears, and withdrawal, to the point of even suicidal moods (*imagines to see obstacles in his way everywhere, occasioned partly by contrary fate, partly by himself; makes him feel desponding*).

But when in balance, the *Aurum* person is a true individual; most of the great liberating deeds in world history originate from a leading personality like *Aurum*, never from the masses. Becoming an individual is reaching the gold in life; it is an act of high courage, a supreme realization and the achievement of the greatest possible freedom one can realize. It also means paying a steep price, as isolation from the unconscious masses is inevitable (*forsaken; delusion, he is unfit for this world*). The battle to become an individual is, therefore, not a particularly popular undertaking, but people like *Aurum* have embarked on this path of liberation from childhood on. When keeping his composure and equilibrium, *Aurum* represents the seeds of the tree of humanity. Rather than following the collective beaten track, he urges forward in the narrow path leading to the unknown. What drives such people from a young age? It is an inexplicable vocation, an irrational factor, a need to be different from the herds. *Aurum* is called upon by an inner voice and cannot resist his fate and destination: it is a mandate he must obey.

No doubt, *Aurum* unknowingly and involuntarily becomes a leader. In his ascent to power, he will become a personality; he can, however, also succumb (the negative syphilitic side) to the increasing load of responsibility, expressed by his numerous abovementioned delusions, as he progresses in life confronted by many obstructions and challenges. But at least *Aurum* has the opportunity to realize life's meaning, which is becoming a personality. Most people fail in this mission, but Nature is merciful and never puts the question "Did you become an individual?" in people's minds. And so it goes: where no one asks, no one needs to answer. In their search for gold, the alchemists discovered other things—medicines, gunpowder, the laws of Nature. The balanced *Aurum* is the true alchemist of the materia medica, one who never ceases to search for new ways to improve the conditions of his fellow men while finding optimum happiness in doing it.

Causalities

Financial Loss

As exemplary as an *Aurum* person is, he is not always necessarily a spiritual person, one who is not interested in amassing money and material goods. For some *Aurum* types (a minority) money plays an important role as their whole life is focused on one single goal: amassing riches! Stockbrokers on Wall Street are a perfect example. Margaret Tyler, who lived through the world's greatest financial crisis, wrote, "Some of us could tell tale after tale of patients, who, reduced to despair by anxiety, threatened suicide and yet were rapidly restored to life, to hope, to renewed effort by a few doses of homeopathic gold."[15] A common *Aurum* causality and pathology is *depression due to financial loss in the family or business failure* (stock market losses of '87—brokers committed *suicide by jumping from the window; loss of home or property, loss of job* especially of the father). Financial loss in the family also can be accounted for as the #1 stress factor for the pregnant woman who is overwhelmed by the loss of security for herself and the unborn fetus. For the *Aurum* person himself, the thought of disgrace, of falling from the throne, is unbearable. He tends to put all his eggs in one basket, and when he loses his financial independence, he takes stock of the balance of his life. Knowing he cannot make up for his loss because of older age or a bad economy, **if** this is the case, he begins to have suicidal thoughts. If the pregnant mother has suffered such a mishap, the child can be born in an *Aurum* state through mystical participation. Parents' unemployment, pay cuts, or reduced hours yank many children out of their comfortable cocoons as they are forced to deal with material downgrades, moves, and parents in turmoil. Economic recession can bring a sense of siege, and the collective emotional tone of the family, even of the world, seems to revolve around it. Stigma can also be caused later when an excellent teenage student, because of family bankruptcy, must transfer to a lower-quality school or cannot attend the college of his dreams. Some have to let go of ambitions; I knew of a tennis prodigy who had to give up his

15. Margaret Tyler, *Homeopathic Drug Pictures* (New Delhi: B. Jain Publishers, 1996), 106.

dream of becoming a professional tennis player when his father lost his job and, at fourteen, it became the boy's responsibility to augment the family's meager income. Adolescents should learn in a gradual process to become more independent, but if it happens all of a sudden, as they see a parent's loss of status and sense of identity crumbling, the teen may feel deeply disappointed and frustrated. In *Aurum's* case, a parent's loss of fortune and position, which often, under the guise of "protecting" the child, has gathered under cover of darkness hidden from the child, reveals itself all at once. Such a scary moment rattles the child's belief about basic things: "Am I safe? Will I have a roof over my head? Will there be enough food?" For this child it no longer seems possible to avoid failing by being *conscientious* and *industrious*—that is the formula his parents and their parents took to the bank. Such *disappointment and humiliation* (*mortification*) can lead to the most severe of the depressive states with thoughts of suicide because of *Aurum's competitive* and *ambitious* nature. It is also called *ailments from wounded honor*: *Aurum* above all other people has fear of failure because he thinks this will cause him to lose the respect and love of others (*mortification*; *delusion, has lost the affection of friends*).

Loss of a Longtime Partner

Sometimes, it occurs that one spouse dies suddenly and, a few hours later, the other one is admitted to the emergency room, losing consciousness after suffering from intense chest pain along with sweating, nausea, and vomiting. Such cases have long puzzled allopathic physicians but have been understood in TCM and homeopathy for centuries. Dying from a broken heart, the cost of grief and loss, is not just a saying; it is a real physical occurrence! It is very common in older people who have had a long and happy marriage together that, when one partner dies, the other follows in death a few months later (often seen in nursing homes, *ailments from grief*). The death of a longtime partner is enormously painful. *Aurum*, in the depression following such a loss, thinks that the sun and light (his wife, his lover, spouse, or only friend) have completely faded from his life, that there is no hope for him; he even believes he will be lost in the afterlife (*doubtful of soul's welfare*; *despair of religious salvation*). Such a loss of psychic balance occurs because he has lost a loved one around whom his life revolved, and now *Aurum* wonders whether his own life still has meaning. *Aurum* seems unable to take the blow of fate, and he is unable to strengthen his soul, finding himself with no moral reserves left. This is the often case for a person whose unconscious life is completely fed by the unconscious of another. Fed through the soul of his partner, *Aurum* remains like an infant in the mother's womb, drawing sustenance through the psychic umbilical cord. If this is suddenly snapped, it is as disastrous to the older person as it is to the newborn. When the unconscious is suddenly deprived of its emotional food, there may ensue a feeling of being utterly lost and cut off from life, a form of hopeless grief.

For the *Aurum* child, having very few friends, a "longtime" partner takes on another meaning when a particularly meaningful friend leaves him. It is *deception causing grief and mortification* and always considered the loss of a longtime partner even if he has known his friend only for a short time. When he starts a friendship, *Aurum* (at any age) is convinced it will last a lifetime! The serious *Aurum* adolescent dreams of ideal love at a very young age and takes any relationship very seriously: the first partner is his soul-mate. Even being lightly teased by this partner mortally injures his soul (*he is easily offended* and *takes everything in hard part*). Such emotional vulnerability can even lead desire to avenge against those who leave him (*deception causes grief and mortification*), and after an unsuccessful suicidal attempt, he will make sure to make his ex-partner feel guilty. He might even start the relationship again and break it off after a short time: having the last word is important for the *Aurum* person (*hatred and revenge of persons who had offended him*)!

Ailments from Retirement

When *Aurum* retires (especially if he has had an important function as a CEO or a general) he might lose all purpose; he thinks no one cares about him anymore, no one appreciates him anymore. This sudden "unemployment" leads to a sudden loss of inner structure to the organization of the mind which accompanies the conviction that life is now meaningless, leading to an early psycho-physical deterioration. All of a sudden, in the mind of the retired person, old age emerges very rapidly. Homeopathic *Aurum* will abolish the depression of such a person in an *Aurum* state who actually was more interested in having than in being, a rather unbalanced and pseudo-*Aurum*, one who has lost the opportunity of his life as he focused on materialism, power, recognition, fame, and being served rather than on serving others, being humble, and spreading his good will as a quasi-incognito person. So many gates open at the time of retirement. The true *Aurum*, upon retiring, has a chance to live, to be alive, to make living his new business; it has nothing to do with "killing" time. He also has the time to seriously examine spiritual and religious problems and to investigate the real meaning of life as well as the inevitable question of death, something we should not run away from. The balanced *Aurum*, the one that remains in the psoric miasmatic state, can do so, but the *Aurum* personality in the syphilitic phase has lost the capacity to be productive and active in a more spiritual way, as opposed to being merely busy. He must find new ways of being interested in life. "Interested" comes from the Latin *inter-esse*, "to be in," which is to be able to leave the narrow confinement of one's ego and to reach out to that which is in front of him, be it a child, a bird in the yard, or a growing flower; one must become interested in new ideas and, above all, remain interested in those insights that come from introspection in one's shadow side. This is an opportunity for any person to get rid of the professional persona, of the need to be pleasant in order to please a client or patient. Why not at least know that one can be now himself, that one can live more than ever according to his true character?

Disappointment

A common form of disappointment is seen in ailments from failed ambition in work, in business, or at school: the *Aurum* person wants to be number one, the top dog. When he discovers that he can't be number one, it will come to the point that he refuses to go to school; when he thinks he can't get a perfect score, he may refuse to take the test. He suffers therefore from *ailments from emotional excitement* (stress). The *Aurum* adolescent can also be disappointed in society and become a punk or an anarchist. He often dresses in black, as if wanting to hide the fact that he represents the color gold. In dreams, the color black stands for the unconscious, the dark unacceptable passions not yet integrated into the conscious, as well as for withdrawal, contrition and regret.

Ailments from a Terminal or Serious Disease

Depressive disorders are naturally seen quite frequently in people suffering from a painful or terminal disease such as cancer (classic breast, lung and prostate cancer spread to the bones), renal failure, a congenital heart defect, or leukemia. There can be *despair with the pain, thinking everything is lost.* Death is near! There is no better remedy than *Aurum* for this situation, as *Aurum* even abolishes the pain in the bones. However, mental suffering, as covered in some of the previous causalities, often makes man indifferent to physical suffering; it is precisely this that makes suicide easier, since the physical pain loses its importance in those who are suffering from such deep morbid depression and who are tormented by excessive amounts of mental suffering. Indeed, it is not pleasure but freedom from pain, physical and emotional, together with an absence of boredom that *Aurum* will aim for.

Compensations and Consequences

Industriousness

The balanced *Aurum* dares to be himself as he is not interested in what he gets in return or what he can keep (the opposite of *Nux-v*). For *Aurum*, the truth is still sacred, and no energy is spent in repressing it. He is a productive person that animates whatever he touches. Love and labor for him are inseparable. He loves that for which he labors and labors for that which he loves. For *Aurum* at this stage, the energy of hard work is accompanied by vibrancy and a sense of pleasure, purpose and passion. His drive is the engine to his accomplishments. He is a man who expresses humility and is humble and therefore those who listen to him will understand what humility is. He responds to his fellow man because he feels responsible (*conscientious*). What happens to others can happen to him: humanity is not outside, but within him. For *Aurum*, conscientiousness means being prepared and organized, operating independently regardless of others' opinions. It means that he does what he is supposed to do and sticks with it.

But *Aurum* is egged on by an inner voice that encourages him to take this industriousness to new and often Herculean heights. In his beginning phase, *Aurum* shows more of the psoric character: always thinking he does not do enough for other people; *he always thinks that he is neglecting something for which he will be reproached*; *he seems to carry with him this internal restlessness, and it took from him all perseverance and energy*. *Aurum* will initially even persist in a task even when there is no good reason to do so and "tries too hard," pouring all his efforts into one approach. *Aurum* at this stage should be told that in order to lead a full human life, it is perfectly all right to relax from time to time and to focus upon the trivial and superficial parts of life. But *Aurum* beats herself up over everything and holds herself to a very high standard. Some seem to have the fundamental conviction, even from a young age, that they are destined to achieve a superior position in life. "I always believed in giving more to people than they expected from me" is one of their sayings. With serious intent, *Aurum* accepts the task of being a leader of humanity, showing self-sacrifice in the course of obtaining his goal. Aurum remains defiant because he has something noble and great to create. Although he may sooner or later be assailed by those forces within his own depths, *Aurum* is not made for everyday routine.

This child attempts to do everything intensely and perfectly in order to receive recognition as he realizes he is different and superior to others. It leads to restlessness on the mental and physical plane: he shows *restless and hurried impulses, to bodily and mental activity: he cannot work fast enough as to satisfy himself. He is driven to constant activity, and is sorry for his inaction. He desires to be active, to move about.* He cannot do things fast enough. The child, convinced that he deserves the love and respect of others since he is the best, also expects these; unfortunately, he always thinks he has not done enough to excel: he should have studied more, he should not have wasted his time with a friend; he gets very upset about the smallest mistake he makes in his homework and can start weeping from despair about it. He can grieve over such disappointment for hours. It looks like the *Aurum* child sets himself up for failure because of all the difficulties he sees in his way as he is trying to be perfect, to receive the highest score in his class (*he is discontent with all conditions; he thinks that he everywhere finds an impediment, caused now by an opposing fate, then again by himself*). This child is far too hard on himself (*very conscientious*), pushed by an inner command to succeed. As we can see, the *Aurum* personality goes to great lengths to be industrious and conscientious; however, because of his own often unreasonable expectations (overly organized, meticulous, pleasing everyone) and to his great despair, he often fails, which can undermine his self-confidence (*want of self-confidence, and thinks others have none in him, which makes him unhappy*).

Sensitivity to Criticism

The *Aurum* person is initially strong on the mental and physical plane but weak and fragile on the emotional plane. The *Aurum* state is a house of cards ready to fold upon the slightest contradiction. Obviously, when one tries as hard in life as the *Aurum* person does, he expects to be respected, understood, and not criticized. We therefore understand his reaction to criticism: *He is excessively disposed to take offense; even the least thing seeming offensive to him, and affects him deeply and causes resentment. The least contradiction excites him to the greatest anger and he becomes choleric and quarrelsome. He is extremely affected and provoked by the least circumstances, which had the appearance of hurting his feelings; and suffers therefore from ailments from contradiction.* During the interview this patient might be open enough to speak his mind about some things that seem to irritate him quite a bit, but being told not to get upset gets him very angry. This anger has been held in for a long time, so when it is unleashed it is very strong, surprising everyone around him since this person or child has always been known to be obedient and perfect, always doing things for others and never giving anyone trouble: "This cannot be the child I know," exclaims the mother. True to his intense and passionate character, there is violence and even maliciousness in *Aurum's* anger: *passionate and violent; he trembles when he cannot give way to his anger; he feels hateful and quarrelsome* and *he becomes angry at absent persons while thinking of them. He feels he suffers constant vexation and torment.* The *Aurum* personality can therefore change from an introverted, hard-working person to quite an angry and vengeful individual. This often leads to feelings of guilt. To his despair, the bright, precious gold has now turned into a cold and hard ordinary metal. Physical turbulence accompanies this sudden tempest: he shows *excessive anguish with palpitations of the heart, as well as weariness in all limbs and sleepiness. The anguish can drive him from place to place, so that he cannot remain in one place.*

Classical Music

Music is a universal language that can speak to all kinds of people through the heart, while it has nothing to say *directly* to the head. This is certainly seen through classical music in *Aurum's* case which very often moves *Aurum* to tears. As with the *Natrum carbonicum* child, the *Aurum* child loves to listen to classical music. Fast rock-and-roll music (the *Tarentula* child), organ music, and music played by a single instrument (*Graphites* children) are not to his liking. This classical music resonates with the seriousness of this child, often withdrawn on his own, and it brings a calming effect, putting him to sleep. Besides classical music, exposure to sunlight brightens *Aurum's* day. Music and sun are symbols of love, happiness, warmth, and hope, all that *Aurum* needs to rise from his dark state. He despises being cold in the long winter months and sits still in front of a fireplace during cold days, warming up like a lizard.

Depressed

When confronted with depression, one has many pathways in but few pathways out. Antidepressants are now the most widely prescribed drugs in America (there goes the myth of the happiest generation!), and they yield very mixed results. In homeopathy, we have at least 180 different remedies, each for its own variety of depression and with several different etiologies for each remedy (see, for example, *Aurum's* causalities above). How does *Aurum's* depression present? Because of failures to meet his own high expectations, the *Aurum* person initially tries even harder but eventually falls prey, as time goes on, to a slew of more fixed ideas, reflecting the emergence of the kind of depression typical of *Aurum*: *He believes at this point that he has lost the love of others, and this mortifies him even to tears. He thinks he cannot succeed in anything, that he does nothing right and reproaches himself bitterly. He is discouraged and at odds with himself, he is in disunion with himself. He has episodes of crying and wailing and he thinks that he is irretrievably lost. He suffers from the delusion, that he has lost the affection of his friends and that his friends have lost confidence in him*. At this point, *Aurum* feels alienated, like an outsider, and has a hard time making friends. When *Aurum's* consciousness is occupied with such strong fixed ideas, there is not much place left for new positive messages coming from the conscious world, so at this point *Aurum* withdraws more and more and can fall into a deep depression. Depression is a disorder rooted in subjectivity. *Aurum* focuses overly internally on his thoughts, his feelings, and his subjective way of experiencing himself in life. He becomes notoriously bad at engaging in reality testing, gathering information, and double-checking whether his thoughts or feelings actually make sense in the circumstances. Failure for the *Aurum* person is punished with melancholy and even death (*fear with desire for death*). I had an *Aurum* patient who expressed as her only fear open water, especially dark water. She felt there was a tentacle monster with huge teeth, and that it was so large that it was actually the water itself. What does this mean? Dark water represents the personal unconscious, where no doubt many secret and painful memories have been stored, and obviously this woman was afraid to open the door and let this monster escape, or to allow the skeleton3s in her closet into her consciousness. Yet doing just this is *Aurum's* only chance for improvement, and homeopathic *Aurum* will no doubt achieve this, on its own and/or with concurrent emotional work on the patient's part. Integrating unconscious elements into consciousness is always a very positive step for every patient in his individuation journey.

The *Aurum* depression is one of the strongest kinds, and always should be compared with the *Calcarea* depressive state as the two resemble each other closely. *Aurum* in this depressive state sits by himself in a corner, quiet, reserved. *Aurum* feels like a robot emotionally, *sits still, wrapped in deep sad thoughts*, an expression of the syphilitic miasm. He is dejected and seeks solitude. *He imagines that he is not fit for this world and therefore longs for death, of which he thinks with the most intense delight* (all fixed ideas at this point). *Thinking of death gives him intense joy*, and there is a strong inclination to commit suicide; *he is desperate and desires to jump from a height* (usually a bridge or balcony). *Aurum*, when investigating his causalities, feels that he has entirely objective grounds for putting an end to his existence. As seen before, these grounds may include financial loss, painful conditions, or the loss of loved ones. *Aurum* patients can hide their depressions easily, as there can be a remarkable changeability of mind: now impulsive, rash, and very merry, then sad, anxious, and longing to die. It is the principal remedy for the state of *loathing of life*, the desire to die, and the wish to commit suicide. Kent, in his *Lectures on Materia Medica*, embellishes on this theme:

> Taking the mental symptoms in one great whole, you will see that all the affections, natural to healthy man, are perverted. So great in extent is this that one of the fundamental loves, which is love of living, of self-protection, is perverted and he loathes life, is weary of life, longs to die and seeks methods to commit suicide...It is astonishing that one can get into such state of mind, such horrible depression of spirits that there is an absolute loss of enjoyment in everything."[16]

In the unbalanced *Aurum* adolescent, we find two tendencies: those who want to destroy others (revenge) and those who want to destroy themselves (suicide). At this point, some of these individuals start using drugs, become uncaring, and are indifferent to the fact that they are destroying their lives. Others leave school or college and become social outsiders. It is not unusual for *Aurum* teenagers to commit suicide if their loved ones leave them or if their parents forbid them to see their lovers. The teenager or adult at this point may drive around recklessly in the hope an accident will kill him; he may run purposely in front of traffic to be killed. And he starts losing his ambition, which was his driving force in the first place! At this point, he has to be entertained or have something to do. As a rule, though, he wants to be alone. If you can convince him to walk in open air, he feels much better as it lifts his depression quite considerably. Usually, although desire for sun is present, he feels a little better in the evening, because the darkness outside resonates with his dark mood.

---

16. Kent, *Lectures*, 162.

At this point, the person in an *Aurum* state flirts with death, seeking a solution to all his problems and pains (physical pain, like in progressive cancer, or emotional pain). At this point, death often appears as a good thing, as something desired, as a friend. When the terrors of life outweigh the terrors of death, the *Aurum* person will put an end to his life. Worse than physical suffering, as discussed in *Aurum's* causalities, is often spiritual suffering. Spiritual suffering makes *Aurum* insensible to physical pain, for the physical pain associated with suicide loses all significance in the eyes of one afflicted by excessive spiritual suffering. Having encountered insuperable obstacles to his existence and to his extensive efforts, maybe suffering from an incurable disease or from an inconsolable grief from the loss of a longtime partner, the return into the womb of nature is the last resort open to him. Such a return is seen by *Aurum* as the surrender of the physical body. The *Aurum* personality is the most likely of all personalities to commit suicide when he feels of no use in the world. He wants to be put out of his misery as he sees no way out. He blames himself for everything: he is finished; there is no reason to stick around! He had high expectations and they were not realized. It is what we can call a "balance" suicide: Aurum draws a balance sheet of his whole life and decides on the basis of its negativity to dispense with its future existence! He has made the calculation that the business of life does not cover the costs. At this point, *Aurum* misunderstands the role of challenge and hardship in life and forgets that real success is measured by effort rather than life status and positive outcomes.

An *Aurum* individual in such a depressed state without any hope may remain so for several years, thinking continuously of suicide but without talking to anyone about it. Then, if some small incident occurs and upsets the frail balance, he may jump from a bridge. Looking at the causalities that evolve into an *Aurum* state, his act of suicide often moves us to sorrow and sympathy mingled with a certain admiration for his courage rather than with the moral condemnation that usually accompanies such an act. When you try to make contact with *Aurum* in this stage, it is as if you are touching the metal itself: hard, cold, still: no contact is possible anymore! Homeopathic gold, however, can still restore his love of life!

There is a special form of depression requiring homeopathic intake of *Aurum*: **seasonal affective disorder**, in which the blues and feelings of rejection rise in the winter months. The sun represents brightness and splendor, "solar passion," the radiant life energy of the father figure and for primitive people the sun and moon were the eyes of heaven: the Sun was the good eye and the Moon, the evil eye. For them, sun worship was associated with a symbolic promise of protection and salvation; the Sun chiefly represents gold, the most precious metal. The Sun is, therefore, an archetype in dreams, meaning that it is the same basic symbol repeating itself cross-culturally—even among cultures that were not connected historically or geographically. The Sun is symbolic of warmth, vitality, and conscious awareness, the source of one's life energy. As archetypes are the "stuff" that makes up the collective unconscious, it is understandable that such moods transcend the individual: archetypes belong to mankind. As one of these, the Sun is part of the whole spiritual heritage of mankind's evolution born anew in the structure of each successive generation.

Religion

In the final phase of an *Aurum* state, there is another possibility for the *Aurum* person: instead of committing suicide, he turns to religion. This will prevent suicide. When he feels he has not succeeded in doing his so-called duty, he can get the feeling that his soul cannot be saved (*despair of religious salvation* and *doubtful of welfare of the soul*). In the hope of receiving forgiveness (*religious affections from remorse*), he can resort to *religious mania with constant praying* and *involuntary weeping*. At this stage, *Aurum's* world becomes a place of atonement, a sort of penal colony. We see episodes or cycles of working, praying, and weeping. Sometimes the *Aurum* person enters a cloister to save her soul.

Golden Tips from the Masters

- #1 remedy for despair + pain + depression, for instance in terminal cancer patients with pain in the bones as in prostate or breast cancer with spreading to the bones. Also for chronic pain causing suicidal thoughts (also *Nat-s*)
- *Aurum* is very strong on the physical plane but sensitive and weak on the emotional plane. The emotional plane forms a fragile layer which is pressed upon by a strong mental layer. With the least pressure, the house crumbles.
- Great distributor of the cerebral circulation
- Clinically and physiologically related to *Mercury*
- State of great hilarity alternating with depression (manic-depressive)
- Angina pectoris with restlessness, anxiety and violent palpitations and a combination of hypertension, arteriosclerosis, and disturbed fat metabolism (increased LDL, increased triglycerides)
- Numbness in arms and legs upon awaking
- Indicated in heart problems and acute rheuma (*inflammation heart; inflammation endocardium, rheumatic*). With *Arnica* the greatest cardiac remedy.
- Most important remedy for fatty degeneration of the heart (*Phos* also)
- Right-sided orchitis and non-descending of testicle: a pathological remedy like *Lyc* for undescended testicle, provided the testicle is not ectopic (Foubister)
- Indicated in nondescript insomnia since retirement
- #1 remedy to rectify pathology from mercury abuse, as with dentists working with much mercury
- Great action on glands diseased with cystic formations

Baryta carbonica (Bar-c). Witherite

The Cyber Delusion

The Cyber delusion of *Bar-c* is ***he walks on his knees***, also expressed by the delusion *his legs are cut off*. When legs appear in dreams (stuck in the mud, for instance), it is a relatively fixed symbol and reflective of the emotional and physical strength the dreamer has for getting about in life. To have one's legs knocked out from under one or to have the delusion that his legs are cut off signifies loss of confidence and an urge to carry on with life. People enduring such dreams (and certainly this is the case for *Bar-c*) may depend in conscious life upon someone like a partner or parent for support. Ultimately, the legs represent the dreamer's emotional or conceptual support system. Think about the idioms "not having a leg to stand on" or "my legs went jelly" and you know how a *Bar-c* or anyone who has a "leg" dream can feel.

In *Bar-c* we recognize a very insecure, "small" person, a mental/ emotional dwarf, with a lack of individuation, stuck even in adulthood, when he should already possess a dominant function of consciousness. *Bar-c* is a person who never ends the blissful ignorance of childhood to be faced with the never-ending suffering called adult life. He is the backward child characterized chiefly by low intelligence and a general incapacity to understand. A *Bar-c* on the mental/emotional plane is like the child at the theater before the curtain is raised, who sits there happy with excited expectation of things to come. For him, it is actually a blessing that he does not know what will actually come as the curtain is never raised. Growing up, *Bar-c* needs others for protection and guidance in every step of his life. When not remedied by homeopathic *Bar-c*, this creates a permanent handicap due to his lack of individual growth (or individuation). *Bar-carb's* ego has difficulty meeting the outer world and adapting to the demands of daily reality without the help of others. His whole life remains close to the unconscious, even close to the collective unconscious with the Divine Mother archetype, removed from the demands posed by the normal conscious life. *Bar-carb's* ego has a hard time meeting the earthly expectations that would allow him to consciously develop and separate himself from the unconscious. He never severs the psychic umbilical cord from the mother to find his own identity. *Bar-c* leads a shadow existence, reasonably content—out of necessity because of a hereditary low IQ—to cling to his mother or a mother figure in selfless devotion.

The smallness of this person can be expressed on the physical, mental, or emotional plane, sometimes on a single plane, expressed as the non-development of one organ while the others grow; for example, the uterus might fail to mature (infantile uterus). The dwarfishness is most often expressed on the mental-emotional plane, though; society relegates such children to the world of the simple, but in some ways they are very complete and interesting; their quality of mind gives them a poignant innocence, transparency, and dignity. They are the very opposite of precocious children, the unusually brilliant and mentally advanced like the *Lachesis* or *Phosphorus* child. The smallness and insecurity that *Bar-c* feels is also expressed in additional paranoid fixed ideas such as *he is being laughed at; he is criticized; people are looking at him* and *he is being watched.* Such fixed ideas show the small mind of a child who does not understand social nuances and feels very vulnerable in the adult world: "*She suspected that when walking in the street, men found fault with her, and judged her amiss, which made her anxious, so that she dared not look up at nobody and perspired all-over*" (Hahnemann, 1997, p. 394). Her emotional fragility on the streets is clearly indicated by her oversensitivity to noise: *a little noise in the street seems to him at once like a fire alarm, and he is so frightened by it, so that it darts through all his limbs.*

The *Bar-c* person has permitted himself to be born, but he is afraid to take the next step in life: to be weaned from his mother's breast, so to speak. Even as an adult, he remains a person who craves continual mothering, needing to be nursed and protected by any motherly figure; this makes him eternally dependent on someone else so that he can flee from his permanent fear of living. *Bar-carb's* passivity, feelings of inferiority, and lack of confidence make him continually play the injured, ever-innocent being, similar to the *Pulsatilla* child, casting an attractive role for his mother with her natural instinct to protect and nourish (the benign Mother-type complex as an archetype). *Bar-carb's* dependency explains the delusion, *a beloved friend is sick and dying,* expressing the great fear of losing a person so crucial to his survival. If such a person dies, for instance the beloved mother or grandmother, *Bar-c* is full of despair, frozen with grief, as though the rug has been pulled out from under his feet and part of his own self has died, weeping violently over the death of his friend and lamenting, "Why did she have to go?"

A clear sense of identity, therefore, is not yet achievable by the *Bar-c* person: he is alive but does not *live* as he does not make decisions and is not aware of his own potential. Such a person, tied to the mother figure, is not able to say the word "I," nor has he any need for it. He acts like the infant that has not conceived of the world as being different from himself (*childish behavior*). *Bar-c* never has understood Descartes' philosophical question, "Who am I?" *Cogito ergo sum* (I think, therefore I am). Devoid of creative action and a process of feeling, *Bar-c* never conceives of himself as an individual, but as more of a shadow person. More than anyone else, *Bar-c* hides himself (literally: behind the curtains, his mother, or furniture), even behind his fingers, attempting to create a flimsy façade he can hide behind in order to cover up the failure to acquire a sense of identity. The process of individuation has not occurred and has not even started, in spite of the fact that the person is beyond adolescence. *Bar-carb's* world is concrete, vivid, intense, yet simple; because it is concrete, it is not complicated, diluted, or unified by abstraction. Being simple from the start, *Bar-c* has never known or been seduced by the abstract, the conceptual; rather, he has always experienced reality directly and without mediation, often with overwhelming intensity. *Bar-c* is not only a remedy for children and young adults but also for adults, especially for elderly people who have suffered multiple brain infarcts and therefore returned to a dependent, childish state (*dementia senilis with foolish talking; unconscious in old age; prostration in old age*), not a state of imbecility but one in which they behave like two-year-olds, doing and saying things like children with a loss of ego strength.

Causalities

Although *Bar-c* is one of the few *true constitutional* remedies, meaning that it has a genetic makeup, anyone, at any given moment, could slide temporarily into a *Bar-c* phase. I refer here for example to people who, overworked by tests and reading tasks, could fall into "an acute layer" of *Bar-c* (*ailments from mental work*). In these circumstances we need to compare *Bar-c* with *Pic-ac* and *Anac*. *Bar-c* is mainly a remedy of the two opposite ages: the very young and the old; as mentioned before, *Bar-c* elderly can fall into a "second childhood" through an apoplectic attack (*unconscious in apoplexy*). Think about *Bar-c* when you see this *childish and thoughtless behavior* in elderly patients after an apoplexy. All this does not mean, however, that we don't need *Bar-c* for young adults. Kent expresses it as follows: "You will have these patients to treat, where this slow development manifests itself in girls 18-25 years of age, who do things they did when they were children, and say things as they said them when they were children. Childish manner of doing things, playing with dolls and saying foolish things. They have not come into womanhood. They are late in taking on the activities and uses of the woman and they say things just like a little girl would say."[17] The foregoing could have been a description of a child with autism! But usually, we need to refer to *hereditary* or miasmatic factors (psora-syphilis in this case) for the formation of the constitutional or inborn *Bar-c*. *Bar-c* is an undeveloped *Calc-c*, in other words, the negative and weak aspects of *Calc-c* (*stubbornness, fears, mulling things over, indecisiveness, excessive dependency on family and friends, severe hypotonia*, etc.) are accentuated to the point that they paralyze *Bar-c*. The late walking (and even talking) of a *Calc-c* (because only he decides when he is ready to walk and talk) is late **learning** to walk in *Bar-c*, representing a truly handicapped person. The newborn was supposed to be a *Calc-c*, but something (Factor X) occurring at the moment of an important developmental phase turned off the expression of the gene (epigenetics) and changed him into a dependent, clinging *Bar-c* or caused infantile organ formation. That Factor X is usually an intrauterine crime of *anticipation anxiety* in the pregnant *Calcarea* mother's personality, a response to events that normally have a great impact on a *Carbon* person: fears of being forsaken (husband is on a trip); having to keep the pregnancy a secret from her parents; anticipation of pain during delivery (*Carbons* fear pain, injections, seeing blood, etc.) or fear that something might be wrong with the baby when they feel some pain or lose a little blood; and any other little thing the typical *Calc-c* can fuss about, like the smallest injury or innocent cold. Here is an example from the practice of an intrauterine crime:

> During my patient's pregnancy, bleeding started, which of course created great anticipation anxiety. The mother expressed: "I HAD to talk to my family overseas and always felt better after doing so." This anxiety was even further increased when the gynecologist, suspecting something wrong, bluntly said to the patient at a routine exam, where she was all alone without family—and before the sonogram was done: "Your fetus might be dead!" This *delivering bad news* was a grave psychological mistake of the gynecologist (*Calc-c* is a black-type remedy for *hearing bad news*, so intensify that twofold for *Bar-c*). The mother had an immediate, strong feeling of anxiety and helplessness. Never mind that the

17. Kent, *Lectures*, 180.

> sonogram actually turned out to be OK; the intense feelings had already been transferred to the unborn fetus. Furthermore, at home, just before the delivery, the mom could not feel the baby moving. The trip from home to the hospital was a long one, filled with fear, despondency, need for attention, and sheer terror. The end result of this was that these stresses did create a *Bar-c* baby with Autism Spectrum Disorder. One can see that this *Bar-c* state is a deeper form of *Calc-c*: fears are more intense; cares and worries are incessant, and the feeling of helplessness and the need for support are unbearable.

Other examples point in the same direction. Women want to get pregnant at an increasingly older age and often go through many miscarriages or several IVF (in vitro fertilization) treatments. These women are usually more nervous and enter the state of pregnancy with hypervigilance, worries, and cares. The moment something is wrong, some subtle spotting, they are off to the hospital in a panic. The pregnant woman might not even wait for her partner who is at work, preferring to summon a close friend and rush for help. Even when normally very intelligent and rather independent, she now has no direction and is in great need of someone to reassure her, behaving like a child. It does not help, of course, when the physician needs to check her every two weeks. The anticipation anxiety turns into anguish, as she never knows what news she will get. This extreme need for help, reassurance, and professional hand-holding will be reflected by the newborn's behavior as it creates a child who needs the constant attention of his mom.

Compensations

Protection from a Mother

Bar-c starts with the severe handicap of thinking of himself as being smaller (more vulnerable and unprotected) than anyone else out there, so security and support are greatly sought after while growing up is not (*desire to be magnetized*). Unlike a normally developing child, *Bar-c* only wants to obtain only a limited amount of independence; while growing up, *Bar-c* consciously remains stuck in a dependency state. The greatest characteristic is his **dependency** on one person, usually the mom, the one playing the role of the mom, or at least an adult. Even with normally developing children, the most fundamental of the natural ties is that of the child to the mother. Life starts in the mother's womb, and the resulting dependency remains for the first years of the child's life as the psychological umbilical cord remains present long after the physical umbilical cord is cut. But while the libido for independence and natural separation from the family unit should grow from age five on, the *Baryta* child with ASD takes his dependency to a new level. In such a case, the mother has not only given birth to the *Baryta* child, but she continues to give life to him even past puberty. It is as though *Baryta* has not yet been completely born, but is still enclosed in the protective world of a cocoon. Arrested in growth at this point in life, such a child has a permanent craving to be nursed, mothered, and protected; he is the eternally dependent one. Because of his lack of understanding, *Bar-c* immediately falls prey to the first and most prominent human emotion: the emotion of terror! One sees in his eyes the terror of a hunted animal. *Bar-carb's* characteristics are excessive in comparison with those of *Calc-c*. While *Calc-c talks about nothing but murder, fire and rats*, reflecting his fears of a dangerous world, *Bar-c* is even more intense in his fears about his health. Normally indisposed to talk because of bashfulness, *Bar-c*, when and if he talks, *likes to talk about his sickness and injuries*, which amount to nothing. If *Calc-carb's* complaints are "much ado about nothing," imagine how a *Bar-c* sounds. Yet talking about her misery aggravates *Bar-c*. Just *thinking of her complaints make her worse*, and this is only ameliorated by entertainment or diversion of her attention (*occupation ameliorates*).

There is a refusal in *Bar-c* to leave the all-enveloping orbit of the protector. *Bar-c* is the eternally dependent one, who is frightened and insecure when motherly protection is withdrawn but optimistic and reassured when a loving mother is provided. This need is due to *his development arrested*: he is also late in everything: *late in learning to walk, late learning to read, late learning to take in images and form perceptions*. Late learning to walk is not because *Bar-c* has miserably weak limbs with flabby and hypotonic muscles like *Calc-c*; it is due rather to tardiness in the brain, so such children are simply late learning to do things. The dependency takes extreme forms: *Bar-c* will ask mom to do something he can do himself—not necessarily an uncommon trait for many children, but in *Bar-c* we are talking about being fed when he can eat with a fork himself. In other words, for him, when his mom does things for him all the time, it is a sign she that still loves him and that she will not disappear. He often cries and whines and constantly demands that his mom entertain him; she hardly has time for herself. Mom is not able to have a life of her own, and if she talks to other people on the street, the *Bar-c* child can resort to biting her or pulling her hair—whatever works to get her attention and support. Such an episode of anger is nothing but reactive anger rooted in fear because of disappointment and frustration when a need or wish is not fulfilled, and also, often, because of an inability to understand social cues and the needs of other people. This child may also appear to be overly jealous, but this is not the case; rather, a great fear of losing his support is the drive behind this behavior. Such a child, older than age five, puts glue anywhere on the floor, puts baby powder all over his body, urinates on the floor or in his pants, and puts his face close to the face of other people—in other words, things we can expect of a fifteen-month-old but not of a seven-year-old. At home, he needs to have mom constantly in his sight. If he needs to get a toy in another room, he will take mom by the hand and pull her along with him; there is no way that he will go alone to a room that is upstairs while she is downstairs. When falling asleep, he needs literally to feel a person; he loves putting his leg against the parent's body.

The infantile regression and arrested development is easily seen at bedtime. Another *Bar-c* child in my practice slept in mom's bed up to age ten and woke up constantly to see if she was still there: he would always put his hands on her face or his leg across her legs or chest. He is able to sleep alone but, overcome by his intense fears, he prefers to be in his parent's (or parents') bed (*fear in children; fear of evil and something will happen*). Even in fantasy parks like Disneyland, his mom is not allowed to go on a ride without him: he needs to hold her hand all the time. His lack of identity is visible everywhere. You ask the *Baryta* child what his favorite toy is and the verbal *Bar-c* child answers: "I don't know; can you choose one for me?" (That is, of course, if he has all these words.) Or you ask her, "What is your favorite food?" and you get the answer, "I don't know." In every aspect of his life, every choice he needs to make, this dependency and irresolution (much worse than in *Pulsatilla*) are always at the fore (*irresolution in acts, about trifles, and in projects; he proposes to himself a brief journey, and as soon as he is to make his preparation, he is sorry for it, and prefers to stay at home; long wavering between opposing resolutions; she is very anxious and solicitous about things quite trifling*). And he loves to be read to for hours (also *Calc-c*).

An eight-year-old girl, whom I treated, never had her mom out of sight; even when someone else was feeding her, she constantly looked at her mother. During sessions with therapists, the mother could not be present because the child would pay attention only to the mother and not to the therapists. On her own, this *Bar-c* child just flapped through the pages of a book without reading or paying much attention. Dressing a *Bar-c* child in the morning takes at least a half an hour with constant prompting, and the parent may have to set a timer, although often to no avail. The moment you ask the older *Bar-c* child a question, she responds in a two-year-old soft baby voice, though she has had no problem talking normally to her mom when behaving moodily that morning.

Ego Contents Remain Sparse

In a normally developing child, the ego grows from islets of consciousness through a constant interchange with the outside world. But because of a lack of such interchange without a filter, *Bar-carb's* ego contents remain sparse, almost resistant to growth (*childish behavior remains*), so he is frightened and insecure when motherly protection is withdrawn! There is a want of clear consciousness. There might be physiological changes, but there remains a mental/emotional retardation with *no sense of identity*, not being aware of himself as an entity separated from his mother. The *Baryta* child remains one with his mother for too long. As a result of not having a sense of his own identity, he cannot orient himself in the world intellectually; being joined to mom's hip, usually the problem starts, for instance, when the mom starts working again after her postpartum stay with her baby. And if, in such cases, the father should leave to work in another state or country, the "small" mind of this child translates this into a situation in which "Mom kicked out Dad." As with all *Carbon* personalities, the harmony of the family is of great importance, and separation is a great trauma to the simple mind of this child. When you take such a child to the barber to have his hair cut, or when you want to cut his nails, he screams from the top of his lungs as though he will be murdered: in his mind, people with scissors have dangerous intentions! *Baryta's* weakness in the conceptual and abstract can also tend in quite an opposite direction: towards an obsessive preoccupation with particulars. I have seen such children putting water in a small cup and then pouring it out, or shifting objects from one part of a room to another over and over again, all day long.

Aversion to Company

Bar-carb's behavior leads to a lack of individuation, a high degree of immaturity (*childish behavior in old age children covering their face with their hands, but looking through their fingers; development of children arrested*), and difficulty in connecting to the outside world which is shown in further provings of her reluctance to leave home. Strangely enough, as dependent as he is, *Bar-c* has an *aversion to company, to the presence of other people* and *ameliorates when alone. Bar-c*, being an extreme version of *Calc-c* (who usually has at least one good friend), is very *bashful and timid*: *Bar-c* children are *indisposed to play* and *sit in a corner doing nothing* and *shrieking*. Play never evolves to parallel play or symbolic play as it does with normally developing children. Being clumsy and ill-coordinated in all his movements, *Bar-c* can be painfully shy and withdrawn, feeling intuitively that she is, and always will be, a "comical figure" (*delusion, being laughed at, mocked*). *Aversion to strangers*, to the point of *misanthropy, especially men*, is peculiar in *Bar-c*. *Bar-c* children typically hide from strangers (*child hides behind the furniture and thinks all visitors laugh at her*). The approach of a stranger, even a harmless one, revs his body up into overdrive; as a result, the nervous system that is designed to prepare him for social encounters often overheats, short-circuiting his resolve and thwarting his best intentions. In addition to hiding behind a parent or furniture as an expression of his extreme *bashfulness*, the child will also hide his face behind his hands when in a setting such as a new classroom, or when having lunch in a cafeteria, because now there are many more children he does not know. Once he is back in his own small classroom, he feels okay and there is no more reason to hide.

While superficially a mass of handicaps and incapacities, with the intense frustrations and anxieties attendant on these, *Bar-c* is capable of warm, deep attachments to certain persons and is very fond of animals, music, and nature. *Bar-c* persons literally and figuratively have to "lean on someone": even walking in the street, they hang on to someone or something, not only because of their emotional immaturity, but also because of their fear of fainting. So his supporting cast is reduced to a very close family member or, as an adult, to a very intimate friend entangled with him in a codependent relationship (*desires to be magnetized by them*). It is this strong degree of *bashfulness* that **supersedes** any other trait in *Bar-c*! If such a child goes to a gym and there are a lot of people there, she will refuse to perform her gymnastics routine, in spite of normally liking it very much and in spite of the fact that gymnastics usually greatly motivates her to enjoy herself. The more people are present, the shyer the child is, and when pushed to perform her regular routine in such circumstances, she will throw a tantrum. Her timidity further leads to *a vanishing of all self-confidence*, even to *cowardice*. It goes so far that the child *becomes extremely discouraged, even peevish and cross* and *indisposed to work or play*. Encouragement to change *Bar-carb's* disposition can be met by bursts of irritability: *sudden excessive, but quickly transient bursts of anger and wrath, even to rage, even from slight causes*.

Due to the lack of self-confidence, anxiety is another hallmark of the *Bar-c* child: *anxious apprehension about things quite trifling, while all self-confidence has vanished.* His dependency grows in direct proportion to his anxiety. *Bar-c* exhibits anxiety in malls or places with a lot of commotion and people, even more so if the place is entirely new for him. Before he even enters such a place, even if he has been there before, he starts showing his anxiety right away through flapping, shrieking, hitting, and striking his head against the wall. He will clutch at mom, start crying and want to get out of there. I have seen such behavior starting at the age of four months! Even when his mom talks to his teacher, someone he knows, he still becomes upset and runs away (*runs away to escape*) to get mom's attention. It is perplexing for a mom to grasp why her child, on whom she dotes, only hits **her** and no one else. But Mom, in such a child's eyes, is the only person he can depend on. In homeopathy, we call this "his beloved friend is dying," the beloved friend being the one he totally depends on (his mother). When she leaves to do an errand, he gets upset as he experiences great separation anxiety.

I remember a father who unknowingly sabotaged his pre-verbal eight-year-old *Bar-c* child with ASD, refusing to accept his disability (which was that he had the mental function of a two-year-old) and insisting that, because he was eight years old, he should be able to do what was being asked since all eight-year olds could perform the task. It was one humiliation after another, effectively canceling the homeopathic therapy that was given. Such a child pays little attention to what his father says, but he intuits what his father is. Far from being a model parent, he is a father who wants to use his child as an excuse for his own lack of fulfillment in life. Only when the father started analytical therapy and homeopathy could the burden from this child be removed; then, progress was seen in the child.

More resources should be allocated to play, not just to benchmarks of academics—for all children, and definitely for *Bar-c*. When a child is not ready (a *Bar-c* is always delayed), pushing him into academics can send him further into the paralyzing state of fear and worsen the ASD condition if it is present. Parents, teachers, and caretakers need to be aware of these most insidious situations—the ones that leave no physical scars but injure the victims inside, violating something in the child's soul. Physical abuse is most often preceded by psychological violence (deliberate neglect or pushing a child beyond her mental capability). Countless children live in fear, humiliation, and total withdrawal because of a verbally brutal person in their life who has never hit them. I am talking here about the verbal and psychological treatment that is characteristic of abusers vis-à-vis their victims. There is a clear difference between mental cruelty, or deliberate neglect, and having a row over homework that still needs to be done.

The greatest separation anxiety is always experienced with the mother or the one playing the maternal role, such as an aide who is shadowing the child at school: she needs to be present all the time. Even if the child just sits there, doing nothing or watching TV, the mom needs to sit next to her and is never allowed to do something on her own. This can be seen as a form of jealousy. I knew one child who would throw something at any person with whom mom was engaged in conversation. Even if his mom sat next to him, holding him, while telling me his story, he would throw an object at me; then, when his mom asked, "What do you want,?" he would say "Mommy"—although she was holding him. So he wanted her continuous, undivided attention. Often, this is reflective of the great need that mom had for attention when the child was intrauterine. Interestingly, in this case, everything came to a crashing halt when he was three years old and his grandparents—who, for an entire year, had cared for him every moment of the day—left. The next day, he was sent to school for first time. As he had been getting attention moment by moment from his grandparents, there had been no reason to be jealous or needy; all of his needs were fulfilled. As a result of this, the expression of *Bar-c*, the true picture underneath, had not yet appeared. The departure of the grandparents, coupled with beginning school (a time at which many children require extra attention), caused him to go ballistic, throwing things and hitting children and teachers (*rage, leading to deeds of violence*).

I remember an anxious call I received from the mother of a *Bar-c* child I was treating. Her child was suddenly demonstrating a fetish for people's feet. Even if a stranger came into the room, she wanted to kiss and touch his feet. While this was disturbing to the mother, the behavior had started after treatment with *Bar-c* began and therefore represented a step forward to the cure. What we need to remember is that if a child wants to be part of a relationship but feels shy, rather than talking (and she was delayed in talking like many *Bar-c*), she will lean into the person and seek closeness through touch. This interest in peoples' feet was a step forward, because now she was seeking active engagement, even with a stranger; she was beginning to take part in the external world!

Safety

Safety is a big issue; I knew one child who, up to age nine, would take his blanket, hide in the cupboard at home, and stay there. Unlike the *Stramonium* child, *the Bar-c* child is not afraid of the dark; he even wants the light off when he goes to sleep. But I have noticed crying in a *Bar-c* child as young as four months old when going to a new place or a gathering of new people. Interestingly, a *Bar-c* child, as he improves under homeopathic treatment, makes contact with adults sooner than he does with peers. He will talk to adults or older siblings, yet he will not play with his peers. This is understandable when we recognize the Cyber delusion or essence of *Bar-c*, that *he walks on his knees*: he feels so small that only a person bigger than he is (an adult or older child/sibling) can provide the support and protection he craves.

As is usual with any child with an impaired developmental state or delay, this backward behavior exacerbates around puberty as the miasm flares up. If mom, at any given moment, starts saying, "If you are going be like this I will have to leave you," the remark will only fuel the separation anxiety. Long before puberty, the *Baryta carbonicum* child will pick up masturbation, but he can be gently redirected if this behavior persists beyond an expected age (unlike the *Bufo* child, who will seek isolation to masturbate). Like *Calc-c*, *Bar-c* craves junk food, dairy, and sweets, although he aggravates physically from them. Due to malabsorption, he will suffer from yeasty stools or gushing diarrhea alternating with constipation.

The smallness and dwarfishness which is the essence of *Bar-c* is most often seen on the mental plane rather than the physical one. We see *great forgetfulness; he does not know what he just had said before* or *he forgets the word he is about to utter. In the middle of her sentence she cannot think of quite a common word.* The child in school is left quickly behind as *there is dullness and stupidity in the head. There is total aversion to mental work. The child simply cannot be taught for it cannot remember and has great absentmindedness*! Such a child simply cannot comprehend or maintain a thought. The mother goes over it and over it and the wonders if the child will ever learn anything. These are children who can bankrupt the family with endless speech therapy, but only well-adjusted doses of *Bar-c* will bring such children out of their isolation.

Golden Tips from the Masters

- *Bar-c* is the #1 remedy for the formation of chronic recurrent swollen tonsils with induration: strong affinity for the lymphatic glands all over the body
- Is of great benefit in toning up the nervous system, especially that of old men or those in premature old age
- Down syndrome
- Child is timid with teacher but can bully other children (*Lyc*)
- Arterial hypertension due to extreme arteriosclerosis with loss of sexual desire and loss of erection
- Senility after apoplexy or after drugs
- When growth stops: sometimes first give pituitary 3x or 6x and then follow with *Bar-c*, as it will work better
- Sudden disgust, no interest in food though hungry
- In Alzheimer disease due to arteriosclerosis of the brain with multiple brain infarcts: they become prematurely senile and behave like children
- A differential diagnosis with *Calc-c*, *Pulsatilla*, *Hyoscyamus*, and *Bufo* is necessary

Calcarea carbonica (Calc-c). Impure Carbonate of Lime

The Cyber Delusion

The helmsman of the *Calc-carb's* boat, the one that steers the life of this person, is the fixed idea or delusion ***he is about to sink into annihilation***. This Cyber delusion, reflecting the fragility of the *Calc-c* person in spite of his usually impressive bulk (*Calcarea* children are always born with a weight and length in the 90th percentile), is expressed in another, similar fixed idea: that *his body is being dashed to pieces*. This, again, represents a sense of brittleness in spite of his layers of protective fat. The size of such a baby inevitably leads to a prolonged or delayed labor, symbolizing this infant's wish to remain in the maternal womb, that paradise-like pool in which he effortlessly floats and enjoys the availability of constant nourishment and protection. While the *Calcarea* child starts his life this way, the *Calcarea* person, regardless of age, seems to always want to remain close to the mother, anxious about discovering the world with all its challenges. Driven by the Cyber delusion of falling to pieces, this child is overdramatic when he falls, showing a great sense of exaggeration as though he were close to dying. If someone bumps into him by accident, he will yell a big "OW" and say, "That really hurts," a completely inappropriate intensity for the situation (*despair with the pains*). For such a child, a "hit" is almost any physical contact, by accident or not. Forget contact sports (soccer, American football, rugby, and hockey) or team sports in general: with the slightest contact, he will cry out and weep as though having suffered a grave injury; obviously, this brings mom to him, and she must now acknowledge this great hurt. Such a child prefers legos, reading books, and watching Walt Disney films (not horror films). He is prone to severe nightmares, after which he will call upon his parents, and is startled at the slightest noise in his sleep, often falling into a *Stramonium* state (*Calc-carb's* acute). He inevitably needs a little night lamp as he is scared of the dark, and he is always affected by *hearing bad news* like the death of a friend, family member, or pet, or by seeing emaciated children on TV. Many times, if a

Calc-c with recurrent nightmares can talk of his repressed emotions through the homeopathic remedy, temper tantrums break out in the day and the nightmare gallops out of the window of the night.

The person needing *Calcarea* is always convinced that there is something wrong with him, and he is concerned about the smallest inconvenience and distress (*hypochondriasis, imaginary illness; delusion, he was about to die; delusion, he has an incurable disease, of having a heart disease; delusion, being sick and therefore will not work*); he faints upon seeing blood and flees at the slightest suggestion of getting an injection. *Calc-c* has a great sense of exaggeration; Hahnemann called him a nuisance to those around him because of his complaints about trifles and because he *torments those about him, day and night*: "I have this white spot, what does it mean?" "What is the meaning of this?" These are the questions with which *Calc-c* tortures. Kent describes: "When the Calc-c patient relates to his friends how he feels they all naturally say to him, 'Why don't you put that aside, it does not amount to anything,' but to him it is a big thing, and he cannot put it aside; all these little things combine to convince him that he is going crazy and he is very sick."[18]

This peculiar characteristic might give the impression that *Calc-c* changes the subject all the time like a *Lachesis*, but it is like telling a story backwards, completely filled in with details. No wonder the *Calcarea* person is an avid reader of medical books: he is looking for urgent answers regarding his imagined ills (*mania to read medical books*). This sense of vulnerability and danger creates other fixed ideas in *Calcarea*: that *he will be murdered*; and *he has horrible visions on closing his eyes,* and delusions, *of animals*. He is the most childish character of the hypochondriacs as *he weeps for trifles*! What makes him even more powerless and exposed is that he is convinced that everyone can see this fragile state, an inevitable meltdown (falling to pieces!) about to happen, expressed in other fixed ideas such as *others will observe his confusion* and *he is being observed* and *delusion, people think her of becoming insane.*

If it is not an illness that will befall *Calcarea*, there is always that *fear that something terrible will happen*. Who hasn't been swimming in the water and heard the *Jaws* theme song play in their head, or boarded an airplane with a flicker of fear that it would crash? Whenever faced with the possibility of a tragedy, less paranoid people calculate the risks and tell themselves

18. Kent, *Lectures*, 281.

they will be OK. After all, what are the chances that it will happen to them? Not so with *Calc-c!* Arguments about the odds don't fly with *Calcarea*, even if such an event (lightning strike, plane crash, shark attack) happens to only one in a million. *Calc-c* has the feeling that he could be the one! After all he belongs to Jung's **sensation** conscious function type, which means that only anything coming through his five senses is real; it tells him that something **is** there, but not what it is (for that, one needs the **thinking** conscious function). The sensation type sees an astounding mass of details: how is it constructed? What does a thing look alike? How to take things apart? Feeling and sensation must not be confused as they so often are in English. In French, the distinction is clearly indicated by two entirely different concepts of *sentiment* (feeling) and *sensation* (sensation). As seen before, and as expressed by the CD, the sensation type, *Calc-c,* is subject to repressive intuitions like anxieties, intuitive fears, and forebodings.

Causalities

Ailments from Anticipation and Bad News

His *ailments from* (*A/F*) include, in the first place, *ailments from hearing bad news* and *ailments from anticipation* (*apprehensive mood, as if some misfortune was about to happen, about his health*; *that he might have an organic disease of the heart*; *aggravation from mental emotions*). It has everything to do with his health, and we see right away that *Calc-c* easily falls prey to a depression similar to an *Aurum* depression when his fragile sense of stability breaks down: for instance, when *hearing* or *seeing* or *reading about bad news.* Although this hearing bad news can be triggered by outside events not at all related to himself, *Calc-c* has an uncanny ability to relate horrible incidents to his own person. It is as if all these events will or can happen to him (or a very close member of the family): sickness, poverty, worst of all hunger, tragedy, tsunamis, hurricanes, wildfires, earthquakes... everything has to do with, and is thought of as, a possible threat to his own health and environment, which he discusses extensively with every conceivable individual he knows, even with sympathetic strangers. It is expressed in *talks about nothing but murder, fire and rats.* We find also in the provings: *fears excited by reports of cruelties.*

Pregnancy is always a period of great anticipation anxiety. There are always worries when something seems to go wrong: spotting, lack of fetal movements... of course, anticipation anxiety increases when the pregnancy follows three miscarriages or when it has taken a long time to get pregnant. There can be constant anxiety of losing the fetus throughout the pregnancy, and the mother-to-be can get caught up in the world of numbers: in this month, this and this are supposed to happen; then, there is measuring of the amniotic fluid, the fundal height, the thickness of the nuchal fold, and eventually, in delivery, the number of contractions, the time in between... no wonder some *Calc-c* children exhibit obsessive behavior about numbers!

Cares and Worries

Calc-carb's worry is always personal and close to home, not for the rest of the world (the "world" being anywhere beyond his own neighborhood, indicating *-affectations from egotism.* He avoids bad news on TV and in newspapers, but when something happens to any of his family members or close friends it hits him with a vengeance (*ailments from grief*)! And, of course, in these days of ubiquitous communication, it is difficult to avoid seeing bad news, as the *Calc-c* person stays in close contact with friends and family. For example, he posts endless pictures on Facebook: of his baby when he smeared his food in his face, of reunions, of parties with family and friends, as if life were nothing but a never-ending party. It is easy to see that a depressive situation (again, similar to an *Aurum* depression) can arise due to excessive worry and excessive responsibility (on a small, family-oriented scale versus that of the larger worldview of the *Aurum* and *Causticum* mentalities). We find *Calc-c* simultaneously under the rubrics *duty, too much sense of duty,* related to her worry about domestic issues only, and *duty, no sense of duty* regarding world issues or even any matters beyond those affecting immediate family and close friends.

Pregnancy for a *Calc-c* leads to another kind of worry. Upon hearing she is pregnant, the first reaction of a *Calcarea* mom is happy and excited yet nervous and worried: *ailments from care and worry* feature greatly in the story of the makeup of a homeopathic constitutional *Calcarea* disposition. Mom might run to the doctor every ten days. More than ever, such a mom needs her partner's support; if support is not forthcoming, anxiety increases as harmony in the family is very important to her. Even arguments with in-laws followed by a lack of contact, leave such an expectant mother in a state of great worry. She will inevitably turn to all of her friends for the needed support; if she is away from them, however, her whole world can crumble, reflecting *Calc-carb's* Cyber delusion. The worries can be about anything: how she will combine motherhood with her job, whether she will be a good mother, whether the child will be normal, whether her partner will be as happy as she is, whether the partner will be able to keep his/her job, the family home, etc.

As one can see, the *Calc-c mind is full of concern about imaginary things that might happen to her. A rush of thoughts prevents their sleep and the mind is confused to what she has read or heard. She thinks she is sick to death, nevertheless she could not complain about anything; there is melancholy about the heart, without cause.* It can become so intense that she *feels she would lose her senses* and *that people will observe her confusion* (*fear, her condition being observed*). Often this leads now to withdrawal of *Calc-c* into his shell, his home (*desire to go home*), which in extended meaning is translated into going to live with the parents or in their close vicinity. The expectant mom may move in with her family during the last months of pregnancy and may make more visits to her trusted physician. It is also important to her to have a burial place in the family plot as, even in death, the vicinity of family is a consolation. *Calc-c* is not averse at this point to seeking to dull these anxieties with alcohol, although often it fuels her delirium to talk about all the calamities that can happen to him: *mania-a-potu with delirium about fire, rats, mice and murder.*

The newborn *Calc-c* child is always the giant among his peers: big head, highest weight, large and hypotonic, and always successful in delaying the delivery as much as possible: it is symbolic for his desire to stay in the intrauterine swimming pool, not to be taken away from that peaceful and quiet place and put into the precarious and painful position of the birthing process.

Grief/Fright

I had a patient transfer a worried *Calcarea* state to her child because she had been mourning a brother who had committed suicide; her whole pregnancy was immersed in thoughts such as "What does it mean? Why did it happen?" In homeopathic language, this can be translated into *religious affections, alternating with metaphysical concerns.* A *Calc-c* person is always highly sexual (*ailments from sexual excesses*), but she is even more so in pregnancy. If her partner does not want to be intimate, it will bother her as she perceives it as rejection and experiences sadness. But certainly, her excitement after grief can be strong; Kent provides a vivid picture of excitement after grief in his Lectures on Homeopathic Materia Medica: "The mother loses her child or husband **[or, I should add, her dog!]**; she is broken-hearted and greatly excited. It is a hysterical state. And yet I have seen the same in men. I remember one. It came upon him from business cares. He had the same feeling, he would walk up and down the house, he said he felt as if he must fly or jump out of a window **[compare to Aurum]** or do something that is analogous to the mental state found in hysteria, or a great state of nervous excitement."[19]

Of course, once *Calcarea* persons are in this state of excitement, and with the power of their obstinacy, nobody can convince them that they are not gravely ill, and we return to the Cyber delusion that they are disintegrating. All this leads quickly to depression, where we see now *disinclination to any kind of work* (where at least *Aurum* with some stimulation will do something), and *he does not care to get well at all or do anything to assist in his recovery. He is despairing and hopeless of ever getting well, with fear of death, tormenting him day and night. There is a despairing mood, with dread of disease and suffering. There is indifference and inertness.* Inertia (mental and physical) is one of the greatest enemies of conscious choice! Inertia describes *Calcarea's* depression well as it reflects his immobility; one could almost call it his paralysis and total apathy. This might also explain why *Calc-c* is not inclined to commit suicide (< > *Aurum*): *Calc-c* is characterized by a *weakness of will*, a black type remedy. They don't have the courage for suicide; they have no stuffing so to speak (*fear of the pain* and *fear of suffering*, both provings also to be found in *Aurum*). *Calc-c* often will state: "Why should I do something, as my fate has already been determined? I just don't give a damn about anything anymore. What is the use of life anyway? Why can't get I as much out of life as others?" It is often the hidden desire for a lazy, self-indulgent life which cannot always be fulfilled.

Here is a description of such a *Cal- c* depression; one can see the similarities with an *Aurum* depression. I have put the corresponding rubrics in italics after the patient's expressions:

> I have sunk now into a level of depression where I am now even entertaining thoughts of death (*suicidal thoughts*). I am not actively suicidal, but I am not taking care of my health (*indifference and inertness; he does not care to get well or to do anything to assist in his recovery*, Hering; *despair of recovery; discouraged, indifference about recovery*). I get to the point of being non-functional, especially when I have lost confidence in the efficacy of the remedy and give up (*delusion, is about to sink into annihilation*). My sleep is OK but I have *many dreams* involving family or

19. Kent, *Lectures*, 283. Emphases added.

just processing the stressful events regarding my business (*ailments from worry, cares; anxiety about business*). Anxiety is less severe (*ailments from anticipation*) [had taken another remedy before, *Sulphur*], but still causing early morning diarrhea (*morning diarrhea*). I always feel guilty when I don't accomplish enough and I have started praying (*religious affection; wants to read the Bible all day*) again for help with this miserable state. I seem to have lost all ambition (*indifference to duties*). I still have no contact with my child and I grieve for the loss of my family (*home, desires to go; homesickness*), for the loss of what I grew up with, a strong family unit and the sense of contributing to society through my children; I must have failed as a mother (*reproaches herself*) [this reflects more the idea of not being a nourishing force in the family, certainly a *Carbon* theme: family comes first; this is certainly the most important duty, if not the only one, for which she is responsible]. My main worries now are the following: the keloid, which is painful to the touch, itches and burns and is relieved with cold applications. I want to excise it before it becomes malignant, which is my worry (*fear for cancer; fear of impending disease; fear of misfortune; despair with fear of death*). [For the homeopath more important is the fact that she puts this as her #1 concern, above the depression, typical for the *Carbon* person who focuses on physical complaints first; the itching and burning shows psora active.] The depression renders me a useless human being (self-depreciation; want *of confidence; delusion, she is disgraced* (*Sulphur*); *delusion, being sick and therefore will not work; delusion, is ruined*).

Calc-c rather than *Aurum* was the remedy that saved this patient's life!

Compensations

Familiarity to Relieve Anxiety

Unity with other living beings is an imperative for any human being. Of course, different people achieve unions in different ways. For the constitutional *Calc-c*, an attempt to become one with his limited world is to submit to a person or a group (family) and most often to God. In this way he transcends the separateness of his individual existence by becoming part of something bigger than himself (the family unit and God), strengthening a perceived need for protection.

What is this anxiety all about and how does the child deal with it? Anxiety becomes very clear when the child needs to separate from the parents (typically starting at age five) to start his own individual journey; the separation will affect him in many aspects, as social and physical skills are usually delayed. More than any other type, *Calc-c* needs familiarity, which translates into security for such a child: there is anxiety about undertaking new things; it is difficult for this child to watch any new TV shows or play any new games. He is very rigid about this and will play according to a very limited storyline; he can become very angry if the storyline deviates from his idea of how the story should go. The story can only have one path, and he always plays the good guy. When he plays with his friends, he is very black and white about who is his friend. If someone he knows is friends with someone he doesn't like, then that person is on the wrong "team" and the *Calcarea* child will not want to play with him, even when the third person (the one he dislikes) is not around.

He is cautious about making friends. It is not that he does not need or want friends, but the anxiety, insecurity, and fear of rejection (*falling to pieces; forsaken feeling feels of not being beloved by his parents and friends; offended easily, takes everything in bad part*) constantly obstruct his ability to bridge the space between him and his peers. In fact, this child has an easier time connecting to adults than he does relating to his peers: such a withdrawn, cautious child easily stirs up the sympathy of an adult, especially a woman with her natural nourishing anima. He also connects more easily to much younger or much older children, with whom the roles are more automatically defined. *Calcarea* has great fondness for food and drink. He tends to overcome anxiety (which is everywhere!) and depression (always looming) by eating and drinking. The mouth is a prominent feature, often the most expressive one: lips tend to be thick and open, as if in a state of continuous expectation to being fed. This is a symbol of being loved. He is always nibbling on something; even more, he is driven to eat. He has to eat to quiet his anxieties about being unloved or about the calamities that are so visible in this world (these are avoided at all costs by the *Calc-c* person as they belong to that "foreign" world, too calamitous to consider). Food is like a drug for him, acting as a tranquilizer: a refrigerator full of food and drink is his medicine cabinet in case of worry and/or depression (to which he is quite prone)!

Calc-c is much happier engaged in a one-to-one conversation in a quiet corner of a restaurant than he is flitting from person to person at a noisy party. Unlike a true extravert, who is energized by the social stimulation of a crowd, *Calc-c* becomes exhausted in these circumstances.

The *Calcarea* adult (besides hanging on to childhood characteristics) is the person who still believes in the greatest marketing slogan of all time: "the pursuit of happiness"—a happiness in which the nuclear family is the psychological and economic basis for this whole grand experiment in living. He expects his marriage partner to be his best friend, a great lover, an excellent cook, a great parent, financially secure, who subscribes to the *New York Times* and loves dogs—a soul mate with a great sense of humor who believes that having kids will increase the joy in life. *Calc-c* has these impossible expectations for marriage, but he tries very hard to fulfill them in any case. In the name of love for the kids, the norm is that his life is out of control as he spends every weekend going to 61 birthday parties after speeding the kids from the soccer game to the ballet class. It's a treadmill locked on the highest setting that never lets *Calc-c* catch his breath or consider how he started running this fast in the first place. *Calc-c* might complain that his kids always entertain themselves on the Wii with games, but he himself is interested in playing games on his iPad at every free moment rather than using his legs for walking or any other form of exercise. This child-centered style of parenting results in an adulthood divorced from extra-professional relationships. The adult *Calc-carb's* life is ceded to his children, with possible boredom, stress, fatigue, depression, and unhappiness as an outcome, especially when the children leave home. The anticipation of the overflow of bliss that *Calc-c* believes is the certain outcome of every birth rarely materializes: children don't always guarantee a life filled with happiness, excitement, contentment, and pride. But for *Calc-c* it remains a quest to dream the American dream, and he is probably the only one who can make it happen, at least in his mind!

Quest for Safety

The *Calcarea* child's fragility and fear of getting injured is easily seen when he is invited to a birthday party. He always will stay at his mom's side, observing the situation, for quite some time. He is not the one galloping into the crowd and claiming his spot. Mom has to encourage him constantly, and even then, he will look for toys he is familiar with and will prefer to sit by himself, close to his mom and away from the ruckus that is so much a part of the typical world of children. You might think of him as the quiet child or the gentle giant. He seems unsure of himself, very shy even when he has been more outgoing in the past. The more his ego grows, the more he becomes cautious (*timidity and bashful*). Sometimes his family thinks he is just too bashful or, worse, questions whether he is mentally weaker than his peers. A good school (one in which he can adjust for many years so that it becomes a second home) and a sensitive teacher (who becomes the ersatz parent) provide a structured environment in which he can find peace; outside of the classroom structure, though—even on the playground—the teacher can find him in the sandbox by himself, doing the same limited things like pouring sand in his hands, digging for rocks, swinging, and avoiding the commotion and noise on the playground (*aversion to certain persons*; *sensitive to shrill sounds*).

A quest for sameness and consistency will remain throughout his childhood: whenever he finds a kindred soul, that child becomes his only friend, whom he must have around all the time. He does not wish to dominate his friend as does the *Lycopodium* child; rather, this friend becomes part of his close family. Unfortunately, he becomes very possessive of this person, which is understandable when we acknowledge how difficult it is for him to make new friends. He wants the same friend, the same type of games to play (the safe, nonphysical ones), and the same bland foods. It really is his Cyber delusion that, as usual, explains all this behavior. Part of his makeup is also the fixed idea that his peers are laughing at him and that they can see how confused he is (*delusion he is laughed at* and *fear, that his condition is observed*). Very often, especially when in the deeper state of *Calcarea*, which is *Baryta carbonicum*, he can become very unhappy, irritable, and even angry whenever anyone laughs in his presence. This is because he cannot distinguish laughing at something funny from laughing at him, and he does not like to be teased at all. All this can lead to screaming and angry outbursts. Obviously, such a child is not very good at reading such social cues, getting jokes, or understanding the nuances of social/peer play. His ego growth is also hindered by difficulties in gathering information from the nonverbal communication that goes on around him.

It is just not emotional weakness that the *Calcarea* child suffers from and that creates his Cyber delusion; he is saddled also with various bodily attributes which limit his physical capabilities. Reluctant to leave the womb, and feeding until the last moment, a *Calcarea* is always a gentle giant, from birth to adulthood. He is born, so to speak, "off the charts": big head, big weight, big everything. He is always in the 90th to 100th percentile on the charts, except for that low muscle tone (hypotonia): not a lot of bounce to the ounce! It is, therefore, not uncommon for the *Calcarea* child to have an *unsteady gait*; he often falls, apparently being somewhat *clumsy. Ascending stairs can be difficult.* Low muscle tone is also responsible for the difficulties he has with fine motor skills, such as holding a pen to write or holding firmly to an object. At the age at which all of his peers can do the monkey bars, his muscles lack the tone and strength to achieve the same result. Additionally, his hands sweat profusely, making it hard to grip the monkey bars; and then, he cannot figure out how to swing his body to help him with momentum. And even when, much later, he is finally able to manage the monkey bars, he will forget how to do it if he does not practice it for a long time. Even climbing stairs or riding a tricycle is frightful. There is a constant anxiety about getting hurt: he will breathe hard and his palms will continue to sweat. Because of lack of tone in his muscles, the *Calcarea* child also has difficulty generating any physical strength in his body. He can barely open a water bottle because he can't seem to get any strength in his hands to hold the cap tightly and turn it. If he is about to try skiing, he can't get his skis onto his bindings; though it might look like he is pushing down on his skis, he is generating no force. When he does learn to finally do things, after a lot of direction and encouragement from his frustrated parents, he doesn't remember how to do them again the next time. Since he cannot easily access the creativity or ability to think of how to do something in a different way, he will continue to try to open the bottle in the same way every time even though it's not working. This lack of physical ability disappears when the *Calcarea* child wants to fight. He can throw a hard punch or land a hard kick when he is angry. So he does have the ability to generate physical power and strength, but can't seem to do it for everyday practical things. It is desirable for him to expend the minimum effort: although he should exercise his flabby muscles, he prefers that mom push the tricycle for as long as she is willing to help him. This inertness goes along with an awkwardness that is reflected in difficulties buttoning his pants and shirts, zipping his jacket, or tying his shoes. When parents insist that he try these things on his own, it only increases his anxiety.

Anger

His anxiety makes him a very angry child with a very short temper. He will have loud, angry outbursts at school if he thinks he has been wronged in any small way. When he is unhappy with something at school, he sighs very loudly and disrupts the class. He becomes easily frustrated with tasks in class, causing him again to make some noise or dramatically throw his head down in class in great demonstrative frustration. This child gets very moody and dark when things/events do not progress as he expects, especially when he makes mistakes in homework or is trying to assemble a toy.

In general, he is a very sweet child: he is affectionate, generous, happy, and good-natured. But when his anxiety level rises, he becomes the opposite of his true self: *anger with red face*; *consolation aggravates*; *aversion to family members*; and *irritability from trifles*. He is not mean-spirited, self-centered, spiteful, abusive, or bad-mannered in any way, and the homeopathic *Calcarea* will balance him out so that he can become again the well-adjusted, smart, funny, independent, and loving person that is underneath the hard, stubborn shell. In the safety of the home (*desires to go home*), *Calc*-c remains *active and full of fun*. The outlook of a typical *Calcarea* person is optimistic and friendly. But he becomes anxious when his source of support (parents, friends, family) and his castle or home is threatened. Even the family photo album is a support tool, and it is constantly brought out to reassure him that his family is still close. The *Calcarea* person demonstrates genuine warmth and wishes to help others, but doing things for others is also done in order to secure favor with them.

Inertia or Non-movement

One only has to think how *Calc*-c makes nice coral reefs and provides a home for thousands of fish. Speaking of inertia! The idea of inertness comes often sooner to *Calc-c* as it is part of his innate character; in other words, it can set in **before** depression starts. Inertia is one of the greatest enemies of conscious choice. *Calc-c* is a person tending to receive things from the outside, not to be very productive on his own. He is a good listener (can be an excellent psychotherapist), but his talent lies in receiving ideas, not in producing new ones. *Calcarea* always expects everything from an outside source, even in religion: God is the almighty protector (*religious affections, in children*; *religious affections, alternating with metaphysical concerns [black type, only remedy]*; *religious affections in puberty*) from whom he expects everything; it does not occur to him to put forth an effort. Faith allays *Calc-carb's* deepest fears and mitigates unbearable losses. He is always searching for the magic helper, as in the fables and dream worlds that he likes so much. He has many friends simply because he needs many hands to feel secure, so he has a hard time saying "no"; therefore, he loves to say "yes" to everything and everyone, resulting in a paralytic mind, unable to make decisions (*irresolution*) which makes him more and more dependent on others. Of course *Cal-c* feels lost when alone, even frightened, as he feels he cannot do anything without help, or take responsibility for himself; he feels too helpless to make decisions and take responsibility (*responsibility, lack of*)! The parent of such a child has to tell him to brush his teeth, to pick up his clothes, to get his glass of juice, to pack his backpack for school, to put his shoes on, and yes, to keep on going! Inertness translates for *Calc-c* into procrastination, often caused by a childlike impulsiveness which is also a measure of how easily he is distracted. *Calc-c* always has a hard time resisting temptation. He is keenly responsive to immediate stimulation, prompt rewards, and present-moment distractions like playing a game on his iPad, not to vague future plans like an exam that is months away. The more readily he succumbs to distraction, the greater chance there is that he will procrastinate. If there is homework to be done for the Monday, he waits to do it till breakfast on Monday morning rather than dealing with it on the weekend. Modern technology has not helped him: there is the iPad with games, there is email, voice mail, Twitter, Facebook, web surfing, YouTube—you could not design a worse working environment for *Calc-c* if you tried! Hence *Calc-carb's* tendency to give in to what feels good, seeking immediate emotional relief, leaving tasks for later. If and when he formulates some grandiose plans for the future (like losing weight but not liking any diet plan well enough to stick to it), they must not be too hard to achieve. In fact, they need to be easy!

Calcarea (*magnetized, desire to be*) gives up his inner independence and submits to an authority, so he readily starts thinking and acting what the domineering hypnotist makes him think and feel. All the characters in the rubric *magnetized* (*Lach, Sil, Phos*) are often in a state of semi-hypnosis, gladly giving up their powers of critical thinking and submitting emotionally to the speaker. Rather than disagree with the ideas of the speaker, *Calcarea* often submits to an authority who seems to have magical powers with which he can seduce his semi-comatose audience. This way, *Calcarea* and the other characters mentioned become part of someone or something bigger than themselves. Once I asked a *Calc-c* teenager, "What do you like most in school?" The answer was: "Recess!" Speaking of inertia! One woman, when I mentioned the "enjoyment of inactivity," reported that her husband's mother had told her that "it took ten months to create him, not the usual nine." Only a well-chosen dose of homeopathic *Calcarea* makes the stone of inertia roll away from the tomb.

Non-movement in a child is also expressed in the *Calc-c* gastrointestinal tract. Bowel movements remain a mystery and a seventh world wonder at the same time. The *Calcarea* person might not go for three days and experience no apparent discomfort, but then he makes stools that clog the toilet. Perspiring is something he does in abundance: especially from the head (Mom finds his pillow soaking wet in the morning) but also from the body, although dry heat is equally possible; it is not uncommon for him to need to get fresh clothes, even more than once during the night, because of heavy perspiration. This night perspiration is worse than perspiration during the day. At night, according to Traditional Chinese Medicine (TCM), the Yin has to be preserved; the Chinese called this kind of perspiration "rob sweat" as it is robbing the person of essential nutrients. Even during the day, the child is rather chilly, perspires upon the slightest exertion and has clammy hands.

Water: The Other Home

Water, the relatively fixed symbol for the unconscious, the motherly womb, is another place of protection and comfort. *Calc-c* would live in water if he could. He feels naturally at home and can float in a pool for hours, dive in it, and remain submerged longer than anyone else; in other words, the pool is his home. Certainly his great protest when it is time to go home (his other castle) testifies to that. But don't ask him to do laps in the swimming pool: he will do a few laps, and then lay there like a stranded whale (while encouraging his dad to do laps: "Way to go, Dad!"). If he does swim in a race, he always will be dead last; he is distinguished by his slow, awkwardly moving arms. He is rarely an athlete and abhors exercise in general. If anything, he prefers table tennis, with its limited movements, and he will pretend that he plays soccer and tennis when you ask him. He may tell his parents, "I played soccer," but in reality he watched, and for him that **is** participation!

Stubbornness is his Name!

Stubbornness is the hallmark of the *Calc-c* boy or girl, whether trapped in a state of autism or not. That means, inherently, that *Calc-c* will walk and talk later than other children: it is an expression of their stubbornness to decide when they will talk or walk; statistics do not decide. It is not uncommon for a *Calc-c* child not to speak a single word yet at 13 months and then to suddenly speak in sentences at 14 months. Of course this would make an early diagnosis of Autism Spectrum Disorder (ASD) difficult; there are, however, enough *Calc*-c-peculiar ASD characteristics to recognize such a fellow. Stubbornness is shown everywhere, but especially with his parents, who dote on him. I had a seven-year-old *Calcarea* child with ASD say to his mom when he got spanked, "I didn't feel anything; I wiped it off!" You have to admire that tenacity! Stubbornness is also shown in *delayed closing of the fontanelles* and *delayed dentition*. And when the speech or behavior therapist pushes him a little beyond his limit in performing, he will exclaim, "I don't need this anymore!" and nothing can change his mind. Another *Calc*-c child will decide to stand in the middle of a busy market, having determined he has had enough of walking, and refuse to budge another inch in spite of any motherly encouragement. You can't move a rock!

One *Calcarea* child I knew took this to an unexpected extreme. When I say "unexpected," it is because this boy loved eating (like any Calc-c), especially carbs and sweets. So when his health-oriented and loving mother made him drink a concoction with all those "delicious" natural greens and ginger before each dinner, he suddenly stopped taking dinner until mom stopped giving him the healthy drink. That is stubborn, knowing how much such a child loves eating! While he likes any food, pasteurized milk is hard for him to digest; this is one of the characters who will give his parents a "wow" moment when milk is omitted from his diet. Milk causes distention of the stomach, loose mushy stools (in contrast to that obstinate constipation), and painful cramps.

Stubbornness is also used as a tool to ensure his security. He likes to stay with the same style of food, and if he practices a sport, he always uses the same tactics and is not open to a change. One *Calcarea* child chose fencing as his sport (to my surprise). But the mom told me that he chose it only because it was considered a safe sport. And when she watched him during a tournament, he was excellent at defending himself, always using the same style, but rarely attacked! It reflects so much the nature of the *Calcarea* child: putting up excellent defenses but rarely going on the offense!

Stubbornness is maintained, even to his detriment. I had a patient who liked playing on the swings at school; although there were five swings, he always sat on the same one. When someone else wanted to sit on his preferred swing, he decided he would rather fight than simply go to another swing. He did not change this routine for the entire year, even when he was abused daily by the other child.

Focus and Food

Calc-carb's attention span is always short—except when it comes to food, with which his mind is constantly busy. For him, the pleasures of food, drink, rest, and sleep are paramount. He has a constant, voracious appetite and is always scouting for food as though he had some extra antennas guiding him to food, any food. In my office, I always had a snack hidden for unforeseen moments, but even the most secret place in the office is no match for the laser eyes of such a child. He has great fondness for sweets, *boiled eggs, ice cream* and even eats indigestible things like pencils and play dough (*craves indigestible things, chalk, coal,* etc.). When it comes to non-preferred activities like schoolwork, the *Calcarea* child needs to be constantly reminded that he needs to focus more and continue to work at it. The whole world is competing for his attention, and just about anything can distract him: noise, radio, the refrigerator, the iPad, games, and the TV with marketing designed especially for him. It is personal, seductive, and distracting. He finds any possible excuse as he has trouble staying focused for 30 minutes, let alone for an entire school day. He seems to wait for the missing muse to inspire him and for the right mood (which rarely comes) to motivate him. The behavior is a combination of curiosity and restlessness. He is one of the *restless* children—not as much as the *Tarentula* child, but enough to drive you crazy. Coloring does not last more than a few minutes. It all has to do with the short attention span, but there is also a degree of laziness present. One child usually did a few rolls of a ball with his parents and that was it. After treatment with *Calc-c,* he did it for half an hour and was the initiator, getting everyone in the family involved.

Only at the table with food will these children remain seated for more than 10 minutes. Even as young children they like to bake and help out in the kitchen, be signed up for cooking classes... usually to make a mess. *Calc-c* can't remember to bring home all his homework even though his teacher writes it all down for him to copy, goes over it verbally, and asks him to check for all his things before he goes home.

The Search for Permanent Protection

I have already mentioned that the *Calcarea* child did not want to leave the maternal womb (that warm oven with a swimming pool). As he has been forced out anyway—much to the relief of his mom (long labor!)—protection and safety remain a priority. He prefers to interact with other children on a one-to-one basis. Groups of children are approached with great care, and before he will mingle with them, a long observation is done from a distance, often from the safety of a parent's immediate vicinity. From a distance, he watches with excitement, but a trusted adult needs to bring him gently into the circle of the other children. He often struggles more than the average child to join in play with peers during unstructured play time. He plays well with his siblings as long as he can dictate what game will be played. He initially gets excited at the prospect of an upcoming social event like a birthday party. Then, however, he gets anxious, leading to a meltdown (*fear in a crowd*; *fear of public places*). He readily admits that he is scared, contrary to the *Lycopodium* child who instead becomes bossy, a displacement for his fear. *Calc-c* needs constant reassurance from a parent or from any adult: it boosts his ego and allows him to face the dangers of the world. Contrary to *Baryta carbonicum* (the deeper state of *Calcarea*, who can be afraid of any animal), he loves dogs; he can, however, show his enthusiasm too strongly, thinking that jumping on the dog and pulling his tail is playing. The *Calcarea* child has numerous fears: fears for noise (when toilet is flushed), for mice, for thunder, bodily harm, suffering, *for his condition being observed, for disease* and *infection, for evil,* etc.).

To deal with these fears which seem to disturb his balance, he looks for something that provides constant security, something that he can count on. So he may get upset when Mom leaves home to do an errand, even if Dad is home. On the other hand, his father leaving while his mother is still there provokes no reaction. Of course, generally, Mom comes first; a mother's love never fails as she is infused with anima, which stands for food, empathy, unconditional love, protection, and warmth: mother is earth. What Mom sometimes does have to compete with, though, are numbers. The *Calc-c* child has an obsession with numbers to the point of OCD-like behavior. Numbers are secure: one is always one; it can't be anything else, and it is always exactly what he expects it to be. One plus one is two: there is no other solution. He likes numbers more than letters: letters form different words, with different meanings and pronunciations. Therefore, they are less reliable.

When the *Calcarea* child becomes anxious, he will get into conversations, citing numbers: I am ... years old; my birthday is... He is smart enough to be able to direct conversations towards numbers. In class, when he sees a calendar, he will get engrossed in it and forget everyone and everything else. He cannot have a clock in his bedroom or he will obsess over it and become an insomniac. He gets very upset if this security device is taken away. When one of the moms in my practice asked her *Calcarea* child whom he loved more, numbers or her, he thought about it and said, "Numbers." Seeing her sad reaction, the next day he declared, "I love you more than numbers, Mom." One sees the need to create this protective environment everywhere: this is a child who will group even his toys. He creates a harmonious world with cars, soldiers, and animals because harmony is equal to security and family. Don't forget the essence or Cyber delusion of this remedy: *he is about to sink into annihilation and his body will fall into pieces.*

The *Calcarea* child is rather shy when it comes to expressing himself; even if he knows the answer to a question, he prefers to remain silent. He hates it when attention is drawn to him, as he is convinced that everyone sees how confused he is (*fear of, his condition, being observed*). Even when he is ten years old he will ask his mom to phone his friends to come over—or, more accurately, his one good friend. He does not like to be laughed at, although he is the first one to tease others. If attention is drawn to him in a classroom setting, he does not know where to hide. It feels very uncomfortable to the *Calc-c* child to "be observed." But he chuckles when someone else takes the risk of doing something naughty, although he is wise enough not to get involved. After all, he cannot handle any kind of punishment: it would crush him.

Religious and Metaphysical Questions

And then there is the ultimate protector: God. No one asks more religious and metaphysical questions than the *Calc-c* child (*religious affections, alternating with metaphysical concerns*). He prays for anything: health, protection, food, an animal... Heaven becomes that other wonderful environment of love and security. However, one *Calc-c* child asked: "But what if I want to leave Heaven?" This demonstrated the ever-present *Calc-c* fear that he would get hurt. "When I die is it going to hurt?" They can appear to be preoccupied with suffering and death, even at an early age; I have seen many such four-year-old patients. The greatest of all evils, the worst thing that can happen to anyone anywhere, is death; his greatest anxiety is focused on death. He has a boundless attachment to a protected life. Voltaire, in his wisdom, questioned this objective value of life when he stated: "We like life, but all the same nothingness has its good points. I do not know what eternal life is, but this present life is a bad joke." It does not help that *horrible things affect greatly.* He delays falling asleep because he could die: the fear of death is indeed extreme. When it thunders, he shivers, as Nature's force is a threat to his safe home. If he has siblings, he might ask: "Where was my sister before? Was she in heaven and why did she only come down now?" The root of *Calc-carb's* curiosity is fear, and fear is the expression of a neurotic introversion that can potentially hinder the development of a child with such a constitution or in such a state.

This child loves reading—but only fiction, as he is rather afraid of reality. The *Calc-c* child, on his numerous rounds to doctors, is fascinated with patients coming in. When he can observe something visible like a limp, a scar, or any disfigurement, he asks a lot of questions loudly: "Why does he have trouble walking?" "Why is his head bandaged?" And he will ask others: "Do you have allergies too?" He just feels that if someone has an ailment, he needs to know the details so he can avoid the same fate. After all, he thinks always about *murder, rats and fire*; in other words, he is worried that something bad can and will happen **to him**.

Golden Tips from the Masters

- Relates to the F's: fat, flabby, feeble, fleshy, fair, faint, and fears
- The #1 remedy for hereditary psora (*Sulphur* #1 for acquired psora)
- Follows *Rhus-tox* and/or *Ruta* when they stop working
- The corpulence of the patient, which at first gives the impression of being a constitution, is in reality a sign of illness
- Covers the three miasms: often polypi (sycosis) and often exostoses (syphilis)
- Loss of appetite when overworked (mentally or physically)
- #1 remedy for children with nightmares about monsters
- A *Calc-c* child can go to *Belladonna* or *Pulsatilla* in acutes; a *Calc-c* adult can go to *Rhus-tox* in acutes
- Excellent indication in leg and foot cramps at night in the elderly
- Obsessive list-writers
- *Calc- c* favors absorption of pus (< > *Silicea* which hastens suppuration)
- Sweating on head and hair especially, but also in genital area, with inclination to uncover (< > *Silicea*)
- Great impairment of nutrition: especially great desire for or aversion to milk, a product which the patient's system has difficulty digesting
- Lack of vital heat
- Coldness and perspiration of the feet
- Secondary effects of strain or overexertion and also from dampness or becoming wet
- They desire order in their world (not fastidious!). They know where everything is, obsessed with their bookshelves. Down-to-earth people, the "mother" type, responsible for everything, but easily are overwhelmed and will go to a *Pulsatilla* state
- Menses: three P's: profuse, prolonged, always premature
- Hypothyroidism, arthritis with same modalities as *Rhus-tox* and dizziness in the elderly
- Shortness of breath ascending stairs
- Irregular bone development (open fontanelles, late dentition, curvature of the spine) because of imperfect or irregular nutrition of the bones, while the soft parts (muscles, skin) are suffering from overnutrition
- Teeth cannot endure air or any coldness

Causticum (Caust). Caustic substance

The Cyber Delusion

The dominant fixed idea in this person is the ***delusion, about criminals***. It does not mean that the *Causticum* person *is* a criminal, but rather that, in his view, crimes are being committed all around him, all the time, in the past, present, and future. It is all about injustice, perceived or real. Who are the criminals? Who can they be? People who steal from him (*Ars*)? People who don't want to listen to his advice (*Chel*)? People who try to get rid of him in relationships (*Hyos*)? People who want to undermine his business (*Ferrum-met*)? None of the above! Is the criminal the justice department (murderers are walking the streets and often have more rights than victims) or the medical system pushing inhumane cancer treatments for instance, or Big Brother (invasion of our privacy by government)? Indeed, the "crimes" are committed by these and other agencies.

This Cyber delusion is further linked to injustices and crimes committed against Nature (destruction of trees and animal habitats), animals (medical laboratory experiments and eradication of animal species, whale hunting and clubbing of seals), and underdogs among people (the vulnerable and defenseless ones, especially children, the poor, and victims of natural disasters). Above all, the target for *Causticum* is to destroy the worldwide industrial system and to break the domination of the environment which has resulted from consumerism. It is often not limited to monkey wrenching against timber companies, factory owners, road builders, farmers, retailers, and oil and gas producers (in fact, virtually anyone who can be considered involved in industry); *Causticum* is fueled by an apocalyptic vision and is driven to deeds of destruction. Wherever he looks, he sees suffering humanity and the suffering animal world. *Causticum* finds the world's callousness towards the poor and the underdog, as well as the drift toward the destruction of Nature and animals for the sake of individual egotism and greed, unbearable. Many Causticum people may start with earth-friendly steps like tree hugging, living in a sequoia tree, displaying such decals on their bike as "100% vegetable powered" or wearing a T-shirt that says "Kiss me, I compost." Maybe they voice their concern over pollution and global warming by calling their senators to quell the powerlessness they feel over large global issues, but few among them progress to become true active environmentalists driven by that desire to save the earth. Many of these *Causticum* people were originally the most idealistic and sensitive of their generation, but at some point they became desperate and began trying to achieve the impossible by the use of force. They form so-called revolutionary groups and expect to save the world and avoid imminent apocalypse by acts of terror and destruction, failing to realize that they are contributing to the general tendency toward violence and inhumanity. They have lost their capacity to love and have replaced it with the wish to sacrifice their lives, indignant at the great outrage that they have experienced or witnessed and overcome with the desire to take vengeance on the perpetrator of that outrage. Their *delusion, of fancy illusions* is that they can create a world where there is justice, peace, and equality for all living beings and creations of Nature—if necessary, by force.

Is there another delusion that reflects the Cyber delusion? Yes, there is. *Delusion, is going to be robbed.* The question is: robbed of what? Look at the well-known sequence of remedies: *Causticum-Colocynthis-Staphysagria*. This tells us about situations of *indignation and injustice* and the fear of being robbed of one's dignity! One of my patients, a young child, arrived home with a torticollis, or stiff neck, after being humiliated by her soccer coach in front of her teammates (*injurious effects from vexation*). The *Causticum* person, as sensitive and sympathetic as the *Phosphorus* person, has this sentiment of indignation even if it stems from situations in which others have been robbed of their dignity (rape is another circumstance raising such emotions of indignation, as is suppression and domination by big corporations, powerful people, and the establishment). There is even a kind of transference of pathology when indignation or perceived injustice is inflicted on someone else. We find this sentiment clearly in the following provings: the *Causticum* child is overly sympathetic *when hearing the stories of others, and about the cruelties they have suffered, she is besides herself and cries and sobs and cannot contain herself.* In my practice, I have seen children begin to display nervous tics after seeing another child in a wheelchair (*twitching and clonic spasms; spasms after a fright*). This is expressed also by the proving *after seeing a case of chorea she gets it herself.* A child whose mental age is far below his biological age can be pushed to indignation when the parent demands that he act according to his biological age, which is impossible. This further creates another fixed idea linked to the CD, a *delusion, that he is unfortunate* and *on closing his eyes he sees frightful images,* instilling fear in the *Causticum* person to which he has to react, even proactively, often with violence.

If almost everyone is perceived as a criminal, what is the state of mind of the person in a *Causticum* state? *Very suspicious and distrustful*! The *Causticum* person does not trust society easily and strives to form small groups of like-minded people. Only after an exhaustive battle, reminiscent of David's against Goliath, is *Causticum* overcome with a sense of despair and a *delusion, he is sick and therefore will not work,* supported by the provings *he feels defeated, exhausted and disillusioned. There is persistent silence, difficult to overcome. There is great melancholy from care, grief and sorrow* and *she looks upon the dark side of everything.* It is an astonishing turnaround for this person, usually a troublemaker and activist and now in the darkest of moods. *There is great melancholy from care, grief and sorrow and he looks upon the dark side of everything. There is hopelessness and despair, with a weeping mood. He will have great apprehension whenever anything happens and becomes despondent, depressed with the most excessive exhaustion and prostration.* In this depression, he is also likely to *have an irritable temper as he has a disposition which takes everything in bad part.* Again, this reflects the Cyber delusion that everyone is a criminal!

Causalities

Repetitive Grief

Ailments from *repetitive grief and long-lasting grief and sorrow* are the main triggers for a *Causticum* person. The *Causticum* child will not express grief any more but will hold everything in: it is as if his feelings are dead! I am reminded of the sad story of one of my patients. This story demonstrates the devastating effect such a trigger can have on the central nervous system, often resulting in chorea and involuntary jerking of the muscles, convulsions, *tic nerveux* or nervous tic, and even paralysis such as torticollis and Bell's palsy on the physical plane but also paralysis on the mental (*confusion; forgotten something, feels constantly as if he had forgotten something,* a person who always has to go back to check on things) and emotional planes (*indifference to welfare of others,* the opposite of the normal *Causticum* state). My patient was a grandmother and was on an outing with her family. She was feeding the baby and, in an unfortunate moment, the baby suffocated after the food that was swallowed caused an obstruction on the passage of the bronchial tract. This first enormous grief was compounded by a second one when, a week later, the mother of the child accused her own mother of having been neglectful and caused the death of the child. When this grandmother came to me, she could barely function as she was forgetting everything and needed the constant help of her husband; he did not understand the situation and thought he was acting correctly when he did not want to help her find things, thinking "she could find them herself"; he did not want her to become dependent on him. So this was yet another source of grief for the woman: not receiving the support of her husband. The incidence of these kinds of examples of grief felt by such a highly *sensitive and reserved* person is often related to the *death of a child, a parent, a friend or a pet* and can even be caused when such a child sees a handicapped child (*after seeing a case of chorea she gets it herself*) or *when hearing about or seeing cruelties* against children and animals (*weeping from sympathy with others*). Being sympathetic is a wonderful virtue, but not when it will hurt the sympathetic individual. A *Causticum* child is *excessively sympathetic and easily beside herself, with weeping and sobbing and cannot be contended when listening to accounts of the hardship of others*. There is *fear something will happen; that others should be harmed*. *Causticum* children should not look at TV images depicting the suffering of people, especially children, or at pictures showing the ravages of war and its destruction of society, or at those detailing the clubbing of baby seals and the killing of whales. Regression to a form of autism or pervasive development disorder not otherwise specified (PDD-NOS) can occur as a result of seeing any of these! Unbalanced *Causticum* adults, on seeing these same things, will react with boiling blood, a mixture of rage and anguish, unable to keep still and answering the voices of their consciences, ready to act to set the wrong right (*irritable temper; disposition to take everything in bad part; anarchist; sensitive to oppressive influences*).

Injustice

Many grief-causing incidents are considered by this *compassionate* person to be acts of injustice towards themselves or others (*cannot support injustice*). The *Causticum* person expresses idealistic views from a very young age on, but is also prone to act on this idealism, to try to correct injustices. Unfortunately, this is not attempted peacefully but with aggression: "An eye for an eye" is his motto. This is, of course, different for a child and an adult. As the ego in children under age five is still undeveloped and archaic, an "injustice" in the child's mind might also refer to moments at which Mom or Dad doesn't find time to play with him, or when the parent doesn't want to buy him a present every time he goes into a store, or when a friend chooses to play with someone else. The *Causticum* child reasons: "You are mean to me, so I will pay you back with the same kind of meanness." Again, this desire for justice could have been transferred to the child through mystical participation if his mom suffered from an injustice during pregnancy. The strong sense of righteousness of the *Causticum* state easily leads to excessive introspection in children as they already tend to feel guilty (*anxiety of conscience, as if guilty of a crime*). The adult, with a greater consciousness, must have suffered before from an injurious injustice strong enough to create the Cyber delusion. Crimes against oneself or against others can create a crusader mentality like that of *Nat-m*, although with *Nat-m* the state comes from having experienced acts of outspoken deception, betrayal, or loss of a child. As discussed before, for *Causticum*, injustice is not just personal injury but includes crimes committed against society and Nature. While *Nat-m* joins support groups, does volunteer work, or becomes a psychotherapist, *Causticum* is a loner and *anarchist*, the only sheriff in town, ready to right the wrong with blazing guns as *horrible things affect him greatly*. Together with *Nit-acid*, *Causticum* aggressively uses the law to plead his case (*litigious*). We recognize already the syphilitic nature of *Causticum*: he is hardened and resolves to take actions which, if necessary, will be as brutal as those he has seen committed. The word "caustic" also means bitter, sarcastic, vicious, *malicious*, contemptuous, *censorious*, *defiant*, etc., all words that might describe *Causticum* at one time or another.

Worry

The *Causticum* person is full of worries, especially *from hearing or seeing bad news*, that the same *or something like that will happen to her*. This *fear that something will happen, to her or her family* (*she is full of worries about others and about relatives*) often changes *Causticum* into an introverted, serious, and obsessive person and is responsible for incomprehensible behavior such as temper tantrums and fits of violence. The fears are all *about misfortune, of being alone at night, fear of the dark, fear for strangers, fear of death, fear of evil, and fear from noise* as well as *fear for people*, so we see the need for hypervigilance. *Causticum* is also full of worries about what should have been done. "Did I forget to close the door when I left home? Did I turn off the stove (*feels constantly as if he had forgotten something.*)?" *Causticum*, ever preoccupied, is the first one *to forget purchases, goes off and leaves them behind*. This can easily lead to obsessive-compulsive behavior in which, for instance, the person returns to the office, fearful that she has forgotten something, or does the same when leaving home for the office. "Did I bring everything I need for work (*cares about his business.*)?" Worry is a common theme of all the *Kalis*, and *Causticum* has *anxiety for others*;

cares, full of worry about others; full of worries about relatives and *weeping from sympathy with others* (only *Causticum*!). Clearly, *Causticum* is very worried about family, meaning close family as well as extended family, which includes everyone who has suffered a similar injustice or has been subjected to the same emotional trauma that he has. *Causticum* is less worried about herself, in contrast to the other *Kalis*, who place restrictions on the immediate family to stem their own anxieties. *Causticum* is more like *Phosphorus* and therefore inimical! But the sympathy goes much deeper than it does for *Phosphorus*, as is expressed by the following proving: *excessively sympathetic; she is beside herself, with weeping and sobbing and cannot be contended when listening to accounts of the hardship of others* (T.F. Allen).

Compensations and Consequences

Dictatorial and Dogmatic Behavior

The following provings express the *Causticum* mentality: *they can be hot-headed and vehement. They are furiously opinionated and quarrelsome.* There is rigidity in his reasoning, a tenacious holding to principles, ideas, dogmas, and rules. *Causticum* people are harder and more convinced, perseverant, confident, and fanatical than *Kali-c*, the other great member of this group, who is more overwhelmed with anxieties regarding his own person and loved ones (*Kali-c* has that carbon element in its name!). *Causticum*, again, has the greater vision and expands his concerns to encompass the rest of the world rather than focusing on his own person. Being *obstinate and headstrong* can be positive, but obstinacy often leads to negative characteristics in *Causticum*, who cannot stand a dissenting opinion: *he is defiant and has a disposition to contradict* everyone not siding with him. *He is easily offended and takes everything in bad part* as he is convinced that he is fighting for what is right. Criticism is, by definition, something that no one wants to hear. At best it is annoying; at worst it threatens a person's identity and even survival. But for *Causticum*, any criticism is a scorching harangue which evokes not only defensiveness as a first natural response, but the desire to strike back with a vengeance. It is hard to discuss issues logically with a *Causticum* person unless you are of his opinion. He is not always open to logic and reasoning and will not invite constructive criticism or harmonious interaction. With his fighting spirit and hawkish, anarchistic nature, he is not particularly diplomatic, which makes him a tough negotiator. Resistance to authority seems to be in the genes of such a person, and he can be considered unruly, difficult to control, always finding fault with things, and therefore hard to deal with in business and daily life; he plays the roles of the anarchist, the fearless leader, and the crusader at the same time (*furiously opinionated, enraged dogmatism* and *inclination to quarrel* and *great excitement when talking*). How he could benefit from a dose of *Causticum* is seen in the curative action in a proving: *although political disputes were brought to him, still he remained quite calm, though indeed he felt sensitive, yet he avoided speaking of it and subdued his emotions.* Otherwise, *Causticum* remains *furiously opinionated leading to inclination to scold and easy violence.* This shows how *Causticum* can be the extravert thinking type, easily losing control with an appeal is made upon his archaic feeling function.

Why, then, do we see *Causticum* as an *amativeness/amorous* black *type*? It is reminiscent of *Nit-acid's* sympathy, both remedies prominently present in the rubric *sympathetic.* Only for like-minded people is there sympathy, love, and passion. "You are either for me or against me!" For the souls of his crusade, there is plenty of sympathy (*excessive sympathy for others' suffering*) and many tears as he is easily moved by their plight (*weeping easily, even at trifles* and *even in sleep* and *involuntarily*). For those with a dissenting opinion, there remains nothing but contempt and sarcasm.

Disobedience

The word "disobedience" comes from the Greek word *dis* or "separate, apart, two" and the Latin word *ob* or "reversed, against." Disobedience, therefore, means being separate, not agreeing, referring to two parties against each other. In the case of *Causticum*, disobedience is nothing but having the courage to stand alone, to err and to sin and to stick to his opinion. However, courage is not enough. The tragedy for *Causticum*, and many other individuals, is that one has to live in a system which proclaims freedom yet stamps out disobedience, a system in which one cannot speak the truth or have a dissenting voice. Throughout the centuries, disobedience has been considered a sin, while obedience has been considered a virtue. But one can only speak of rational authority when the interests of both parties are not mutually exclusive. *Causticum* says "no" because he obeys his conscience and the principles he has chosen: he is a revolutionary activist, not a rebel or terrorist. Most people have become one of the numerous sheep, that is, have succumbed to brainwashing from day one and have respect for conformity, rules, and regulations. Hence, they remain blissfully unaware that they are obeying simply because they do not feel forced to obey.

For *Causticum*, however, disobedience is an affirmation of reason and will. It is man's capacity to see, to say what he sees, and to refuse to say or do what he does not see. Acts of aggression and injustice are just called that and not sugar-coated or politicized! But *Causticum* is convinced that there is no other way to disobey than through aggression and rebellion. He is convinced that he will open the eyes of those who are half-asleep through acts of violence, which often turns the public against him, no matter how many noble goals he has written in his manifesto. Killing and destroying evoke repulsion and condemnation. There are other ways of being disobedient. Hahnemann was not a *Causticum* person. His act of disobedience was to abandon the then current trend of medicine, to disobey the authority of the traditional thought of his time when it came to the treatment of the insane and the sick in general, to disobey the rules that only pharmacists could prepare remedies (of course not his!), and to decline the honors bestowed on his colleagues (if only he had stayed the traditional path!) rather than find himself in conflict with their methods of treatment, with the clichés that they believed and taught. Hahnemann brought light to darkness, as reflected in his epitaph: *Aude Sapere*, or "Dare to know." *Causticum* is a person who fights against slogans such as "Long live death" and against the medical/scientific "progress" that can only be made by sacrificing members of the animal or human population (called "collateral damage"). *Causticum* fights against collateral damage and disobeys rules not because he is an anomaly in society but because he is a man who loves life.

Paralysis

Anyone dedicating his life to the defense of the underdog and in spite of unrelenting energy and great opposition is bound to run out of energy at some point—to the point of paralysis. Paralysis can take place on the mental, physical, and emotional planes. Because of longtime grief and injustice, concentration can become difficult. This can create great anxiety. The person *becomes absent minded* and *feels constantly that he forgot something*. There is an *absence of ideas*. He is *inattentive and distracted*! Paralysis leads to a *loss of ideas, weak memory and using wrong words* (*dyslexia*). *He understands things only after repetition*. This mental paralysis also reflects his dogmatic nature and his immovable points of view. Paralysis on the emotional plane is seen in *persistent silence, difficult to overcome; child is full of fears to go to bed alone because he constantly thought of anxious things*. If there is also constant and continued suppression of his own feelings, he appears very stoic about his own suffering until things get out of hand. Such strong emotional suppression leads to severe physical symptoms like deformative arthritis with paralytic stiffness. *Causticum* is equally indicated for paralysis on the physical plane, which can be seen after a person suffers severe grief or indignation. He can be *clumsy and drop things*, or there might be a sudden appearance of right-sided Bell's palsy in the face or sudden retention of urine when he keeps his urine in for too long. It can also be indicated in bedwetting in the first half of sleep as well as *loss of urine when sneezing, coughing or blowing the nose*. I have already mentioned sudden occurrence of a stiff neck, but sudden appearance of tics and *stuttering* in a child, when he is under stress and excited, must make one think of *Causticum* before any other remedy. As the reader can see, physical consequences will go straight to the nervous system, the deepest physical level, with chorea, paralysis, twitches, and restless legs in sleep, toothaches, headaches, and stitching pain in the chest. We find in *Causticum* one-sided *paralysis of vocal chords, of tongue, bladder and eyelids. This is a gradually appearing paralysis of single parts, also caused by exposure to cold wind or draught.*

Golden Tips from the Masters

- When exposed to cold dry weather, *Causticum* will show neuralgias (facial paralysis) and >in wet weather for rheumatic conditions! This is exceptional! (Like in rheuma cases >dampness #1 remedy and in asthma cases >in dampness!)
- Symptoms in children: stuttering, tics, restless legs in sleep, disease through imitation of others.
- *Diabetes insipidus* remedy
- Keynote: especially indicated in warts of eyelids, fingers, and nose
- *Causticum* is full of contractures (#1 remedy in Dupuytren disease or claw hand) but less so than *Cuprum*. Just remember: in spite of being a chilly remedy, amelioration of symptoms in cold damp weather! (<in dry cold wind, resulting in paralysis of parts like Bell's palsy)
- It is one of the plain cystitis remedies, which should be used **before** *Cantharis* in simple cystitis. There is great and frequent urgency without being able to pass anything at all, but then when they sit or talk to someone, they might have an involuntary loss 15 minutes later.
- It is the #1 remedy for *involuntary loss of urine* when laughing, sneezing, coughing, blowing the nose, or doing anything strenuous. It is certainly the #1 remedy for *postoperative paralysis* of the bladder.
- There is painful retention of urine brought on by the slightest exposure to cold. Also retention of urine in young children. A peculiar symptom is shooting pain in the rectum when the patient tries to urinate. Also, sometimes, complete insensitivity to the urination; in the dark, he can scarcely believe he is urinating until he makes sure with the sense of touch. As a rule, *Causticum* is a cystitis medicine and not a kidney remedy. Formation of excess of uric acid. Itching at the meatus. Paralysis of the bladder from retaining urine too long.
- Bedwetting remedy in first half of sleep
- #2 remedy for torticollis (*Lachnanthes* is #1)
- Paralysis of face (#1 remedy in threatening chronic Bell's palsy after *Aconite* is given in the acute phase), of right hand, torticollis, paralysis of upper eyelid, and gradual paralysis of extremities, all preferential on right side! #1 remedy in carpal tunnel syndrome.
- Cerebral Vascular Accident (CVA) with hemiplegia on right side: #1 *Causticum*!
- Argumentative after a divorce. Messy relationships with a lot of fighting
- Major remedy for stammering

- Lack of sleep from nurturing a loved one (*Cocculus*)
- Deep hacking cough with the feeling that he cannot cough hard enough to clear the mucus
- Sensation as if the parts/tendons are too tight, constrictive feeling
- #1 remedy for erysipelas (*Ars*, *Rhus-t*)
- Menses are slow by day and cease at night and leucorrhea flows at night and never in the day
- Loss of voice after exposure to cold or during coryza
- Chronic problems with vocal cords such as progressive paralysis
- *Causticum* feels anxious **for** others, *Phosphorus* feels the anxiety **of** others
- Morning nausea: thought, sight, or smell of food takes away the appetite (*Colchicine*)

China (Chin).
Cinchona officinalis. Quinine tree or Peruvian bark

The Cyber Delusion

China's dominant feeling is that ***he is persecuted***! The word *paranoia* comes from the Greek; it refers to a distraction of the mind caused by the false belief that someone is persecuting the person. *China* has this persecution complex: he always thinks someone is hindering him from achieving what he wants to do or become. Someone is stopping him from realizing his ambitions (resembling *Nux-v*, who suffers from *A/F deceived ambition*), and he thinks that he is the target of a vast conspiracy, that people will come and get him. This Cyber delusion is also reflected in other similar delusions: *delusion, being obstructed; delusion, pursued by enemies; and delusion, he considers himself unhappy* and *thinks he is hindered at work* and ***tormented*** *by everyone* as well as *delusion, thinks he is unfortunate*. The notion of "torment" really reflects the essence of this remedy: **an over-irritation or over-stimulation of the CNS due to a perceived obstruction by others and circumstances in her many plans.** One can compare the *China* state to a nerve that lies open on the surface and is irritated continuously so that, after some time, the person is exhausted and irritable (*irritability with weakness*), on the verge of a nervous breakdown. Possessed by such abnormal sensitiveness, *China* often alternates a predominating melancholy with periodic fits of unrestrained liveliness.

In general, delusional ideas are a mixture of wish-fulfillment and a sense of having been injured or persecuted, a feeling sometimes compensated by megalomania (*haughty*); in the case of *China*, though, the compensation more typically involves very violent reactive fears. The idea of persecution stems from a relationship infected with mistrust. It shows the paranoia of *China* leading to delusions of reference. What are delusions of reference? Driven by his Cyber delusion (CD), *China* can grossly misjudge any small acute circumstance, gesture, word, or perceived slight. Often, during the first moment of anger when *China* meets with a mishap, he immediately jumps to the conclusion that he has been deliberately injured or insulted or treated maliciously (*delusion, he is hindered at work; she thinks she is very unfortunate and constantly harassed by enemies; fixed idea that he is unhappy; delusion, he is persecuted by enemies*). A patient in my practice once said: "I feel like people are trying to get me mad. Almost like people are intentionally trying to get under my skin or push my buttons, like they are just out to see if they can get me upset." Another patient, a menopausal woman, spoke to me about her husband, who was used to a very active and excessive sex life with her: "I wanted to tell him that he needs to slow down a little as in reality I do not want to get aroused all the time." He interpreted this to mean: "She doesn't love me anymore; she despises me; she rejects me and just wants to be left alone." He needed *China*, of course. *China* has restored many crippled marriages when the two partners have seemingly irreconcilable needs.

Whatever negative things happen to a person in a *China* state, she has a very particular interpretation of the situation. For instance, a *China* patient applied to a summer writing class, but unfortunately the class was already full. Upon hearing this, the person was not able to see the obvious, that the class was filled; she drew her own "obvious" conclusion: that she was being rejected! *China's* reaction will be intense and defiant ("I'll show them!"), leading to feverish activity to prove how unjust it was to reject her. Instances of non-recognition and jealousy about others often impel the person needing *China* to work even harder. To another student, it might be a passing disappointment, but not for *China*! Hearing bad news creates an intense unrest in her. Art in any form is the real passion of *China's* life; it is the love to which all other loves are as marsh-water to red wine. After all, *China* is married to her Muse! Such fixed ideas might not be present in *China's* early life, but once exhaustion sets in, due to his ailments from (A/F), *China* puts a wall between himself and the other party as he *feels misunderstood* and *wants to avoid further injury and dejection*.

Such a patient is not an easy client for a homeopath or psychotherapist. With her wounded soul and *suspicious nature*, *China* will test them to see which side they are on. Each initial question of the homeopath is perceived as a threat, even as an insult, from which the patient needs to protect himself (*suspicious; delusion, of vexations and offences*). The homeopath may be one of the enemies to be avoided, one among many people who are out there to stop him in the many plans he has formulated in his dreams (*delusion, pursued by enemies*). The result is even further withdrawal, in which state she can dwell on her bad fortune (*disposition to be alone; company, aversion to the presence of other people, desire for solitude*). It is interesting that *Hyoscyamus* and *Lachesis*, two of the most jealous characters in our materia medica, also have many delusions of reference. Prejudices of this kind may establish themselves and inevitably lead to delusions of strange machinations, such as the delusions of *Lachesis*, *will be sent to the asylum* and *the medicine is poison.* The latter delusion also belongs to *Hyoscyamus*, who is now also convinced that *his lover is faithless and will not marry him*. This road will lead straight to paranoia, with respective delusions of *being sold* (*Hyosc*), *being poisoned* (both *Hyosc* and *Lachesis*), and *being sent to the asylum* (*Lachesis*). For *China* it will only lead to a road of *despair with the pains, lamenting* and *delusions, of being forsaken.*

Ailments from Sexual Excesses

In general *China* is very sensitive to a loss of fluids, be it from diarrhea, perspiration, vomiting, or excessive menses, but one cause stands out: loss of fluids through excessive masturbation. Due to his great sensitivity on all planes, but especially on the emotional plane, *China* as an adult is often a loner (*aversion to all people*). Satisfying hunger and thirst, sleeping, and taking bodily exercise, as well as satisfying sexual desire, are rational pleasures rooted in the chemistry of the organism; satisfying these demands, though, is perceived as a desire. If desires remain unsatisfied for some time, a painful tension is felt. The word satisfaction is derived from the Latin *satis-facere*, "to make sufficient," and the satisfaction of these rational pleasures (due to the physiological changes that take place) relieves tension. However, in *China*'s case, the intensity of these desires is not due to the demands of the body; it is, rather, determined by psychic needs, and is often the result of a psychic dysfunction. The delusional ideas of persecution, unfortunately, sometimes lead to a *disposition to hurt the feelings of others. China* is quick and sensitive in her relationships with others, which often can lead to much heartbreak. Because of the Cyber delusion and the suspicion created by it, as well as physical exhaustion due to loss of fluids, *China* becomes a loner later in life and is not erotically or sexually active. He remains in isolation, as it were, with his sexual instinct, and the expression of this isolation is masturbation. That is the form that the sex lives of lonely people take. Sexuality is experienced in an indirect way; the act of masturbation entirely lacks any object outside of the self, any direction towards a partner. But masturbation is known to create pathology (ailments from loss of body fluids); Traditional Chinese Medicine (TCM) warns against the **unregulated affairs of the bedroom** with which the precious energy located in the kidney organ, called the Essence, is depleted with each orgasm. This notion is very old and can be found in the *Yellow Emperor's Classic of Medicine* (or, as it is also known, the *Book of Simple Questions*). Masturbation, if practiced too frequently among the young, will certainly decrease not only future sexual potential, but also the amount of Essence present at the time of conceiving a child (*consequence of excessive and long continued seminal losses).* Other early symptoms of deficient Essence or K-Qi present in the adult are *premature or too quick ejaculation*; *seminal emissions at night or pollutions,* and *softening of the penis in the middle of intercourse,* all of which *China* can suffer. Then, of course, besides the physical impact of masturbation, there is also the psychological impact. The hangover which follows the act of masturbation comes from the guilt (*anxiety as if guilty of a crime*) that arises when one flees from the normal, active, directional experience of sex to the passive, non-directional experience of masturbation. This will detach the shy *China* person even more from the world, isolating himself in his world of silence.

Anger with Silent Grief

A *China* person is often shaped by a single important event, such as death of a parent at a young age. It leaves such a child with feelings of grief, guilt, and anger that often haunt him for life; this can lead the child to adopt a profession such as that of an artist, but even more typically, that of a poet, allowing the person to deal with these overwhelming emotions in writing (*desire to write*; *makes verses*). When growing up, the *China* child looks well-adjusted and is usually an excellent student who dazzles her teachers with her writing and creative abilities; with her peers, though, she is considered weird, naïve, and dreamy (*intelligent but very naïve*; *sentimental*). When growing up, *China*'s dominant function of consciousness is feeling, with sensation as a secondary function, as all her *senses are acute*: *vision, hearing, smell are acute* and in general *China* has a sense for beauty. These are all characteristics that destine *China* people to become artists, writers, and poets and that set them apart from the masses. For *China* people, withdrawal from the world is voluntary, even sought after: as much as they are inclined to be *taciturn,* paintings, sculptures, and poems become the mouthpieces and outlets of their pent-up emotions. Irritability is a defense mechanism and also a natural outlet for *China.* For a person who is so touchy and misunderstood, such a jump to negativity is not rare. We are not surprised to see *excessive irritability with despondency* and *intolerance of noise* and *inclined to vex others.* Being a true individual, something most people can't be (as they are unwilling to explore their unconscious) puts *China* in the position of being very opinionated and self-assured, as well as misunderstood by the masses (who have sacrificed their individuality to live a more conforming life). Therefore, *China*'s plans (*makes many plans at night*) are not always understood, and her work is not always appreciated until after her death. A real artist does not make art for others but first and foremost for his own pleasure. He is a supreme individualist with a unique temperament, one who does not try to supply and produce what other people want; in this way he would cease to be an artist, and would instead become a tradesman. If the *China* artist had to write, paint, or sculpt for the amusement of others, he would be forced to suppress his intense mood of individualism: in other words, to surrender everything that is valuable to him. Individualism makes the *China* person *sensitive during labor* and *to moral impressions* and *intolerant to contradiction* as for him it only fuels his CD (*he is persecuted* and *hindered at work*). For *China* to be truly appreciated, the audience must be receptive. The spectator is the violin on which the master (*China*) is to play.

Angry confrontations with others are common: *he is peevish, ill-humored and easily angered; he seeks every opportunity to being angry*. With a well-fixed, assured ego and aware of her standing in society or where she thinks she should be recognized by everyone for her talent, *she can be contemptuous to everything* and *intolerant to contradiction* (this is the *Nux-v* part of her). *China* absolutely believes in himself, because he is absolutely himself; she can fly off the handle at the slightest provocation when others disagree with her. She is convinced her perspectives, beliefs, and values are right and therefore has a hard time tolerating contradictory conversations. *Depending* on the force of her CD, she can be so angry that *she could have stabbed anyone*; when a sudden tempest comes up from the depths of her being, she is ready to destroy any opposition (*disposition to hurt feelings of others*). What *China* most fears is failure (*fear of falling*). As one can see, *China* is not always an easy person to live with; often she cannot escape tragedy taking over her personal life: her soul mate may well leave her, as he is overwhelmed by the stark, oversensitive, and brooding character of the *China* spouse!

Compensations

Aversion to Company

China is a person who, for at least two hours a day, needs to lock herself up in her room to work on her art or to write in a diary or blog. (Though sharing with others is not on every *China* person's list, writing a blog for readers can be a catharsis to clear her mind.) Artwork is a form of meditation; *China* is a loner (*aversion to all persons; talk, indisposed to talk; talk of others aggravates; company, aversion to the presence of others*). Immersed in her self-imposed cocoon, *China* exhibits the artistic temperament, which is concentration of vision and intensity of purpose (*conscientious about trifles*). The only people she cares to be with are other artists and people who have suffered like she has: those who know what Beauty is and those who know what Sorrow is. To those, like *China*, who are preoccupied with the beauty of form, nothing else seems of much importance. She does not want to be touched (*aversion to be touched*) and aggravates from light touch like *Hep-s* (*hyperesthesia, renewing pains when not present by merely touching*), but at same time she likes *deep and hard touch* on every plane: mental, emotional, and physical. On the emotional plane we see that, if during the inquiry you touch the emotional plane ever so lightly and superficially, then the patient aggravates, even explodes in *rage*. The patient is delicate and edgy. (Think of your porcelain dishes and how easily they break.) *China*'s touchiness means that he expects you, as his homeopath, to have great interest in his case; he expects much love, warmth, understanding, and friendship, and if he does not sense this, he will not come back (*Nat-m*). The adult *China*, with her strong emotional antennae, rather likes intense and **deep, probing** conversations, not superficial chit-chat. Children, on the other hand, because of their lack of individuation, are very irritable when questioned. They *don't want to be looked at*; rather than answering, they tend to look at and to a parent (but they are not as sweet as *Pulsatilla*!). If you insist, they are irritated and angry and just will answer with a yes or no or not at all (*answering, refusing to answer; answers unintelligently; talk, indisposed to, desire to be silent*). When you insist on a more elaborate answer, they turn to Mom and ask: "Why did you bring me here?" or give impolite answers (*rudeness of naughty children*). They may say to Mom: "I don't want to be here; everyone looks at me and bothers me with their questions (*cannot bear to be looked at.*)."

Imagination and Creativity

China is an individual who seeks the pleasures of sensibility; these consist in observing, feeling, intuition, writing poetry, painting, playing and listening to music, and meditating. One should always be drunk. The only question for *China* is: drunk with what? For some people it will be with love, with compassion *(Phosphorus)*; others will become drunk with ambition *(Nux-v)*, and hopefully the search for meaning in life *(Sulphur)*. For *China*, it is being drunk with poetry and introversion. To *China*, expression through the arts is the only mode in which she can conceive life at all. As the introvert type, *China* is inclined to explore the themes of death, self, and nature in artistic works that express his uncertain attitude toward the universe. Even as a child, she is powerfully aware of the beauty and terror of nature, so both love and fear of nature are present (*fear of animals, even domestic ones; fear for noise; fear of people*). *China* is often the voice that, through her work, teaches us how to go on living in a destructive, materialistic world as she expresses her need for faith in the healing power of art. *China* does not hesitate to use his personal voice in his work, which stands out in its dramatic structure and is marked by the exploration of highly personal themes. If *China* becomes a poet, her poems will be personal accounts of her anger, insecurity, fear, and often her tremendous sense of loneliness and death, finding the voice she has sought to cultivate for so long. Her greatest moments of creativity come at night, when the muse speaks to her (*ideas abundant and clearness of mind at night—he has a large number of projects and he makes many plans and reflect upon their execution* [T. F. Allen]; *full of projects and ideas, especially in evening and at night*). If a poet, she will write feverishly throughout the night, continuously, almost as though possessed, bringing her exhausted body to the brink of destruction—but the muse's voice can't be stopped. Even when sick, such a person would force herself to get out of bed to write, convinced that she is a genius of a writer, that she has it in her, and that the flood mustn't be dammed up. *China*, who is born with a talent that she is meant to use, is indeed happiest when she is using it. But such exhaustion for a tender soul easily brings on depression, which causes her to see life as chaotic and civilization as barbaric. Even as a child, writing is the biggest outlet; she often keeps a journal to narrate her struggles and aspirations with life beginning at a young age. Initially, those poems are innocent distillations of daily life, but as time goes by, the subjects of poems and novels reflect the emerging tragedies that are inevitable in anyone's life. Evenings are the best time for *China* people, as they feel they can resolve everything then, while in the daytime they have difficulties communicating with people and feel misunderstood (*delusion, is forsaken*). Art, writing, and poems are therefore positive tools used to escape his troubles, but often art isolates him even more as he appears an eccentric. It makes him feel that *everyone is persecuting him* since he speaks a "different language"; when the pathology goes deeper, he starts making mistakes in speaking (*mistakes, using wrong words; mistakes in speaking, misplacing and reversing words*).

Planning

Planning is an integral part of the *China* person's life. Even as a child, ambitions and aspirations are outlined in a journal, and the steps to be taken are usually written down in detail. However, it is rare that life goes as planned:

> I remember one of my colleagues whose main complaint was "irritability"—which had been present for about 30 years when he met me! It began at the time that he finished his residency (in psychiatry, not a coincidence) and started his practice. He lived in Puerto Rico and was concerned about the future of his family. Things were out of order bureaucratically, and he was frustrated. He would pay his taxes and then he would get notice that he had not paid them. Out of frustration he took

his family to the U.S. His irritability abated after re-establishing himself in the U.S., but it flared up again five or six years later. At this point his children had grown up, and so he made plans to move back to Puerto Rico, lying awake at night, theorizing how life would now be much better in his native country, thinking of the wonderful things he would do there (*thoughts, rush, flow of thoughts in bed at night*). Then his son got sick, and in addition, his wife was not keen on moving again. He was used to planning everything well, to approaching everything intellectually, and even then things went wrong. He got irritable when things were not going his way: when he had to wait for a late patient, when people cut him off in traffic, when he had to be somewhere by a certain time and things kept him from arriving on time, etc. One sees the Cyber delusion in all these incidents. His second complaint was "worrying." When I ask him what it meant, he said that when he made a wrong decision—even about something as minor as not going to see a film—that for days he thought about it and couldn't let it go. He even lost sleep over it (*cares, full of, about trifles; thoughts, disagreeable, foolish thoughts in the night*). Even when he rationalized it he still could not forget it; he was always asking himself, "What do I need to do to make it better? What could I have done differently?" First he was hard on himself, and then he *reproached others*. All his life, he was *irresolute* in his vocation. He had many different interests but was especially drawn to the arts. He played guitar, piano, and accordion, and had had artistic talent since youth. He had never wanted to be a regular doctor. Here again we see a person who betrayed his dominant feeling function (not following his artistic, feeling vocation), a person who had too much "plain living and high thinking." He had been raised with an intense focus on the thinking function, on intellectual performance, which was not in his nature. Among Jung's psychological types, he was a feeling-intuitive type; violating one's dominant conscious function always leads to neuroses and physical ailments. He had all kind of digestive problems like constipation, diarrhea, bloating, regurgitation, and borborygmata. He felt heaviness in the abdomen and felt full either immediately after a meal or one hour later. He even had to take his clothes off after spicy and fatty foods. He *had aversion to fatty and oily foods, < milk* (diarrhea) with a tendency to constipation and incomplete stools.

One sees easily the emerging picture of *China,* with many delusions visible: *delusion, he is tormented; delusion, he is unfortunate* and especially *delusion, he is hindered*

> *at work*: my psychiatrist colleague always planned everything very carefully in his mind, and he was ready to move on, but something got in his way: his wife did not want to move, his son got sick... he thinks that, after all his theorizing and planning, everything should turn out all right (*intelligent, but very naïve).* Other symptoms were clear too: *making many plans; serious; anger at trifles; anger and incline to vex others; dwelling on past disagreeable occurrences; full of cares; discouraged; reproaching others,* and stagnation of thoughts, as he was unable let go of some silly thoughts for days!

China brought great improvement in this patient's physical problems and in his life on all levels.

Depression and Suicide

The *China* person, isolated and often admired at the same time, always considered "most likely to succeed" or "the golden girl" in school, can easily tire of this image, feeling pressure to excel intellectually; combined with a great sense of responsibility, she often suffers a serious mental breakdown, as a result of which the sensitive, scholarly student can commit suicide. Fueled by her CD, *China* is frequently brooding, overcome with a sense of danger and a lurking feeling of horror about man's place in the universe. A divorce, the death of a loved one, or the tragic loss of a parent can crack the foundation of any child's personality, but such an event pushes disillusioned *China* to an act she would normally fear: suicide (*suicidal disposition, but lacks courage; suicidal disposition with fear of death*). Seeing no way out, and overcome by the callousness she perceives in the world, she often kills herself by means of carbon dioxide inhalation, putting her head in a gas oven: a death that comes quickly, painlessly, and cleanly, the only exit for such sensitive soul (*inconsolable anxiety, even to suicide*). When looking at the life of such a person, one can almost see that she is doomed from early on. It is not that she has a death wish, but that someone immersed in language, poems, and art, and often equally in recurrent tragedy, uses her talents to describe the societal problems of isolation, grief, and unfaithfulness. She describes her own suffering thus, often in a well-kept diary or in poetry. The *China* person needs the diary as an outlet; fed by the CD, though, she feels hopelessly abandoned, often not understanding *why* all this is happening to *her*. And when the "why" finally emerges, that this is a foreign world to her, such a person does not hesitate to leave her miserable existence. *China's* death can be tragic, but her life often is a triumph; this is a person who, from a young age, is driven by a vision of life that guides all her powers toward the creation of beauty. She is finally overwhelmed by the ugliness of the world.

Golden Tips from the Masters

- Think of *China* when you see **periodicity** (every other day; every week; every two weeks), loss of fluids, food poisoning after bad meat, history of quinine intake in malaria (*enlarged spleen, painful, especially in chronic malarial poisoning*—compare *Ceanothus* and *Cedron*) and the great fear of animals, especially of innocent animals like cows).
- *China*'s picture is **physically *Lycopodium* and mentally/emotionally resembling *Nux-v*.** It also resembles *Nat-m* and *Phosphorus* because of its sensitivity. So often we have prescribed *Chel, Lyc, Lachesis, Nux-v, Phos,* and *Nat-m* with deficient results. Think of *China*!
- It is a great remedy for **gall bladder stones,** which can even be dissolved. Often obstruction of gallbladder with colic.
- Their abdominal complaints are worse from *eating fruit—**fermentation from fruit*** (*abdomen flatulence from fruit*). *Constipation with dark, greenish stools. Colic with shivering.* Eructations do not relieve!
- Liver problems are accompanied with an enormous distention across the whole abdomen so that they cannot stand the slightest pressure (*pain liver, when touched; pain liver, pressure aggravates*)
- Peculiar symptom: when the mother places the child to her breast she gets a toothache (*Silicea*: has discharge from uterus when nursing the child; *Borax*: pain in the opposite breast while nursing the child)
- #1 remedy for acute hemorrhages and #1 for heavy menstruation
- Ill effect from overuse of quinine
- #1 remedy for food poisoning from bad meat or food
- Ill effects from drinking tea
- NWS fever, perspiration, and diarrhea, leading to Chronic Fatigue Syndrome (*Ph-ac*)
- #1 remedy to restore the patient after an attack of influenza where chilliness and weakness remain (DD with *Gels*, with feeling of heaviness)

Cocculus indicus (Cocc). Indian Cockle

The Cyber Delusion

The Cyber delusion is ***everything seems unreal***; *Cocculus* is a person being thrown into an unreal and confusing world. It is one of the few italic remedies in this rubric (no black type present!), together with *Alum*, *Anac* and *Med*. *Alumina* and *Anac* states are created by *ailments from domination*, causing an inadequate persona. *Medorrhinum*, with its extreme sycotic state, creates an excessive persona who loses his foothold on reality and suffers from *A/F anticipation*; this is triggered not only by emotional excitement (because everything seems unfamiliar and new) but also by severe suspicion (*delusion, someone walks behind him*). *Cocculus*' loss with contact with reality is of a different character. Its CD is confirmed by the delusion *familiar things seem strange*, expressing *Cocculus*' disconnection from the real, familiar world. In such a state, the person experiences a break with reality, with the adult world, as a degree of disconnection is present; this is an ominous indicator of approaching dissociation, either as protection or as a direct consequence of a splintering of the ego (difference between neurosis and psychosis). Full psychosis may not be present, as we don't find *Cocculus* in the rubric of dissociation (*wills, two wills*—*Lachesis* and *Anac* as main remedies), but we do find it under *weakness of will*. There is definitely a gap between reality and the exhausted, *absentminded* and *absorbed* state of *Cocculus*, as this person seems to be on the verge of a nervous breakdown because time goes too fast and she has a hard time keeping up with her life (*delusion, time passes too quickly, seems earlier*). As everything seems to happen so quickly to her, she loses the sense of the meaning of time: "Is it already so late? I still have so much to do. I can't keep up with it all." There is so much to do for *Cocculus*, and there is so little time in her day! Twenty-four hours in a day hardly seem enough for *Cocculus* to attend to all of her chores.

The question is: what causes the gap between reality and *Cocculus*' frame of mind? And what causes such pressure in this person? The Never Well Since (NWS) must answer this! *Cocculus*' is a rather strong defense mechanism. We will find out what motivates her so strongly in the NWS. There is a going back and forth between consciousness and unconsciousness. When the pressure becomes too much, there is withdrawal to the unconscious. But then the call to duty comes, causing a constant vacillation in her mood (*mood, changeable, variable; changeable, hypochondriacal humor; melancholy reflections*). As a protective reaction, *Cocculus* shows a tendency to escape into an illusionary world (*delusion, of fancy illusions*), away from a hectic life, but both the reason and the kind of illusionary world in which refuge is sought should be different from those of characters like *Nat-m, Nat-c, Hyosc, Plat, Sulph, Ignatia, Stram, Bufo* and *Lachesis*, all of which are also found in this rubric. What could *Cocculus*' delusion, *hollow, being hollow in organs* mean? It symbolizes the sense of depletion felt in her body (*sensation of emptiness*)! It is a loss of Qi or Vital Force, mentally, physically, and emotionally, both during her ordeal and at the end of her ordeal. Sometimes we say, "My heart is full of love." What if the heart is hollow? There is nothing there, no emotions. Such a hollowness in the brain will affect memory: *head readily fatigued by mental work; easily forgetting things what he had just thought; answers slowly, needs a lot of time to recollect.* Exterior stimuli cannot penetrate as there is the creation of a vacuum in the ego consciousness, an emptiness or hollowness allowing for a delusion to fully occupy the ego consciousness. When one says "I feel hollow," it means that one has nothing left, no more substance. Imagine that one is like a balloon with no resistance arising to any slow breeze or challenge, easily pierced by obstructions. Will this be the fate of *Cocculus*?

A differential diagnosis needs to be made with *Sepia*, and one of the ways to do it is to compare their delusions. For instance, to what in *Sepia*'s delusions do you compare *delusion, hollow organs*? It is interesting that *Cocc* has a feeling of hollow organs whereas *Sepia* has the delusion, *feels every fiber in her right side of her body,* the right side symbolizing the male or sword side, the one taking command and doing things. No doubt the energy reserve of *Sepia* is greater than that of *Cocculus*, which is why *Cocc* more quickly takes refuge in a dream world. Certainly, *Sepia* seems to be stronger when she sets out to do her daily duty, and it takes much more time before *Sepia* wants to disconnect from the adult world and take a vacation. How a *Cocculus* person feels at the end of her rope is expressed by the other delusions: *sees dead persons, sees specters and visions on closing the eyes.* Ghosts and dead persons refer to herself! She feels dead, and feels like she is already living in the world of dead people, disconnected from the real world. Familiar things seem unreal; she can't recognize them anymore: it must reflect the lack of Qi in her mind, and the Mind, according to TCM, is located in the Heart organ (called *Shen Min*)—so one can now understand that some of the NWS must be related to the emotions of the Heart organ. Its dominant emotions have mainly to do with family relationships! So we will see if indeed the NWS shows this. Of all the themes expressed by the delusions, the desire to escape is the strongest, as most of *Cocculus*' delusions belong to this theme; a particular hint about her refuge in the unconscious or dream world might be expressed by another delusion: *delusion, about criminals*. In *Causticum*, these "criminals" are well defined as perpetrators against the oppressed, the poor, animals, and nature, while for *Nux-v* and *Ferrum*, also found in this rubric, enemies are any competition in business; none of these, however, seems to be the criminal in *Cocculus*' world. Here, too, the causality of a *Cocculus* state will bring more clarity about the nature of the criminal.

Causalities

Grief Combined with Loss of Sleep

In *Cocculus*' case we always must have a **combination** of emotional and physical exhaustion, much like that of *Sepia*. This will bring us *to Cocculus*' two most outstanding causalities: grief and loss of sleep. Grief, in this case, has to do with taking care of a sick relative or friend, expressed by *ailments from care and worries over a loved one* (only remedy). The nursing of a loved one during a protracted illness or a terminal illness (for instance, cancer or amyotrophic lateral sclerosis [ALS]), with obvious emotional and physical involvement, takes a toll on every level. There is always that thought that this loved one will pass away while she is not watching, while she is just doing an errand, which creates *A/F anticipation* and *emotional excitement*: "My loved one might die while I am asleep." Even when working at the office or in school, *Cocculus*' thoughts are never far from his loved one, whether child or adult: "I hope everything will be OK today;" "I hope no crisis will occur while I am not there;" "I hope my child with autism will not have a meltdown at school," etc.

The autism epidemic may have created another legion of *Cocculus* sufferers. For many mothers in the autistic world, this *Cocculus* state has become a grim reality. Their grief reflects an aspect of the loss of *Cocculus*' personal life and, in the case of a child with autism, for instance (translated in the rubric in extended meaning, *A/F death of a child*), the loss of the possibility to lead a normal family life. What started as a great joy has turned into a great tragedy.

Cocculus is a person who continuously must keep her own life on hold as all attention goes to the sick loved one or the child with special needs (*anxiety about health of relatives; anxiety about night watching*). No vacations are allowed: God forbid that the loved one should die while she is gone, as it would create *anxiety as if guilty of a crime*. At the end of the day, no more energy is left for anything or anyone else, especially not for her own needs. It is no surprise that continuous insomnia can transmute into depression with *mental exhaustion*. The sleep deprivation and the necessity of putting aside personal pleasures in order to care of an infant or child with special needs make it far more likely that these parents will go through periods of depression and find their marriage on the rocks. Nonetheless, raising a child is one of the most rewarding and meaningful of all human undertakings. The short-term sacrifice of happiness is outweighed by other benefits, like satisfaction, a meaning of life, altruism, and the chance to leave a significant legacy. These parents are often willing to admit that they are not been able to live the life they'd always hoped for; they are, however, usually fully committed to the life they lead. The job of night watching is a constant one and is far more demanding than any regular job one can hold. This is readily seen in parents caring for a child with special needs; they often have their sleep interrupted with shrieking or are called for in the night; the child may sleep between the parents in their bed, asking for a bottle of milk several times a night; the child may urinate in bed daily, or start playing in the middle of the night. All the while, the alarm clock prepares to issue its vengeful cry. For such parents, especially in the case of Autism Spectrum Disorder (ASD), this is a never-ending process with seemingly little hope for change!

Although the *Cocculus* person always dances on the rope of a nervous breakdown, often, she becomes ill when the family member for whom she has been caring either dies or recuperates and her caretaking role has come to end. While this is surprising to many around her, the adrenaline rush that kept *Cocculus* going during her watching period is not needed anymore; *Cocculus* now starts to recognize that caretaking has undermined her constitution; this shows on the physical plane, possibly having caused an adrenal gland and/or thyroid dysfunction. In the present ASD epidemic, night watching has taken on a different meaning, and it affects countless more parents worldwide. This can be considered an extended and prolonged *Cocculus* situation: the immediate mortality of most children in such a state is not a factor, but their needs are often greater than those of the dying person! There seems to be no end in sight! To the question "When will my child recover?" no one can give a definite answer! The exhaustion in *Cocc* is a slow-growing but inevitable process: it is an insidiously working poison undermining the VF. How many patients diagnosed with CFIDS and fibromyalgia would benefit from Cocc (*weakness from nursing the sick; weakness from loss of sleep*)? Many, I suspect, if you combine grief over their lost vitality with loss of sleep!

Indeed, the other outstanding *Cocculus* causality is prolonged **loss of sleep for any reason,** not just for night watching and grief (*sleeplessness nursing the sick*). A *Cocculus* situation is also created in the student who has lost months of good sleep preparing his final exams (*sleeplessness after mental exertion, Cocc, Nux-v, Lyc, Lachesis).* Another example is the mother breastfeeding her baby several times a night for months, especially if she does not have enough milk or if the baby is a sycotic and voracious eater, often not latching on while breastfeeding. And countless parents of children with ASD wake up continuously because of the child's insomnia, bedwetting, anxiety, fears, and compulsive behavior. For such parents, this combination of lack of sleep, coupled with the grief felt because the child is not normal and may never be, and because they themselves cannot live a normal life, would possibly require *Cocculus* rather than *Sepia*. We have now a growing legion of mothers deprived of sleep, and there is no solution in sight as long as their children do not recover from the suffocating grip of ASD.

Another example of prolonged sleep deprivation coupled with grief is found in families who have troubles with family members (on drugs, in prison, etc.), or in people caught in a war, or those suffering after breakups. Then we have those who must adjust to a night job rather than a day job and now suddenly complain of headaches and forgetfulness. Twenty percent of American workers are night-shift workers, and the number is growing. While the rest of society sleeps, police officers, security agents, truck drivers, hotel desk clerks, office cleaning crews, nurses, doctors, pilots, and many others keep patients alive, streets safe, and packages moving. But going against the body's circadian rhythms causes a kind of biological revolt! Consider the frequent world traveler, the professional tennis player, and the businessman who cannot adjust to the many different time schedules; with *Arnica* and *rescue remedy*, *Cocculus* is wonderfully effective against jet lag (one remedy, not the combination of all three!). Loss of sleep can also be caused by a myriad of other situations in which Cocc is indicated: worry about one's job and about the economy in general (*sleeplessness from fear; from activity of thoughts, especially of business)*), (*Nux-v*, *Ambr*), or sleeplessness caused when losing a home or a relationship that has gone south (*Lach*, *Nat-m*, *Ign*, *insomnia from grief*—Cocc should be added to this rubric!). *Cocculus* is found in many other rubrics of sleeplessness. Sleeplessness *during heat;*

from menopause; from anxiety; from nausea during pregnancy (morning sickness); *after loss of sleep* (only remedy), and from *slightest noise* (Hahnemann: *a slight noise goes through all his limbs*). It is surprising that not everyone needs *Cocculus* at some point! *Cocculus* cannot be found in the rubric *grief, undermining the constitution,* where we find *Phos* and *Carc,* but it should be there! The empathetic *Phosphorus* suffers grief from any disconnection with friends and family, in spite of or because of continuous efforts and lack of stamina, eventually leading to the exhausted *Ph-ac* state. *Carcinosin* is very demanding of herself; her overwhelming anticipation anxiety prevents her from loving herself enough, so the family's haphazard doses of love (only received after a good performance) are insufficient for her existence. But *Cocculus*' situation is a combination of the two abovementioned remedies: disconnection from family and friends because of dutiful behavior combined with another highly demanding job. There is only an endless giving and expectation and outpouring of love and care without much emotional return as other family members often turn their back to the situation, either from indifference or inability to help due to geographical distance.

To many, the apparently self-sacrificing *Cocculus* looks like a saint, but is she? Like many others who are pressured in hopeless and demanding situations, *Cocculus* initially tries to maintain a mask made up of "contrasting moods." The mask of the contrasting moods is the mask of the clown who performs the day after her child's death as the show must go on. The tears of the clown are often unseen on the painted smiling face. A *Cocc* person must hide her true feelings in a benumbed state in order to stay upbeat for the sick relative: *asks for nothing; cheerful; dancing; jesting; spasmodic laughing* and *vivacious.* But how long can this last? The parent of a child with ASD, for example, must show continuous optimism, an upbeat nature, and immense patience and effort to guide her child in the right direction—and the path often has many dead ends! One can see that this behavior is awkward and not real. While acting like this, in a state of apparent and forced optimism, it is only human that the *Cocculus* person will need to find a dumping ground somewhere else (work, relationship, recreation) to unload her pent-up feelings of frustration: *anger with silent grief.* There is only so much a person can endure and suppress in the unconscious (*anger at trifles*)! Therapists advise hitting the bed with a pillow or shouting out in anger to release these suppressed emotions. The homeopath orders *Cocculus*! Not surprisingly, *Cocc* suffers from *A/F homesickness,* which in this case can have two meanings: first, a longing for nonexistent close family support and her own lost life, and second, reminiscing about the good old times she has had with the person she is taking care of, about the days when life seemed to be easier and simpler, before this demanding role was thrust upon her.

Sometimes a *Cocculus* state is not due to a loss of sleep but is triggered by a **greater demand on her daily activities**, draining her energy, especially when the demand takes the form of caring for someone else. It is like a loss of sleep, too, because in order to recharge her batteries, the patient requires now far more sleep than the usual amount; she suffers loss of sleep even if the number of hours slept remains the same. There is a greater continuous demand than supply! Night watching, indeed, now takes place even during the day, outside of the home. An example would be the housewife who visits her dying father in the hospital every day but still manages to finish her work. And if her partner criticizes her for neglecting her children or him because of it, causing more grief, a *Cocculus* situation develops even more quickly. *Phos, Carc, Ign, Nat-m* and *Cocc* are mainly female remedies for the simple reason that they belong to Jung's feeling conscious function types; in spite of emancipation (which did not entail an increased feeling function in men), more is expected from women than from men in terms of caring and providing a source of emotional support, as the female symbolizes love, compassion, nourishment, feelings, and anima. How often have I heard men say to their spouses when raising children with special needs: "This is your job, not mine. My job is to earn money." In *Cocculus*' case, grief is very intense; I have seen cases of Ménière's syndrome—tinnitus, deafness and vertigo (*vertigo from grief*)—develop in such states. One of my very first homeopathic cases was like this, and to my utter surprise the case was cured with a 6C potency. It was pure beginners' luck! But it sure got me hooked on homeopathy.

Anger with Silent Grief

Cocc is a 1 for *A/F anger suppressed* but a 2 for *anger with silent grief*: it looks as though there is more anger aimed at the fate that has forced her into this role. But there is no blasphemy (*Nat-m, Nux-v, Anac*), no religious expressions or anger with God or becoming agnostic (*Lachesis*). Looking at the provings, it seems that *Cocc* considers herself more the criminal for not doing enough (neglecting duty), as seen in *great apprehensive anxiety of conscience and feeling at heart as after committing a wicked deed, with desire to escape; constant desire to escape*... What does this express? She is torn by her sense of duty (*little concerned as to his own health, he is very anxious about other's sickness; thoughts fixed on one unpleasant thing and observes nothing about her; when her mind is turned away from herself her sufferings are forgotten*), but there must be moments, as expressed in the other provings, that it is all too much—so she wants to run away and is then plagued by guilt that she even has such ideas, considering herself a criminal for even thinking this (*anxiety, of conscience, as if guilty of a crime*: Cocc)! If she could, *Cocculus* would withdraw more quickly from her duty than *Sepia*. How do we know? See the rubric *too much sense of duty, Sepia*. Cocc is not there! Cocc is also not in *aversion to duty*. It looks, in *Cocculus*' case, as though fate, rather than duty, has imposed on her; since it is a family member or very good friend calling on her, she can't refuse to help, but the pull is more coming from the heart and feeling function (Eros) than from the thinking function of conscious or Logos.

Compensations

Sympathy

Starting *Cocculus*' story, I wondered how such a selfless person copes with his situation; how much energy and time is left to even have **one** positive compensation, and what contradictory emotions (contrasting moods) might run through this caregiver and be part of her makeup? Suppressed anger? Resentment? Hatred? Frustration? Forsakenness? Despair? Irritability? Hopelessness? Impatience? Isolation? Even wanting to kill the object of care? I would not be surprised if all of them were present at some moments in her ordeal!

The innate character of *Cocculus* seems to be appropriate for a caregiver: there is *mildness, introspection, serious and earnest, sympathetic and compassionate, timid and bashful,* and *sentimental* with a rather *yielding disposition*. No wonder *Cocculus* is a remedy for extreme sadness, particularly in females, the bearers of nourishment. As Hering expresses it, *Cocculus* is *sympathetic* and *has reverence for those around her* (<> *Platina*). In other words, *Cocculus* respects and honors others and thus gets drawn into a demanding situation. So at least initially, before weariness sets in, the Cocc person can be *cheerful, and mirthful, even dancing* (compare *Sepia* in its first stage) with *irresistible inclination to sing* (DD with *Nat-m*), a kind of mania, forming *Cocculus*' contrasting moods and representing the underlying nervousness and adrenaline rush. However, depleted gradually by too much external stimulation, worry, and her great sense of responsibility, *Cocculus* thrives on reflection and solitude as solitude quite literally allows the serious *Cocculus* to hear herself. Enough stimulation already!

Oversensitive Nervous System

Anxiety sets in quickly as the caregiver is constantly preoccupied with the ill person, and lack of sleep starts undermining *Cocculus*' constitution: *anxiety during sleep* and *loss of sleep*. It does not take long before *Cocculus* turns into a *brooding, busy person, full of cares and worries about others. She has thoughts about business at night* (the care-giving business, that is—DD *Ambr-gr* and *Nux-v* where it is a more selfish business), and she is *haunted by nothing but unpleasant thoughts* (DD *Sepia/Nat-m*), all thoughts about grief and the precarious future of the one she watches and how she will cope with all of this (*she indulges in sad reveries*). The primary concern, though, remains the sick one she cares for. *She is little concerned as to her own health but very anxious about other's sickness.* This last proving is a good summary of *Cocculus*' state of mind, one which we find nowadays in so many situations. I can only think of the many dedicated mothers of children with ASD for whom the recovery of their children can become the primary and even the only goal in their lives. Loss of sleep is one of the major gateways to ill health and mental breakdown; unsurprisingly and, in fact, inevitably, the conscientious *Cocculus* person—who always sleeps with one ear open—turns into an irritable, contrary individual (DD with *Sepia* again). This proves that those quiet creatures walking among us are not as mild-mannered as they appear to be. *Cocculus* resents, and will even lash out at, those who encroach upon her personal comfort zone: *censorious; intolerant of contradiction; contrary and intolerant of interruption. Exertion from mental work aggravates; head readily fatigues by mental exertion* (DD *Calc-p* in schoolgirls is necessary). Slowly, the toll of overexertion sets in on the physical plane as well, making *Cocculus* run around like a zombie (*stupefaction with sleepiness and hysterical fainting*). *Cocculus* is a great remedy, found in many rubrics of *generalities, faintness: generalities, faintness, from suppressed menses; from pain of menses; from pain in abdomen; in uterine complaints; during palpitations; accompanied by nausea* (think morning sickness); *on excitement; with vertigo; after vomiting; from weakness.* But this is also a black type remedy for *hysterical fainting.*

Suffering from anxiety and increasing physical and mental fatigue, and now on the verge of a nervous breakdown, *Cocculus* shows *easily angered at trifles* and *from contradiction* and *she is very easily affronted.* Initially, because of her innate good temperament, ridden with *guilt, anger alternates with cheerfulness and jesting, and jesting alternates with vexation,* but this is only temporary. The time bomb is ticking, exhaustion sets in, and *Cocculus* finds herself on a very slippery slope. Like the exhausted *Sepia*, there is *a sensation of emptiness* and *aversion to being disturbed.* Hence *Cocculus* now *takes everything in bad part* as brain fag sets in. A nervous breakdown is near! Patience runs thin and *Cocculus* becomes *intolerant of contradiction*, but violent acts are rather rare as she is utterly devoid of energy. A conversation between an introvert like *Cocculus* (*serious*) and an extravert like *Nux-v* can result in a series of misunderstandings. As *Cocculus* struggles to follow multiple conversational threads and sort out his own thoughts, she remains quiet and appears to be just listening. The extravert reads that as engagement, a cue to keep talking. The introvert *Cocculus* struggles with the continuing flow of input and soon starts to shut out the extravert, just smiling and nodding as the conversation becomes too challenging. *There is dullness and difficulty of thinking* and *she becomes forgetful of words while speaking* (DD *Thuja*). *The confusion of mind is accompanied by vertigo.* Cocc now sinks into the depths of a dark world. Cocc *is absorbed within herself and observes nothing about her. She appears imbecile and at other times acts like a maniac, is wicked and talks constantly. Often reflecting and answering takes a long time. There is tearful chagrin about the least trifle. Melancholy and sadness set in with weeping and profound absorption in sorrowful thoughts. She feels great apprehensive anxiety of conscience as after committing a wicked deed with great desire to escape. And she is vacillating and cannot accomplish anything at her work or finish anything.*

Alcohol Use Leading to Further Breakdown

What do you think some people do when their minds become so frazzled that they can't sleep, and when they have that sinking feeling that they are becoming insane? To calm her mind, the bottle of alcohol becomes a source of relief, the calming and sleeping pill for *Cocculus* (*dipsomania*), but mental symptoms (*confusion*) strongly *aggravate after drinking*. Like in *Sepia*, stress causes trembling (*excitement with trembling*) in *Cocc* as she increasingly loses control of the situation, and alcohol is no help. She has to spend more and more energy to do her daily work as her memory starts failing: *memory, weakness of expressing oneself, for what has happened and for what he has read. She is distracted and easily forgets of what he has just thought. It is also great trouble for him to pronounce words so she mumbles.* *Cocculus* has a hard time finding the right word when asked a question: *answers abruptly; answers difficult; answers hastily; does not want to answer when questioned; reflecting long, and answers slowly*! As her frail nerves abandon her, and *Cocculus* looks in vain for relief and a peaceful place, her sensitivity to external impressions only increases: *over sensitive to all external expressions and starting easily from noise, during her sleep or when touched. There is intolerance of noise or any disturbing influence. She is excited by loud talking or least increase of temperature.* Everything bothers her!

Masturbation

Ailments from sexual excesses play a role, as they do in *Sepia*, but whereas in the dutiful *Sepia* these ailments refer to her many pregnancies/miscarriages, with *Cocculus* it is due to *masturbation*, another supposed stress reliever like alcohol (DD *Pic-ac*). Such a person is neither erotically or sexually active. *Cocculus* remains in isolation, as it were, with his sex instinct, and the expression of this isolation is masturbation. But TCM knows very well that such "unregulated affairs of the bedroom" lead to a depletion of vital energy (Chinese medicine calls it Essence), leading to further exhaustion on all planes. Then, a person with a broken-down constitution experiences the hangover that follows the act of masturbation. The homeopath should not be surprised that, in *Cocculus*' case, this can even lead to *insanity*. Preceding such insanity is the kind of depression *Cocculus* presents. Totally withdrawn (*great sorrowfulness with constant inclination to sit in a corner buried in thought—sits still, wrapped in deep sad thoughts and notices nothing* (*Puls*!), and *indisposed to talk with talk of others aggravating*), *Cocculus* ends up in the same exhausted state as *Sepia*, running around as if in a daze (*pale, prostrated* and *full of despair*), which brings us back to her CD.

Golden Tips from the Masters

- Sensation of hollowness in the head and the belly, giving rise to nausea and causing one to faint, the same feeling one has when moving forward on a swing or going down in an elevator
- When bending down, he feels as if he is about to fall backwards and has to hold on something or someone quickly
- A "sinking" feeling and metallic taste in the mouth are keynotes
- #1 remedy for travel sickness (cars and trains especially) as well as jet lag: the patient wants to vomit but can't, there is just *nausea because of dryness in pharynx* and *nausea on rising from bed* and *nausea from cold*
- Twilight sleepers: they have no recollection that they slept
- Weakness and stiffness of all joints
- Ménière's syndrome after grief (*vertigo, lying down necessary; tendency to fall sideways; vertigo warm bed ameliorates; vertigo with nausea,* and *vertigo night watching and loss of sleep*)
- *Cocculus* is also indicated in cases of multiple sclerosis and paralysis, when we see the illness developing from weakness to numbness to paralysis in the lower extremities (*weakness, lower limbs, paralytic, especially in the knees*). Also indicated in trigeminus neuralgia (*face pain, opening the mouth, eating and talking*) (Mezereum).

Conium maculatum (Con). Poison Hemlock

The Cyber Delusion

Conium's Cyber delusion is ***he is pursued by enemies***. Who are these enemies? Family? Friends? The government? Others? Everyone? Does it have anything to do with *Mercury's delusion, he is surrounded by enemies* (as he tries to hold on to his dictatorship)? We have to look for other provings to find out. *Conium* feels that he needs to be on guard all the time, and this constant watching when people approach (*shyness at the approach of people and yet dread of being alone*) has to take a toll on such a person. The **paranoia** creates hardness or induration to produce a shell for protection on all levels (mental, emotional, and physical), as will be discussed further, also fostering **superstition**—another reason to look at people as possible enemies (*Arg-n, Med, Rhus-t, Mancinella, Stram*). *Conium* suspects that something can happen to him at any given moment, recalling *Kali-carb's* anxiety-provoking CD, *an abyss is behind him*. We know that *Kali-c* tries to obtain order and control in his life through rules and regulations. It is interesting for the homeopath to see what compensations *Conium* chooses as survival strategies, engulfed as he is by his suspicions about people, and what pathology it will create on all levels. It is also interesting to learn why *Conium* has to be so alert in the first place, joining remedies like *Stramonium, Lycopodium, Arsenicum, Lachesis,* and *Hyos*—all, of course, suspicious and watchful for the enemy for their own reasons. What other delusions support *Conium's* CD? *Delusion, animals dancing on bed; someone was coming in at the door at night; someone is entering at night; house is full of people; he is persecuted; he sees people at his bedside in his room* and *sees thieves,* and *illusions of hearing*! These fixed ideas all point to a single threat: that someone will enter his "house" and try to take something away from him, usually at night and when he is in bed! A house usually is the relatively fixed symbol for the Self, the dreamer himself. The bed, in turn, is the symbol for sleep, the unconscious, place of birth and creation of life, where sexual activity takes place. Looking at this relatively fixed symbol, we see a fear of someone robbing *Conium* of the ability to create life, of the place of birth, linked to sexual activity. This symbol (and its creation of the CD) should be somewhat connected to *Conium's* NWS. It also includes the *delusion, sees dead corpse, brother and child.* The brother is the shadow side in the case of a man and the *animus* in the case of a woman; it seems to reflect the death of the characteristics of the animus: will, decision, activity, courage, authority, initiative, planning, sexual activity/aggression... The death of a possible child refers to a renewal of life, a rebirth of life. These translations have to be found back in *Conium's* characteristics, in his losses and weaknesses, as we will discover. *Conium* also has a *delusion, of fancy illusions*: why this retreat into the unconscious? Is he looking there for what he has lost? It is most likely the search for the restoration of the animus, the loss of sexual creativity and procreation reflected by the delusion of the death of a possible child, the renewal of life. There is a desire to return to the womb and to the Great Mother, a symbol for the collective unconscious. What caused this situation? How can procreation and renewal of life have come to a standstill? The NWS will tell us. So *Conium's* delusions reflect paranoia about a threat with a retreat into the unconscious as defense mechanism.

Causalities

Reversal of Fortune

The greatest ailment from (A/F) seems to be NWS *reversal of fortune.* The question is: does this refer to financial loss (*Aurum, Arsenicum*) or to a reversal of fortune in work (*Ambra, Lycopodium*), relationships (*Lachesis*), or health (*Arsenicum, Stannum*)? *Conium* has a great desire for two things: **material** possessions (*haughty, likes to wear his best clothes*; *insanity, makes useless purchases*) and **sex**, which continually roams in his mind (*sexual thoughts intrude*; *satyriasis*; *lascivious*). *Conium* is, therefore, very sensitive to the loss of a partner and to any economic or financial loss. But *Conium* has less grief than *Ignatia* after the death of a lover and is less melancholic than *Aurum* after a financial disaster. What the homeopath observes instead is that *Conium* will produce a cancer (right-sided breast cancer, uterine cancer, prostate cancer) six months to one year after such an emotionally stressful event! So think first *Con* when you see cancer after grief or financial loss; this is due to the suppression and non-acknowledgment of his emotions as he has an *emotional indifference* and hardness. Originally he has *ambition for fame,* so a reversal of fortune can certainly be linked to monetary loss or loss of position. But in most cases, reversal of fortune has a totally different meaning for *Conium*, as it is linked to his second desire, sex. Regarding sex, it is interesting to note two important A/F that seem at first contradictory: *ailments from continence/celibacy* and *ailments from sexual excesses.* At first they seem to express opposites; continence refers to the suppression or abstinence of sexual desire, the opposite of sexual excesses, but in *Conium's* case the two are closely connected. They are expressed in Hering as one unit, *hypochondriasis and hysteria from suppression of, or too free indulgence in sexual instinct* and *bad effects from suppressed sexual desire or from excessive indulgence.* It refers to people who at one point in their life had normal or even excessive sexual activity or who react very quickly to any excitement with a sexual response, and for whom such activity has now come to a sudden halt for any of a number of reasons: loss of spouse through death or divorce; sudden conversion to a religion in which sex is taboo and sinful; joining a sect in which the guru now forbids sexual contact; or becoming spiritual with renouncing of sex. Celibacy is, of course, seen in priests and nuns, which puts them at risk for cancer of the prostate and uterus, all links of which TCM has great knowledge. Hunger, thirst, and the need for sexual satisfaction are physiological necessities, and if they remain unsatisfied for any length of time, a painful tension is felt.

Satisfaction comes from the Latin *satis facere*, "to make sufficient or enough," as when these physiological needs are sufficiently met, the tensions will disappear and the person will derive a form of pleasure from the activity—a pleasure often unequaled to that experienced at other moments in his life. Intense sexual desire in *Conium* is a combination of physiological and psychological needs: because of the absence of a partner for any of the abovementioned reasons, the physiological needs are not met. At the same time, the grief experienced as a result of the sudden halt of these normal natural expressions causes the development of the kind of pathology seen in *Conium*: a malignant indurated cancer, a severe "punishment" for violating Nature's laws. *Conium's* situation is different from, say, *Lycopodium's*, in which the insecure and often domineering person has an intense need to prove himself: that he is still as virile as before, that he is still loved by his partner, and that he is still the one "in power," demanding what is owed to him in the marriage. In *Lycopodium's* case, the painful tension and the intensity of his desires are due not to the natural demands of his body but, in reality, to his psychological needs, which can be called irrational desires as they are entirely on one side of the spectrum (hypersexuality). This corresponds in the *Lycopodium* person to his irrational desire for power and wealth, as well as his passionate craving for fame, domination, and competition, an expression of envy and jealousy. In well-balanced people, physiologically conditioned sexual desire is satisfied with the removal of the physiological, sexually conditioned tension and will only reappear when this physiological need arises again.

For the *Lycopodium* person, by contrast, the irrational sexual desire is insatiable, except at the brief moment of the act itself. Greed, like lust for power, is a bottomless pit, and the idea of the relief derived from its satisfaction is nothing but a Fata Morgana. Greed and love for power are rooted not in man's nature, but in his distorted mind and imagination. The *Lycopodium* person, incapable of loving himself and never able to love the other person for who she **is** (not how she looks), is always stuck in this irrational desire that has become part of his life. In *Lycopodium's* case, the Chinese would have called the circumstances an ignoble misfortune (evitable and blameworthy), as opposed to the noble misfortune (inevitable and immutable) of *Conium*, in which *Con* is forced to give up sex through circumstances mentioned before (lack of partner). While *Lycopodium* derives brief joy from any sexual conquest, he never experiences the continuous joy that we call happiness. Typically, the hedonist *Lycopodium* person, through excessive sexual activity and loss of fluids, will burn out, leading to impotence and erection disturbances later in life (*too early ejaculation*, to which the Chinese in old times referred to as "delivering newspapers" as this person never sticks around after delivering the newspaper), and even at a young age.

But one who has sex in response to a purely physiological need and as an expression and result of love increases his powers: he burns without being consumed. In *Conium's* case, belonging to both sides of the spectrum (too much and no sex), he is a victim of continence or celibacy, so there is no more satisfaction of the sexual physiological necessity. Inevitably, in the long run, this prolonged continence leads to many psychological problems: *anxiety, sadness and even hysteria from prolonged continence* or *sexual abstinence* or *from suppressed sexual excitement.*

Stress

Secondary for *Conium* is stress in general or *A/F emotional excitement: he cannot endure any kind of excitement; it brings on physical and mental depression, with weakness.* Repetitive stress has brought the patient into this paralyzed, chronic *Conium* state. In *Conium's* case, *ailments from care* have nothing to do with others but rather reflect loss of money and loss of his sexual outlets;

he suffers ailments from *care with aversion to company* like *Nat-m*, who wants to withdraw to contemplate his fate (*indisposed to talk* and *talk of others aggravates* and *dwells on past disagreeable occurrences*).

Compensations

Escape into the Unconscious

Escaping from reality can take different forms. Meditation is one form, and for *Conium* it is not equal to deep introspection and seeking an understanding of the self. Rather, as Hahnemann states in the proving, *Conium is lost in deep meditation and anxiously thinks over the present and the future, and therefore seeks solitude*. Isolation, loneliness, and anxiety are the only consequences of this introspection. It is interesting to note that deeply meditating individuals with much animus and less anima are "hard-feeling" with cancer as pathology (*Carbo-an, Sep, Con*). *Conium* indeed retreats into the unconscious, a search for the Great Mother, part of the collective unconscious and shunning conscious life, expressed by *shuns light; quiet disposition, bright light is intolerable*, light being a relatively fixed symbol of the conscious. *Conium* prefers to dress in dark or black clothes, representing the unconscious. It is not just light but also noise that *Conium* wants to avoid; *Conium* is *intolerable to noise with a painful sensitivity to noise and startled by it*. How difficult it is to connect with consciousness is also seen in the rubrics *confusion of the mind after siesta and sleeping* (Lachesis), as even a short nap seems to hold *Conium* captive in the unconscious. *Desire to be magnetized*, for Conium, therefore reflects the desire to connect not to people but to the self-created dream world.

Gradual Induration/Paralysis or Hardening on All Levels

Induration on the Mental Level

Mental and emotional induration takes place **before** the physical repercussions. The *Conium* patient *has an inability to sustain any mental effort, creating tired and weary sensation in the brain with physical as well as nervous prostration. His memory is feeble with excessive difficulty of recollecting things, particularly dates. He has difficulties of correctly expressing himself nor can he rightly remember and there is such stupefaction that he has difficulties in understanding what he reads. There is obtuseness of all senses and he is wandering about as if half asleep.*

Induration on the Emotional Plane

Conium's lack of emotions is clearly shown in the way he treats others and even himself. As this process gradually continues, *Conium* goes from being a high-anxiety person to exhibiting *indifference, especially when walking in open air,* remarkable in view of the severe pathology he suffers from (cancer). He also *becomes discontented with himself.* He is *easily disturbed by trifles, moved to tears and anxious.* The slightest stress seems to bring *Conium* totally out of balance: *cannot endure any kind of excitement, it brings on physical and mental depression, with weakness. He has disinclination for business* and *indolence* rules! *He is timid* and *cannot be persuaded to work; want of proper will.* In fact, provings show that he takes a rather careless, indifferent approach to life: *likes to wear his best clothes, makes useless purchases, cares very little for things, wastes or ruins them; does not want to work and prefers to play. Complete indifference and takes no interest in anything, with a paralyzed feeling in all the limbs as though a great grief weighs upon him with inclination to sit still. There is disinclination for business and unsympathetic from indolence yet is he worse from being idle.* This makes him a rather difficult patient to deal with, as the "enemy" might also be the homeopath with his inquisitiveness. This is an introverted person who is not very forthcoming in the inquiry, but often the homeopath can find a past history of many tremendous emotional sufferings (*Nat-m* events!). *Con* can look like a *Nat-m* person, but usually we have a *Conium* layer on top of a *Nat-m* one. A complement is *Tuberculinum*. Pregnancy is not a good time for *Conium* as her delusions seem to flourish: *aversion to friends during pregnancy and mental affections. Conium is averse to being near people, to be talking or dressing himself, taking food* or *see his children. She is discouraged, despondent and dissatisfied with herself and her surroundings* and *is inclined to cry, sobbing aloud when alone. And the least spirituous liquor intoxicates her.*

Induration and Gradual Weakness on the Physical Plane

Conium comes from the Greek word *konos,* which means dizziness. Normally, *Conium* is resilient on the physical plane. First we see mental/emotional symptoms, while physically *Conium* remains strong. In *Conium,* everything is slow and gradual. Therefore, a *Conium* patient only shows up for a consultation when he already has severe pathology. For this reason, we see *Conium* pathology rarely in children, since there has not been enough time for it to develop. The gradual hardening on the physical level leads to a slow-forming malignant cancer. The following rubrics indicate the kind of cancer: *cancerous affections, epithelioma, glands; ulcers lips cancerous; genitalia male, cancer; gen, female cancer of the ovaries; gen, female, cancer uterus*. *Conium's* urinary symptoms are also peculiar: a keynote is *constant urge to urinate with little or no result*. The patient gets up at night because of his strong urge, but he has to push hard to urinate a little. This can be so serious that he becomes anxious and desperate with perspiration, headache and vertigo (*bladder, urging, ineffectual, with headache*). After some time the patient is exhausted and returns to bed. After a while the whole cycle starts again. Other prostate symptoms are found in several rubrics: *loss of prostatic fluid by merely touching a woman; discharge of prostatic fluid on every change of emotion, without voluptuous thoughts; emission prostatic fluid, while fondling women; seminal emissions, during caresses; seminal emissions, while frolicking with a woman; loss of prostatic fluid with stool.*

Golden Tips from the Masters

- Think of *Conium* when there appears the combination of headache and ineffectual urging to urinate. Also when ineffectual urination and vertigo. The typical triad of vertigo in *Conium* is: <from lying down, from getting up, and from turning in bed. Therefore, the patient keeps the head perfectly still. Dizziness disappears on closing the eyes!
- Right lobe of prostrate is hard as a stone, firmly fixed and much stinging or biting (like flea bites); a weight like a stone in perineum
- #1 in prostate cancer with spreading to the bones
- #1 in cervical cancer (you can manipulate the pap smear result with 30C to 200C *Conium*)
- #1 in hard right-sided breast cancer
- Recent cases of gonorrhea with orchitis and severe nocturnal pains.
- Usually there is a layer of *Conium* on the top of a *Nat-m* layer (in case of MS, breast cancer, prostate cancer)
- Ascending paralytic symptoms as in cases of MS (from the legs upwards while the brain remains clear)
- Grief from death of a loved one
- Dryness in throat on a small spot
- Pains and aches are relieved by letting the limbs hang down
- Perspiration as soon as one sleeps or even when closing the eyes!

Cuprum metallicum (Cupr). Copper

The Cyber Delusion

As usual, we try to discover the essence of the remedy by examining the corresponding Cyber delusion; the *Cuprum* state is well represented by a delusion of grandeur (*pompous*), in particular that of *he is an officer*. This Cyber delusion, ***he is an officer***, represents an excessive persona, and is definitely supported by many other fixed ideas: he is not just an officer, *he is a general*; *he is a person of high rank*; *he is a great person* and *he is being a commander*. This all sounds like a so-called high-ranking position, but it is true only in his eyes and maybe in those of a few admirers. The next delusions tell us how high-ranked he really is, and what the delusion *he is doing business* stands for: *he is repairing old chairs*; *he is selling green vegetables*; *he is gathering herbs*; and *he is engaged in some occupation*. So *Cuprum* feels important for having reached the zenith of his modest profession, but in reality it is not one leading to worldwide recognition or earth-shattering changes. He is like the master shoemaker I used to know below my practice, who would pound on shoes all day long until late evening; people from the city would flock to him. He is like the great car mechanic who always finds the best solutions for your car; he is like the top-notch craftsman in anything except for a job requiring mental work as expressed in *ailments from mental work* and *disinclination to intellectual work, yet idling is burdensome to him*. This can be called a benign form of narcissism, as these personalities have a narcissistic pride in their work as shoemakers, attorneys, or physicians: often we find them dominating the conversation at gatherings, and when one pays attention, it is all about them. But at least this kind of narcissism is the result of effort that people have put forth in their lives, and of what they have achieved, contrary to the malignant side of narcissism which is only about what a person **has**: an attractive figure, great jewels, nice dresses, a nice car, etc. The reader might also recognize *Platina* in this category.

Cuprum and *Ferrum* are both cramped individuals who look over their shoulders constantly. While *Ferrum* exhibits a certain degree of paranoia, as he thinks that everyone is out to push him off of his throne (*delusion, sees thieves, sees devils; suspicious*), *Cuprum* is distinguished by the *delusion, he is about to be arrested* and *delusion, a police officer called on him.* Somehow there are even fixed ideas in *Cuprum* that allude to some half-criminal behavior (some business ethics that might cross the legal line to stay ahead of the competition), as he is continuously alert: this is not a relaxed person or someone who serves humankind; rather, *Cuprum* is someone who strives for recognition and perfection in his little world. But the striving for this position comes with a heavy price: at no given moment can he let his guard down; he needs to be vigilant and aggressive towards competition (*desire to bite*)!

Causalities

Mental Work and Holding on to a Power Position

How did he become, literally, such a *cramped* individual? As mentioned before, this is the person who is exhausted from *mental work* and has a *deficiency of ideas with weakness of memory for words,* so he discovers that his future lies in the mechanical professions or sales jobs and other tasks that do not require a constant drain on his limited intellectual powers (*prostration of mind; exhaustion and brain fag with sleepiness*). This can be the case of the regular physician whose daily practice work is routine and automatic, not brain work. *Cuprum* suffers also from *anger with anxiety:* this might have well to do with the degree of paranoia he has about the possibility of being bumped from his "high" position at any moment. There are thousands of others that do what he is doing, so he feels the stress of competition. He is not a *Wunderkind* who will receive the next Nobel Prize; at most, he is just a master of his trade. There is a need for this individual to be high-strung and to be always on guard to ward off competition. *Fright, excitement,* and *hearing bad news* all are parts of his causalities, but they also all have to do with losing his hard-earned "power" in business, and we see in the provings that he can be *deceitful.* No wonder he feels cramped and tense: he must be constantly on high alert mode in order to keep his standing. In the extended meaning, *Cuprum*'s *fear of misfortune, fear of accident, fear of falling,* and *anxiety about the future* represent worry about losing that coveted position. Everything in his life serves to maintain the sacrificial, almighty, and valuable professional persona he has created (*cautious*).

Compensations

Industriousness and Aggressiveness

Besides his industriousness, there is also *Cuprum's* attitude, which he thinks serves him as a positive tool. *He acts like a dictator; he speaks with a voice of command* and *is pompous* as he is convinced that this will maintain the excessive persona with which he wishes to impress people. In fact, he can *bark* or *bellow* his orders to underlings. *Cuprum's* further behavior shows *ridiculous or foolish gestures; he covers his mouth with the hand; he feels important* and *grimaces*. Criticisms or questioning are seen as attacks on his safely guarded authority, just as the allopathic physician, hiding behind the white coat, does not want to be challenged about something he knows little about (for example, diet or alternative healing methods). As he feels himself to be some kind of authority, this feeling of being attacked is not a constant one (*anxiety in paroxysms; rage in paroxysms*); he always will have some followers among the masses who will never challenge him and who swear he is the best person for the job at hand, someone who always thinks in the box. But his rage comes in spurts, in "cramps," demanding that he react in a rather violent, cramping way. *Cuprum* is very well known for clenching his thumbs in his palms, ready to strike.

A *Cuprum* child has an archaic ego and therefore looks to achieve his power position as part of his Adlerian complex, by *a desire to pull hair, spitting in faces of people* and *biting*, a rage in which *he does not recognize his relatives* and *shrieks before convulsions*. Such a child is also *restless at night, tossing about in bed* and has a *desire to play at night*, which is also seen in some children who are in an autistic state. *Cuprum* always reacts in a sudden, attacking way. He is all about defense and attack, with *delusions, of being a general, an officer, or a person of high standing* who does not want to be challenged! In circumstances where his authority is questioned (he has a *disposition to contradict*), *Cuprum* can be *besides himself* and *spit in the face of people*. This last proving expresses the fighting spirit of a rather unsophisticated being to win his battles against competitors by using intimidation. This might secure him some victories, but in the long run it will come back to haunt him. He will win some battles but lose the war.

A Loner out of Necessity and Misplaced Pride

Paranoid about others (*suspicious*), he only listens to his own advice: *he has a great disposition to contradict. He can be mild* (only when you don't contradict him), but *mildness easily alternates with obstinacy, screaming and shouting.* It has to be his way! This makes me think of the allopathic physician who sends registered letters to his patients when they refuse to follow his advice to the T with messages such as: "If you don't do what I say, you are not my patient anymore" or "If you refuse these vaccinations, then look for another pediatrician (*malicious, spiteful and vindictive*)!" Questioning his authority leads to a perpetually anxious state, even *anguish at the end, especially that he is always dissatisfied with everything*: *there is anxiety with fear, anxiety about the future, profuse perspiration from anxiety* and *anxiety with congestion of the head.* There is never time to let his guard down; someone might conquer his business and he might fall from his throne! Not even his sleep provides him with an oasis: *he is restless and tosses about in bed.* This anxiety also leads to *difficult concentration* and *confusion of the mind,* surely not helpful in maintaining his position. And children only are obstructions to his ambition and a hindrance to his work: *he cannot bear to have children near him.* At first, *magnetized ameliorates* seems to be a positive tool, as in general it means deriving support from and being influenced by a stronger personality, but in reality he *avoids the sight of people, as the presence of others aggravate his symptoms* and *he has fear of strangers.* He even has *aversion to company when sad.* He is industrious at what he does (*idling is burdensome to him*), and *occupation and diversion ameliorates* as it makes him feel important in society. So the magnetizing is more about being totally engrossed in his profession, a one-dimensional state to hold his well-guarded mask on his face. Because he cannot trust anyone and thinks he is the king of his territory, he becomes a lone commander who wants full responsibility for all actions taken in his own life; this leads to anxiety and becoming a cramped individual with an *aversion of being touched* in the literal and psychological sense (don't ask probing questions or *he runs away and attempts to escape*). It is the rather pathetic, primitive defense of an insignificant position by an immature and insecure individual to control the little world he has created. Behind the mask, he is an insecure individual who *weeps after slight emotions* and *when making speeches.*

Golden Tips from the Masters

- Massive spasms, blue fingers and face, thumbs clenched across palms of hands >with cold water
- Violent cramps at night in bed in the elderly (*Calc-c*)
- The strongest anti-nausea remedy in the materia medica, stronger than *Ipecac*
- Suffocating asthma attack that comes on suddenly, ceases suddenly, and improves by drinking a small amount of cold water
- Elderly people can't make a speech without crying
- #1 remedy for convulsions aggravated during menses
- Hacking cough until face turns blue; threatens to suffocate, >drinking cold water
- Severe spasms after fright and from vexation/anger
- Another remedy for chorea with *risus sardonicus*
- #1 remedy to ameliorate dry cough in measles
- With *Camphor* (first stage, extreme coldness, dry skin and collapse, wants window open during coldness; with cyanosis of nails, hands and feet), *Cuprum* (terrible cramping pains) and *Verat-a* (>with warm drinks and hot applications, with copious diarrhea, vomiting and sweat) are the immortal remedies for cholera both in the past and now!
- #1 remedy for whooping cough in which the child's face becomes blue, the fingernails become discolored, and the child is seized by a spell of violent, suffocating coughing until he loses his breath and lies there as in a coma until a violent spasmodic action in breathing brings the child back to life. Drinking a little sip of cold water will also relieve the cough! (Kent)
- Cramps in soles and calves when attempting sexual intercourse (*Graph* during the act)

Fluoricum acidum (Fl-ac). Hydrofluoric acid

The Cyber Delusion

What is the *Fl-ac* Cyber delusion? ***Delusion, betrothal*** [engagement, vow] ***must be broken*** (only remedy)! This CD is confirmed by almost all of the other delusions: *delusion, he must drive children out of the house, delusion, he must get rid of his servants,* and *delusion, marriage must be dissolved.* It looks as though we have here a very self-centered individual, an escapist who pays no attention to his closest family, not even his children (*aversion to his own family, bordering on insanity but talks pleasantly to others*). "Duty" is not a word in his vocabulary! What is the driving force behind this indifference to his family? He *shows indifference towards those he loves best; he has no objection to their presence but does not care to converse with them; he has a great disposition when alone, to repulsive fantastic imaginations, particularly in regard to persons with whom he stands near relations, or with whom he is connected; it seems, for example, as though he must get rid of all the servants, children must go out of the home, a betrothal must be broken off, a marriage should be dissolved,* etc. Obviously, for *Fl-ac,* communication with family is strictly reduced to a minimum; with his immature ego, though, he still wants to be connected to the protection provided by his home as he has also the *delusion, of impression of danger.* But his main desire is connecting to others, to strangers, to whom he appears the most charming, upbeat personality (*desire to leave home and if strangers or mere acquaintances come in he will enter into an animated conversation*). From his fixed ideas, it is clear that *Fl-ac* is not the most faithful or dedicated family person. He wants to get rid of everyone, wife, children, servants and nurse (*irritability, sends the nurse home*), as all his connections are only for self-serving purposes (*self-gratification and fantastic, repulsive delusions*). Certainly *Fl-ac* does not follow the saying "There is no place like home," except in that he views the home as a resting and protection place after his escapades. His fixed ideas are the expression of the only things he has on his mind: sex, drugs, and glitter! He is waiting for the high of drugs, the high of sex, and the high of rock rhythms that hypnotize him, carry him off, and sweep him away to that land of abundance and promised joy. But

Fl-ac never loves a person for what he **is,** only for what she **has** (beautiful hair, money, great body), characteristics which, with time, all are eventually lost, creating the desire for new victims. In the old Chinese times, they would have called *Fl-ac* someone who "masturbates on someone else."

Causalities

Ailments from Debauchery

The main and practically only NWS of *Fl-ac* is *ailments from debauchery, a debauched life style* (*dipsomania* is another aspect). We have here a highly stimulated individual, sexually speaking, so the last things we can expect are loyalty and closeness to his family; this is confirmed by his Cyber delusion. Entertainment is sought in the outside world as he is driven by that other set of secondary delusions: *delusion, of fancy illusions.* We are not referring here to the fancy illusions of *Nat-c* or *Nat-m,* who flee into a magic world because of heartbreak or an inability to connect to the real world. *Fl-ac's* world is the real world all right, but a limited version of it: *he has repulsive fantastic delusions.* "Repulsive" refers to the sexual attitude; *Fl-ac* as a remedy has become a modern polychrest due to the introduction of Internet porn sites. The real world for *Fl-ac* is right at his fingertips, and he does not have to satisfy his *lasciviousness, ogling women on the street. Fl-ac* has become one of the major remedies for the sex addicts who are going to fill our waiting rooms (*sexual thoughts,* and *thoughts intrude and crowd around each other*)! The person in a *Fl-ac* state is a sex addict who will spend all his available time pursuing his obsessions, day and night, whether he is shopping with his wife at K-mart or driving to the office. When people are obsessed with things, whether sports, cars, or work, then those things fill their minds and days. For a sex addict like *Fl-ac,* everything revolves around sex. He wants women. Now, please—although tonight will do. At worst tomorrow. *Fluoric-ac* wants women like that old Army poster ("I want you") with the finger pointing outward. He calls upon women constantly and urgently (*lascivious*). Have you seen a *Fl-ac* man walking though a crowd? Then you will witness the spasmodic necks and detoured eyes and high-pitched whistled salutes that form together the grand choreography of *Fl-acid's* desire. He does not care that he exaggerates his overtures; he has everything to gain from a sexual encounter and very little to lose, so he might as well try. Any score supersedes people's opinion of his moral attitude and life style. A rebuff does not touch his pride. *Fl-ac* is *industrious:* he constantly seeks to improve his success rate with charming behavior, drawing attention to himself by a boisterous laugh or spreading his arms wide (*buoyancy; cheerful, gay, mirthful; excitable*). Reliable data on the incidence of sexual addiction are difficult to find because of the enormous shame surrounding its admission. Contrary to popular belief, only a small percentage of sex-addicted adults are the pedophiles and rapists whose stories appear in headlines. *Fl-ac* personalities are not easily distinguished from others. They are men and women, gay and straight, with children, families, and steady jobs. The great majority of *Fl-acid* people do not have to "ogle women on the streets," as was the case in the past. They engage primarily in legal or at least culturally acceptable sexual outlets; they amass secret collections of pornography, call sex lines on the phone, pick up prostitutes, log on to sex chat rooms and porno sites on the Internet, or cruise bars. They often date friends, neighbors, and acquaintances with whom they have consensual adult sex (*with whom they enter in animated conversations*). *Fl-ac* explains the lack of control over his sexual behavior as a "constant itch one has to scratch." Part of the NWS can be an ignoble misfortune following seduction of the child or teenager by an older person, even a parent. An early introduction to sexuality is characteristic of many sex addicts as it was the trigger that fell on the fertile sycotic soil present in the family. Or the outcome is the opposite: saddled with the stigma of abnormally introduced sexuality, often at the moment of puberty ("the unbearable age" and moment of psychological revolution), the person does not even want to be alone with a woman or child for fear of losing control over his sexual desires!

Compensations

Increased Activity

"Acidum" represents increased activity followed in a secondary phase by exhaustion. The essence of *Fluoric acid* is that there is a great effort neglect and to break off contact with his entire family, connecting rather with strangers (*feeling of indifference towards those he loves best; has no objection to their presence but does not care to converse with them, yet if strangers or new acquaintances come in will enter in animated conversations*). In other words, family members are ghost figures whom he tolerates, but he comes to life only when new people enter his world. In other words, the notion of industriousness is used in the wrong way. He is industrious all right, and he spares no effort to put all his energy toward achieving his goal: the creation of his own fantasy world, which for *Fl-ac* is dedicated to only one topic: *sex* and anything that helps him get it, like fast cars, nice clothes, and plenty of money! In other words, the *Fl-ac* person wants to feel free to fulfill his fancies of ogling women on the corner of the street (*lascivious, lustful, ogling women on the street,* and *libertinism,* and *libertarianism,* which means love of freedom). This is a person who wants his absolute freedom, unfettered by any duty, to fulfill his fancies and especially to take sexual liberties (*delusions, repulsive, fantastic, only remedy; nymphomania; satyriasis*). We should find *Fl-ac* under the rubrics *duty, aversion to domestic duty* and *under, duty, no sense of,* but we do not! We only find it under *unable to take responsibility*. It is very hard for *Fl-ac* to think of anything but sex (*lascivious thoughts now and then so that he must force himself to think of other things*). Intercourse is the ultimate goal, and elderly men have equally strong desires at night in their sleep (*highly excessive enjoyment and pleasure during coition; sexual passion strong, with violent erections all night, and desire to cohabit; elderly persons had often attacks of venereal desire and erections*). This is a person who dehumanizes everyone else, especially women, who are just objects of love and nothing more.

Great Physical Stamina

Fl-ac is always on the move, a hunter *driven by his desire for company and aversion to solitude* and by his high sexual drive; he is restless, looking at and ogling his prey and exhibiting great stamina (*increased ability to exercise his muscles without fatigue, regardless of the most excessive heat; generalities, sensation of strength; less affected by excessive heat in the summer or cold in the winter*). Here we find also *Nat-phos* (a remedy well known for worms and arthritis), another remedy who wants to connect and communicate with others, but, being a *Natrum*, has far more difficulties in doing so. She does not possess the charms of the *Fl-ac* person, as the *Natrum* element makes her more closed and hypersensitive. *Fl-ac* often needs only a short sleep (*sleeplessness from the time he has gone to bed until the next morning, when a very short and light sleep will be sufficient to refresh him, as if he had slept all night; a short sleep suffices and refreshes him*). The abovementioned rubrics reflect how *Fl-ac's* energy is boosted by the thought of what he sets out to do: "I can't wait to start my day and leave the home and make all these new acquaintances!" It is really a self-destructive and destructive process, luetic in nature. Flirting is second nature for *Fl-ac,* but he consciously disregards his partner's inner personality as he really does not want to know the other person. A lack of closeness to his family often manifests itself in flirting with others. Missing happiness in life, he must compensate by assembling the maximum number of sexual trophies. Rather than real love, sexual pleasure becomes an end in itself. The relationship with each new partner ends once the pair had sex, because the idea of sexuality is purely mechanical and un-psychological, while with most women sexuality is associated with feeling. The thought of sex stimulates him like street drugs would stimulate someone else. Sex is his drug and job. But for all the sexual pleasure and the number of sexual partners he can accrue, he remains inwardly empty. His world is far emptier than that of the real lover, and his life is unfulfilled and senseless.

Creation of an Excessive Persona

Fl-ac, a charming Casanova, seems to have no problems attracting others. His *excessive hilarity, his great buoyancy of mind* is of course attractive to people; *he looks happy and serene and is vivacious in the morning*! *Everything seems satisfactory* to him. Who would not respond to such an apparently jolly fellow who seems to be full of life and is such a smooth talker? We find in *Fl-ac* also a characteristic of *Lycopodium*, *Nux-v* and *Platina*: *being kind with strangers but not with his family and entourage* and ***indifference to loved ones*** *but animated to strangers*. As usual, we have to seek the reasons for this behavior to understand the nuanced differences among these remedies. *Fl-ac is always ogling women on the street* and his mind is occupied with sexual activities as the ultimate goal is to get the target in bed with him; *Lycopodium has love for power* and wants to be recognized by his peers and get ahead in his business; the haughty *Platina* only has respect and awe for someone more intelligent and famous than she is; and *Nux-v* might need that person to further his career or business (*ambition increased*)! This sentiment of *Nux-v* is also expressed by further provings: *avarice as regards his family but generous too much towards strangers*. *Fl-ac* dresses the part, because he knows that "the feathers make the bird." *Fl-ac* is certainly represented among many pimps. He also flip-flops, never hesitating to change his opinion about people he really does not like if it will serve his purpose and hopefully bring him rewards (*hatred, which he vents in words, but a suddenly altered view as soon as he sees the people*). So he can speak badly and hatefully about people, but as soon as he sees them, he changes and greets them with pleasure. In other words he is simply an opportunist with an excessive persona who is only out to make very *superficial* connections to serve his sexual purposes only (*indifference to relations*). His advertisement in the newspaper reads: "Wanted, **overnight** meaningful relationship" (just like *Lycopodium* and *Med*).

Irresponsibility

Another positive tool ("positive" in his sick mind, because everyone else considers it negative) for *Fl-ac* to achieve his goal of creating a fantasy world is ***his neglect of his duty*** towards family (*aversion to members of family; to his wife*) and work environment. He is one of the most warm-blooded *remedies*, obviously, with sensations of heat and a desire for cold baths and showers and a need to walk in open air for relief. His only way of making contact with other people is through an endless stream of fleeting sexual encounters or, at least, attempts at those. He is focused on the *material world* (with *Conium* being the most *materialistic* remedy in the materia medica) and is, naturally, not particularly interested in exploring the spiritual world or any serious conversation (*conversation aggravates* and *mental exertion aggravates*). He has little respect for conventional norms or for the mores of society. The *Fluorine* person does not want to commit himself to his home or business. He has an *aversion to his business*, and an *indifference to business affairs*, with *Sulph* and *Ph-ac*. However, in *Sulphur* and *Ph-acid*, this indifference represents the **end** stage of the remedies, while in *Fl-ac* it is present almost from the **beginning**.

Fl-ac might be *industrious*, with a *mania for work*, but this quickly ends as his lustful behavior takes over; in addition, "work" here is not always what the average person has in mind (*mental work aggravates* and *mental weakness*). Besides his "industrious" side, *Fl-ac* has only one goal: sex and glitter. It is like the rock star (many *Fl-ac* guys) who does not look at his work as business but as a way to indulge (*libertinism*) in all the available material goods and sex. *Ph-acid's* indifference is due to a weakened Vital Force resulting from a longtime illness, grief, or homesickness. *Sulphur's* indifference, on the other hand, results from burnout or invalidation of his deeds, embarrassment, or simply from being cut off from his successful world (*Aur, Arg-n*) upon retirement. With *Fl-ac* it is an *inability to realize responsibility*. *Fl-ac* becomes irresponsible and immoral, while feeling greatly enthusiastic about his existence (*indifferent, takes no interest in a very sick patient; buoyancy; uncommonly gay disposition of the mind, the next morning*). His dreams seem to be the only moralizers. Following the compensation law of dream interpretation, *Fl-ac* has dreams about what happened during the day but also compensating ones about his indifference towards family and loved ones: *dreams of distant acquaintances dying; dreams of sudden death of his little son, and also of the son of one of his friends; thinks in both cases that he is to blame because he has neglected physical examinations and mechanical remedies; reproaching himself very much and weeps bitterly and on waking is very happy that it is not true.* It is clear that guilt in the case of *Fl-ac* shows up first in the messenger of his unconscious, his corrective dreams, but as so many characters do, he dismisses those dreams as nonsense ("It was just a dream") and continues with his debauched lifestyle, *alcoholism* included. At the end, *Fl-ac*, a Casanova who always tries to prove his manhood, becomes a failure by concentrating on the vices of humankind: sex and glory. Rather than giving to life, he always thinks first of what to take from life, therefore missing the opportunity for self-development.

Fl-ac is the true sexual addict, and his four cornerstones are:

1. Lack of morality
2. Increased sexual activity
3. Indifference to family
4. Indifference to his job

Golden Tips from the Masters

- Remedy for gonorrhea (*gleety discharge with swelling of the prepuce*).
- Similar remedy to *Mercury* and *Calc-fl*
- Delayed dentition and recurrent dental caries
- Big keynote: <from heat and ill from warm drinks
- Remedy for *alopecia areata* (*hair falling in spots*)
- #1 remedy for painless varicose ulcers (*Lach*) relieved by cold as well as for bedsores (*Ledum*) and caries of long bones (osteomyelitis)

Gelsemium (Gels). Yellow Jasmine

The Cyber Delusion

Gelsemium is a great remedy for strokes, as well as for other CNS diseases such as multiple sclerosis and transverse myelitis; this remedy has a great affinity for the brain, spinal cord, and motor nerves. *Gelsemium* also has an affinity for the eyes, causing *diplopia and slow accommodation with blurred vision and objects fading away and then reappearing* as well as *droopy eyelids,* so the homeopath knows that this is a great anti-syphilitic remedy to address the miasm that always targets the precious organs! Therefore, the Cyber delusion of *Gels,* that ***of being double*** covers this same idea, and in identifying this we see a delusion that draws our attention because it fits the syphilitic background! There is the *delusion, she is someone else identity,* another syphilitic expression. This corresponds to a split personality or dissociation of the ego, a kind of mild schizophrenic state: there is loss of control of the ego over the conscious life, which will reflect into a dreamlike state of the *Gelsemium* patient. This semi-unconscious state will cause other fixed ideas, reflecting a distortion of the reality conception, especially in that everything appears larger: *delusion, distances are enlarged; the head is enlarged,* and *objects are enlarged.*

As the *Gelsemium* state evolves from neurosis to psychosis, there are times that the danger line is transgressed, and now visual hallucinations are possible: *delusion, he is in his grave,* symbolic for continued regression into the unconscious and loss/disconnection with one's conscious life. The grave is the first place that the soul goes after death. Then there are delusions about snakes: *delusion, sees snakes in and around him; delusion of white snakes.* In order to understand the meaning of these delusions, we need to know the relatively fixed symbol for snakes. The snake can have different meanings depending on the person and the situation; it is the symbol of healing/spiritual awakening, healing/transformation, and resurrection, the shedding of old persona. It stands also for femaleness, the darkness, night, yin, death, and fear. Whenever a snake appears in dreams or delusions, it symbolizes a piece of the instinctive psychology in us, something of tremendous power. It represents the vital, the instinctual, and the drives stirring in man, his unconscious dark side in contrast to brightness (the conscious side of his nature). The serpent in Oriental psychology symbolizes the treasure of wisdom. It can also be a symbol of danger, of being caught in coils, swallowed, or poisoned. A snake is also an anxiety symbol; monkeys and horses, for instance, are instinctively afraid of snakes. When a snake appears at the sickbed in dreams it can indicate foreboding of death. The snake is also a symbol of time: the idea that the snake represents time is probably connected with the fact that it sheds its skin. Some aboriginal peoples interpret this as a reincarnation and infer from it the snake's immortality. The three most important aspects in snake dreams are that of an earth demon, a savior, and a time symbol.

In the case of *Gelsemium*, looking at his NWS, the snake is most often a symbol of danger and anxiety, with a recoiling in the unconscious as a defense mechanism. *Gels* can therefore become a socially anxious person that wants to bond but feels self-conscious or paralyzed (*timidity, appearing in public*). What about the *white* snake? A black snake represents evil, a demon which creates a sense of danger; the integrity of Man is threatened! All of the symbols/archetypes possess, however, a positive as well as a negative meaning. Likewise, positive symbols can be translated the other way around. The womb that creates life can also create death. In one case it is white magic, and in another, black. These images are symbolic of different psychological situations (our individuality law in homeopathy): dreaming of a snake may have different meanings for different people. In *Gelsemium's* case, it seems that the white snake symbol creates life, not death—in other words, a rather good prognosis. Indeed, white stands also for purity, innocence, and the beginning of a new life, the place where new things are born or started. In the case of a *Gelsemium* person whose CD is ***delusion being double***, it is the union of this being double that needs to take place to create the new being, the regaining of his own identity that was disturbed by an event or causality (NWS). This is reflected by the rubric *desire for light*, the coming into consciousness again after being temporarily locked up in the unconscious, represented by the typical five D's of *Gelsemium*: drowsy, dopey, dizzy, dumb and dull. It is a constant struggle for *Gelsemium*, hindered by fears in the unconscious, to be reborn again: the person exhibits *fear appearing in public* and *fear, the child holds on to the mother*, the mother proving symbolic for rebirth, protection, and nourishment.

Causalities

Bad News

In order to find the cause of such disruption of the ego control in *Gelsemium*, we must think of a shock to the person, an ego shock, most likely of a severe mental/emotional nature. Indeed, we see NWS *bad news, anticipation, emotional excitement* and *silent grief,* all to a high degree, as the main causalities. It is really all about hearing bad news, being involved in an earthquake, a tsunami, the loss of a child, a public rejection, a professional failure, a failure in an exam, hearing one has been diagnosed with terminal cancer, all about *ailments from mental shock, even from reproaches*. Provings about its causalities tell us more about this: *bad effects from fright and fear; every exciting news causes diarrhea* (Arg-n); *from anticipation of any unusual ordeal and effects of grief in which she cannot cry (silent grief)*); *after losing a son, she is inclined to brood over her loss and becomes rapt in imagination as she thinks herself at the grave*. Because of *Gelsemium*'s syphilitic nature, such calamities lead almost immediately to a great loss of control of the ego over the conscious life if not to a split of the mind, resulting in a disturbed, quasi-comatose state. Bad news is the worst when it is first received as it bears the weight of surprise. Yesterday you were healthy; today you are a cancer patient. It is doubtless the anticipatory stress that causes most of the initial suffering and anguish. The way *Gelsemium* reacts to a sudden ego threat is often to go numb and paralyzed: just for an instant, time stops, the mind goes blank, and the world suddenly seems unfamiliar. At such moments, our sense of invulnerability is pierced, and the self-protective armor that normally stands between us and our perceptions of the world is torn away, creating a *Gelsemium* state. This loss of control creates the typical *Gelsemium* symptoms: *cataleptic immobility with dilated pupils, dullness of the mind, incapacity to think or fix the attention, sensation of intoxication with diarrhea,* a sense of being paralyzed as *muscles refuse to obey the will when attempting to move and a desire to be quiet; she does not wish to speak nor have anyone near her for company, even if the person is silent*. There is also *shivering and trembling from fear*. One can see the perfect storm created from hearing bad news, reducing the person to a shell of what he was before, naked and unprotected, incapable of doing anything as the intensity of the trauma goes to the deepest levels of the human being, creating a huge vacuum in the ego where her CD will settle down and rule!

Compensations

Hanging on to Familiar People

It should not come as a surprise that *Gelsemium*, a person lost in the unconscious and trying to escape the darkness and regain consciousness, looks to familiar faces for support. Overcome by weakness in his struggle, he *clings to persons and furniture and grasps the nurse when carried and in his fear the child holds on to the mother*. At the same time *there is strong aversion to the presence of others and he desires solitude* and shows *great irritability, and does not want to be spoken to*. *Gelsemium* does not have the guts or spine to confront any situation out of the ordinary such as an appointment with the dentist or an academic test (*cowardice, anxiety anticipating an engagement; complaints from anticipation before going to the dentist, physician and before going to examination*). Inevitably *Gels* is seized with diarrhea (*diarrhea from fear*). Being the complement of *Arg-n*, there is a strong fear of leaving the home as evidenced by *fear for crowds* and *public places, agoraphobia* and *fear appearing in public*: with the perceived weakness and *fear of losing self-control*, *Gelsemium* needs to be assisted by a close relative or friend to move away from his paralytic state. And yet he *needs* to move, as he is overcome with great *fear of death* (remaining in the unconscious): he believes that his *heart will cease to beat unless he is constantly on the move*.

Saving Energy

When unable to gather support, *Gelsemium* will do anything to preserve her small energy reserve so as not to sink deeper into annihilation. *She wants to be quiet, in half reclined position*, and in response to your solicitous questions you can only expect *slow answers or monosyllable answers*, a yes or a no. There is *fear of being touched* on the physical and emotional plane: don't try probing questions with *Gelsemium*; all he can muster is maybe a nod of the head. He is averse to being spoken to, and his speech is confused and incoherent as if intoxicated. It is not for nothing that *Gelsemium* is a complementary remedy to *Arg-n* and *Sepia*, reflecting respectively the anticipation anxieties and fear of losing control of *Arg-n* and the burnt-out state of *Sepia*. However, it is obvious that, in spite of trying to conserve energy, *Gelsemium* slips increasingly into a syphilitic state of semi-consciousness to unconsciousness, almost into a paralytic state on all levels. The brain is so much affected that everything not only seems to happen in slow motion, but also often indicates a disconnection between the signals of the brain and the rest of the body. As we see, the dissociation takes place on the emotional plane (*indifference, apathy; sits still*) and also on the physical plane. This rupture of the ego and the consciousness is reflected in provings such as *when attempting to move, the muscles refuse to obey the will; stupor, cannot open the eyes; the muscles obey feebly or muscles refuse to obey the will when attention is turned away*. The paralysis on the mental plane completes this somnambulistic state: *cataleptic immobility, closed eyes; incapacity to think or fix the attention; unconnected ideas, cannot follow any idea for any length of time; if he attempts to think consecutively, he is attacked by a painful, vacant feeling of the mind; dullness of the mental faculties*. *Gelsemium* indeed is the great paralyzer!

Golden Tips from the Masters

- NWS the flu, when the patient feels as though run over by a truck and cannot muster the strength to even lift a finger! Other flu symptoms: **thirstless**, aching on moving the eyes, shivering up and down the spine and slow pulse. Wiped out and listless, so tired they can't sleep. Head is so tired and heavy that it can't be lifted from the pillow. Flu of mild winters. Lies still like *Bryonia*, but there is more congestion in the head.
- Nervous dread of appearing in public for singers and speakers
- #1 remedy for fear of the dentist
- Remedy for hysteria during pregnancy and labor
- Another possible class 1 remedy for stroke besides *Arnica*: a remedy to restore bleeding as well as to restore consciousness. *Gelsemium's* indications: stroke is characterized by drowsiness, slowness in movement and thick speech leading to unconsciousness; pupils are dilated and there is no stertorous breathing; face is dark red.
- #1 remedy for neurogenic bladder: *no urine flows during effort.* This creates a distended bladder up to the navel; constant dribbling of urine but not a drop flows on making the greatest effort, no pain, not even upon pressure. Total paralysis of bladder.
- Essence: Stupefaction and sluggishness on every level: **the D's:** down, drowsy, droopy, depressed, dizzy, dumb, diplopia, dullness, dropsical, diuresis, delirium, dysphagia, drooped eyelids (ptosis), <downward motion, <damp weather
- NWS mononucleosis (*Carc, Merc*) and flu vaccinations
- MS remedy with diplopia and paralytic weakness
- If a patient has all symptoms of *Gelsemium* but is thirsty, *Ph-ac* is indicated
- Relief of the situation is indicated by passing large amounts of urine
- Insomnia: complete physical exhaustion with the mind brightly awake
- Acute poliomyelitis remedy (*Lat-sativus*)
- Is rarely indicated in superficial affections of the eyes but especially adapted to diseases of the fundus and paralysis of the eye

Graphites (Graph). Mineral carbon

The Cyber Delusion

The Cyber delusion of *Graphites* is ***everything is strange, familiar things seem strange***. What does it reflect or express? What does it mean and where does it come from that, in a *Graphites* state, everything looks unfamiliar, looks foreign? It means that the *Graphites* person is confused and in a daze (*cobweb sensation in face*), not recognizing familiar things, and never feeling surrounded by familiar things or persons. Cobweb sensations belong to other insecure, dependent, exhausted, and dense remedies: *Bar-c*, *Mag-c* and the exhausted *Sul-ac*. The CD reflects a sense of isolation and density. In Jung's typology, *Graphites* would be an introvert sensation-feeling type! Some *of Graph's* characteristics are roughness and hardness, which might be contributing to this sense of strange and unfamiliar surroundings. This roughness and hardness makes it difficult for external stimuli to get through the filter of the ego, and since *Graphites* is a sensation type, this person needs to feel first what the object/subject is before they can explore it further (feeling in the terms of the French word *sensation* and not *sentiment*). This rough outer shell makes it difficult for *Graphites* to connect to others. Having feeling as his secondary conscious function, and with that feeling remaining somewhat primitive and leading to hysterical behavior, it is difficult for *Graphites* to deal with the delusions pertaining to health which always seem to preoccupy his mind: *delusion, of having a heart disease* and *delusion, being sick* at times overwhelm this confused person, leaving him at a loss as to what to do about it (*irresolution*). Withdrawal into the unconscious is expressed by the *delusion, of water* as well as *delusion, sees dead persons* and *delusion, of fancy illusions*. Water in dreams is the relatively fixed symbol for the unconscious, the feminine, the eternal Mother, the womb, or protection for the person. *Graphites*, being the complement to *Calcarea*, has the same need for the Divine Mother's protection, which without he feels very vulnerable in spite of the rough, hard shell—which is also similar to *Calcarea*.

Causalities

Discords

It is the first remedy to think of (together with *Sulphur*) for ailments from *discords between chief and subordinates* (parents and friends), and more notably, from *ailments from discords between one's friends* and *discords between one's parents* (also think *Mag-mur*). This is even more important for *Graphites* than for *Sulphur* since *Sulphur* has more adequate tools than *Graphites* to deal with such discords. *Graphites* is pure carbon, which means that home, friends, parents, and the stability of the family are a source of support and safety for *Graphites*; she needs a peaceful place where she can be nurtured, so discords (especially fights between parents) transform her familiar surroundings into a strange, hostile, and scary place where she can no longer thrive or find peace and security.

These discords are a great source of *grief* and *anticipation anxiety* for the *Graphites* person, two more NWS for this individual. The anticipation anxiety is, rather, a secondary NWS following her confused state as she witnesses the fights between parents. This might also be the main reason for her flight into her illusionary dream world. *Graphites* is not a simple soul like *Bar-c*, but there is a kind of vulnerability, innocence, and transparency about *Graphites*. The *Graphites* person deals with reality directly and without mediation, often with overwhelming intensity. Such discords, the main causality of *constant and chronic grief*, tug at her heart and more often than not release a floodgate of tears, which *relieve her mood*. It is strange that even *organ music*, crude and simple and rather harsh, *makes her cry*, but no doubt it is this type of music that resonates with her mood, just like classical music does the job for *Aurum* and *Nat-m*. But any other kind of *music aggravates*!

Compensations

Inert During the Day, Active at Night

Being besides herself from anxiety, discouraged with anxiety and anguish, Graphites is held like a prisoner during the day. Beset by this host of largely groundless daily concerns (*anxiety about trifles; preoccupied with trifles*) which start the moment she wakes up (*anxiety on waking; easily frightened upon waking*), she does not want to wake up from her dream world to fall into a strange environment, especially one that is confusing and puts so many requirements on her. Even *when sedentary employment and sitting increases her anxiety, she is too occupied with trifles* to do any groundbreaking task (*averse to business with dread of mental work and indolence*; although sometimes very intelligent, *mental or scientific work fatigues*). The *Graphites* person demonstrates an inability to stick with any challenging intellectual task. *Graphites* seems to have an inner voice telling her to get through the day (*inclination to sit still* but also *fidgety while sitting at work*) as the evening will bring relief and energy into her life! Not much gets done during the day, as this *restlessness while at work)* disrupts her concentration with dashes to the refrigerator for "emotional" food (*excessive hunger)*. She gets distracted by every little noise or *other sensual impressions,* anything to bring some relief from this overwhelming emotional anxiety and *strong exhaustion of the whole body,* which prevents any form of exercise and leads to *obesity* (physically akin to her complementary alter ego, *Calcarea*). The only other thing that resonates with *Graphites* is the evening and nighttime. Through Traditional Chinese Medicine (TCM), we see indeed that this dense Yin person will resonate with the most Yin time of the 24-hour daily cycle: midnight (*excitement at night*). So *Graphites* students are like *Medorrhinum* students: they operate mentally best at night but forget everything in the morning, which makes them fearful and irritable (*full of fears in the morning*). Of course this mental excitability at night will also prevent her sleep: *thoughts of many things at night prevent sleep and unable to fall asleep before midnight.* This is especially because the thoughts are not always pleasant or stimulating, but rather depressing ones: *at night, thoughts full of care, from which she could not free herself and which were so distressing that the blood became excited, and she could not sleep the whole night.* In TCM, worry is the main emotion linked to the Earth element—the element to which *Graphites* belongs.

Weeping

We can rarely expect from a *Graphites* person (or from *Carbon* people in general, unless their secondary function is thinking, and even this is limited and rather undifferentiated), that he will be able to connect his physical ailments to his psychological problems. The only tool or reaction that comforts a *Graphites* person is weeping: *extreme apprehensiveness so that she did not know how to overcome it, disappearing after weeping. She was obliged to weep, without cause. She was obliged to weep at music*! As you can see, *Graphites* does not know **why** she weeps; the only thing she knows is that she feels better after weeping! And music will always make her weep and improve. We are not talking about classical music (*Aurum, Natrums*) or rock and roll (*Tarentula*), but very simple music like organ music, one flute and a drum, etc. Even a *Graphites* child in school, in her confused and dense state, will weep and confuse the teacher since she cannot give any reasonable or conscious explanation as to why she is crying. All she knows is that it makes her feel better. Just as other people are puzzled by her behavior, *Graphites* is herself disturbed by it and cannot make any sense of it. Don't ask *Graphites*, "Why are you crying?" This leads to easy *confusion and irresolution*, not helpful in trying to connect to one's inner Self. We see in the provings *extreme hesitation; she is unable to make up her mind about anything, coupled to timidity; weakness in head with dim recollection of recent events; slowness of purpose and carefulness.* Her worry and anxiety, as in any *Carbon* person, is mainly directed at her own person: *solicitude concerning her spiritual welfare; she thinks her end is near and the greatest misfortunes are impending.* The pure *Carbon* has only one world—his own little space—and the homeopath will not find *Graphites* in the rubrics *care, full of, for others or relatives*!

Eventually these emotions lead to the typical *Graphites* depression. Remembering the NWS anticipation anxiety, we are not surprised that *Graphites*, like *Calc-c* (for whom *Graphites* is a great complementary remedy), falls into a depression *from over worry about the simplest things and excitability about trifles.* There is *grief about the slightest occurrences, even to despair* and *sadness with thoughts of nothing but death.* Her dullness in the head, her *weeping without a cause,* and her *irresolution* all lead to a dull depression. *Sad and despondent, she was obliged to weep. She feels miserable and unhappy.* The only favorable thing about *Graph*'s depression is that, because of her blandness and thickness, she never goes into a very deep depression like *Aurum*; rather, she lives to a ripe old age without degenerating into any deep mental pathology such as dissociation of the personality. From there, the secondary delusions are rather infrequent; her lack of comprehension does not produce them, and *Graphites* remains stuck in his CD.

Nature

The other consolation is contact with Nature and trying to connect to the Earth (*Graphites* belongs to the Earth element in TCM). While we cannot expect mental and refined work from *Graphites*, she does like to get her hands dirty in the soil, as if to reach out to something that resonates with her: *indolence, aversion to work, air, in open, ameliorates.* Philosophy is too much for them, as one of my patients, looking at a book on my desk called *Inner Work*, said, "That is too deep for me!" Though an investigation of her shadow side would certainly be beneficial, the unconscious world remains closed to *Graphites*. If *Graphites* ever resorts to painting landscapes, don't expect more than mediocrity; there is nothing of the refined spirit of the *China* artist in her works. She is a dilettante who mainly dabbles in the arts to keep herself busy.

Golden Tips from the Masters

- For gastric and duodenal ulcers relieved by food or drink and by lying down. Predisposition to skin eruptions alternating with duodenal or gastric ulcers
- Premenopausal remedy with onset of weight gain (unhealthy corpulence), uterine fibroids, perspiration, profuse acrid leucorrhea coming in gushes, and low sex drive: *Graphites* is to menopause what *Pulsatilla* is to puberty
- Sterility due to hypofunction of the ovaries
- Cancer regrows in scars: *cancer of mammae, cancer in old cicatrices of mammae*
- #1 remedy for keloid scars
- Restless feet and legs, even hours after retiring. *Graphites* is in deep sleep but rubs his legs
- Eczema with sticky honey yellow discharge (glutinous) and cracked skin, especially behind the ears. Other locations: bends of joints and eczema *capitis* forming massive, dirty crusts which mat the hair. Eyelids of babies are stuck together in the morning.
- #2 remedy for impetigo and intertrigo (*Antimonium-crudum* #1)
- *Graphites* is the *Sulphur* for women!
- Aversion to fish, salt, and sweets
- *Nux-v* and *Graphites* are the best indigestion prophylactics
- Constant constipation in obese people (*Calcarea*)
- Great remedy for anal fissures (*Ratanhia*)
- Sense of smell abnormally acute (such as for flowers)

Helleborus niger (Hell). Christmas Rose or Black Hellebore

The Cyber Delusion

Helleborus' CD is ***everything is new***: *Hell* feels doomed, lost, and dull as everything appears to be different to his senses, as though he must learn even the simplest things anew like a newborn baby or like someone who has lost all past memory after a head trauma (for which *Hell* can be an indicated remedy: *head, internal, concussion*), delivery trauma, or car accident. *Helleborus* is supposed to know how to do these basic everyday things, and yet he does not! *Hell* is the only italic remedy in this delusion rubric, in the company of *Stram* and *Asarum*. *Stramonium*, in his delirious state, is obviously *lost and alone in the wilderness* and everything appears new and scary to him. *Stramonium's* senses, however, are hyper-acute, not dull (*sensitive to light and noise*; *convulsions from light*, and *convulsions from noises, from running water*, reflecting the excitability of the brain < >*Hell*); his reactions are at first psoric in nature (*seeking company and light*). *Asarum*'s CD is *he is incorporeal light*, which reflects the discovery of a new world as he is dissociated from the real one (*his body was lighter than air*; *he is floating in air*) and his sensory senses are extremely acute (*hearing, sensory, acute*; *sensitive to slightest noise*; *scratching on silk, rattling or rumbling of papers is unbearable*). In *Asarum*, there is over excitability of sensory nerves; his nerves are on edge! Only *Theridion* is close to *Asarum* in this excitability, as he is *sensitive to noise aggravating* (hurting) *the teeth and causing nausea*!

Helleborus has its own etiology and picture, different from these previous remedies. Why does everything appear new for *Hell*? Could it be the desire to escape from grief into a fanciful, desirable world (like *Nat-c*, *Nat-m*), or is it that the person wishes to flee from a dangerous and frightful world (*Stram*, *Op*)? Could it be an escape from a real world in which it is physically intolerable to live, therefore making a split necessary to escape harm (*Asarum—sensitive to the slightest noise, striking of clocks and ringing of bells*)? Is it an unbearable psychological trauma whose harm can be avoided only by going into a trance? I had a sweet young *Pulsatilla* girl who was forced to have biweekly visits with her divorced father, who was a sociopath and totally neglected her when she had these visits. Every time she returned to the loving home of her mother, the next morning she would wake up "as if in a trance," not connecting to anyone, family or friends, and this would last for a whole day! These absences were never seen unless she had paid a visit to the father. *Puls* has *delusion, of fancy illusions,* and as sub-rubric, *when falling asleep* (*like Calc-c*). It is an escape for her, and she does not want to wake up out of fear and great anticipation anxiety that she will be returned to the father. Another rubric expressing such absences is *delusion, he is separated from the world,* in which we find *Anac, Anah,* and *Thuja*. At the same time, such inexplicable and cruel treatment must create the delusion *she has done wrong*. How else can an innocent child justify this treatment? A temporary *Helleborus* state was the result of being exposed to the inappropriate environment of her father's home.

In *Hell* there is **dulling**, rather than a hypersensitivity of the senses (in all the previous remedies, initial hypersensitivity on all planes has taken place). *Hell* remains on the other side of the spectrum, numbed and semi-comatose. Hering gives us an apt description of the essence of *Helleborus* in his Materia Medica: *stupor, blunting of general sensibility; vision unimpaired, nevertheless sees imperfectly and does not regard the objects he sees; apparatus of hearing intact, yet hears nothing distinctly nor comprehends; organs of taste in working order, yet finds not the proper taste in anything.*

The above reflects the essence of this remedy very well: in all cases of *Hell*, **stupefaction and numbness** occur to a greater or lesser degree. Sometimes it is complete stupor and sometimes it is only partial, but it is always stupefaction and sluggishness causing *Hell* not to recognize even familiar faces and things. Such a person can sit in a chair for the greater part of the day, gazing fixedly before him or plunging into the absorbed contemplation of a tiny spot, a spot that could hold him for an hour without any urge to shift his eyes. He also acts like the slightest movement requires extraordinary effort, particularly to overcome his initial inertia. To make matters worse, whatever is new in *Helleborus*' world is not positive; rather, it seems horrible for *Hell*, as other delusions express: *delusion, sees devils; pursued by enemies; horrible delusions in the dark; talking with dead people; and sees ghosts; a multitude of fantasies are* ***forced*** *upon him* (*Hell* only remedy; emphasis author's). So it is not desirable for *Hell* to fall into this "new" world: all of the new things referred to in his CD seem scary and incomprehensible to *Hell*. It is this last word, incomprehensible, that truly reflects the essence of *Hell*: not only does everything seem strange, but also *Helleborus*' behavior is incomprehensible and seems rather hysterical to everyone else. How else can one interpret the fact that *Hell* pretends not to be able to hear, yet his hearing is found to be perfectly normal? And that it is the same with the other senses? Is *Hell* a con artist, the class clown, prankster and mischievous guy playing practical jokes on everyone like *Tarentula*, who feigns a disease? Or is *Hell* like *Verat-a*, pretending to be *pregnant, blind and deaf,* just to become or remain a "somebody" in society? *Hell* might look like someone who reacts hysterically or feigns disease (*feigning to be sick, Tarentula, Verat-a, Puls*), but that is not the case, as we will discover.

In his Materia Medica, Kent describes the case of a young child, coming out of a coma with the help of *Helleborus*, suffering tremendously from tingling in the extremities (a sign of the awakening of the central nervous system as well as following Hering's observations).[20] Of course, application of the 5th Edition split method would have reduced this suffering to a great degree. *Hell* is a personality that has seemingly, but not truly, lost his sensory functions (*senses are dull and blunted*): upon physical examination, nothing abnormal can be found. Many children with Autism Spectrum Disorder (ASD) exhibit this symptom and are sent for vision and hearing tests. Is *Hell* a hypochondriac, or is he one of those mystery cases in which a physical exam fails to inform the physician of any causality? As usual, the CD and the NWS must give us an answer! There seems to be another delusion in the second degree: *delusion, he has done wrong*. Is it possible to find this in the NWS? Hering describes a case of hysteria mania:

> "An old woman was accused of theft by the women around and took it so much at heart that she hanged herself. This suicide produced a profound effect upon the women in the village. One after another accused herself of having caused the death of the old woman by their insinuation; they wept and howled, ran about day and night wringing their hands and despairing of salvation on account of their sin; they became quite deranged. In this way 25 women were affected, every fresh case being followed by another."[21]

---

20. Kent, *Lectures*, 517.

21. Hering, Vol. V, 529

One can see the dissociation that took place and the transition from a neurosis to psychosis in these women seized by a form of mania. In modern terms it is called somatic conversion neurosis, and when it leads to uncontrollable twitching of muscles and other Tourette's-like symptoms, it can require either *Helleborus* or *Hyoscyamus*. Such an occurrence of mass hysteria is not uncommon at present: in January of 2012, twelve teenagers in the same high school in New York State were attacked by similar symptoms. Rather than just calling it "conversion syndrome," it would be interesting to find a common emotional etiology, just as in Hering's example above, rather than examining an environmental toxin (which was in fact ruled out). Homeopathy understands better than any other medical modality that susceptibility varies from person to person; if the trigger had been an environmental toxin, more students in such a large school would surely have been affected.

A woman can fall into a temporary *Hell* state when pregnant and, through mystical participation, trigger a *Hell* state and ASD in the child. One such example from my practice:

> The night the child was conceived, the parents-to-be were barged in on by a family member (an aunt) after lovemaking and told they should "Stop it!" The mother-to-be felt angry and guilty, as if she had done something wrong. She felt a black cloud over her ("doom," yes!), and during her entire pregnancy she "did not feel vibrant." When the couple tried to share their joy about the baby's imminent arrival, they were met with negativity on both sides of the family ("How could you get pregnant again so soon? How can you afford it?"). Again the pregnant mother felt she had done wrong. Then, the birth was treated allopathically in a way she did not agree with, and she felt she had done her baby wrong. When I saw her, she still blamed herself, and cried while recounting the story. One can clearly see the formation of the delusion *she had done something wrong.*

Causality

Disappointed Love

Hell mostly suffers *ailments from disappointed love.* The disappointed love can have an extended meaning: it can be a disappointment in any relationship, usually personal, but also professional (for instance, in the case of betrayal by a business partner). Working closely with someone is like creating another marriage or being part of a family as much time is spent together! I remember such a case in my practice: a well-functioning MD, after betrayal by his colleague, went in only two months' time into a very deep *Hell* state, with atrophy of the brain as diagnosed by MRI. He showed all the *Hell* signs, but the damage had become irreversible in a very short time due to the presence of a strong syphilitic background. A *Hell* state is also possible during the aging process (a loss of Kidney essence in TCM), especially in those in whom the syphilitic miasm is strongly present in the family history: *slowness in old people* (caused by multiple brain infarcts; differentiate with *Bar-c*). This different kind of disappointed love is also seen in the corporate world. CEOs of big companies take big bonuses while regular people are laid off. Outsourcing jobs is a common occurrence and company loyalty is rare (from the employer as well as from the employees). *Grief*, therefore, is a rather common *Helleborus* occurrence. Even when *Hell* is suffering from noble misfortunes, he blames himself for the situation he is in: *delusion, wrong, he has done wrong; reproaches himself and anxiety of conscience*, which only increases his growing *despair of recovery*.

Homesickness

One NWS closely related to the previous ones is *A/F homesickness* (*homesickness; forsaken*). Although *Helleborus*' homesickness lacks the intensity and frequency of indicated remedies like *Ph-ac* and *Capsicum*, the homeopath needs to observe the consequences of such an event. With *Ph-ac* it can lead to a very deep depression and indifference to everything; with *Capsicum* it creates insomnia; and with *Hell* it will rapidly destroy the brain, or at least dull the senses and create forgetfulness, bringing the patient into a temporary trance as an escape (as seen in the previous example of the girl in a *Pulsatilla* state). Homesickness relates mostly to young people who move away from their neighborhoods, especially for *Phosphorus* and *Calc-c* types, or even in those away from their protected and loving environments for a weekend. There are also cases in which the child is caught between divorced parents. Suspect *Hell* when such an event is present and when it occurs around puberty (*mental affections in puberty*)! There is also *depression in girls before puberty, in puberty* (*Lachesis*, *Nat-m*) *and during the first menses or menarche* (only remedy) as well as *sadness, quiet, in menarche*, *Hell*, only. *Hell* should be added to the rubric *silent grief from disappointed love* (*Ign*, *Nat-m*, *Ph-ac*).

Head Trauma

One A/F not mentioned in the repertory is *A/F injuries from head trauma* (*head, injuries, of the head, after*). It is very important to remember the possibility of trauma during delivery as the head (often too big like in *Calc-c*) tries to descend in the birth canal and gets stuck. *Hell* should be added to the rubric *head, injuries of the head, after, in children from delivery* (Nat-s, only remedy). One mother of a child with ASD described this process to me as "the head protruding many times in the canal and then receding and finally the baby coming out with a long cone-shaped head, which remained this way for quite some time." Forceps in the past, and now vacuum extraction, can be a real trauma for the rather porous skull of the baby. While allopathy only recognizes a certain percentage of subdural hematomas in these circumstances, it has not acknowledged or recognized this trauma as possible etiology for ADD, ADHD, and other challenges experienced by children. But *Hell*, as a complementary remedy to *Arnica*, remains the main remedy in chronic ill effects of head injuries in children, especially when a slow and gradual decline is seen in the child since such head injury. The connection between the presenting clinical state and the previous head injury can easily be missed and should always be investigated by the homeopath when treating children with special needs (CSN). The homeopath must always inquire about the birthing process and its duration, which, with dullness of the mind, might point to *Hell*.

Compensations

How will the homeopath recognize children and adults alike who need this remedy? Will they be able to explain themselves well enough? How do they present, and how can we get these victims out of such an unfortunate state? Every remedy has compensations, and unfortunately *Hell* does not possess very many positive tools. We would all like to see some possible psoric compensations. At least that would give *Hell* a chance, if not to avoid, at least to delay the descent into the abyss of destruction (*has no more desires*), presenting the homeopath with an opportunity to remedy *Hell* before he reaches such a dull state that finding the simillimum becomes more difficult.

Occupation

Helleborus' psoric and sycotic phases are very short, and the patient falls quickly into an abyss of unconsciousness and symbolic darkness. *Helleborus*' etiologies (disappointed love, grief and head trauma) must be of such intensity, and striking individuals with a strongly inherited syphilitic tendency, that a break occurs rapidly (< > to *Plb*), completely and suddenly, leading to blunted sensory perceptions. There is no time for the *Hell* person to form defensive psoric and sycotic compensations. Only trying to get the patient's attention for a while, engaging her and keeping him preoccupied (we call it "redirecting" for CSN or ASD patients) seems to ameliorate; *but the muscles refuse to obey the will when the attention is turned away, and therefore Hell will drop things* (*extremities, awkwardness*).

Company

Is company a positive tool? It certainly looks as though this individual needs company to get through life. No! *He has aversion to the presence of others and desires solitude yet at night he has fear of being alone*! The patient fears being alone because of his extreme helplessness, and usually it is the family that needs to explain the patient's situation to the doctor because the patient cannot express his ideas. (*Reflects long before answering and answers slowly. His answers are confused as though he is thinking of something else.*) A *Hell* patient has difficulty making contact with his homeopath: *thoughtless staring* (also *Puls*) and *he is suspicious*. The patient can be roused as the homeopath tries to engage him, and the *Hell* patient will attempt to say something, attempting to move, to gesture; but *Hell* simply stares at the doctor with eyes partly open, with a dazed expression on his face. When questioned he is not able to tell you what is on his mind (*dullness, says nothing; deficiency of ideas*). The homeopath sees the suffering in his eyes and facial expressions; only a few audible tones are heard, silent tears are present and there is a silent plea for help (*blank; automatism; as if in a dream; feeling of helplessness*).

Further Breakdown

In TCM, brain formation depends on the Kidney organ, and the short-term memory is also a function of the Kidney. This is well expressed in the homeopathic provings regarding *Helleborus*' break: *weakness of memory for what he has heard; for what he has said* and *for what he is about to say* (all black type). Hahnemann says: *Hell could not retain what he had read one instant*. When such a child starts a new school year, he has forgotten everything from the previous year: it is as if he has learned nothing! As the breakdown evolves, *Hell* can't remember his name, birth date, or address (*Cyber delusion, everything is new*), as if the mental level has split off from the physical level. At first, *Hell* realizes this and is very annoyed by it. At this point, he asks for sympathy (*consolation ameliorates*) and help but is unable to explain what is wrong with him. There is even *sadness on seeing others happy* (*Hell* only remedy!), as if he is totally removed from such happiness. In this stage at which sympathy and occupation ameliorate, *Hell* appears more like *Phosphorus* or *Puls*. For a short time, he even has the impression that he can function well again, and he is full of grandiose and delusional ideas and plans, but shortly afterwards he becomes forgetful and confused (*deeds, feels as if he could do great, Hell* only remedy*)* and is unable to accomplish anything. It was only a glimmer of hope and lucidity, a small flame that died quickly. Contrary to *Plumbum*, there is not much violence at all in this remedy (*seeks to escape but is not violent*), because rapid brain destruction changes him into a rather stuporous, helpless, and indifferent person with *bruised pain in the head with stupidity, in one and now in another part of the brain* (Hahnemann). Only for a short time, violence is possible (*Hell* is found in the rubric *striking, and rage, fury).* And then comes the total indifference: *indifference to loved ones, to pleasure and to relations,* all black type; *indifference, has no action of the will* and *indifference to suffering* are not so much the expression of a burnt-out person like *Sepia* or *Ph-ac*, but rather the reflection of a non-functioning, destroyed brain; the patient slips away into a world of darkness, reflected in a deep depression, somewhat different from *Ph-ac*: *dull and indifferent to all external expressions; will not speak and sits quietly in bed and seems lost in brooding; will take food when offered but never expresses desire for anything.* It is a condition in which true depression and weakness is present and in which the patient is governed by fixed ideas. A six-year-old *Hell* child in my practice presented as follows:

> He was a very sweet, docile, taciturn, eerily content child. When he wanted to play with his Play-Doh (he responded to sensation on his palms and feet) but could not (if it were time for him to eat or something else intervened), he hit his mom (*striking, and rage, fury).* He had no remorse, but I don't think he understood (*indifference to loved ones*). He felt no empathy, nor did he feel his own pain (*Generalities, painlessness of complaints usually painful*). He was totally shut off. He never made eye contact with his mom and lived completely in his own world. His needs and his responses were very primitive. The mother was told that his functioning was like that of a four-month-old. We see clearly the *Hell* picture emerging. How did the boy react to *Hell*? He made progress after just a few doses LM1, though he always spit out most of the dose. Then, he got his

> first full dose—one teaspoon from the RSB, one teaspoon from the cup. The mom reported "regression" for three days: three nights in a row, he was "stirring, kicking in his sleep, like he couldn't get comfortable, couldn't relax." He cried inexplicably, and even urinated several times during the night, including one time on the floor. (He usually slept soundly.) Then, after the three tumultuous nights, he woke up, smiled, and said, "Happy!" His first real communication ever! He made eye contact, and his mom said, "Now he's reaching out to us!" He had become interactive, understood questions, and was performing appropriate imitation. He began to sleep well again! He continued to progress for several weeks, with no repetition of the remedy, until later when an adjusted dose was given, a smaller amount, with drops instead of the teaspoon. This is highly reminiscent of Kent's *Hell* case in his practical Materia Medica.

Mind work becomes impossible: *mental work is impossible; Hell has no more desires; there is difficult concentration, deficiency of ideas, and even imbecility*. Hering calls it *a perfect picture of acute idiocy*! *Hell is dull and says nothing; there is stubborn silence* and, at this point, *consolation aggravates. There is diminished power of mind over the body, he cannot fix ideas.* No wonder that, if not remedied, *Hell* returns to his CD. He has sunken into a new world, separated from everyone, and he is hopelessly lost. The homeopath recognizes a kind of Alzheimer and ASD situation in this helpless and absent-minded person.

Golden Tips from the Masters

- Melancholia in girls at puberty before menstruation has been established or if menses have appeared and then failed to return
- *Hell* is useful in affections of brain and spinal cord. *Hell* is mainly indicated in **inflammation** of the brain (meningitis, encephalitis, hydrocephalus, after typhoid fever, ecclampsia with convulsions, cortical blindness) but also after concussion of the brain when *Arnica* fails. One warning: the remedy acts slowly (compare to *Gels*) when given in these cases of brain and spinal trouble. When a reaction appears (perspiration, diarrhea or vomiting), do not interfere. This is a sign of the CNS coming back to life. If the patient has vitality enough to recover, he will do so now. If you stop the vomiting, the *Helleborus* action will be antidoted! Leave it alone; it will pass and the patient will be cured!
- In case of brain bleeding, *Hell* could be a complementary remedy to *Arnica*. *Hell* is indicated in the case of stupor remaining after a brain operation.
- What is amazing is his very high threshold for pain: *generalities, painlessness for complaints usually painful* (*Op*, *Stram*)
- Late learning to walk because of loss of power of muscles; weakness of gait; can only walk slowly; can walk but slowly on account of weakness of feet. Sudden relaxation of muscles; great debility. Muscles refuse service when not governed by strong attention and will
- Similar to *Opium* in coma
- For cases of hydrocephaly and epilepsy

Hyoscyamus (Hyos). Black Henbane

The Cyber Delusion

The *Hyoscyamus* child seems to be overly dependent on one single person, usually the mother. Without that person, *Hyos* cannot function; that one person is his lifeline! The very peculiar delusions of *Hyoscyamus* will tell us what drives him to do and think as he does. In the mind of this child, or adult, he has served his purpose and is no longer needed or wanted. In other words, his welcome has worn out! The *Hyos* child has the paranoid delusion that he will be sold: a newcomer (which can be a new baby in the family) is receiving (at least in his mind) his mother's entire attention, and now he feels he has been reduced to the status of someone who is disposable. *Hyos* feels threatened by the arrival of a new sibling, and in order to defend his position, he is willing to destroy life around him. He thinks that his mom only has eyes for the newcomer, and he therefore believes that he will be given away, as expressed in his Cyber delusion: ***he is being sold*** (*jealousy, when the newborn gets all the attention*). The psychological compensations and consequences of the acceptance of this belief are the same whether the threat is imagined or real: *Hyos* is fighting for his very survival, the greatest human instinct!

This Cyber delusion of *Hyos* has been nourished and preceded by another delusion: *he is going to be married,* and *delusion, of a wedding* (*Oedipus/Electra complex*), which shows how important this very intimate relationship is for him and how many expectations *Hyos* attaches to the beloved person (*delusion, of fancy illusions*). So in the mind of children with the *Hyoscyamus* Cyber delusion, just as they start feeling confident of the love of their parent, someone else displaces them. A common trigger is the birth of a sibling, and the *Hyos* state can also be fueled when another relative comes and lives with his family, or even a new pet that gets some attention, thus creating in the mind of a child in this state that his Mom is not true and faithful in her love for him (*delusion, wife is faithless*). Or Mom decides to resume a job after a long period of being at home, and the message the child receives is that of being cast away, whether he is sent to a nursery or saddled with a babysitter! The fixed idea that he is going to be sold will intensify in the *Hyos* child when the well-meaning parent subsequently takes his little security blanket or his pacifier away, which is usually done to signal to the child that he is now a "big boy." Furthermore, *Hyos* is very alert to every step his mom takes, and as soon as she leaves bed in the morning, he follows her everywhere she goes (*desire for company, aversion to solitude*). He doesn't want to share her with anyone! The *Hyos* person, child or adult, has an immature ego which does not allow for anyone to take away the attention of the subject of his love (mother, father). He swears, he hits, throws, kicks, and screams when angered, especially when he perceives that the younger sibling has interrupted his time with his mother (*cursing; desire to break things; desires to bite; mania with rage*). *Violent anger, playing antics* and *childish behavior* symbolically reflect an expression of *greed, where he grasps greedily with both hands anything that is offered to him*. It is the Oedipus complex described by Freud: the struggle of the son to overthrow the father and possess the mother. In the case of an adult who has been stuck since childhood, it is the immature, codependent person who lives and breathes through the other person (lover, best friend, even you as the homeopath). All these events can be translated into the *delusion, he was in the wrong places*!

This child thinks that, at any moment, he will be sent away to school and never allowed to come back, or that the family might move away in the middle of the night and leave him alone. Nightmares are therefore common occurrences and can be used as a handy excuse to go to the mother's bed at night. The child is possessed with fears that show his deep insecurity in the domain of love, which should be his natural emotional home. But once such a fixed idea has gotten hold of him, no reasonable amount of reassurance can still his relentless need for constant proof of love. He wants to know: "Do you really love me?" This excessive reassurance-seeking occurs when people experience self-doubt and desire strong relationships; in order to feel more confident and connected to his mother, *Hyos* asks for signs of love and acceptance. There is nothing wrong with asking for reassurance now and then, and most people are happy to provide it. But *Hyos* goes overboard and asks over and over again. He winds up pushing people away or aggravating them, and the reassurance stops, which creates even more self-doubt and the conviction that he will be sold! Ignoring the desperate pleas of this child only leads to a reinforcement of his delusion of abandonment. It is here that the indicated homeopathic remedy will bring great relief to the whole family and dissolve the mother complex described by Freud.

To some extent, we all have ambivalent or mixed feelings towards others, especially for those who are closest to us (parents and siblings). For instance, being in love with one parent and feeling hatred towards the other (an Oedipus/Electra complex) is something we have all felt at some point in our lives (if we want to be honest with ourselves) and something that will always be part of the material of psychic impulses. Unlike most people, who try to release themselves from the prenatal psyche at the age of five, in the case of *Hyos*, the person is totally stuck in this complex. What Freud intended to posit with the Oedipus complex was **not** that little boys normally have fantasies in which they have sex with their mothers. What they want, according to Freud, is sole possession of their mothers, while they experience their fathers as rivals. Like one of my patients said, "If Daddy dies then I will marry Mommy." Another said, "I kicked Daddy out of his bed and gave him mine" (after which he moved into Mom's bed). Thanks to Freud's explanation, we can better understand why we don't have to feel guilty about these mixed feelings. Sex is natural and innocent. Freud called the sex drive *libido.* From age five on, an integration of sexual aspiration takes place, and for boys, the mother is the object (Oedipus complex). This comes to an end and is replaced by a period of more or less complete latency during which restraints are built up against the Oedipus complex. During puberty, the Oedipus complex is revived in the unconscious and starts a fuller transformation to include the other sex in general. However, a *Hyos* person never reaches this stage; in *Hyos*' case, the Oedipus complex remains firmly in place way beyond puberty!

Once these two delusions are present (*delusion, he is sold* and *delusion, he is going to be married*), the impetus is provided for other fixed ideas to arise; an immature ego and arrested psychological evolvement easily produce more delusions than a mature ego. What is in store for him? Now he starts imagining the ways in which people will dispose of him: *delusion, he is about to be poisoned—Lach, Kali-br and Rhus-t; complaints of having been poisoned; believes himself poisoned*); *delusion, he will be murdered; delusion, he will be bitten; delusion, he is about to receive an injury; he is injured by his surroundings,* and *he is pursued by the police.* No wonder we see such statements about *Hyos* in Hering's provings as *she received her physician, conversed intelligently, but would not wear a single garment of any kind; refused medicine and cunningly evaded all strategies to receive it.* Of course, in *Hyos*' mind, there exist good reasons that people want to dispose of him. *Hyoscyamus*' fertile yet infantile mind has no difficulty creating more delusions: *delusion, thinks he is demoniacal; delusion, he is a criminal; delusion, he has neglected his duty; delusion, he has offended people* (the object of his desire) and *delusion, he has done wrong.* We see clearly here the expressions of *guilt* and *self-reproach*. The depth of his grief about being left and about a perceived break is so extensive that it produces an array of new delusions: from *fears to be left alone* to *delusion, he is forsaken* and *delusion, he has lost the affection of his friends*; he is convinced that he is *injured by his surroundings* (similar to *Lachesis* with regard to the rival for his love subject), *that he has suffered wrong* and *that he is persecuted*: *he complains of the injustice that he imagines has been done to him* (*Staph*). These delusional provings express *Hyos*' sense that everyone is out there to deceive, cheat, and trick him—in other words, a fixed idea of *being wronged*! From all the delusions discussed above, we can see that *Hyoscyamus* is a promising remedy for cases of persecution mania, the simplest form of a schizophrenic state!

There is of course another reason, besides having an immature and primitive ego, for being so clingy and dependent: this is a very dependent, naïve, and insecure individual for whom the world remains a place of great danger. We see this in the delusions *of animals, of crabs; seeing devils*; *people are swine*, and *delusion, devoured by animals*. In such terrifying circumstances, in such a threatening world, who would not want to be hanging on to a dependable source of nourishment, the mother, expressed by the *delusion, he is away from home and must get there*, (home being the relatively fixed symbol off the womb, the mother, the Divine Mother)! In children suffering in a *Hyoscyamus* state, these fixed ideas are often the source of parallel dreams about monsters (*fear, of waking from a dream*; *frightened easily on waking from a dream*).

Hyos' dreams reflect his conscious attitude: there are dreams *of war* (with rivals) accompanied by the jerks of fighting arms and legs, *lascivious dreams* (parallel to conscious attitude), *and anxious, frightful and threatening dreams*. As these are all dreams of an immature ego, they possess a parallel nature, reflecting the present daily conscious nature rather than a compensating one.

Causalities

Jealousy and Disappointed or Unhappy Love

The greatest trigger is *jealousy and grief about a faithless lover*. The faithless lover is, of course, the parent, the subject of love, around whom the Oedipus/Electra complex is created. The prenatal psyche is formed mainly by the mother before the age of five after which a separation needs to take place. When this does not take place, the manifestations of imbalanced behaviors from the undeveloped ego are called regressive infantile behavior. Rather than stimulating the formation of a growing ego, the ego remains archaic and primitive, and the path to becoming an individual is obstructed. Here is a proving of an **adult** in Hering's Materia Medica that reflects also the attitude of a *Hyos* child. *A gentle, lovable woman became extremely jealous of her husband and although fully realizing that she did him injustice, she was so filled with grief that she found no rest day or night, and could neither drink nor eat.* With *Hyos*' primitive, regressive infantile ego, this jealousy leads to rage and a desire to kill the competitor (younger sibling, pet, or rival) so that he can marry his mother. *Hyos*' hostility is aroused by the frustration of seeing that another person (Dad) is loved by someone (Mom) whose love he desires; or, in the case of an adult *Hyos* person, someone else is chosen by the beloved.

This child always thinks that the other children are favored, and that not only his parents, but also his teachers, are partial to others; he feels that everyone is out to deceive him. He has a strong desire to be close to someone and always feels like an outsider. How can such obstruction to the ego formation occur? When his mother has suffered an incident during the pregnancy, the shock of an event prompting a jealous fit (which is not uncommon for a woman who has been overcome by state of insecurity) will be transferred through the psychological umbilical cord to the unborn fetus; very soon after birth, possessiveness can be seen in the clinging and demanding behavior towards the mother. The young child needs to be held or rocked to and fro all the time, or starts crying and moaning even in his sleep. *Hyoscyamus* is mainly a jealous remedy for **men** and male children. Its female counterpart is *Apis*! *Apis*' essence is of pent-up sexual feelings inadequately expressed, leading to inappropriate actions such as *nymphomania* (erotic insanity), *lewd behavior, salacious talk* and *foolish behavior*. We see much of the same behavior in *Hyoscyamus* (*dresses indecently; wraps up in fur in the summer; gestures, makes gestures like an actor; imitation, mimicry*). *Hyos*' jealousy leads to dangerous dimensions in adults as there is *a desire to kill with a knife in their rage* which often leads to stalking of their victims. Short of the death of a loved one, the end of a long-term relationship is one of the worst emotional blows one ever experiences. But *Hyos* reacts to rejection like a drug user going through withdrawal. Days and weeks after the breakup, he only can think of his lover and his behavior is like those addicts that are deprived of their substance of choice. This romantic rejection creates an intensity of pain, which compels the spurned *Hyos* to stalk his ex-partner; he is willing to do just about anything to make the pain go away, killing included! *Hyos* believes himself to be disrespected and disliked. *Hyos*' defense against pain is refusing to acknowledge that the relationship is over, which precludes healing and requires homeopathic doses of *Hyos*. He continues to pine for the lost love with little hope of relief. Many stalkers need this remedy to cure them of their unnatural obsession!

Fright

When one feels or perceives that he is all alone and forsaken with no friends or family caring for him, fright becomes a great trigger for the enhancement and perpetuation of the state of neediness and jealousy (*fear of being alone; fear of being betrayed*). The child who has been saddled with this unprocessed weight is one that is easily frightened upon waking, even from a short nap, when the transition from unconsciousness to consciousness occurs; he will subsequently submerge himself in the controlled world of *fancy illusions* that he has fashioned (*antics, plays; gestures, ridiculous or foolish*). The tension in his unconscious life is illustrated by *strong grinding of teeth, moaning, clenching the fingers, shrieking, babbling* and *muttering and twitching* and *jerking of the extremities*. He also can suddenly *start as from a fright* in the middle of his sleep, which relates to the fright that reigns in his unconscious; in the unconscious, the absence of inhibitory actions leads to his strong fears. When fright or grief is strongly present, it can trigger *convulsions* and epilepsy in the child with *enuresis, shrieking, grinding of the teeth* and *purple face with projecting eyes.*

Fright in general, and also in *Hyos*' case, can lead to a sudden loss of speech (regression), for instance after witnessing violent quarrels between one's parents. Or the seed can be planted in the embryo or fetus if the mother-to-be is left by her partner during the pregnancy, or if violent actions occur between them (for instance, rape of the mother leading to the pregnancy):

I remember a *Hyoscyamus* patient, a child, who was so intensely afraid that not only could he not discuss fear, he did not want think of it! As with any *Carbon* personality, there is intense fear of being injured and suffering pain. I had another young *Hyos* patient who was traumatized by his experience of 9/11: he obsessed over it and talked about it constantly. He had a picture reminding him of the incident in his room and looked at it often. This went on for about two years! His mom was understandably exhausted by having to constantly talk about the collapse of the towers, yet her son was truly fascinated by it (*mind, talk, dwells on one subject*). *Hyos* fears scary movies, going to the physician, or sticking his head under water.

These all make him feel unprotected (*constant fear of everything*). *Hyoscyamus* likes one-on-one contact and withdraws when a lot of people talk at the same time. *Hyos*' biggest *fears are for people* and *being alone*; he is not particularly afraid of the dark. The mother of a child I was treating for ASD reported to me that she had initially thought that her child had a fear of the dark since he refused to go upstairs at night (when it was dark), but when she asked him what he was afraid of, he said, "There could be someone there who is going to stab me with a knife!" (*Hyos* has the strong desire to kill with a knife, and he thinks everyone else is like him!) So it was not an overwhelming fear of the dark but *fear of people* and the delusions *he will be murdered* and *he is about to receive an injury*, as well as the *delusion, people are swine* that roamed in this boy's unconscious! This is an important lesson for the homeopath to always ask one more question in order to arrive at an understanding of the real rubric! This same boy had a toy man in the basement that he had stabbed numerous times with a toy knife, a warning to take very seriously the mind of this youngster! He also would send all of his little toy animals to the slaughterhouse where a toy man slashed them with a knife, and he loved helping his mom cut watermelon by stabbing it. *Hyos* was successfully administered to this young man before the unconscious dark forces led him to despicable acts!

Compensations

Regressive Behavior

How does *Hyos* recapture the attention of the beloved person and tie her to him in permanent union, his ultimate goal? Regressive behavior (such as thumb-sucking, bedwetting, talking with a baby voice, and escaping into a dream world) is one path toward successful compensation. Jealousy when Mom is talking to some other person on the phone can also lead the child to pass stool in his trousers: *Hyos* has *involuntary stool from excitement*. In order to gain back the adoration of his mother, he will resort first to infantile behavior: since the newborn baby seems to get all the attention from the parent, it seems logical to desire to be a baby again, as this seems to be the ticket to receiving the unconditional love he so much hopes for. And if that does not work, violence and jealousy towards the younger sibling erupt; there may even be murderous attempts (*violent rage, tries to kill people*; *jealousy, between children, when the newborn gets all the attention-abusive*). I had a little patient who for years convinced his little sister that she had been bought at a farm in Texas; he even drew up a certificate of purchase! Without any prompting from adults, this emotionally charged boy turned everyday family life into a daily drama for his sister, competing for what he saw as the starring role in the family. Feeling that he was short of maternal affection (which was completely unjustified), he became destructive, rebellious (*violent anger with red face*), abusive (*children insulting parents*), depressed (*sadness from disappointed love*) and anxious as the perceived experiences of deprivation became incorporated into his own self-evaluation (*delusion, he is forsaken*). It did not help that his grades dropped while his sister got straight A's, was conscientious, well behaved and cared about school. This all changed when homeopathic *Hyos* relieved him of his demons. Children only *seem* to share the same home and parents. In reality, they inhabit different microenvironments, influenced by miasmatic inheritance, maternal emotional traumas during pregnancy, constitution, temperament and sensitivity. In his fertile mind, *Hyos* creates a world for himself in which he is married to his mother (*thoughts of marriage*). Any rival needs to be eliminated (whether younger sibling or father), and *Hyos* can act on his fantasies with violent deeds. Sometimes such a child either regresses or gets stuck on his path of development, remaining a "mama's boy" for life.

Sexual Misconduct

If a child is convinced of the "unfaithfulness" of his parent, or if an adult is convinced of the unfaithfulness of his partner (*fear being betrayed; wife is faithless*), besides obsessively controlling the unfaithful one, he may use the most primitive of tools—sexual behavior—to turn the tables in his favor again (*erotic mania accompanied by jealousy*). As Jung knew, most of the troubles in a "marriage" (which is also the perceived love union of the child to the parental figure) consist in a cunning invention of irritating topics which have absolutely no foundation. The primitive *Hyoscyamus* will resort to extreme compensation and, as we expect, to rather crude behavior which is as old as humankind: sexual expressions! Few characters are as cunning as *Hyoscyamus* (except, perhaps, for *Tarentula*, who also uses his sexual powers to attach his victim to him): thoughts, trickery, and behaviors are routine for *Hyos* to catch the attention of the "unfaithful lover" (parent or spouse). From the moment the *Hyoscyamus* child is aware of his sexuality, this becomes his main weapon, and we can speak of an incestuous tie to the mother. Such a tendency to remain bound to the mother is in constant conflict with the normal development of a child: to be born, to progress, and to grow. When can we normally see this sexual awakening? Jung divided the development of the libido into three periods:

first, a pre-sexual phase which ends at about the age of three; the second stage is one at which boys normally develop the Oedipus complex and girls develop the Elektra complex. In the third phase, beginning at around age five to six, the child should direct his libido *away* from the family. If it leaks incestuously backwards, regression and neurosis ensue. This is what happens to the *Hyoscyamus* person: libido-wise, there is no turning away from the mother or father figure. More than with any other remedy, overt sexual behavior is evident. "I give myself fully to you" is the message. "I want to be on the most intimate terms with you, and no one should come between us." *Hyoscyamus*' ways of sending not-so-subtle messages to her lover are manifold: *lies naked in bed and prattles; loves smutty talk; sings amorous and obscene songs; erotic mania accompanied by jealousy; masturbation since childhood; has always been attracted to the opposite sex and prematurely busied himself with thoughts of marriage* (*delusion, of a wedding*); *lascivious mania, uncovers body, especially sexual parts; goes about nearly naked, will not be covered; constantly throwing off bedcovers or clothes; entire loss of modesty; he lies in bed nude and walks in a fur during summer heat; desires to be naked and especially inclined to unseeing and immodest acts, gestures and expressions; amativeness, nymphomania* and *erotomania*.

This is a child who loves to walk naked at home. Besides an expression of sexual behavior, Kent explains this wish to go naked also as an expression of **hyperesthesia of the skin:** he cannot bear clothes on him not because he is too hot but because he cannot bear the touch of clothing on his skin. Hence, even when it is cold, he tends to undress and be naked. But sexual misconduct is a powerful tool for the child. He will come into the room where his mom is talking to a friend and touch her breast and kiss her on the mouth. He is constantly playing with his genitals and grabbing at his sibling's butt. He wants to remain in bed sleeping with Mom, as this is his "right." Unfortunately, a divorced mothers or widow can unconsciously encourage this behavior by allowing the *Hyos* child to sleep with her. Some mothers allow their children to sleep with them when Daddy is on a trip: wrong move with a *Hyoscyamus* child! I even had one young male *Hyos* patient telling me, "I sold my bed to my daddy!" Children in a *Hyos* state often touch their genitalia in presence of others (*genitalia, handles*), have their hands continuously in their pockets handling their genitalia (*Bufo*), drop their towels in front of Mom when coming out of the shower, play sexual games with other children (straddling a friend, for instance) or curse with sexual words. *Hyos* is shameless and exposes himself outside (urinates constantly in public). Of course, a differential diagnosis with *Medorrhinum* and *Fl-ac* is necessary with this behavior.

As long as the *Hyoscyamus* patient finds a sexual outlet, he is protected from a total psychic breakdown or psychosis and paranoia, which is a more advanced stage. One can imagine that this sexual and foolish behavior starts annoying parents and others alike, especially when it is very much in the open, seemingly without any shame or inhibition (*entire loss of modesty*). I treated young male *Hyos* patients who would try to force themselves into the shower with their mothers or would talk continuously about sex and wanting to marry their mothers in the presence of others. Some threatened to kill their fathers and little sisters so that the way would be free to marry their mothers. *Hyoscyamus* boys often grab their mothers' breasts constantly or put their heads on her chest. Cuddling in bed, as innocent as it might appear, is a come-on and provides confirmation for *Hyoscyamus* that **he** is the husband.

Foolish Behavior

Sexual misconduct is not the only trick up his sleeve. What if this compensation to garner all attention does not work? Are there any other available to *Hyoscyamus*? Certainly, attention is obtained by talking constantly to the source of affection; if it is not about sex he is talking (*lewd talking*), it is more like *constant unintelligible chattering and talks about imaginary wrongs and makes abrupt, short answers to imaginary questions*; *there is talking in sleep*, and *also sings constantly* and *talks hastily, but indistinctly*. *Hyos* becomes a show-stealer, spinning riveting scenes out of dull moments and stirring up tempests during peaceful times (*antics, playing*; *mind, makes gestures, like an actor*). Of course it looks like foolish behavior, another compensation in which the *Hyoscyamus* patient excels in order to draw attention: *foolish laugher*; *does foolish things, behaves like one mad person*; *comical alienation of the mind and performs ludicrous actions like monkeys*; *makes ridiculous gestures like a dancing clown, like one who is intoxicated*. Such a character might add a welcome splash of color to a black-and-white scene, but *Hyos*' insatiable hunger for attention looks more like a symptom of arrested development, which is just what it is! If he does not keep his need for an adrenaline rush and a captive audience (besides mom) in check, he risks spinning himself into a caricature—resented for the chaos he creates and inevitably labeled in school as having ASD, OCD, or ADHD (or, when older, a histrionic personality). He can become an extreme drama queen. This child makes noise, flails around, and possibly throws temper tantrums in order to get others focused on him and his needs, fearing that otherwise he will not be taken care of. The live case of a 12-year-old *Hyos* child was presenting during one of my seminars, but before we commenced the intake interview he used the lights of the projector to make all kinds of gestures to amuse himself (*makes gestures like an actor*). In addition to his generally foolish behavior, there was also sexual innuendo seen during the evenings, as he pleaded with his mom to kiss him on the mouth and was constantly talking about marrying her.

Violence

If sexual and foolish behavior does not work, this child will resort to violent outbursts, threats, and temper tantrums provoked by jealousy, suspicion, and disappointed love, especially when interrupted or disturbed while playing on the computer (*malicious, spiteful and vindictive*) or *contradicted*. He will *strike bystanders in the face without provocation. He wants to kill somebody or himself*; he demonstrates *ungovernable rage with exhibition of unusual strength*; he *is violent and beats people, hits his head against the wall, bites, scratches and nips everyone interfering with them* and *tries to injure those around him*; he has *convulsions after trying to swallow*; he *strikes at bystanders and can scarcely be restrained, looking very wild. In these fits he has a desire to break things*. One of my *Hyos* patients was filled with rage when a boy flipped him off at the playground. He told me that he wanted to do something to this boy, at the very least flip him off in return (*delusion, he was wronged*). These fits of passion are often followed by *melancholia, lack of appetite, restless nights, timorous, hides himself, being speechless* and *exhibiting a loss of strength*. Such sudden fits, especially in a pre-verbal child, can also stem from recollections from the past, even intra-utero: *involuntary recollections of past events*. This can be a strong emotional or violent event that affected the mother and imprinted itself on the child's memory (like the rape of the mother leading to his existence), released from the unconscious suddenly when the original painful event is touched upon by a word, gesture, or event. And then we can see *weeping and whimpering in his sleep*. Violence can even be evoked by hearing someone chewing and swallowing food (*sensitive to noise*).

The *Hyos* child loves to pester and annoy his dog or cat, another competitor for the love of his parent. If the dog chews up his toy, the child wants to "hurt him," often with a knife! The same child who stated the foregoing held a kitchen knife in his hand at one point, saying, "I want to kill something." And when playing with his toys, he pretended he was using a knife to chop his dog's head off.

A *Hyoscyamus* person is usually quite cheerful, gay, and happy unless provoked. He is also is quite shy (*timidity*) when around others, so much so that other people have no idea how angry and violent he can become. Overall, the *Hyos* child is less violent than the

Stramonium or *Belladonna* child, but what sets the *Hyoscyamus* child off when he strikes out is the perceived lack of total attention, and even more commonly feeling disappointed or being denied what he feels he deserves. If he sees a FedEx or UPS truck and there is no package delivered for him, he goes bonkers! Also for example, let's say that the library is closed. The child is begging his parents to go and is taken there, only to confirm that it is indeed closed; he starts crying and, once in the car on the road home, he lashes out in total despair; he can hit, pull, or bite. It can even happen if he is not allowed to do something he wants to do, or if he does not receive an expected present when going out (he always expects to get a present). He is very sensitive: if, when helping him to write or type, Mom misunderstands and chooses the wrong word; he goes berserk.

Restlessness

He *runs about in the room, wants to get out of bed at night, tossing around,* and *climbs on furniture. He touches everything out of restlessness* and wants to leave home, yet when outside, he wants to come back home (*wants to get up and attend to business or go home [Bry]*). He picks at his fingers and makes *automatic gestures, grasping or reaching at something, as if intoxicated. He imitates spinning and stamps the feet* (makes gestures). He always has to do something; he is always in action: one of my young *Hyos* patients was continually riding his tricycle in circles inside the house, and it was almost impossible to stop him. This degree of physical or mental restlessness leads to *weakness of memory for what he has heard* or *what he has said* or *for what he just thought.* He is extremely impatient and cannot concentrate at school; he has a horrible time waiting for his turn! Restlessness can be provoked by *violent headaches from exposure to the sun or noise, which improve by walking in open air.* This child has great difficulty paying attention in class and will not do any schoolwork unless the teacher is standing over him telling him what to do, step by step. He can be a bright boy with lots of potential, but he does not apply himself unless he is one-on-one with a teacher.

Religious and Suspicious

When he is sick, he is clingy and wants his mom to sleep with him (*desire for company, fears to be alone*). The one thing that sticks out that he always refuses to take any medicine; even when he is sick, he puts up a battle (*refuses to take the medicine*). He is very sensitive when he is one-on-one; he weeps when he hears soft music and worries about his family. He prays every night with his mom, especially if he knows she is mad at him; he will do it for her (*religious affections* and *remorse*). Just as in *Verat-a*, one can even observe religious insanity in *Hyos*, as seen in the proving: *as in a priest's cassock, put on over nothing but a shirt and in fur boots, he wishes to go to church, in order to preach and to perform clerical offices there, and furiously attacks those who try to prevent him.*

Here is an example from my practice:

> A boy was two years old when his sibling was born. On top of that, his little blanket was taken away because he was now a "big boy" (*delusion, he is going to be sold*; *delusion, he lost the affection of his friends*; *delusion, he has suffered wrong*). He had many ear infections for five years, all treated with antibiotics. Jealousy and mild anger had been present since age two, but this anger increased after using a nebulizer for a recurrent cough. He showed incredible anger and rage towards his family, especially the younger sibling. He swore, he hit, threw, kicked, and screamed when angered and also sometimes without cause, but especially when he perceived that the younger sibling had interrupted his time with his mother (*cursing*; *desire to break things*; *bite, desire to*; *rage, fury, tries to kill people*; *mania with rage*). He could not stand the attention being taken away from him; he loved attention more than anything (*jealousy with rage*). He laughed when someone else was being reprimanded (*laughing at serious things*). He talked inappropriately for his age (seven). He asked if his uncle slept with his girlfriend and made sexual comments in conversation (*smutty talk*; *lewd talk*). He walked around naked, especially in front of his mom to aggravate her (*shameless, exposes the person*; *lascivious, uncovers sexual parts*). He told his mother constantly that she did not love him, that she hated him. The mother reassured him that she loved him, but he replied that she was a liar (*delusions, lost the affection of friends*). When he played with his little brother, he told him that he would kill him. When I was talking to his mom, he quietly came in to give her a kiss and whispered in her ear that she was stupid and stuck his tongue out at her (*foolish behavior*). He was possessive of his friends and did not like it when they played with someone else (*jealousy*). When he was sick, he became clingy and wanted his mom to sleep with him (*desire for company, fears to be alone*). He had been sad lately (*sadness, despondency, from disappointed love).* Hyos finally came to the rescue for this boy!

Golden Tips from the Masters

- Jealousy is based on feeling forsaken
- Convulsions in children after fright (*Op*)
- Manic depression after grief
- Dilated pupils (*Bell, Stram*)
- For epileptic attacks with erratic behavior before the attack
- Good remedy for certain cases of Alzheimer disease
- Passive insanity as distinguished from the violent insanity of *Stramonium*
- Indicated in post-operative hiccough, <at midnight, with involuntary urination
- Melancholy gradually develops into true madness
- The keynote of the remedy is **non-inflammatory** cerebral irritation (< >*Bell*). Produces a picture of delirium and mania of a paranoiac character, often with sexual excitability, also convulsions always with great weakness, tending to stupor
- Indicated in old arteriosclerotic people who show jealousy, paranoia, and twitching of single muscles everywhere
- Chorea in which every muscle twitches from the eyes to the toes

Ignatia (Ign). St. Ignatius Bean

The Cyber Delusion

The peculiar Cyber delusion of *Ignatia* is ***she is married***! *Ignatia's* state has evolved further than *Hyoscyamus*' she believes that she is already married, not, like *Hyos*, that she is **going** to be married (the latter having also the *delusion, of wedding bells*)! We are not talking about a lover in *Ignatia's* case (as with *Hyosc*), but something more intimate and deeper, more a feeling about a perceived spouse (not real), already having an unbreakable and permanent bond, or at least belonging to one family! It is a symbiotic relationship in which the attached person (*Ign*) is a part of the "host" person to whom she is attached. She cannot live without that person, and great anxiety occurs when this relationship is threatened. For a child, this means sharing an unseverable bond with a parent, but she also perceives this bond to exist with her best (and often only) friend. Of course, in *Ignatia's* case, such a bond is essentially one of feeling and fantasy. This CD explains her hysterical behavior, and *Ignatia* is therefore also a remedy of codependency in children *and* adults. The delusion that goes hand in hand (at least in adults) with the CD is the *delusion, she is pregnant*. What better proof of being married to the subject of love than carrying his child? Indeed, *Ignatia* has these kinds of *delusions, of fancy illusions* more than anyone (also *Verat* and *Puls*); they reflect the fantasy world she is creating, a world that is often far removed from reality. *Ignatia* people are very romantic and sentimental (*Plat*), fall quickly in love, or cultivate deep friendships with total abandon, mind, and spirit, even—and especially—when they are not married to the person. This is so well expressed by Hering: *delusion, she is married and desires improper things and cries aloud when they are refused.*

Ignatia's romanticism is bound to conflict with reality, just like *Platina's* world fails to materialize with her intense and incompatible desire for sex and spirituality at the same time. *Ignatia* always speaks in exaggerated (sycotic) and hysterical terms when she falls in or out of love. Here are some of the things I have heard in my practice: "My whole world turned around when I found out that he did not love me…" "I feel I am falling apart and I can't cope with what I have been forced to face." "The pain is too great for me to bear now." "My whole life has suddenly and unexpectedly fallen apart." Or when the relationship feels good: "I am in the most satisfying and joyful relationship, a deeply mutual one with the deepest and most tender love, passion, understanding, and pure joy, more than anyone can dream of." "My partner's arms feel like a home that I have never known." Unfortunately, the other party is often completely unaware of the real feelings involved, and *Ignatia* is equally unaware that her feelings are not always based in reality. In order to keep this platonic love story going, other delusions are created like *brooding over imaginary troubles* and *she is breaking her vow* (if she thinks she still has not done enough to serve the person or secure his perceived love), which also reflects the delusion, *she has neglected her duty* or *she has done wrong*. So at first there is self-reproach (*reproaching himself*) and self-castigation based on the fallacy that there will be a better return from the other party with just a little more effort on her part. This effort, of course, is exaggerated and rather pathetic. Then, when the other party does not return the "love" in an equal manner and with equal intensity, other fixed ideas cram in her consciousness, turning now to the partner too: that *she is doomed* and *her soul cannot be saved* and *she cries and rages* and *that she is insulted*.

Causalities

Unrequited Love and Hearing Bad News

We all know the saying "love is blind." However, it is infatuation with a person and the projection of our soul mates (anima and animus) that makes us blind, while real love in fact enables us to see. *Ignatia's* sentiment is perfectly expressed in the proving *the pain and penalty of unrequited love* (also *Tarentula*)! This proving is self-contradictory: if one truly loves another person, there can be no pain or unhappiness, whether or not the love is returned. A person who really loves is always enriched by the enrichment of the beloved, so this proving does not reflect the true meaning of loving someone! Most victims of unrequited love have only fallen in "love" with some part or character trait of the other person, but they have not gotten beyond the outer appearance to discover the spiritual core of the other person, to connect with the most secret and most rewarding part. And, therefore, such a person is never enriched by the experience when it turns out unhappily. There is so much self-pity in *Ignatia* that she, as we will see, has a hard time recovering from this unhappy experience (*brooding, chaotic, confused behavior* and where even *kind words aggravate*).

As does anyone, *Ignatia* has some tools and character traits beyond her romantic nature that can keep her on a positive path in the psoric phase, trying to avoid the inevitable fall into the depths of despair! But the ultimate trigger that will bring about these delusions (as well as a chain reaction of emotional and hysterical symptoms) is deception, betrayal, or disappointment, often a new one. For a child, we talk about *ailments from deceived friendship* when, for example, the other party (her "best" friend) betrays her by having a sleepover with someone else (also *ailments from disappointed love*). Sometimes it is ailments from the death of a loved one (which can include that of a pet!) that make this child a difficult one (*great grief after losing persons or objects very dear,* including *death of a child*). *Ailments from the death of a child* may be the single worst thing that can happen to people—or to any mammal. To understand this, it is sufficient to see an elephant mother standing above her dying baby on TV, staying there a long time even after its death before joining her herd again. Ailments from the death of a child have taken on new meaning in the epidemic of autism: having a child with autism can often be translated as *death of a child,* as this certainly is not the child one was expecting (*Cocculus*). To overcome the acute grief and shock upon hearing such a diagnosis, *Ignatia* has helped many parents cope with this cruel fate, with possible feelings of guilt (*anxiety as if guilty of a crime*), and with their increased worry (*cares, worries, full of*) so that they can go on with a clear head to proceed in the best possible manner to secure the future of their child.

As usual, it is intrauterine trauma that very often triggers the fixed state of a morose *Ignatia* child. I think about the expectant mother, pregnant for the first time and now feeling very much left alone, even betrayed, by a partner who is traveling much of the time for his work (*aversion to being alone*). An *Ignatia* person already has an *unusual tendency to be frightened (for thieves after waking after midnight) and fright is often followed by grief.* But worse, there are things actually happening to the pregnant mother: being abandoned, or separated, or her partner's death or illness! All these incidents can be called *hearing bad news.* These are a few of the many possible triggers that can create the *Ignatia* situation in a pregnant mother, planting the fertile seed of codependency and clinginess in the unborn child. It is interesting to see how the nursing *Ignatia* mother, while grieving, will exert a negative influence on her baby (*infantile colic after taking breast of mother or nurse, who suffers from grief*). It is like feeding grief directly to the baby!

Ignatia is also the adult who falls in love with an unobtainable partner, for instance, a married person (just like its chronic, *Nat-m*). Things get even stickier if children are involved. How often have I heard that story that the other party "is just days away from starting his life together with me" (the *Ignatia* person)... *Ignatia* is absolutely sure that her beloved will divorce his spouse (with whom he surely has nothing in common), and that he is looking forward to starting his life with Ms. *Ignatia*. This situation usually reflects a longtime relationship or affair; when it really comes down to making the ultimate decision of divorce, though, one party (the one with children) often backs out. It is at this point (*ailments from emotional/mental shock*) that the other person falls into the hopeless *Ignatia* state; it is the ultimate betrayal: "You shared everything with me, you promised me, I did everything for you," are the exasperated words of the "victim." Often this is followed by a nervous breakdown, because it recalls her feelings of abandonment in her youth by mother, father, or previous lovers. *Ignatia* either locks herself up in a dark room or becomes more sycotic and wants to go out to bars and drink all the time. If a real cure is not offered (through homeopathic remedies and/or introspective psychological analysis), the person goes from one "close," longed-for relationship to another, repeating the soap opera scenes in her life over and over again. The painful complex of betrayal and abandonment evokes sentences such as "The world is cruel to me; I am crying out for help but people turn a deaf ear to my desperate pleas; there is no soul available to me to talk to and I am all alone in this sad world of deafening silence (*Puls*); my life in reality has ceased to exist and I am unable to eat or sleep (*sleeplessness from grief*). I am paralyzed and suspended in the nightmare of my pain; my insides are shaking and my mouth is dry," etc. One can see the exaggerated and neurotic tone of this person, as well as the tendency toward hysteria.

Mortification

Humiliation is another common causality for *Ignatia*. We can understand the humiliation a wife feels when she discovers the unfaithfulness of her husband: usually everybody else already knows the facts before she does. This, of course, can cause *ailments from anger with silent grief* as withdrawal from society is a normal defense mechanism for this person (*desire to be alone so as to give way to her real or imaginary grief; weeps bitterly*). There are, however, other instances of indignation that have nothing to do with love affairs but, rather, with sudden changes in the person's social life. I am thinking here of losses suffered in the stock market that can reduce one's standing in society (*ailments from pecuniary loss*), the loss of a job (*A/F loss of position* and *A/F shame*), or failure in examinations (*A/F literary and scientific failure*)—even circumstances in which one has been ridiculed at work for something one did not do (*A/F reproaches*). *Ignatia*, in all these circumstances, can help resolve the mental shock in a patient in whom we see hysterical reactions; *increased or no appetite, globus hystericus, sighing* and even *convulsions* occur after such incidences.

Compensations

Delicate Conscientiousness

Ignatia's *finely sensitive mood* and *delicate conscientiousness* are positive tools to tie people to them, as others can be attracted to this, but at the same time they reveal a certain vulnerability that leads easily to a hysterical outburst. What helps *Ignatia* to strengthen her Cyber delusion even further is *her mild and quiet disposition through which she bears suffering, even outrage, without complaining. She has an amiable disposition if feeling well.* She is idealistic, highly romantic, perfectionistic, and driven: a very loyal and yielding friend indeed—to a fault. *Ignatia* is a martyr in fact, just like its chronic, *Nat-m!*

The pregnant *Ignatia* already has a *great inclination to fixed ideas,* so she remains stuck (*thoughts persistent; thoughtful thoughts*) and influences her unborn child through mystical participation by *tears that are wept inwardly, and desiring solitude at that moment so that she can nourish inward grief.* There is *aversion to any amusement as well as indifference to everything, while living without the usual good humor.* All these sentiments can easily transfer to the fetus, who will now also become a person of *sensitive disposition and hyper acute feeling, a serious child.* That does not provide an easy start in this harsh, complicated world.

Commitment to Duty

Ignatia slides easily into sycotic behavior to solidify her "marriage." The *Ignatia* person exhibits *a restless activity, busy, with a great memory for mental work; she is industrious, exhibiting a mania for work,* doing everything possible to please that other person, even to the point that she has *the delusion, she neglected her duty*: *I am neglecting my duty and breaking my vows.* It is the kind of great "unselfishness" which is worse than selfishness. If someone tells you that he loves you more than he loves himself and that he wants to sacrifice himself for you, your next question should be: "How much does such a love cost? What will you want afterwards?" *Ignatia* is playing exactly this trick on the unsuspecting victim. "I am only happy when I can do everything for you to make you happy," she says, since *occupation for the loved one ameliorates. Ignatia* shows *affection and amativeness in this stage*, but she betrays her own soul by being utterly devoted to the friend, boss, guru, parent, or lover. She is a person *full of cares and worries,* an approach that suits the receiving party for as long as it lasts. It looks, indeed, as though the *Ignatia* person does not demand anything in return; she seems to be the person that can offer unconditional love effortlessly and perpetually. But what a charade, what a deception she is playing! Without knowing it, *Ignatia* exercises emotional blackmail through her fixed delusion. In reality, the other party will never be able to recompense her devotion or even come close to matching the ceaseless efforts she makes in the course of a day. Remarkably, *Ignatia's* only desired reward (and an amazingly sufficient one), is acknowledgement of her devotion as she suffers from the pain and penalty of unrequited love.

Foolish and Hysterical Behavior

If pure devotion does not work, there is always foolish, hysterical behavior to draw the attention of the beloved one! There are *incredible changes of moods; at one time she jokes and makes merry, at another she is lachrymose, alternating three or four hours. She laughs and cries almost in the same breath. She sighs and sobs and will not be comforted. She isolates herself so as to give way to her real or imaginary grief. There is even twitching of muscles or sudden onset of torticollis (stiffness of the nape of the neck). She might utter remorse about imaginary crimes. Or she shrieks for help with suffocating constriction of the throat. There are hysterical spasms of the throat and she cannot swallow liquids or solids! There is senseless staring at one object with remorse about imaginary crimes.* If only Jung had known about this magical remedy for many of his hysterical patients! Of course, hysteria draws attention only momentarily and, if her attempt is unsuccessful, it will only fuel her grief and fright, which takes her back to the Never Well Since (NWS). The border between neurosis and psychosis is rather blurred, as *Ignatia* is overcome with *anxiety and disquiet as if she had done something wrong, or as if some great misfortune were about to happen; this so overpowers her, that she can only with difficulty refrain from weeping and has great inclination to fixed ideas.* Other hysterical physical symptoms are vocal tics, cramps, spasms, chorea, and the feeling of a ball or globus in the throat that prevents swallowing.

Self-reproach

Ignatia is also the child who suffocates her best friend by demanding reassurance of her friendship and loyalty (she wants this friend all to herself!); even when she is reassured, it is never enough as *she broods over imaginary trouble,* initially convinced that she must be blamed for the breakup (*remorse for imagined crimes; reproaches herself*). *She becomes more serious, still, melancholic, withdrawn with moaning. She has melancholia from suppressed mental sufferings with much sighing. Appetite and digestion leaves her. She becomes bilious, has trembling of hands disturbing her writing and would scarcely move from the fire for days. There is sleeplessness, anxiety and severe palpitations.* The child also becomes very sensitive to *kindly admonition* (sycosis): *spasmodic affections (convulsions) of children, consequent on being put to sleep soon after punishment. She now dreads every trifle leading to irresolution and inertness.* There will be *crowding of thoughts* as she rehearses her life story, even in bed, a life that starts resembling a soap opera (*nightly fancies which fatigue the mind; contrary to his will, thinks of vexatious and peevish things and dwells upon them*) in which she *howls, cries and is besides herself on account of trifles.*

Golden Tips from the Masters

- *Ignatia* is the S's: sighs, sits, sobs
- It is the female counterpart of *Nux-v* (both contain Strychnia): *Nux* indicated for anger and violence, *Ignatia* suitable for alternating moods, laughing and weeping
- Sighing is getting relief from taking a deep breath
- *Ignatia* women hold their frustration until they are premenstrual; at that point, they can show twitching and spasms and become combative
- Is a fragile person who snaps like a string under pressure
- #1 remedy for changeable and contradictory moods: no remedy equals it!
- *Ignatia* works for the typical spoiled girl who has everything in life, and who, for lack of true hardships, is unable to bear any challenge or difficulty. Such a person, no matter what you say, is not reasonable. You cannot be rational; it is always a love-hate relationship
- Voracious appetite to relieve grief
- Hypersensitive to smoke of tobacco
- It is a great insomnia remedy and the rehearsal remedy; patient can't sleep because she thinks about what she should have said or done. There is often a conflict situation, relationship problem or frustration. Also dreams full of disappointment and unfulfilled expectations
- Numerous anal and rectal problems: hemorrhoids, pain, itching, etc.
- Administer in the morning as it causes restlessness when taking at night

Kali bromatum (Kali-br). Bromide of Potash

The Cyber Delusion

"For rulers hold no terror for those who do right, but for those who do wrong. Do you want to be free from fear of the one in authority? Then do what is right [...] But if you do wrong, be afraid, for rulers do not bear the sword for nothing."[22] *Kali bromatum* lives under that sword, believing that he *is singled out for divine vengeance.* The problem for him is that he thinks he has done or is about to do wrong, so rulers do hold terror for him! Indeed, the CD of *Kali-br* is ***he is the object of God's vengeance*** (*imagines he is singled out as an object of divine wrath*). What does this most painful delusion mean? The fixed idea certainly reflects some feeling in the person that he must have done something wrong for which he now needs to be punished by the highest authority (*delusion, she has moral deficiency*). The essence of *Kali bromatum* is a concern about one's character, morality, about how one is seen or judged by other people. She tries hard to do what is right in the eyes of her family and others. In her struggle with (her perception of) morality vs. immorality, she ends up feeling worthy of punishment. **The *Kali bromatum* state is created from the conflict between a strict moral code and what she fears she has done wrong or will do wrong.** Essentially, the CD expresses a deep sense of *guilt,* and the guilt seems to carry a *religious* overtone, different from the guilt of *Aurum,* who thinks he deserves reproach from all (not just from God) because he has not done his duty. This is also different from *Nat-mur's* guilt, which stems from failed relationships or the death of a child, and from *Chelidonium's* guilt, based on her perception that she failed to give adequate advice because someone did not listen to her. In the case of *Nat-m,* "death of a child" also has the extended meaning of death of a close relative of whom *Nat-mur* took care for many years during a severe illness (*Cocc*).

From *Kali bromatum's* Cyber delusion, we see immediately the idea of religious conflict that is part of the *Kali bromatum* picture. This conflict will be found especially during the

22. Rom. 13:3-4 NIV

tumultuous period of burgeoning sexuality (puberty), but also in times of additional duties and responsibilities towards the family (which can include simply obeying the rules); the *Kali* theme of family obligation remains firmly in place. This patient, in her religious belief, fully believes that she deserves the harshest punishment for her perceived mistakes: *she desires death; she desires to escape; she reproaches herself as having feelings of moral deficiency* and *has especially suicidal thoughts to be run over by a car* (*Alumina, Aurum*). God must punish her, because *Kali-br* has been found guilty in her own court of law!

This feeling of guilt and, consequently, of deserving punishment as expressed in the CD is confirmed by many other fixed ideas: *brother fell overboard in her sight; he had committed a crime; she is about to be arrested; she is about to murder her husband and child; and he is pursued by the police for robbing a friend.* This CD, as is often the case, will lead to secondary fixed ideas ("If I am this bad, I deserve punishment, and it is certainly waiting for me"): *delusion of being doomed; impending destruction of all near her* (family theme again); *he is a devil; his life is threatened; he will be murdered and persecuted; and he is about to be poisoned*! All these delusions reflect a picture of someone who views herself a person with evil inside her; her eroding confidence shows that she is certain that she must be punished for his perceived horrific deeds, creating a great sense of anxiety, suspicion, and even paranoia. The last of these is another theme we find in a person needing this remedy. *Kali bromatum's* paranoia also leads to a conviction and *delusion, that there are conspiracies against him.* While this is irrational and false, brought on by his Never Well Since (NWS) (death of a child is one of them: God conspires against him), the thought process on which the premise is built often shows a remarkable amount of intelligence. *Kali-br* makes logical connections and deductions based on real facts which are difficult to disprove, so for this paranoid person, fear of conspiracies have become a fact and a reality.

Causalities

Death of a Child

What are these horrific deeds that *Kali-br* accuses herself of? They can reveal various themes. One should not be surprised to find this causality in many intrauterine "crimes"; these often carry a great stigma of guilt:

> I recall the case of a woman carrying twins, of which one died intra-utero; the other suffered from autism and respiratory distress from an early age. She wondered if she could have caused the death of one twin (*A/F death of a child, Kali-br, Ign*) and the illnesses of the surviving child by carrying defective genes. She had also showed extreme anxiety about the remaining baby during the pregnancy, to the extent that she asked to be hooked up to the heart monitor (*delusion, child* ***is*** *dead,* only *Kali-br*). She said she feared that if anything happened to him, she would not be able to go on (*A/F fright; suicidal disposition, to be run over*). She also carried a great burden of guilt about having left the hospital when the baby suffered respiratory distress, thinking that he must have felt abandoned by her in his hour of greatest need (although the doctor had advised her that everything was all right and that her presence was not required).

This story reflects *Kali bromatum's delusion, of impending destruction of all near her* and *the fear something is wrong with a sense of doom.*

Another example is when the death of a child occurs—when, for instance, the mother or a sibling walks with the child, waiting to cross a road, and suddenly the child gets away from the mother/sibling and is killed in front of the mother. This expresses quite literally the *delusion, brother fell overboard in her sight*! Imagine the grief, the guilt, the horror! Such a person is often overcome with tremendous feelings of guilt for many years, and often this issue is only resolved in a dream, the messenger of the unconscious. Under the influence of *Kali-br,* the dead child may appear in a dream and tell the surviving person that she is forgiven for this misdeed, that the child is happy where she is. No message can be more powerful, releasing the grieving person from the yoke of guilt.

Another example in which *Kali-br* was indicated shows that this guilt can even be carried over from one generation to another. I had a patient who had undergone eight abortions, and now her adult daughter could not get pregnant:

> They were both convinced that it was "God's revenge" for those past misdeeds of the mother (*reproaches herself*). They felt that this had to happen, as God always punishes such terrible acts. The mother's fear and doom created a kind of inter-generational guilt. In this case there was no death of a child; the child was not even born!

I have seen other cases in which people accused themselves of "horrific crimes," for instance, a married woman having lunch with a male colleague and feeling that this was an act of disloyalty towards her husband, that she had committed a heinous crime. In this case, think also of *Chelidonium*, with its delusion, *has committed the unpardonable sin*, although religious undertones are far less present in *Chelidonium*. A truly heinous crime, though, is the sexual abuse of a child:

> A mother, watching her child descend into the depths of autism, found out that he had been molested at school. Now the mother was overcome with guilt: "Why was I not there to protect him?" She even cursed God for giving her two "imperfect" children (she had another child with special needs), although she was very religious (*delusion, forsaken, is forsaken by God; delusion, God, he is the object of God's vengeance* and *delusion, neglected, duty, he has neglected his*). This indicated that her remedy was *Kali bromatum*, which relieved her from those fixed ideas!

The crime of sexual abuse is disastrous, an evil that cannot be undone: *her child is dead*! Be it the worst crime or the worst punishment, the worst pain has come upon her; she is *helpless* with *grief* and *despair of recovery*. It is arguably the most painful experience to lose a child to death; it is worse yet to feel responsible for his death. And, in light of the *delusion, brother fell overboard in her sight, Kali bromatum* likely sees the death of her child as her fault. Almost equally tragic, and equally painful, is for moral guilt to throw a soul into the torment of believing her child is dead when he is not, berating oneself for not having been there to protect the child! However, the spiritual death, the death of her child's soul through sexual abuse, is unbearable. At any rate, in a *Kali bromatum* state, the delusion *her child is dead* arises from and reveals tormenting psychic pain over morality, a crime that she feels she has committed, and ensuing guilt.

Sexual Excesses and Sexual Emotional Excitement

If one is raised in a family in which sexuality is taboo, one may develop a *Kali bromatum* state during the surge of hormones and awakening sexuality of puberty. This sexuality can lead to masturbation or other sexual thoughts or practices for which the adolescent will feel exceedingly bad: *fancies, lascivious; nymphomania; satyriasis; thoughts, sexual; amativeness. During the partial slumber, especially if in bed, there quickly arises a greater or lesser degree of sexual excitement, usually accompanied by erections and emissions, which awake the subject and of which he is perfectly conscious.* The person may end up experiencing *want of moral feeling*, but at other times suffers *religious melancholia, reproaching himself.* It is against this backdrop that *Kali bromatum* suffers many *delusions, about persecution and violence*. Sexual feelings and guilt may bring on the *delusion, his mother's house is invaded by lewd women*. This is mainly a secret thought and reflects the teenager's struggle as he is confronted with his sexual awakening at puberty, inviting "God's vengeance" for such sinful thoughts caused by the hormonal avalanche (*sexual thoughts wandering*). This awakening sexual libido, with the force of a Category 5 hurricane, is hard to subdue; it is, however, suppressed in many families in which the topic of sex is taboo—either for religious reasons (most commonly) or from shyness or modesty. What a mistake for parents to let the teenager find out for himself how to deal with his natural libido, as this hurricane force can cause devastation from which one needs much time to recuperate! In general, the male teenager will have different compensations or displacements than the female, whose anima and feeling function of consciousness is more attracted to religion and other rescue missions (volunteering in hospitals, pet stores, etc.) rather than the active, sword-wielding animus in young men who displace the sexual pressure, if they are able to, with thrill-seeking behavior. We see a *Kali-br* state appear not only at puberty, but also in other circumstances in which the hormonal balance is changed; all its symptoms express themselves more forcefully during pregnancy and in menopause as well (*anxiety of health during climacteric period*; *complaining during climacteric period*; *nymphomania during menses*; *frightful imaginings in a pregnant woman during latter months, they are under the impression that they have committed a crime, or about to commit, some great crime, such as murdering their children or husbands* (Sepia).

Sexual excesses, unfortunately, do not occur only in teenagers. Many adults are overwhelmed by loneliness in their lives, for which masturbation seems to offer momentary pleasure and satisfy the sexual libido. But contrary to what happens in a happy, loving relationship, where sexual intercourse is a consequence of love (not the other way around), the tension in the loner is not relieved at all after masturbation. Worse, the feeling of a hangover is created, mixed with guilt feelings and fixed thoughts that God will punish him for this horrible deed. There is indeed a saying, "Post coitus omne animal triste est praeter gallum qui cantat," translated as "after coitus all animals are sad, save for the rooster who sings." The animals referred to here are human beings! *Kali-br* is prone to *sadness with impotence* and *sadness with pollutions* from these sexual excesses. And after some time the unsatisfactory non-directional libido returns with a vengeance and needs to be satisfied, so the cycle of sexual libido—masturbation—hangover—guilt recurs again and again; the victim sees no escape as he sinks into the quicksand of hopelessness.

Compensations

Religion

We will always see that a remedy like *Kali-br* seeks a source of displacement. It will be difficult to uncover the real complaint in a consultation. She comes to a consultation with small, innocent physical problems, because a *Kali* person is incapable of introspection or of making a connection between her physical chief complaint and her "misdeed." Such understanding has been buried but, as usual, can come up in revealing dreams, stoking the guilty fire. A favorite displacement of *Kali-br*, as we have noted, is excessive religion (*religious delusions*) and thrill-seeking behavior, often equal to the degree and intensity of guilt (be it sexual or related to a misdeed in life) that the person feels (this is sycosis, the miasm of excess!).

Amelioration with Occupation

Among so many mental/emotional expressions of this well-proven remedy, it is extremely difficult to find a single positive compensation. Even if one is observed, it is only in the first degree: a sign that it will soon be overcome by doom and gloom. *Kali bromatum's* fixed idea is so strong that **psoric** compensations seem to be impossible. Yes, we see *amativeness, busy and occupation ameliorates*, but the proving picture is full of stronger negative emotions. Being busy and ameliorated by occupation signal, in fact, a sycotic nature: *restless and fruitless busy* (*Verat, Lil-t, Kali-br*). Though mixed with an overtone of anxiety and restlessness, *occupation ameliorates* is still her best compensation as it keeps her away from the wandering thoughts of her perceived horrible deed. Her strong degree of anxiety, bordering on anguish, is seen clearly in the constant wringing of her hands while she tells her story: *gestures, grasping, plays with his fingers, wringing the hands* and *gestures, picking at fingers*, Kali-br. The *hands* are constantly *restless*; this person must continuously do something with her hands, like playing with her fingers, with her glasses, with a cigarette, keys, or a pen (*constantly busy, tying his shoes, fumbling in his pockets, picking threads*, and so on). In children, this hereditary (*stemming from intrauterine trauma*) anxiety is quite commonly seen in the form of nightmares: *anxiety in children at night* (*a nightmare of children, not from indigestion, with screaming and unconsciousness of what is occurring around them; cannot recognize those around them and cannot be comforted by their friends*—compare with *Stram*: *delirium, recognizes no one*). We must not forget that severe anxiety in children leads to *stubbornness*, a defense mechanism ("No, I am not going to bed. I want to sleep with you!"). It also explains the *high shrieking voice* we see in these children (often diagnosed with ASD), the vocal equivalent of the emotion the pregnant mother must have felt upon hearing bad news (of disease, death of a twin in utero, or the like).

Superstition

The pronounced psoric manifestation of anxiety moves easily and quickly into its sycotic phase, as sycotic fears become outspoken and numerous in a *Kali-br* case to the point of superstition and paranoia. These include *fear of being poisoned* (the latter to be seen as a punishment for the great crime he has committed), but involve anticipation fears in particular. Such fears can be observed in all the *Kalis*: *fear something will happen; impending fear of destruction to all near her* (as a result such a mother gets very upset about trifles in her children); *fear of something wrong* and *fear to walk past certain corners.* When such fears are added to her guilty delusions that the police are pursuing her and that God is punishing her with a life of doom, *Kali-br* nears the point of a nervous breakdown, behaving increasingly like a trapped and wounded animal. First, irritability shows: it is *irritability from grief and with sleeplessness. There is muttering in sleep and then sadness comes from sleeplessness. There is constant brooding over the loss of her child. She is almost crazy from fretting, loss of rest and want of nourishment* (*Cocculus* and *Ignatia* come to mind too). Her anxiety and fixation on doom will make her impatient, irritable, and sleepless!

Mental Breakdown

On the mental plane, due to sleep deprivation, *Kali-br* becomes like an *absentminded* and insane person (*feels as if she would go out of her mind; thinks she is becoming deranged*): *she has difficulty expressing herself and finding the right words in conversation, in other words deficiency of ideas; she had to be told the word before she could speak it; she makes many mistakes in her speech as she uses the wrong words and says the opposite of what she wants to say since her senses are dulled; she repeats words and makes mistakes in writing while her writing is indistinct. She is unable to concentrate her mind on anything.* Imagine a *Kali-br* child in school who, no doubt, will fall under the ASD label! Who will understand this child? But the insanity always has a religious overtone (*religious delusions*), a common trademark of *Kali-br*: *religious madness; melancholia in religious affections. Concentration is difficult and confusion present on waking,* even to the point of not knowing who she is (*confusion as to his identity*). Of course, *mental work* in these circumstances *becomes impossible. Her answers are either slow* or *she repeats the question first* or *answers monosyllable, answers no to all questions.*" We see here the extreme poverty of *Kali-br* on the mental plane.

Golden Tips from the Masters

- Another physical symptom stems from her Cyber delusion if she feels guilty, for instance, that her child has died: *sleeplessness from grief* (*Nat-m, Ign, Gels, Kali-br, Lach*). Often *Ignatia* is indicated, but if it does not work, consider *Kali-br* in such cases—especially when you see hand-wringing.
- Great remedy for nightmares in children with no recollections after waking up
- Insomnia and depression due to embarrassment, loss of reputation, financial loss, and mortification (*Aurum*)
- #1 remedy for chronic unsightly acne on face and on back with scarring, associated with puberty and hormonal changes and before, during and after the menstrual period
- Epilepsy and insomnia with an aura of *sensation he is swelling*
- Antidote for lead poisoning
- For cases of schizophrenia and manic depression if they fit the picture
- Main remedy for aphasia
- #1 remedy for asthma in sailors only better at sea

Kali carbonicum (Kali-c). Potassium carbonate

The Cyber Delusion

The Cyber delusion of *Kali-c* is ***an abyss is behind him***, referring to the chronic anxiety and invisible threat that a *Kali-c* patient feels. *Kali-c* feels that she has to be on guard against all those unknown but (in her mind) real ordeals that may threaten her welfare and that of her family. She is not sure **where** and **when** it will hit, but there is always that looming doom, that deep pit or abyss behind her, so every step in life must be taken with great care. Great hypochondriac that she is, *Kali-c feels her emotions in the epigastrium* and *has anxiety about health* and *the future*, her most prominent anxieties.

Kali-c is never at peace! Preoccupied with the future, she has not figured out that the present alone is true and actual and that she should enjoy every present moment that is free of pain, physically and emotionally. But *Kali-c* forgoes the present hour of happiness by spoiling it with uneasiness about what is to come, about the future which lies beyond her power. As Mark Twain said, "I have known a great many troubles, but most of them never happened." *Kali-c* is unable to find the peace of mind which is the foundation of human happiness; she forgets that every day is an irreplaceable portion of life, a day which comes only once and never returns. *Kali-c* is a person who is confined in an emotional straitjacket. At the same time, the anxiety about health invites (because of its permanence and intensity) her numerous physical complaints; hence, what *Kali-c* fears so much does come to pass: failing health. So many happy hours are wasted for *Kali-c* in hypochondriacal anxiety, when she lets pleasant times slip by unenjoyed. *Kali-c* is caught between the abyss behind him (the past) and the anxiety of going forward (the future), which eventually results in a spastic paralytic stiffness that is symbolic of *Kali-carb's* struggle in life. To try to control his health and avoid future calamities, a *Kali-c* person becomes a health fanatic. *Kali-c* is always seeking the right foods and the right drinks; she is a drug store's friend. People who always take such care of themselves always have a tendency to become morbid and hypervigilant. That amazing faith in drinking a certain kind of water, for instance, comes from a continuous fear of death. It is something in them that says: "For God's sake, don't let me die, because I have not lived yet!" (Think of *Lachesis*, too.) Although *Kali-c* looks anxious but not unhealthy, she easily imagines that something might go wrong—and if not with her, then perhaps with her husband or children. *Kali-c* frequently passes this health mania on to her children, so those poor beings are sometimes made extremely ill through the fears of the parent. What the *Kali-c* mother fails to see is that human needs and longing, in her children, are not only for food, physical comfort, and protection; they are also for social dignity, interpersonal connections, and some form of authentication. Her conduct will only lead to unfulfillment and feelings of frustration in her offspring.

The essence of *Kali-carb's* Cyber delusion, a hypochondriacal anxiety, is also expressed and supported by other delusions found in further provings: delusions such as *he was about to die, his bed is sinking, he is sinking, he will be murdered,* and *he is being sick.* When many delusions express the same theme (in this case, a delusion of impending doom and personal demise), they reflect the Cyber delusion. All these delusions point to seemingly inevitable catastrophes and pending dangers which don't appear to be under *Kali-carb's* control. The figurative sword of Damocles is hanging above her head, and she never knows when it is going to come down on her! She is talking about an abyss "behind" her, not in front of her; she fears, then, a danger which she cannot see but of which she is very well aware: she can sense it. So she feels the need to be hypervigilant, always on guard! This is different from the situation of *Nat-c,* who faces the Cyber delusion *there is an abyss between her and others,* an acute separation anxiety, an inability to connect to other people even when she wants to. *Nat-carb's* major concerns are relationships, while *Kali-c* has more personal anxiety (which is transferred to everyone else in the family).

There are some other delusions reflecting a sense of naivety and vulnerability but, above all, a distrust of others (even family): one is *delusion, her whole body is hollow,* meaning that she senses that her body is insubstantial and feels a need to reinforce it through compensations in order to survive all the ordeals in life. He also experiences numerous fearful delusions stoking the fire of unrest, which make *her scream* (*shrieking about imaginary appearances*): *delusion, sees dead persons; sees hideous faces; sees figures during sleep; sees thieves* and *delusion,* creeping *of worms.* What a world of terror and perceived danger! Now that we have entered the mind of *Kali-c* and know the fixed idea that tortures her, we must ask: why is she thinking this in the first place? What causes her to be a constant nervous wreck, always seeming to be on the verge of a nervous breakdown?

Causalities

Sexual Excesses

One of *Kali-carb*'s principal etiologies, and one of the most surprising ones, is ailments from sexual excesses. Is *Kali-c* a nymphomaniac and hunter like *Hyos, Fl-ac, Med,* and *Lycopodium*? It would be hard to make such a case for *Kali-c*. Certainly there is a hormonal component, as we see *nymphomania before and during menses,* but it is not very prominent in comparison with *Phosphorus, Plat,* or *Verat*. For *Kali-c,* there is a great need to be part of a relationship in order to exist. This wish to connect to others, and her spontaneous and rather naïve behavior, adds to a desire for a cohesive and united family, explaining the sexual excess. Part of it is her duty to her family (*duty, too much sense of*), and procreation is a big part of the family program (also *Sepia*). Link this characteristic to her great family connection, and we can see that she might not refuse sex to her husband—just like *Sepia* in the initial state. This mental/emotional state also parallels *Nat-mur*'s first-stage behavior: *Nat-m* also looks desperately to connect to someone, anyone, to relieve her feelings of loneliness and forsakenness. The difference between the two is that *Nat-m* tries to attract the opposite sex with singing, laughing, and hysterical behavior, while *Kali-c* is more serious, intensely controlling, and critical in her approach (*censorious; contrary; conversation aggravates; impetuous*). Where *Nat-m* in the initial stage tries to establish a good emotional relationship for personal reasons, *Kali-c* is mainly concerned about her relationship with her own family. In older males, this leads to a weak constitution and sexual prostration with nightly pollutions as the sexual desire is excessive, but all his symptoms aggravate after sexual intercourse.

Disappointed Love

Kali-c, being set in her own mode of thinking and determining how things in life should be approached, suffers many heartbreaks (like *Nat-m,* but for different reasons). Being a self-centered, abrupt, and harsh individual, she is overbearing and difficult for most people to tolerate, which inevitably will lead to many events of *hearing bad news, disappointed love* and *excitement after bad news.* As a result of these heartbreaks, *Kali-c* suppresses her emotions, appearing stoic and stiff in public so that no one can guess what is going on behind the walls of her home (*indifference while in society*—a syphilitic trait) but, as always, the price of denying one's feelings is very high. It will create a flurry of neuroses and physical complaints: stiffness and rigidity of the spine, *stitching* pains in joints and lungs, sciatica, and stomach ulcers, the last being particularly unsurprising as we see in the provings *feels her emotions in the epigastrium.* Much of all this can be blamed on *Kali-carb's* attitude. *Kali-c* is a person who is rarely capable of true conversation, which comes from the Latin words *con* or "with, together" and *vers* or "turn, change." In the strictest sense of the word, this means: "You talk and then I talk"—taking turns, in other words. *Kali-carb's* conversation is, rather, a monologue (for which *Sulphur* and *Lachesis* are also well known). *Kali-carb's* social behavior demonstrates poorer communication (*speech hasty, incoherent and wandering*) than that of these two other intelligent personalities, driven as she is by her Cyber delusion. There is not much *intellect* in her conversation (she has *weakness for expressing herself*). There is no room for negotiation or exchange of opinion between two or more parties (somewhat like *Nit-ac*): "You must be of my opinion, and if not, I will try even harder to convince you." However, as William Penn said, "Right is right even if everyone is against it; and wrong is wrong even if everyone is for it." In conversations with the dogmatic *Kali-c*, you will hit a wall: her dominant conscious function is sensation, with a mainly introverted attitude. But, because of this, *Kali-c* brings her painfully nervous condition upon herself (*easily startled from fright, during sleep* and *from noise*).

Compensations

Looking for Company

Let's not forget that her fixed ideas have brought her to a constant state of anxiety (*anxiety with fear; timid and apprehensive of future and about her disease*). What will she do to alleviate this? First of all, she will look for company *(desires company and aversion to solitude)*! I wonder if it is the proverbial "misery loves company," the wish to commiserate about her anxieties like the *Arsenicum* person, or if there is something else behind it? That she wants company is indicated in the provings *she does have great aversion to be alone, fear of being alone, fears she will die* and *desires to be carried.* This last proving seems to explain the need of the *Kali-c* person to be able to communicate her anxieties to someone—anyone—just like the person in an *Arsenicum* state. However, *Arsenicum* and *Kali-ars* will show their anxiety readily as they have no control over it, and they will make sure not to offend anyone (*delusion, she has offended people*); in *Kali-c*, though, the controlling *Kali* element will mask the anxiety to some extent. For that reason, the anxiety usually appears later than in does in *Arsenicum* and *Kali-arsenicum*. The other big difference is the way she treats her company (family): *desire for company, yet she treats them outrageously*! So there must be another reason that she is looking for company, not just to heap her burden on her company like *Arsenicum* does; this reason will become clearer further on in our analysis.

Home Sweet Home

The second place *Kali-c* looks to still all her anxieties and avoid perceived dangers in the world is, of course, the home (the *Carbon* part of her): *desponding in open air, disappears on entering the home*. We see clearly in this last proving that the world is a dangerous place for her and that the home is her only refuge, her castle. The *Kali-c* person is greatly attached to his family just like *Calc-c* and *Pulsatilla*. In the case of *Calc-c*, this is because of insecurities, an immature ego, and his constant thoughts about all the cruelties in this world (*he talks about nothing but fire, rats and mice*). Above all, *Calc-c* needs a home to call his own. *Puls* is a homebody (home can include the school) due to her emotional dependency and need for attention, but she also likes to be in the open air and ameliorates there. *Puls* can be like a leech or an octopus, with her arms hanging constantly around the desired person. Dependency does play a role in the attachment of *Kali-c*, but *Kali* persons (children included) are more demanding of their family members than are *Calc* and *Puls*; they also have a greater hoarding instinct due to their underlying anxiety and feelings of gloom and doom about the future (*Arsenicum*).

Dogmatic Rules

If one is in constant fear of losing control, in a state of permanent worry about the future, feeling vulnerable and insecure with a great *fear of impending disease*, one may turn to dogmatic rules in order to create some stability and order in life. Others, like *Silica*, with an excessive persona, resort to paying exaggerated attention to trifles or details (*conscientious about trifles*). With *Kali-c*, conscientiousness about trifles is not an option (*ailments from mental work*), but rules serve to express her dogmatic ideas about what **ought** to be, as well as to voice her opinions about people whose attitudes she feels to be entirely wrong. This is a ruthless, animus driven, powerful, steamroller dogmatism, a devil of an opinion and quite a conscious one—and all of this exists in the name of righteousness, truth, "motherly love," and "angelic goodness," as *Kali-c* proclaims. Her dogmatism encompasses opinions, moral/ethical discipline, routines, and conformism: rights and wrongs with nothing in between, in which the *Kali* parent pushes her "virtues" on her children for the sake of their "welfare." *Kali-c* rejects the live-and-let-live attitude, revealing her own rigidity. Being so highly conscientious, she takes rules very seriously. Her high anxiety and not very agreeable nature add up to a tendency to be severely critical of others. She wants to be valued by her family; she engages in a social power grab within the family, trying to gain respect while holding others to impossible standards. She often wears a smug mask of moral superiority, which only betrays her excessive anxiety. Her harsh discipline and the repression of desire only lead to her family's frustration, resentment, and a sense of emptiness. Yes, it is true that children cannot be raised without learning discipline and responsibility. Yet if stigmatizing rigidity is to be avoided, value judgments and rules will have to be offered as models, not inflexible prescriptions and blind hostility, to be observed in spirit and not followed by rote to the letter. Children need to find their own standards and emotional values with minimal physical and emotional punishment; otherwise, emotional security, self-confidence, curiosity, and autonomy will be the first victims. Shielding them from failure does them no favors: without the trial-and-error learning from gradual exposure to risk, children become vulnerable to anxiety disorders. *Kali-c* does not consciously harm her children in any obvious way, yet she slowly strangles the family's joy in life; her negative attitude towards living is contagious and infects her family like an insidious illness. It should not come as a surprise to us that children at the mercy of such saintly mother, to their horror dream of "killing the witch," compensating for their helplessness in real life.

Any change in routine causes undue anxiety, aggravating *Kali-c* and making an escapist out of him (also *Lycopodium*, which is complementary). *Kali-c* likes to work like an efficient, automatic robot. Therefore, a person with a *Kali-c* personality is likely to gravitate toward the military, with its "family" spirit and its strict rules and code of conduct. Let's consider, however, the effect that such a mother has on her children.

A mother figure must possess great anima in order to create harmony in the family. Anima (a natural and defining component of a woman's soul) stands for embracing, enveloping, devotion, happiness, protection, nourishing, and loyalty: in other words, the domain of happiness. However, the picture of the domineering *Kali-c* mother, especially in relation to the male child, is one of a mother who is not concerned with her child growing up and marrying. With her strong animus (her masculine component), the controlling *Kali-c* mom and the chained son help each other to betray life. As a result, the mother's attitude, unbeknownst to her, prevents her child from gaining a foothold on his island in that vast ocean of unconsciousness. Life makes demands on the child's conscious side, the masculinity of a man, on his courage, decision-making abilities, and resolution. It is as though *Kali-c* has inoculated her son with too strong a dose of anima in order to still her own anxiety. Such a son might have a strong anima, but this will not always be good for the man if he wishes to pursue a traditional societal role. A *Kali-c* mother creates a field, or atmosphere, of dogmatic, oppressive restraint, a disabling barrier which keeps her children from establishing a conscious individuality of their own. Age-inappropriate over-parenting causes children to become aimless, irresolute and prone to depression; as adults, they suffer from diminished self-efficacy and lack the ability to put plans in place to achieve their goals. By not letting children stumble over little things, a *Kali-c* parent prevents them from developing coping skills. Failing to acquire a sense of mastery and self-confidence fosters long-term dependence on parents, but unconsciously, that is what the *Kali-c* mother wants and demands.

The *Kali-c* mother is full of strong opinions, and she does not reflect on the possibility that other opinions may be valid. The beliefs of a *Kali-c* mom are priority assumptions that claim to be the absolute truth. She never believes in exceptions. She is an animus possessed woman, which is expressed in her unshakable opinions, in order to overcome her adversaries. With the *Kali-c* mother, it is a question of power and control. Such a mother often has tremendous potential that has not been realized in her own life (the life unlived). While deliberately tolerant in her conscious intellectual convictions, she is quite rigid and tyrannical in her unconscious emotional demands and reactions, which permit no deviations from the way in which she has planned, arranged, and reasoned every detail of her life and those of her children. It is her way or the wrong way! She is truly a rigid mother and one who presents her children with a constant, profound dilemma: to either develop complex and constricting coping mechanisms to maintain a relationship with her, at great cost to their own outlooks, opinions, imaginations, and values, or suffer ridicule, criticism, disapproval, mortification and rejection at her hands. Everything has to be just so, and the result is that her child is not able to catch his own breath, which is symbolized in the asthmatic oppression and right-sided base pneumonia for which this remedy is so well known. "Breath" in Greek is *pneuma*, which also means "spirit". The spirit of *Kali-carb's* victim is oppressed. *Kali-c* refuses to acknowledge her developing child as a person with independent thoughts and feelings. The undeveloped creative power of the *Kali-c* mother always threatens to destroy the individuality and the life of her child. No matter how friendly and obliging she appears, she is possessed by *Logos* (Thinking) rather than *Eros* (Feeling), and nothing on earth can shake her or change her dogmatic opinions! In other words, *Kali-c* (and *Sepia*) women are fiery warhorses! Their exaggerated animus always draws the sword of power. Such mothers are capable of engaging lovingly with their children; however, they place fixed conditions on their love, approval, and appreciation, setting up a coercive relationship. In women, such an exaggerated animus expresses itself in the form of opinionated views and interpretations, of insinuations and misconstructions. Another sad result is that this pathogenic complex in the mother will be transferred to her daughter, who will identify with her mother's complex. Aping the mother's behavior, she will become, as an adult, another female who "knows best," continuing the chain of ruthless mutilation and castration in the name of love. Even worse, when such a child cannot break her ties to the *Kali-c* mother, she cannot escape from suffering intense fears of being destroyed by this archetype of the negative mother figure.

According to *Kali-c*, her rules are proposed out of concern for her family members, but our task is to understand the why and what for of such behavior! *Kali-carb's* concern for the family is not expressed in *cares about relatives*, where of the *Kali* family we find only *Kali-s—but also Sulph*! *Kali-c* is a black-type remedy for ***too*** *much sense of duty*, just like *Calc* and *Nit-ac*. It should get our attention that his rubric does not say "Great sense of duty" but, *too much sense*. These three strange bedfellows (*Kali-c, Calc-c* and *Nit-ac*), the only black-type remedies in this rubric, are all psoric-syphilitic remedies, and it seems unimaginable that they would appear there. But then again, all the *Kalis, Causticum* included, as well as other anxious remedies such as *Arsenicum*, are in this rubric. Indeed, we have here three remedies whose egos are not well formed in the sense of maturation and individuation. Each of these fellows, as nice as this rubric sounds and as much as we might wish for it to refer to a great and noble characteristic, possesses a limited scope of duty (not like an

Aurum!) and is driven, rather, by a more personal agenda. We shall investigate this further in order to clarify.

Nit-ac (a psoric-syphilitic remedy) has only a sense of duty toward the underdog, a little like *Causticum*. But *Nit-ac* is driven by that CD of *engaged in lawsuits,* and he feels that only people of his same mind and opinion can be trusted and supported—so his is a rather distorted sense of duty. *Calc-carb's* sense of duty is only skin deep, and in fact, *Calc-c* is found at the same time in the rubric *no sense of duty* (black type)! This is no contradiction. *Calc-carb's* duty is towards himself in the first place, and then towards his immediate family and friends, but it goes no further than his "village," so to speak. Everything else upsets and drains him too much (*hearing bad news aggravates; sad stories aggravate*). The rubric "*no sense of duty*" refers to *Calc-carb's* syphilitic, final, exhaustive depressive state (in which she refuses to help herself to get well) and also to his indifference towards—or, should we say, fear of learning about—suffering in the world (*horrible things affect her deeply*). *Calc-c* feels no duty to come out and help, overcome as he is by fear of bodily harm.

Kali-carb's sense of duty is also limited, and she is steered by the fixed idea that not only does she herself need to be rescued from the abyss behind her, but so does her immediate family; she therefore keeps a tight rein on them. "Mother knows best" is her motto, and the rules set out for the supposed welfare and safety of her family members must be strictly followed; otherwise, her syphilitic characteristics will take over: *she is contented with nothing; she is besides herself and gets into a rage if everything does not go according to her wishes, and frequently does not know herself what she really wishes to have, and feels extremely unhappy.* "Of course I have a short fuse," she concedes. "Since when does shouting kill you? Besides, if my children would respect my wishes, I wouldn't have to shout." Such an animus opinion is usually right in a general way, even somewhat reasonable, but most often beside the point. One sees the distorted reasoning of the *Kali-c* person: true love has no place in her heart as she is truly overcome by her anxieties and her inappropriate concern for others. (This is also a behavioral state commonly found in children suffering from autism.) When she feels she is losing control, *Kali-c* goes quickly into the negative cycle, and all of her pent-up emotions will be expressed as great anger towards her children to the point of creating a dysfunctional family life: *impatient with her children; every trifle vexes her; easily aroused to anger, she easily becomes violent; intolerant to human voice; quarrelsome with himself and his family.* These "demon dialogues" that

Kali-c can have with her children (as expressed in the previous provings) engender feelings of panic and being unloved. There is an atmosphere of disconnection between *Kali-c* and her children which is easily understood when one considers *Kali-carb's* rigidity and lack of spontaneity (*averse to being touched*). *Kali-c,* who is hypochondriacal about her health due to high anxiety (*fear of impending disease*), often extends this concern to her children, but the poor subjects are sometimes made extremely ill—and are certainly over-treated and over-diagnosed—because of the parent's fears.

Friends in need can count on *Kali-c,* but her active role is very limited; she tends to assist by formulating rules that work for her and, therefore, should work for the other person too. There is too much anxiety in the whole *Kali* family to take a risky active role and get involved in the problems of others. The only exception in the *Kali* family is *Causticum,* who is driven by his CD *about criminals. Causticum,* as we know, will take a much more active role in fighting injustice (*too sympathetic*), not even hesitating to resort to violence (I think of the group The Weather Underground, a student organization in the 1960s in the U.S. that destroyed government buildings during the Vietnam War). *Causticum* will help out, fueled by his excessive sympathy and compassionate nature (*too sympathetic; sensitive to oppressive influences* and *sensitive to injustice*). *Kali-c,* on the other hand, shuns away from any such involvement.

Depression

As time goes on, when *Kali-c* receives mixed if not fully negative reactions to her oppressive dictatorship and feels that she is losing control, she is easily caught in a tubercular state of mind: changeable! She has an *alternating mood, at one time good and quiet, at another excited and angry at trifles; she is constantly in antagonism (hatred) with herself. She is frequently hopeful, frequently desponded, fretting about everything. She becomes fainthearted and despondent to an extreme degree.* You can see from these provings that she is not in the harmonious and calm state of mind that would help her to be thoughtful and introspective about her real situation. Why, then, does she have *A/F mental work*? Is she an intellectual remedy with thinking as the dominant conscious function? No! She is mainly an introvert sensation-dominant type, with either feelings or thinking as a secondary function. But when she cannot gauge something by sensation (touching something palpable and real)—the way she best approaches her world—she is overcome with uncertainties and the perception of dangers.

At this point, *Kali-c* might be overcome with a kind of depression that makes one think of *Pulsatilla*, as we find *weeping mood; she could at any time burst into tears; she was very much depressed and was obliged to weep much and without cause because it was constantly in her mind that she would die*. We recognize in these provings the annoying *Carbon* trait of pestering others with her trifling, personal, and selfish problems. This brooding will become so bad that *at night, after lying down, forebodings overtake him, on account of which he is unable to sleep*.

Dreams

Many of her dreams are about water, which is the relatively fixed symbol for the unconscious; this is not surprising for a character who puts all his emotions in the darkness of the unconscious so that her real reasons for her behavior will not come to light (consciousness). Yet, true to the compensation law, *Kali-c* also has erotic dreams as well as parallel dreams about misfortune and dead people. And in the dreams of the poor subjects of her tyranny, there is a desire to kill her, the "witch"; these dreams come as quite a shock to her children, who feel that their mother is a saint who tirelessly watches over them. But the dreams have sent a warning message which must not be ignored: "fight for your own voice!"

Golden Tips from the Masters

- *Kali-carb's* tortured mind will also be expressed in "torturing, painful" physical complaints (stitching, cutting pains) coupled with well-known disease names: pleurisy and cases of pneumonia in the lower right part of the lung, as if the lower lobe of the right lung is adhering to the ribs, and even beginning phtysis; also severe stitching pains in lungs, abdomen, and joints; above all, *Kali-c* is a great remedy to consider for many cases of **stomach ulcers**. Without a doubt, great anticipation anxiety and worry lead to excessive acid production and inflammation as anxiety *is felt in the pit of her stomach and during a cramp in the stomach. Kali* remedies in general, when they fit, are also powerful in normalization of the blood pressure.
- Of all the anxious remedies, the *Kalis* occupy the first spot, followed by the *Calcareas* and then polychrests like *Arsenicum album*, *Nitric acid*, and *Sulphur*.
- *Kali-c* progresses easily to a *Nux vomica* state
- It is the "stitching" remedy *par excellence*: stitches run through every part of the body (eyes, pericardium, ears, lungs, liver, abdomen, mammae, etc.). The pain is independent of movement and <during rest and <lying on affected side (< >*Bryonia*, which presents with the same stitching pain, but <from movement and <from heat). *Kali-c* follows *Bryonia* well when the latter fails to relieve.
- #1 remedy for lower back pain in the third trimester of pregnancy
- The central idea is stiffness on every plane
- It is a backup remedy for *Lycopodium* (and complementary) as it imitates it
- *Kali-c* often ignores her emotional and mental symptoms or minimizes them
- Hypersensitive to noise and touch (especially the feet when ever so lightly touched—ticklishness)
- Bag-like swelling of upper eyelid invariably suggests *Kali-c*! Always examine the kidneys as the swelling is often present in nephritic troubles. *Apis* has the swelling of both eyelids or enormous bag-like swelling under the eyes. *Phosphorus* has swelling all around the eye (Nash).
- *Kali-c*: <2-5 a.m.; *Kali-ars*: <1:30-2:30 a.m.; *Kali-sulph* <4:40-5:30 a.m.
- Excellent PMS remedy where backache precedes the menses with extreme bloating and water retention
- Severe insomnia without an apparent reason
- Wandering arthritis (*Puls, Kalmia*)
- Broken back feeling, sacroiliac syndrome like *Aesculus*

- For the pregnant mother who suffers from a weak back with sharp stitching pains from the back to the uterus. Also one of the best remedies for postpartum bleedings
- Shock, bad news, and fear are felt in the stomach
- Is particularly useful in kidney and uterine affectations
- Labor pains begin in the middle of the back and, instead of coming forward, extend down the sacrum
- Nosebleeds in the morning when leaning over to wash the face
- Nash's **triumvirate** of copious cold sweat, backaches dating from childbirth, and weakness
- NWS pneumonia
- Asthma attack at 3 a.m., >leaning forward with head on knees
- Along with *Arg-n,* it is the other "what if" remedy: "What if this happens? What if I do this?"
- Where *Colocynthis* will palliate the indicated colic, *Kali*-c will cure it, as they are complementary remedies (Kent)

Lac Caninum (Lac-c). Dog's milk

The Cyber Delusion

Lac-c is not an uncommon remedy; unfortunately, because of their low self-esteem, those who have the greatest need for it will rarely consult the homeopath. The low self-worth of *Lac-c* is reflected in its Cyber delusion: ***she is dirty***. It is also expressed in the delusions *she is despised; she is short; she is horrid; that she is of no importance* and *delusion, she feels insulted*. These rubrics are closely intertwined with Hering's proving symptoms: *she feels insulted because she thinks she is looked down upon by everyone; she imagines being dirty; she imagines she is a loathsome, horrible mass of disease and could not bear to look at any portion of the body as it intensifies the feeling of disgust and horror*. One perceives in these fixed ideas the low self-worth that permeates the essence of this person. *Lac-c* is a person who feels isolated in a threatening society in which there is no sense of love and belonging. *Lac-c* is a person whose life, essentially, takes place in conditions of want, distress, and often misery; she has to fight and struggle for her existence. For such a person, the unhappiest moment is that of waking up (*fear on waking*). This is a person who feels that she is at the bottom of the pecking order not only in society, but even more intimately, in her own family. She is the low-ranked servant who is looked down upon and disliked by everyone; she may have a typical Cinderella syndrome, or she may simply see herself as the neglected and forgotten child (often in favor of others). That does not mean that this neglected child is, in reality, an "ugly duckling." I remember a couple that, although both were intelligent and well meaning, wanted a boy so much that upon their son's birth, their first child, a beautiful girl, was neglected as she was an easy child in comparison to her demanding little brother. This alone might be enough to delude a lovely girl into thinking that she must be ugly, that no one wants to pay attention to her, and that she is despised.

When the feeling of self-esteem is dependent on others, each day becomes a struggle as one must convince others of one's own value and worth. As we see in *Lac-caninum's* picture, genuine sadness is intensified and expanded into self-hatred (*antagonism with herself; aversion to herself*) and depression; this sadness can be enacted in her psychotic world through voices (*delusion, hears voices*) and hallucinations that accuse her of being ugly and despised and looked down upon, reflecting her real-life delusions. *Lac-c* feels trapped in an ugly body: *she felt that if she could not in some way get out of her body, she should soon become crazy*. This proving is reflected by the delusion, *body; out of the body* and *the delusion, she is hovering in the air like a spirit*. It is called depersonalization; the person hovers around the danger line between neurosis and psychosis, and will at any time, with the slightest additional stress, succumb to a psychosis. These last delusions really reflect how much she wants to be someone else, how much she is imprisoned by her persona, a despised and disrespected servant to everyone. Depersonalization (*delusion, floating in air; delusion, swimming in the air*) always creates that feeling that everything happens to the person as in a dream (*delusion, everything seems unreal*). *Lac-c* feels worthless, expendable, like garbage heaps and filth (*delusion, thinks she is she is of no importance in life; imagines to be dirty*). Viewing these delusions, we see the depth of bleakness and despair in the person needing *Lac-c* (*delusion, heavy black clouds enveloped her; despair of recovery*).

Just like *Alumina*, from which it needs to be differentiated, *Lac-caninum's* identity has been erased, but in a crueler way than in *Alumina's* case (where sometimes well-meaning parents try to "do good" for their child). But *Lac-caninum's* opinion is never asked, and all her statements and beliefs are dismissed a priori without being heard (*delusion, all she says is a lie* and *delusion, of personal errors of identity*). Just like in *Alumina*, who speaks through someone else's voice, *Lac-c* never feels she is a separate entity from those around her and never reaches the point of taking a single step towards individuation (*delusion, she has someone else's nose*). As she is saddled with such low self-esteem, other fixed ideas take over, reflecting her fragility and fears: *delusion, sees faces in the dark; delusion, falling forward to pieces; delusion, snakes are in and around her* and *delusion, sees spiders*.

Causalities

Parental Domination

Lac-caninum's Never Well Since (NWS) stems from early childhood. The main background is one of ailments from domination and **deliberate** neglect. One or both parents dictate every aspect of the child's life in a degrading way: "You are too dumb to decide for yourself." Often, it is a case of plain neglect, as in the case of a stepmother who favors her own child and pays little if any attention to the child of another mother. Such neglect leaves no place for a learning process or the formation of a dominant function of conscious which is to be reached by the age of eighteen. Poor social training and being excluded from social events inevitably lead to the formation of an inadequate persona, creating a person who suffers from lack of poise, unnecessary defiance and overdefensiveness. Possible dreams of *Lac-c* are dreams of appearing naked in dreams (expressing her vulnerability) or being always seated in a car in the back while someone else is driving and in control of her destination. It might well be that the dominant function of one of the parents, distinct from that of the child's dominant function of conscious, is imposed on the child, creating conflict and always leading to neurosis. "We want you to become a lawyer, not a starving artist; we are a family of intellectuals," they tell her. It is as if we absolutely want to teach someone to be right-handed although he is left-handed, but the emotional impact of derailing the child from her destiny is of course very dangerous. The child remains on the level of poor individuation, dependent and confused. No decisions are taken by the child as the parents "know better" and guide the child in every little aspect of her life. Indecisiveness, confusion, and unpreparedness for life are inevitable consequences! Depending on the child's constitution and miasmatic state, he might react in a positive way, with a compensation that helps him break free. "I never wanted to be like my father!" On another positive note, there might be a silver lining in all this suffering: it can steer the victim to choose a profession in which he will be able to help similarly unfortunate souls: becoming a psychotherapist, a social worker, or a homeopath is often an attempt at self-cure on the therapist's part, and at the same time she is contributing something positive to a cause she knows all too well. This is indeed possible if that child has a different miasmatic background (from the mother if it is a boy) or rebels against the "injustice" done to her (*Causticum, Nat-m*). Such children become the future crusaders against child neglect and abuse. Otherwise, they become adults who have a midlife crisis and feel unfulfilled when they reach the crucial age of 45—when both sexes are confronted in their unconscious and dreams with the animus and anima, and when acceptance of the soul mate is a must in order to go further on the path of individuation. If this acceptance does not take place, they will be among the countless victims of "a life not lived," a spiritual disease worse than any other kind.

Anticipation Anxiety

When a child lives in such a world of terror, where emotional nourishment is not only lacking but distorted into something hostile, it is very understandable that she will also suffer from ailments from anticipation. "What is going to happen when I come home from school?" "Will I be beaten up by my drunken father, or will I have to take care of all the household chores? Will no one pay attention to my needs or desires?" For *Lac-c*, home is not the refuge it is supposed to be, where one can drink from the fountain of love and respect and gather energy. It is a place filled with the unexpected, the not knowing what kind of calamity to expect; such a home depersonalizes a child. Before the dominant conscious function is established at 18, the contradictory emotions hurled at such a child make her lose all sense of self-worth: "I really must be worth nothing to be treated like this!" I have heard these words from adults whose parents would say, "You will never amount to anything! You are good for nothing! You are a failure. You shame our family!" It takes a lot of positive encouragement from somewhere else (often a teacher, distant family member, a grandmother, a friend, etc.) to soften this cruel blow on a child's ego. Forsaken feelings and the absence of a nourishing vessel, the mother, figure prominently in the *Lac-c* person (although *Lac-c* cannot be found in the *delusion, mother is dead*, *Anac*, *Lach*, *Nat-m*, *Aur-m-n*). *Lac-c*, understandably, becomes *sensitive to all external impressions, light and noise*: this is a frail, highly alert person, and she expects no mercy from any corner. With such a degree of *self-contempt* and *want of confidence*, who wants to wake up in the morning to face another bleak day (*grief on waking*)?

Compensations

Connecting to Animals

One should not be surprised if such a person has childhood fantasies of belonging to a different family; this indicates emotional rejection of the parents. Like so many other unfortunate souls, an escape into a dream world in which she creates her own happy family is often the only rescue left: *delusions, of fancy illusions, of beautiful visions in daytime, of floating in the air, as if the feet do not touch the ground* and *of swimming in the air*. These two last delusions are like a symbolic escape from her bleak earthly existence as she flies away like a balloon to better destinations.

Besides retreating to a fantasy world, another compensatory escape may involve connecting to the animal world, especially the world of dogs, the best friends of men who are always pleased to see us and never judge us (*love for animals, for dogs*). *Lac-c* adheres to what Anatole France expressed so well: "Until one has loved an animal, a part of one's soul remains unawakened." Just like *Lyssin*, the essence of *Lac-c* is also being abused by the one he is dependent on, the master, or the parent. An unprejudiced observer will notice an above-average frequency of intense relationships with dogs among those who need *Lac-c*. What *Lac-c* is better known for, though, is an above-average *fear for spiders* and *snakes*: it is the #1 remedy for the latter.

Imitating Others

That *lack of self-confidence* is part of the makeup of *Lac-c* is a given in view of her Cyber delusion and feelings (*anxiety from doubt about success*). This also means that part of her compensation is that she wants to be more like everyone else; the last person she wants to be is herself. In fact, she prefers to **imitate** people in everything what they do (how they dress, what they read, in what recreation they participate) in order to increase her sense of self-value, to feel more like someone else and to fit in. I had a *Lac-c* patient who took on the accent of the person she was talking to and imitated all the habits of the person she wanted to be with: initially she was not a smoker or drinker, but became one in order to feel more like the other, supposedly "better" person. This is expressed by the rubrics *delusion, imagines she wears someone else's nose* and *delusion, errors of personal identity*. Clearly, for *Lac-c*, a more positive approach to resolving her low self-esteem is to give up her identity and try to emulate someone else. Alas, in order to achieve this goal, *Lac-c* often becomes subservient to everyone (*thinking himself too little*)! "As long as my husband is pleased, I am pleased." We don't find *Lac-c* in the rubrics *amativeness, amorous* or *affectionate,* because that is not what she stands for. It has nothing to do with affection (real or false), only with **submission** and yielding *(Puls, Staph)* that can increase her low worth in the eyes of others. In this way, though, she will never be an equal partner in any relationship. Of course, she longs for appreciation or approbation to dull her lament and her *delusion, she is criticized* and *she is ugly*. This longing for approval is not as intense as it is in *Palladium*, who has a stronger ego; for *Lac-c*, simple acceptance as her own person would be enough.

Inconsistent Performance

If no escape to a different world is possible and no connection is established to some other "successful" person, we expect *Lac-c* to react with many negative compensations. Because of her low self-worth, there is a *fear of failure* which will only worsen her self-esteem as she tries to please others (*fear, she will become unable to perform her duties*); paradoxically, she sets herself up for this situation as she *undertakes many things, and perseveres in nothing; she cannot concentrate her thoughts or mind to read; she wants to leave everything as soon as it is commenced.* She tries to overcome this intense feeling of self-loathing, of being dirty and ugly, by *always washing the hands,* but this symbolic hand-washing will never be able to rub out her Cyber delusion.

Destruction of the Ego Control

Lac-caninum's major causality—parental or spousal abuse—is abuse by excessive control like in *Alum*, but the reactions of the victim are different. The anger and rage of *Lac-c* are generally directed at the **self** (still syphilitic—remember *antagonism with herself*) rather than at others (in *Alumina* it is directed at the self—*she cuts herself with a knife*—**and** others). The emotional pain experienced by *Lac-c* can lead to autistic qualities; he may become introverted or exhibit excessive daydreaming, running around as if in a daze. *Lac-c* is stuck in his emotions, leading to irresolution: *she very absent minded; she makes purchases and walks off without them; she goes to post a letter, and brings it home in her hand.* This situation represents the *passive* type of *Lac- c*, which shows great sensitivity (*sensitive, oversensitive*), shyness, reclusiveness, and an inability to express direct aggression or stand up for herself when needed (*lack of self-confidence; lack of character*). It prevents *Lac-c* from having intimate relationships: she is always an unequal partner. She never gets close to a sexual partner or forms a deep friendship. She always remains the "underdog," literally and figuratively, "under or below" the alpha dog in the social hierarchy.

The more *active* type of *Lac-c* individual reminds us of *Phosphorus* with his fears and tendency to feel on the verge of hysteria: he is *very nervous, and feels a constant dread; he has a feeling as if he was going to become unconscious.* These are functional individuals, but they are somewhat off-center and off-balance, with changeable moods as they switch from passive to active states (*mood, changeable, variable*). Like *Phosphorus, Lac-c* has no effective armor to protect herself. There is a certain amount of disorganization, with sudden, unexpected mind changes: *inconstancy; excitement, excitable, extremely nervous* and *irritable, very easily startled.* What differentiates her from the *Phosphorus* type is that crazed look in the eye and the sharp, distorted gestures she makes with her hands (*makes gestures, spread fingers apart*), as well as the sharp expressions in her speech—especially to her best friend (*intense ugliness; writes to her best friends all sorts of mean and contemptible things,* something *Phosphorus* would never do). What sets *Lac-c* further apart from *Phosphorus* is that *Lac-c* people are incapable of expressing happiness and pleasure, leading to a lack of emotional responsiveness: there is a chronic "blue" condition: *everything seems so dark that it can grow no darker. Lac-c* does not express anger either, as she has a lack of character; rather, she feels guilt and shame. Being an unequal partner, she cannot seek relief from her situation by means of demands, paralyzed and frozen as she feels. Her life becomes a struggle for survival, even questioning herself as to whether she has the very right to exist, followed by suicidal ideation. *Lac-c has no desire to live* (*desires death*), *with suicidal disposition,* probably to escape this bleak existence. This might lead her to drop out of society by abandoning her job if she has had one. And now she even feels guiltier, since the money to buy nice clothes and jewelry (in order to increase her value) comes only from her hard-working husband. But a return to work seems impossible as she has the *Phosphorus fears about death* and disease: *fear she will have heart disease and die from it; fear of death with anxious expression of countenance, and mental work aggravates.* She also exhibits a sense of fragility and paranoia: *delusion, of falling forward to pieces; delusion, she has an incurable disease* and *delusion, she will become insane.*

Golden Tips from the Masters

- *Lac-c* is truly is and looks like a cramped individual, even on the physical plane, as she is suffering from physical complaints like headaches, sciatica, cramps in the feet, restlessness of legs, and obstinate constipation. *Lac-caninum's* greatest fame in homeopathic history came from curing **diphtheria** throat with that specific alternation: going from left to right to left, or from right to left to right. This last characteristic is so important that if it is seen in any complaint, eczema, sciatica, rheumatic diseases, etc., *Lac-c* should be tried!
- Indicated in painful finger joints ameliorated by cold. Compare to pain in ankles >cold: *Ledum*; knee pain >cold: *Puls*; hand pain >cold: *Guaiacum*
- Super keynote: alternation of location, mood, and time; symptoms also return to the original side
- #1 for fear of snakes (*Lachesis* is #2); dreams and delusions of snakes
- Pain in opposite breast while breastfeeding; also hypersensitive nipples in breastfeeding
- Vertigo with mental states
- #1 remedy for severe milk allergies
- Amelioration during menses and painful breasts before menses (they can't stand a bra) as well as hysteria before menses

Lachesis muta (Lach). Bushmaster snake

The Cyber Delusion

Lachesis' Cyber delusion is ***about to receive an injury from her surroundings*** and ***she is being injured and wronged.*** As a result, we find *suspicion* (*full of mistrust*) and the trio of symptoms *restlessness, anticipation anxiety* and *hypersensitivity* (*offended easily; sensitive to criticism*). Other delusions that support the CD include: *he is persecuted; he is pursued by enemies,* and *he has been poisoned.* The provings state: *imagines he is followed by enemies, who are trying to harm him,* and *there are robbers in the house* and *he wants to jump out of the window.* The latter delusions often come after the primary delusion has been allowed to run its course and thus will be part of an advanced mental-emotional pathology, making *Lachesis* one of the most frequently needed remedies for all kinds of schizophrenia. As the *Lachesis* state progresses, the vacuum created in the ego continues to grow, while the well-functioning sectors of the ego become narrower and narrower; the dualism (*two wills*) will only disappear when the ego in its entirety has substituted an imaginary world for actual reality, when the victim does not make a distinction between the unconscious and conscious world: a situation called dissociation. The danger of dissociation is always particularly high for a *Lachesis* person: a neurosis is like a car zooming in and out of the right side of the road, creating the possibility of an accident (a psychotic break). When two or three cars are on the other side of the road, the first one might miss you, but the second or third one can derail you. Due to her CD, *Lachesis* cannot relax, and her hypervigilance is seen even when she is trying to mesmerize and charm you. She continually perceives a threat to her existence.

Frequently, delusional ideas are a mixture of wish-fulfillment and a sense of imminent injury or persecution; these feelings are sometimes compensated by megalomania (a protective withdrawal in a cocoon of superiority), but *Lachesis* also responds with very violent reactive fears. The idea of persecution issues stems from a relationship infected with mistrust. It is interesting that *Hyoscyamus* and *Lachesis*, two of the most jealous characters, have many *delusions of reference*. Jealousy is a great cause of delusions for these two remedies, and when driven by that jealousy, any small acute circumstance and/or insignificant gesture or word can produce the grossest misjudgments. T. F. Allen expresses this in the proving *believes himself intentionally injured by his environment, and attaches the most hateful significance to the most innocent occurrences*. Awash with anticipatory anxiety and jealousy, when *Lachesis* and *Hyoscyamus* meet with a mishap, during the first moment of anger, they immediately jump to the conclusion that they have been **deliberately** injured or insulted (*delusion, she has suffered wrong; delusion is injured by his environment*). Both *Lachesis* and *Hyoscyamus* interpret neutral and "negligent" actions (like a delay in answering an email, in texting or in phoning) as intentional slights. The suspicious *Lachesis* always find these situations meant to be harmful to her (*delusion, is about to receive an injury; delusion, is being injured*—also *Hyos*). And no one gets the benefit of the doubt! Seeking constant reassurance from the beloved, even if told repeatedly that they (*Lachesis* and *Hyos*) are loved, they do not trust what they are told—because the affirmation had to be *elicited* rather than being expressed spontaneously! "I had to put these words in your mouth," they shout, "so it is not coming from your heart!" It is maddening for others to deal with these personalities, and living with them is like walking on eggshells. Anticipatory anxiety, anger, and all-consuming jealousy can lead to serious organic disease, given the correlation between coronary health and such emotions as these. Patients possessed by such high-risk temperaments, quick to anger and fast to explode (belonging to the Fire element in TCM and the sanguine Hippocratic temperament), are represented by the archetype of a jealous boyfriend or a vengeful boss (*after a jealous quarrel, she put both hands to her chest and cried out, "Oh! My heart!" Then she fell down and was in an asphyctic state for nearly twenty four hours; no pulse could be felt, breathing was hardly perceptible; Delusion, is going to have a heart attack and die*). Cardiovascular problems increase proportionally to the level of anger and jealousy themselves.

As mentioned before, people with paranoia have often feelings of grandiosity and omnipotence. *Lachesis* is convinced that he possesses remarkable talents as a prophet, scientist, lover, and sportsman. People are just jealous of him because, after all, *Lachesis* is sure that he is smarter than everyone else. That's why *Lachesis* considers himself attractive, irresistible, inspired, and envied by everyone. There is nothing he cannot accomplish (compare with *Sulphur*)! One can readily see that *Lachesis* is the other side of the coin of (and complementary to) *Lycopodium*! Here is a quote from my practice: "I feel like people are trying to get me mad.

Almost like people are intentionally trying to get under my skin or push my buttons, like they are just out to see if they can get me upset." Prejudices of this kind may establish themselves and inevitably lead to delusions of "strange machinations," such as these delusions of *Lachesis*: *I will be sent to the asylum* and *the medicine is poison*. Incidentally, the latter delusion also belongs to *Hyoscyamus*, who is now also convinced that *his lover is faithless and will not marry him*. This road will lead straight to paranoia, with the respective delusions of *being sold* (Hyosc), *being poisoned* (both *Hyosc* and *Lachesis*), and *being sent to the asylum* (Lachesis).

Lachesis' Cyber delusion is even projected on others in his family. Take the example of a *Lachesis* child. This passionate child shows great love and amativeness, especially towards a younger sibling (less often towards an older one), but at the same time, she is in great competition with that sibling for parental love. No kiss can be given to the younger sibling without *Lachesis* asking for one for himself. But, driven by his CD, this child starts crying when his baby sister cries, telling his mom, "Feed her! Pick her up!" In the child's mind, the baby is being injured. He even advises complete strangers when their babies cry. It is *Lachesis*' innate character calling out in his language: "Pay attention! Be hypervigilant; your baby is being harmed!" Such a child always carries something in his hands: a little stick, a stone, a certain toy... they are all part of a defense system, his alertness, and his readiness for the "what if" situation, an expression of a certain degree of paranoia. But he also might refuse to take medication or express fear of the remedy because he thinks *that the medicine is poison* and *that he is about to be poisoned*.

Because of the *delusion, he is going to be injured by his surroundings*, the *Lachesis* child with ASD can have fear of deep water, dogs, and unknown people; he shows great anticipation anxiety (*Lachesis*' *fear of death*). He might have a great fascination with dogs and be unable to take his eyes off of them, but he may scream in fear at the same time. The child is hypervigilant as this dog can injure him—echoing his CD! This hypervigilance is also expressed by high shrieks (even in the pre-verbal ASD child) when the child comes into a new situation such as entering a new doctor's office or a new school; after this initial incident, the child turns to his own world of fantasy and starts scripting something from a video, a sign he has entered into her own safe world of fantasy and imagination. A *Lachesis* child will start scripting whenever she is upset and feels threatened. This scripting and screaming stop once the child is more comfortable in the new place. An example from my practice:

> On the first day of school, a child was assigned a certain table. The child stayed the whole day at this table without moving: this table was her safe place, and it expressed again her Cyber delusion that *she will be injured by her surroundings*. This is rather unusual for the *Lachesis* child as such a child is restless, continuously in motion because he needs to be hypervigilant to avoid *being wronged,* fueling a strong suspicion of *delusion, he has suffered wrong*. One *Lachesis* child expressed this hypervigilance by first needing to examine every room in his school before settling into his own classroom. If this routine was not followed, furious and hysterical behavior resulted. *Lachesis*' CD is also expressed in the following example: a child's foot was hurt by another child's three-wheeler, and whenever that child came close to the *Lachesis* child again, *Lachesis* shrieked and ran. The accident was perceived as an attack and created the fixed idea of *being wronged* and *injured*.

When it comes to Jung's conscious types, *Lachesis* is most frequently the extravert thinking intuitive type. Of course, as usual, according to the circumstances, this extravert type, under the influence of triggers (especially from ailments from disappointed love), can easily become introverted, switching from loquacious behavior to taciturn behavior (*repugnance to society* and *dislike to talk*). For *Lachesis*, having intuition as a secondary conscious function leads to positive consequences. *Lachesis* has *excitement and liveliness in the evening, a kind of fanciful imagination; he sits up late at night at mental work, with great activity*. Indeed, even if he has felt fatigued during the day, *Lachesis* is *impelled to productive work in the evening. He writes with the greatest freedom and increased rigor about everything he knows*. Through his intuitive function, he taps into the unconscious, even to the extent that he feels guided by a godlike figure through which his inspiration comes. Delusions of grandeur, of omnipotence, and of being possessed are the result: *delusion he is charmed and can't break the spell; delusion, he is under a powerful influence; delusion, of higher power; delusion, he is some other person* and *delusion, he is under superhuman control*. These last delusions can prove to be positive if *Lachesis* derives material for her stories from them; at the same time, though, they can put *Lachesis* on a dangerous slope of dissociation (*wills, two wills, feels as if he had; delusion, she is some other person*), leading to incomprehensible deeds if the message of these delusions is followed: *delusion, hears voices that he must follow and confess things he never did and that she must kill and steal*. This latter delusion indicates that the patient has suffered a full psychotic break. I had once a patient who came under the spell of her guru in presence of many other followers; she fell into a trance and started speaking in a language totally foreign to her (*speech, affected, in a foreign tongue*). This person was literally *charmed and could not break the spell and was under superhuman control,* eradicating her own individuality. Where *Lachesis* only sometimes welcomes ESP as a tool for inspiration, *Phosphorus* thrives on it and accepts it with open arms while *Thuja* absolutely avoids it!

Causalities

Disappointed Love and Humiliation

There is no doubt that *ailments from grief* and *disappointed love* play a great role in the pathology of *Lachesis* (*chronic complaints after long lasting grief or sorrow*). *Lachesis* **is** a human being with superior thinking abilities, like *Aurum, Carcinosin, Sulphur, China,* and *Lycopodium,* but her reactions to grief are essentially different from those of the above remedies. The others certainly all possess great ego and great ambition with plenty of delusions of grandeur, just like *Lachesis*—but *Lachesis* is also the extremely passionate person who gets vexed about *competition* (in love and profession) with others. While some men (especially thinking-dominant *Lycopodium* men) might claim that it is "normal" to be able to love more than one woman at a time, *Lachesis* will revolt against such a statement with a definitive "I am a 100% passionate, devoted lover," evoking strong feelings of humiliation (*ailments from mortification*) as her strongest desire is to be loved 100% by one person only! So the CD is understandable: *she feels wronged* and *injured by her surroundings* when the spouse has an affair. The sharp-thinking female *Lachesis* has a highly developed sense of vigilance to test her partner at a relationship's start—acting coy in response to her suitor's attention—but she then becomes obsessive once committed. This situation worsens, of course, upon the approach of menopause, which is a very dangerous period if the *Lachesis* layer has not been corrected and dissolved: she is now easily overcome by paranoia (*delusion, there are conspiracies are against her*). She becomes sensitive to perceived rejection (*easily offended*) as threats lurk everywhere. She may think, for example: "My husband is probably looking for a replacement; my boss is trying to get rid of me, too, in order to hire a much younger and more attractive person." The resulting drop in self-esteem begets an overwrought response to slights, both real and imagined—all of which are presumed to be intentional.

Lachesis, with her Hippocratic sanguine temperament, cannot live without passion; she demands loyalty from her partner, but this demand often borders on foolishness (*ailments *from foolish jealousy*). Anger is never far behind when grief and disappointed love occur. She finds examples among some of her friends who are "spoiled" by their husbands, implying that her partner's behavior does not compare favorably with theirs: "He cut her nails for her," she complains; "He always asks her, 'Can I do anything for you?'" Such examples are markers for *Lachesis* of how much she is loved and cared for (delusions of reference). We see the intensity of *Lachesis* in her emotions: there is no middle path, only the high road! It is like an Olympic flame that burns with desire forever! The flames of this fire indeed need very little impetus to get out of hand, and driven by *foolish jealousy* it can lead to hysteria and compulsion and all kinds of unexpected, spontaneous actions. In her mind, this behavior is totally justified: with her intellect, it is easy to find rationalizations. *Lachesis* is a well-spoken lawyer at heart. You cannot win an argument with a *Lachesis*! To everyone else, this trait is as suffocating as a boa constrictor as well as utterly ridiculous: often there is no real basis for her jealousy except in her great imagination.

A mother can even enter pregnancy in a state of disappointed love and humiliation, which is a circumstance that might have existed for the mother even before conception. This may be especially true if she has not been able to live the life that she had projected for herself. Here is one example of such a situation:

> A woman in her mid-thirties had not been able to reach her potential because of OCD behavior, though she was perceived by the outside world as very intelligent. OCD behavior is often the result of fear of losing control of one's life, and in her case, it was propelled by her own mother's cruel and cold behavior; these behaviors stopped her from following her projected path to a successful profession. To make matters worse, whenever her family came together, her opinion was never asked as she was the "uneducated" one (*ailments from humiliation*). In other words, she suffered with a "life unlived," the essence of the portrait of homeopathic *Lachesis*.

This unlived life can have severe consequences for the *Lachesis* patient on the physical plane, where cancer of the ovaries and uterus feature prominently. From a symbolic standpoint, cancer is a metaphor for life energies finding inappropriate, self-destructive expression in an uncontrolled and unbalanced growth. In this sense, cancer can be considered the revenge of a suppressed, unlived life. Unless *Lachesis* can find appropriate compensatory channels in which she can express herself, she can indeed come to harm, or in other words, get injured—either psychologically (dissociation) or physically (cancer). As too much remains unlived in *Lachesis*' life, feelings of hopelessness, melancholy **(often leading to alcoholism)**, frustration, and even suicidal thoughts overcome the *Lachesis* person when she begins to realize just how much of her authentic life has been neglected and ignored in favor of socially acceptable family traditions. Because she has missed her calling, *Lachesis* approaches midlife with unanswered questions that inevitably turn her glance backward: "What could have been? Why did I not follow my heart?" Thus, the "revenge" of the body and soul creates a midlife crisis: disillusion and regret set in, a terrible psychological letdown comparable in painfulness to physical disease.

> When one of my patients was pregnant, she was not disturbed by her husband's visit to his parents in another country because her beloved brother was by her side. But when she started bleeding at four months, she thought, "I am going to lose the only thing I have in my life," which obviously reflected her lack of emotional support and security, real or perceived. And when later, during a small argument, her husband continued the discussion *ad nauseam* because he wanted to "win" the insignificant quarrel, she could only stop it by shouting at the top of her lungs (*ailments from anger*; *disappointed love*). The next event was one of huge fright when she thought there was an intruder in her house, and in spite of her husband being present, she had to call the neighbor to check as the husband was too afraid. It was, in fact, only a window screen that had fallen down because of excessive wind, but she expressed it to me as a "considerably scary moment" (*ailments from fright*). Her emotions, both long-term and newly formed, created huge scars not only in the expectant mother: they were unfortunately carried over to the unborn fetus. And then the mother, who is very intelligent, reproached herself that she had "ruined the life of her child" (who had ASD). How painful! It was a noble misfortune that came to her, but she was bearing the guilt all by herself (*anxiety, as if guilty of a crime*; *anxiety about salvation*). Weeping became a constant companion (*weeping about former offenses, weeping with the pains,* and *weeping on waking*) until homeopathic *Lachesis* freed her from the shackles of despair.

Anticipation Anxiety

Another patient told me a story that pointed to different causalities belonging to the portrait of homeopathic *Lachesis*:

> For the entire length of her pregnancy, she was in a constant state of anticipation anxiety regarding the health of her unborn fetus, reflecting the fixed idea of *Lachesis*, *is injured by her surroundings*. This fixed idea indicates one's view of the world in a *Lachesis* state, leading to hypervigilance and suspicion. She had to drive herself to buy food and make doctors' visits in an old car that stalled on her all the time in the middle of traffic. Whenever she left home, she was overcome by anticipation anxiety to the point that she would plan a route on which it was more convenient to come to a stop, avoiding busy routes with heavy traffic and greater risk of accidents. At one point she stalled at a traffic light and someone actually did rear-end her. Her anxiety was compounded by having to take a stress test at the hospital three times a week because of low amniotic fluid, again reflecting that Cyber delusion that she and her baby were injured by her surroundings. Upon an ultrasound measuring of the baby, it was shown that he was not growing; the doctor suggested emergency delivery (*ailments from fright;* an injury possible to the baby). To make matters worse, her recovery room was very cold and she feared that the baby was going to be sick, so she checked out early (again fear for injury!).

It was not at all surprising that all of this led to the formation of a *Lachesis* child with ASD and the restlessness and anticipation anxiety so characteristic of *Lachesis*.

Cares and Worries (Stress)

Situations arising from *cares and worries* easily lead to a state of hypervigilance:

> After suffering a previous miscarriage, a woman (who later became my patient) became pregnant at the ripe age of 49, well beyond the age (between 28 and 35) considered favorable according to Traditional Chinese Medicine (TCM). The expectant mother was very happy until a genetic test, mandatory in view

of her age, was done at three months. The doctor told her bluntly that there was a marker that showed great risk for Down syndrome. (What the doctor did not tell the parents, who later researched this issue themselves, was that this marker and Down syndrome were, in fact, very rarely connected). But it started the process of hypervigilance which lasted until the delivery; the pregnant woman went through one ordeal after another. She was always wary of anything that could hurt her baby; as she said, "I prepared myself for anything that could happen!" When her water broke, she was admitted for induction of labor; but her obstetrician had just gone off duty, so her care was taken over by another physician. This physician, against all logic, dismissed her and let her go home. When she showed up days later at her primary care office, her regular doctor was incensed that she had been released and chewed her colleague out in front of the patient. This disturbed the patient so much that she no longer even trusted her original obstetrician! And because of low amniotic fluid, she was now surrounded in the delivery room by a whole crew of caregivers, ready for any emergency, resembling the emergency landing of an airplane with the fire trucks and ambulances on the tarmac. All this did was increase the mother's anticipation anxiety that her "baby was going to be injured." She had endured six months of hyper-alertness and *fear she will be injured by her surroundings.*

Compensations

Religion

In homeopathy, one remedy can easily belong to both ends of a spectrum: this is certainly the case with religion for *Lachesis*. She can pray for guidance through the Bible, where she studies the Prophets in particular: she feels increasingly drawn to those who have lived through struggles similar to her own in order to become more thoroughly human. As seen in some of her delusions, *Lachesis* is drawn to intimate conversations and "direct contact" with Christ. In general, religions provide therapy for the sorrows and disturbances of the soul as well as relief when one is overburdened with responsibility. *Lachesis* searches for protection against injury and attempts to "find answers" via communication with people in high positions, writing letters, for example, to the Pope. It makes one think of *Veratrum album*, who believes he should be received by the most famous people to confirm his so highly sought-after elevated social status (*anxiety about social status*). As usual, we often see a religious compensation when the sexual outlet is either suppressed or unattainable (as, for example, in puberty) (*Kali-br, Platina, Lil-t, Lyc, Verat-a*). It is no different with *Lachesis*: her compensation matches the intensity of the sexual outlet. There is *religious monomania* and *even fear of being damned.* It is especially the female teenager who will follow the religious compensation when sexuality awakens (*religious affections in puberty*), especially if she is being brought up in a strict religious milieu where the topic of sex is taboo. *Lachesis* might go on the streets to preach to people about the end of the world coming nearer (*Verat-a*). Male teenagers have more of a tendency to engage in thrill-seeking, sexual, and dangerous behavior. For *Lachesis*, when life remains unlived, the life that remains often does not seem fair; she consoles herself with tales of an "eternal life" in which wrongs will be set right.

Studying the materia medica, one finds invariably the expression of the dual law, or the law of opposites and complementaries, as symbolized in the physician's caduceus with its dual snakes, supported by the rod of Asclepius. Besides the deep depression and the marked elation, the passion and love contrasted by hate and revenge, and the logorrhea and taciturnity, *Lachesis*' fanatical religiousness can turn into its own opposite, and we find the greatest atheists among *Lachesis* people for whom the promised paradise vanishes like an optical illusion (*godless, want of religious feeling*). *Lachesis* always has compelling beliefs; he is convinced and rejects any dissenting opinion. *Lachesis* is definitely an intelligent person, but, as Aristotle said, "no great intellect has been without a touch of madness." This is clearly seen in the next compensation: jealousy!

A Dark Compensation: Foolish Jealousy, a Voice of the Past

"Go green, save the ozone," is the slogan! Green may be the virtuous color that represents sustainable living in our times, but in the context of jealousy, green is the color of the time-honored serpent. Jealousy is positively associated with neuroticism or emotional instability, and the higher the level of flightiness, the more one is prone to jealousy. Jealousy derives from a complex cocktail of *competitiveness* or *increased ambition,* delusions of grandeur, emotional insecurity (especially the need to be loved unconditionally), and situational dissatisfaction. As mentioned before, *Lachesis* belongs to the sanguine temperament and the Fire element in TCM, which makes her especially prone to pangs of jealousy. She is always on jealous high alert. The root of the torments of jealousy is the attitude toward the object of love as property. Envy is both a vice and a source of misery. It should be treated as an enemy of happiness and banned as an evil thought. Contrary to what *Lachesis* thinks, Jealousy is not the guardian of love; more typically, jealousy is its destroyer. Few people look in the mirror and are honest enough to see green. The jealous person degrades the partner he allegedly loves by treating her like owned property. Such a person claims, "I want to *have* you for myself," thereby expressing that he thinks of his partner as a "possession," as a piece of property, and exhibiting in his claim the classic signs of jealousy: fear of losing his lover, lack of trust, stalking, anger at real or imagined attention to others, and the need to control a loved one. More often than not, feelings of jealousy flare up with such intensity that they obliterate any rational thought and set in motion a host of negative cognitive processes—from doubt to constant relentless preoccupation with a partner's faithlessness and imaged lack of attention. Alas, these behaviors create a self-fulfilling prophecy, pushing away the very person that *Lachesis* desires or needs the most. Jealousy lands with an unexpected and violent thrust, leading to delusions in which one thinks the same thing over and over again, creating a vacuum in the conscious (*compelling ideas*), and the more she does that, the less place there is for other ideas and the more she disconnects from reality. This reaches extreme in many *Lachesis* cases: some have violent reactions to deception such as stalking, and, unfortunately, even murder (*jealousy leading to a crime*; *jealousy driving to kill*; *jealousy with rage*). For *Lachesis*' victim, such "passionate love" seems irresistible, welcoming and flattering at first—until he discovers that she means to have "sole and exclusive rights and privileges" over him. He finds out that lavish presents are nothing but a kind of camouflage, a costly trick for her possessiveness. Most likely, *Lachesis* can use other, less subtle tactics such as yelling at a partner for talking to someone else, cutting a partner off from friends and family, accompanying him on every outing to a store, speaking to him in a derogatory manner, undermining a mate's self-esteem, or threatening violence against a partner or perceived rivals (*jealousy driving to a crime*; *jealousy with rage*; *insane jealousy*; *jealousy driving to strike his wife*). *Lachesis*' jealousy (which is basically a feeling of being unlovable) is accompanied by a sense of deficiency which is hard to bear, and *Lachesis* converts her anger into distrust or *suspicion*—going through his belongings and cell phone logs, cracking the passwords to his email accounts, and if necessary hiring a P.I. to retrace every minute of his day. Jealousy thrives indeed upon doubts! "Was he laughing at that woman's jokes? I think she just touched his arm. He spent far too much time talking to her." Jealousy becomes an overzealous call to arms. No person and no career is allowed to be more important than *Lachesis*; all of the aspirations and goals of her partner must be concentrated on her or she will unleash her rage. And marriage can be the mine that leaves her partner an amputee! Jealousy indeed reveals more about the bearer than about the deeds or misdeeds of a mate. *Lachesis* women are intelligent and can even use jealousy as a test of affection. *Lachesis* does not hesitate to provoke a little jealousy when she perceives that her partner is less committed to the relationship than she is (of course no one can be committed as she is!) Her aim is to alter her partner's perception of how desirable she is. Homeopathic *Lachesis* can stop her on this destructive path; it will make the victim, under the control of her own poison, look within herself and repair her sense of self.

Lachesis, the Bushmaster snake, is so jealous of her territory (her domain) that she will fiercely attack any intruder. It is obvious that jealousy has no place in true love, as Eros is much more than sex (although the French expression *faire l'amour*, or "making love," is a confusing one in this regard). True love acknowledges the beloved's uniqueness, and it is not expressed by infatuation or the pleasure principle and gratification of the sexual instincts. True love is the only form of love that penetrates to the core of the other person; it is experiencing the other person with all his unique features, for what he is, not for what he has.

Lachesis also exhibits another well-known type of jealousy: the jealousy of the partner's past, of previous lovers and friends. He who suffers this kind of jealousy always wants to be "the first," although he does not realize how much more rewarding it is to be the last. I had a patient who married a much older man, and when they had intercourse for the first time, upon hearing that he was not the first, he slapped her and said: "Why didn't you wait for me?" *Lachesis* never wants to hear that he is not the first! This comparing of oneself to others—be it in love or competition—does an injustice to oneself and to others. Investigate your personal life and see how different yours is from every other story! If there appear to be many people who are better off than you are, think about how many are worse off. It should be remembered that no form of hatred is as offensive as the hatred that comes from jealousy.

Even the early intra-utero start of life differs among individuals, and if this start is less favorable and more difficult, it provides the individual with the opportunity to achieve more in the personal realm. We see in *Sulphur* and *Lachesis* that jealousy is always foolish (*jealousy driving to strike his wife*), even when one's partner has cheated (*jealousy from disappointed love*). When *Lachesis* feels unhappy, she cannot bear the sight of anyone who is happy. I had a patient who had a younger sister who became pregnant before she did. She could not be happy for her sister and refused to hold the newborn. Such irrational passions, which compel man to act in a way contrary to his own self-interest, make him suffer the torments of hell.

Jealous characters have not learned that to openly doubt a partner's fidelity without grounds results in what they fear the most: losing the loved one. If one's energy is spent in continuous lawyerly debates and doubts about fidelity, all one will do is drive the other person to someone else as she protests, consciously or unconsciously, this unjust inquisition. Paradoxically, a person who needs constant childish reassurance of devotion and fidelity will drive a partner away and into the arms of a rival. *Lachesis*' demand of *guaranteed* fidelity is unattainable—no absolute certainty of eternal commitment can be granted. The *Lachesis* person who endures these pangs of envy is so consumed with jealousy and resentment that even when he is sure of his partner's love, he seems at times to be carried away by a tempest and cannot think of anything but the fact that he or she must be in an extramarital relationship. This is an expression of crude jealousy, functioning largely below the level of conscious awareness; it is characterized by rage, reproach, brutality, loquacity, foolishness, insanity and despair. When suspicion strikes, *Lachesis*' conversations are belligerent and confrontational, always beginning with "YOU"—did this...looked at her...wanted sex with her...want to leave me...and of course setting off defensiveness in the partner.

This jealousy in *Lachesis* also has a hormonal component: the insecurity and passion evoked when *Lachesis* approaches menopause is well known, and now she feels the need to compete with a real or imagined younger rival. Even before this stage of life, *Lachesis* exhibits strong jealousy *before menses.*

This kind of rivalrous jealousy seems to be almost inherent to the *Lachesis* child. If Mom gives a little too much attention to his little sibling, he will pinch the younger one and will not even hesitate to hit Mom for not loving him "more." Or the **shadow** *Lycopodium* side may order Mom, "Put that baby down!" It really is a foolish form of jealousy, but it is taken very seriously. When his younger sibling has one bookmark and he has nine, he complains that he needs all of them. When riding in the car, he plays the game of who sees a certain car first, and he insists on having seen it first, even when it is not true. Competitive, anyone (*ambition increased*)? Nothing can be done for or given to the sibling without the *Lachesis* child (especially if he has ASD) asking his parents for the same thing—even if birthday presents are being given to his sibling. One *Lachesis* child told his mom to let his dad take his sister to the doctor, because his mom had to take care of him. I heard a *Lachesis* teenager say to her younger sibling in one of her bad moments: "The real tragedy for me started when you were born." *Lachesis* always considers herself the center of the attention. For instance, a teenage *Lachesis* girl, when coming back from a trip on her younger brother's birthday once told him: "Sorry I am overshadowing your birthday (*delusions, of grandeur*)!"

Such jealousy eventually suffocates any friendship that this child has. As a teenager, he will have a passionate friendship with **one** person (passionate mainly from his own standpoint only), considering that friend a true sibling. But if the friend dares to connect to others, *Lachesis*' revenge is swift and extreme. In *Lachesis*' book, this is total betrayal, but he does not realize that his "friendship" was utterly possessive, strangling any possible real relationship. If the *Lachesis* child has money, he will buy his friend's attention, suffocating his friend step by step. This hate-love relationship reflects perfectly the duality of such a person: he has *two wills*, but he never knows which one will win; he feels no qualms about changing around at will. Even as a youngster, if his mom has divorced his dad, he cannot forgive her for trying to find a new boyfriend. "You have me," he might say. "You don't need another person in your life." And he will do anything to sabotage any future relationship that Mom is seeking, making sure that Mom and her new lover pay for such an "injustice." Take, for instance, an example from my practice: a 10-year-old female *Lachesis* child with ASD. She had a quick intuition that perceived the vulnerable spots in other people, and her anger could make cruel use of them; no man in her mom's life was safe from her sharp remarks.

Nothing can withstand such fury! If a friend does not call every day, *Lachesis* feels slighted because he does not feel equal passion coming from that friend. "How could he not think of me every day?" As a teenager, the fire fueled by the hormones of puberty, *Lachesis* tries to get sympathy from others by telling them, "I don't have a mother; she doesn't pay any attention to me." He is being untruthful, of course, because he really means: "Mom doesn't pay attention to me **all the time!**" And some very traditional grandmothers unjustly blame the mothers for neglecting their children if they can't tell Grandma all the time where the child is, what he ate, etc. A *Lachesis* teenager is smart enough to exploit this divide! As one 14-year-old expressed to me, "I am a victim of this world." (Note the sophisticated language, corresponding to *Lachesis*' *speaking in well selected phrases.*)A perfect example of this foolish jealousy appeared in a 2005 advice column:

> "I am constantly accusing my boyfriend of looking at other women and thinking of other women while we make love. Recently I gave my boyfriend a gift certificate for a massage, but I wanted to be in the room, watching everything that happened. When I found out we could not be in the same room, I cancelled the appointment. After hearing him complain about his bad back, I rescheduled. Then after the massage, I yelled at him for having some other woman's hands all over him. I am thinking of leaving him because he has been 'tainted' by someone else."[23]

Of course, the advice given in the newspaper column was "counseling." Indeed, allopathy does not have a single drug for jealousy, while homeopathy has at least 50: each for a specific kind!

The younger a *Lachesis* child is, the more foolish the jealousy. I had one *Lachesis* patient who, at age four, while his mom was on the phone, wheeled the baby out in her crib and put her outside where the garbage was collected. When his mother panicked and asked where the baby was, he answered with a straight face: "I dunno, Mom!"

Addicted to Praise

Lachesis and its equivalent brother, *Lycopodium*, both suffer from an excessive need for the "praise drug." Take, for instance, one of my little patients, bright-eyed, charming, and brilliant and with a speech repertory that would draw people to him like flame-bound moths. He **was** always the star in school performances and loved to be flattered. It was his greatest joy to be the center of attention. However, if he thought no one would be paying attention or that someone else was better than he was, he preferred not even to try out of fear of rejection and defeat. He was *jealous as foolish as it can be.* This poor little child was suffering from something more than the abuse of street drugs, something more insidious than street drugs, something readily accessible through his adoring fans and parents: the adoration and esteem of others that can be called a narcissistic supply. You would never have suspected that he was an addict

23. "Annie's Mailbox," *The New Mexican*, Aug. 30, 2005.

unless you talked to his mom: after glowingly receiving a performance award, he would isolate himself, almost pouting but in reality anxiously looking for the next fix, the next intake of praise. Being praised launched him briefly into manic giddiness and then dropped him into the throes of a depression that made King Lear look like Howdy Doody. He obsessively sought approval, riding increasingly painful waves of hollow elation and overwhelming despair. When such a *Lachesis* child dives into a swimming pool, he wants to be praised for dive after dive! Inevitably, after half an hour, his mother has exhausted all of the words of praise in her vocabulary! I had a 10-year-old patient who stuffed his food in his mouth at such a high speed (it is all about finishing first!) that even his mom found it disgusting. So when she told him to chew every bite very well, he wanted to be praised after each bite. One bite... looks at mom very seriously... praise comes. Next bite and... mandatory praise! In such circumstances, the only one eating at all, obviously, is the *Lachesis* person.

The most common form of narcissism is narcissistic attachment to one's children: parents often believe that their children are the most intelligent and beautiful of all children. Of course, some praise, up to a point, is much better than the continuous put-downs and exorbitant expectations with which some torture their children. But if praise is not based on anything specific, it will cause a sense of insecurity. *Lachesis* and *Lycopodium*, because of their competitive spirit, jealousy, and need to boost the inflated ego behind the mask, know no limit to receiving praise and appear "insatiable." Tidbits of attention are always welcome, if not **needed**, to maintain a reason to live. Rather than being highly suspicious of the vast heaps of praise directed toward him, *Lachesis* seems to be able to absorb astonishing amounts of it with ease, while other people would probably ask: "What is the motivation of this person?" It is not difficult to see that *Lachesis* and *Lycopodium*, in their lives, will look for friends, spouses, and other relationships that will provide them with a never-ending narcissistic supply; otherwise, they will look for the next, "better" partner. One can see the urgency of an intervention with the indicated homeopathic remedy to divert this praise addict from the road to calamity.

Loquacity

Lachesis is a person intoxicated with the power of her mind. To bolster her ego, *Lachesis* possesses something else that makes her superior to *Platina* and *Lycopodium*: her loquacity! *Lycopodium's* speech is more of a dictatorial kind towards his inferiors (*even abusive and insulting towards subordinates, often with anger from any contradiction*). This brings to mind *Nux-v*, who, indeed like *Lyc*, *employs every possible means for his ambition* (also *Platina*!). At the same time, *Lycopodium's* speech changes in the presence of his boss: *he is a flatterer*, because he knows he needs to be on good terms with his boss in order to reach the position he covets. *Platina's* loquacity can be equally abusive and insulting; this is especially seen in children's behavior towards their parents (*Lyc*). *Platina* can be a *braggart and boaster* and *squanders her money through ostentation* (*Verat-a*). Loquacity and boasting are part of her "beauty," which takes the form of an ice maiden rather than that of a warm, sympathetic figure. In her deeper pathology (luetic phase), *Platina desires to be silent and is indisposed to talk*.

Lachesis' quality of speech depends on her state of pathology. When in balance, *Lachesis* is a very witty and brilliant conversationalist. It demonstrates a form of intelligence when one's speech reflects the ability to process information very quickly—and another robust sign of intelligence when one can generate humor. *Lachesis* is capable of both of these. *There is quick comprehension and mental activity with almost prophetic perception*. They stop you in the middle of your sentence as they know the rest already; even worse for you, they know the question before you have posed it. Thoughts, images and emotions pass with the rapidity of a bird in flight across the window of awareness. *Lachesis* talks too much and may realize it when she sees the person's face get rather tired. One mother told me that she promised her *Lachesis* child a toy if he stayed quiet for one meal, but he could not do it! *His ideas are abundant and no sooner does one idea occur to* Lachesis*, a number of others follow in quick succession. She is active, lively and vivacious*. Usually her speech reflects all this: *wants to talk all of the time*; *inclination to be communicative*; *vivid imagination and extremely impatient at tedious and dry things* (Lachesis does not wish to participate in small talk!). *She has the most extraordinary loquacity, making speeches in very select phrases, but jumping off to the most heterogeneous subjects. One word leads into the midst of another story. This exceptional loquacity is marked by a rapid change of subject; she jumps abruptly from one idea to another* (while *Platina* exhibits wandering speech, repeating things), reminding one of the Bushmaster snake darting in and out with amazing rapidity. *Lachesis talks and sings or whistles constantly*. Her apparently nervous loquacity and delusional rambling are used to charm and stun her victim; they are the ultimate means of control and security for *Lachesis*. But when *Lachesis* is convinced of the effectiveness of her own arguments, she can often be ruthless in driving home a point, and she is scornful of her less intellectual opponents (*mocking*; *desire for satire*). She has no patience for stupidity or ignorance (for her time is limited), which makes her quite unmindful of the wounds she inflicts on others (*cruelty, inhumanity*). In a pathological state, her once refined speech begins to resemble the froth and foam on the lips of someone suffering an epileptic attack.

True to her reptilian nature (the Bushmaster snake, master of his territory, pursues and attacks its enemy rather than running away), *Lachesis*' tongue can be used to hurt in a very sophisticated way. Anyone who tries to fling an overly intelligent criticism into a discussion will find himself in an animus battle with *Lachesis* who does not argue to discover the truth, but where *Lachesis*' animus has to win, she has to be right, no matter what happens to the adversary. The venomous *Lachesis* goes for the jugular while being very cynical, *censorious and critical. Lachesis* hurts you with a single word, keeping a smile on her face all the while. She can talk with the tongues of men and angels in order to master the sudden stabs of jealousy that might unexpectedly arise when confronted with truly happy people: people who might not have such brilliant minds or be versed in high spiritual concepts but who are warm, sympathetic, and responsive to others' personal needs. Ugly verbal toads hop out of *Lachesis*' mouth if a colleague gets a promotion ahead of her. "He did not deserve it," she might say, or even "He really has a second-rate mind." *Lachesis* must come, through help of the homeopathic remedy, to see the lack of love that is her arrogance; she must learn that a loving voice rescinds its power to wound. This is not easy for *Lachesis*, as talking and lecturing are the therapy that soothes her Cyber delusion.

Lachesis children usually have beautiful, hurried minds. *Lachesis* children are generally very bright, and language is not really a problem for them, except that they can stammer or speak inarticulately because their speech and thought processes are *hurried*... one thought comes into the mind, and before it can be processed, the next one arrives, pushing the first one aside... but *Lachesis* has a great memory on which she can fall back to support her delusions of grandeur. Parents are often dumbstruck, less because of what the child is saying (although they always *speak in well selected phrases*) and more because of *how* he is saying it. No sooner does one thought come galloping out of his mouth then another one overtakes it, producing a pile-up of words without sequence (the famous *Lachesis* proving: *loquacity, changing quickly from one subject to another*), each sentence canceling out the previous one before it has had a chance to emerge. They speak so fast (to follow the fast train of thought) that they sometimes stammer or cannot be understood; they also may not speak at all if the thought process overwhelms them (*abundant ideas; thoughts crowding around each other; thoughts, rush, flow of*). *Lachesis* often cannot sleep for a long time owing to a continuous stream of flowing ideas.

True to the nature of snake venom (*Lachesis* being made from the bushmaster snake venom), in the unbalanced *Lachesis*, each individual word is like a toxic substance that the child or adult must expel from his body in a hissing, spitting manner. And the longer he speaks, the more incoherent his speech can become (*speech incoherent, hasty* and *foolish*). The speech therapist will tell the parent, "We need to give this child something to slow down her speech." And the adult in conversation overwhelms everyone else so that hardly any true conversation can take place. The *Lachesis* child also gets stuck on one word and asks the parent to repeat it several times before he can let go of the word. Why? When one's thought process is too fast, it is easy to get stuck on a word—any word—and usually, it is one which the child was scripting. The parent, by repeating that word, gets the child "unstuck." The *Lachesis* child can also jump from one topic to another (*delirium, changing subjects rapidly*) rather than talking about one idea or story all day long. Both scenarios are possible, though. Being stuck on one topic is reflected in his playing games: he remains stuck playing with the same train set and seems to have no interest in doing anything else that day.

The high-functioning *Lachesis* child's imagination is fantastic, and he has no shortage of ideas to write into his fabulously original stories. He certainly wishes to be praised and to have his stories read out loud in class to all the other children. The more active a child's imagination is, the less his senses transmit perceptions from without. Protracted solitude in a dream world of his own, silence, and darkness are conducive to the imagination and will work against the libido that wishes to connect to the adult world. When a great deal of material is provided from outside with which *Lachesis* must content, the imagination takes a holiday and refuses to become active even when summoned. Alas, this can be the fate of the *Lachesis* child with ASD: to be the prisoner of his imagination rather than being fruitful for his individuation. He is an avid reader, reading up to 250 pages a day, as did one of my patients. He often expresses delusions of grandeur: "I am a legend," he exclaims. He is a star, but one with a social maladjustment and awkwardness. What he does not like is math: too abstract! Figures are cold, solid, and unchangeable and don't leave anything to the imagination.

What is puzzling is that these children are highly intelligent but socially isolated. How did this characteristic evolve? *Lachesis* can be beautiful and engaging, but she is also given to long spells of melancholy, restlessness and antisocial behavior. *Lachesis* knows that she has a beautiful mind and unusual intellectual gifts, but at the same time she feels isolated by her mind. *Lachesis*' social integration is the greatest problem, as such children with ASD are otherwise excellent students, beloved by their teachers. But they really want to be the ones telling others what to do, because they **do** have the greatest imagination; if the others refuse, they don't insist, but retreat, discouraged. The mother of such a boy always found her child sitting in the sandbox by himself.

The child, with his great imagination, escapes into his dream fantasy world and is very protective of it, even telling others, "It is my imaginary world; you are not allowed in." Such a child absolutely wants to connect to others, but his extensive imagination does not allow him to connect with his peers. Alas, he perseveres with many things (time, dates, and stories, building cities with blocks and legos, linear patterns, drawing maps), demonstrating behavior that resembles OCD. And he keeps reciting the names of highway exits as his mom drives him around; he cannot let his mind rest. Even a *Lachesis* adult's mind is constantly busy and hard to turn off; its shadow side, *Lycopodium*, always keeps the tune of a song in mind all day long. This is also perseverance!

Lachesis' prodigious imagination can make up plays from what he sees in films or reads in books. If such a child is 13 years old, his ideas are interesting for the four- and five-year-olds, but his peers will consider him weird. This is the greatest danger for the brilliant *Lachesis*: it will lead to isolation and being bullied! Five-year-old kids might be transfixed by such an imagination, but the teenage *Lachesis* will receive all kinds of insults and taunts: "weirdo," "geek," "lunatic," and anything else children can come up with. The child's world can be very cruel, and children don't dress their words in a veil: they are uncensored and non-scripted. I had a mom crying on the phone to me as her brilliant child had said to her out of the blue, "All the kids hate me. They call me all kinds of names!" How painful it is for a mother to know that she cannot offer constant protection to her child! This is what is referred to as "hearing bad news" for the mom, a heartbreak! Such a *Lachesis* child will never have an academic problem, and I never worry about that particular aspect of their futures. But it will be hard for him to integrate socially—for his whole life, unless homeopathy comes to the rescue.

When the *Lachesis* child scripts from videos and films, he uses precisely the same language. He sees a yo-yo in the store and exclaims, "Wow, a super-duper spiral yo-yo!" It is the exact language that he has heard on TV. This can be appropriate, but often the scripting is not appropriate. Sometimes children just integrate these sentences into writing about themselves. But when he is asked to describe more than just the facts of what he has read, or when one tries to have a debate with him about what he has read, he actually reasons at two or more years below his age level.

Lachesis children also know maps inside out; they can get you from point A to point B without looking at the map while reciting the exits and numbers of the freeways. The *Lachesis* child loves to build and draw huge intersections of freeways; I treated one kid who used the cracks in front of the garage as his freeway system, using it to drive his cars or simply following the cracks, walking over them as if on his personal freeway. He would lie down on his belly and look at his freeway system with great interest and fascination. Such a child draws buildings with great detail and tells you with perfect accuracy, "This one is situated on the corner of such-and-such street." *Lachesis* creates masterworks with blocks and lined-up cars and, of course, he doesn't want his creations to be destroyed! Hurried behavior also translates in these children to impulsivity, so they have a hard time waiting their turn; they always want to be the first one in line at school, and they grab things from other children without asking first.

Each successful encounter with the adult world adds to *Lachesis*' sense of safety and confidence, which is necessary for this child to steer his passions in the right direction—that of a growing ego, filled with treasures originating from both his own imagination and the outside world. The *Lachesis* child lives in his own extensive garden, where he picks flowers for his burgeoning creative play and stirs his imagination with extensive, lively dreams connected to the collective unconscious. But when society in general, and parents and school in particular, close off this outlet (because it is not socially acceptable, or because it becomes annoying and does not fit in the school curriculum—except for the role he might play in an occasional school play), then there are only a few compensations left on which this child can fall back, most of which are negative.

Lachesis' loquacity is of a sycotic nature, conveying to the homeopath that *Lachesis* is more a sycotic remedy than a psoric one. This is very different from *Calc-c*, a strong psoric remedy, who likes to ramble about all his small sufferings but does not do so eloquently. If anything, *Calc-c* always wants to mull it over before he becomes a nuisance talking about his little issues and ailments (*talks about nothing but murder, fire and rats*). Any compensation of *Lachesis* is an exaggerated one, and its intensity matches its sanguine nature. Initially, at least, for the more stable *Lachesis*, the loquacity outlet is of a rather positive nature: she can use it to be a good lawyer, politician, teacher, or preacher!

Loquacity can also be expressed by letter or email! If you, as a homeopath, always receive lengthy answers to your queries regarding her follow-up—everything about "small" complaints but very detailed—and the tone of these messages is always urgent, pleading, and self-absorbed, you can call it loquacity! Their messages are minute-to-minute events, and are frequently hurled at the homeopath (which makes one think of an *Arsenicum* personality), but *Lachesis* people are consumed with anticipation anxiety and restlessness! *Lachesis* really suffers from the *delusion, is doomed,* and in his panic, reason goes quickly out of the door.

Looking for the Meaning of Life

The essence of *Lachesis* is **the caveat or warning about an unlived life**, or, as the late Whitmont called it in his book *Psyche and Substance*, "the penalty of unlived life."[24] *Lachesis* should be reminded of the fact that death is not to be feared; we have only to fear that we have not lived. Is life worth living? Only if you make it worth living! This should warn us immediately about the possibility of "the unlived life" causing cancer, as the *Carcinosin* state is reflected by exactly the same theme: letting others live her life, having no boundaries to prevent it. The appearance of cancer is the last warning to finally start living your own life. In *Lachesis*' case we are not surprised to see cancer appearing in the ovaries and other sexual organs, as they are the center of repressed libido and sexual urges (*genitalia female, cancer of ovaries and cancer of uterus*). With the presence of **overstimulation on every plane, which requires an outlet**, we should not be surprised to find attendant restlessness, anticipation anxiety, and hypersensitivity. Such a person feels that her life has been barren of opportunities, that people have been overly critical of her, and that she always has been treated unjustly. On good days, she is reasonably pleased with her psychic state. On other days, she has the gnawing sensation that she has not tapped her full potential, that she is not operating on all six cylinders, that she is simply not successful enough or not accomplished enough. "I have much more in me," she says. The feeling of not having reached her potential comes from a discrepancy between the "actual self" (who she really is), the "ideal self" (who she aspires to be), and the "should-be self" (who she thinks others want her to be, the public persona). She is troubled because her actual self does not align with these other visions. Often, as we

24. Edward Whitmont, *Psyche and Substance* (Berkeley: North Atlantic Books, 1991), 151.

will see, this is followed by secondary melancholy and depression. *Lachesis* seems to be unable to cultivate peace in the garden of his heart by removing the weeds of egotism and jealousy. Not surprisingly, peace is not manifested externally either. He talks of "being keyed up" and hard to relax, with a mind that cannot quiet down (*busy; desire for business, restlessness, busy,*). She also has a growing fear of tension within herself, which at times makes her feel that something might give away, and that she might even become insane (*fear, insanity, of losing his reason*). Often, such a mind has long conversations with itself, ranging in topic from vexing past conversations with others to perceived injustices he has suffered (*ideas abundant, compelling; talking to himself, only when alone*). The latter sentiment is definitely born of fixed ideas. No wonder we find *palpitations, insomnia, chest pains, frontal headaches, neck stiffness* and *nocturnal emissions with amorous dreams* in this tortured soul, all worse after sleep, which creates a *great dread of the night*. Kent rightly states *Lachesis*' characteristics as "an improper love of self, a moral insensibility." She may shed tears, but they will be tears of self-pity, not of sympathy with others.

Sexuality

Besides intellect, religion, and loquacity, there is another compensation for *Lachesis*: the sexual outlet. If a sexual outlet is possible, and not suppressed by the family (there is a difference between growing up in a pot-smoking environment and in a strict, religious family), it also takes an extreme form. The male either becomes a Don Juan (*great excitement of sexual desire; lascivious; idea of marriage seems unendurable*) or, more commonly, is so fixated on his partner that he becomes more sexually demanding than even a *Lycopodium* man and easily transforms her into a *Staphysagria* or *Sepia* woman (*Lachesis* has *sexual passion increased; nymphomania,* and *sexual passion violent).* He often will check constantly on his partner, which in his mind is "caring" for her. This quickly leads to a negative cycle, to foolish jealousy, transforming this passionate person into a man who, usually in firm command of all his actions, loses control on the slightest provocation when his archaic feeling-conscious function is called upon. Here, again, is a perfect example of the thinking *Lachesis* person who gets into trouble when the situation calls for the intervention of his inferior feeling side. This superior, thinking individual now is confronted with situations he cannot handle, and his inadequacy shows in very foolish behavior and all kinds of jealous reactions, as seen before: *jealousy with rage; jealousy with saying and doing things he normally would not do; gentle husband becoming brutal from jealousy.* To dull those very painful feelings, *Lachesis,* once he begins to go down this negative pathway, may abuse alcohol (*dipsomania*) (which he can tolerate very well); he may even start to lead a debauched life, which fuels his jealousy and suspicion even more. We must not forget that *Lachesis* is **the** remedy for hereditary familial alcoholism (*dipsomania, hereditary*)! So after suffering heartbreak, a *Lachesis* person often shows self-destructive behavior with drinking and smoking and can become addicted to compulsive gambling as a first resort to calm herself down (*want of control*) and, unconsciously, to desperately cry out to the outside world: "Help me!" (*anxiety about salvation*) before he disrupts his life and the lives of his family.

The female *Lachesis* person looks for love in all the wrong places (as does *Platina*) and takes it one step further (*nymphomania*). She does not hesitate to become a prostitute, with the naïve conviction (remember her feeling function *is* primitive) that she will find love and romance in such a profession. As *Lachesis*' state is worse from the arrest of flow and excretions (for example, during menopause), her sense of having to compete with younger women can openly erupt with the force of a volcano. If there is a younger rival, thoughts and acts of killing that person are not uncommon! And when utterly disappointed by many heartbreaks, she can start a lesbian relationship (*love with one of his own sex, homosexuality*).

An Active Conscious and Unconscious

Both the adult and the *Lachesis* child with ASD often suffer from disturbed sleep: the *Lachesis* person wakes up and starts talking nonstop for a few hours and then falls asleep again. Speech is, again, an outlet, a relief of everything that has been stored during the waking conscious life but not entirely processed and therefore put in the unconscious to be worked on during sleep. The *Lachesis* person does not even wake up while unloading the mass of accumulated ideas; he might use dreams, the messengers of the unconscious, to digest the unprocessed conscious material. Thus, we can understand that *Lachesis* feels worse after sleep or even a nap (*short sleep aggravates; prolonged sleep aggravates*), something he will fight with all his might. One can only feel galvanized by the sheer aliveness of such a child: he is *loquacious day and night*: he is the entertainer during the day and the creator of fantastic dreams at night. It is the homeopath's task to discover the Cyber delusion from both sources (conscious/unconscious); the CD is the key to the explanation of his individual dreams as well as his ever-brewing stormy actions during the day. So there is always *fear of going to sleep* (since this always aggravates his condition and he *fears he will die during his sleep* from a heart attack—*anxiety about the heart; there is seldom a refreshed sleep as their sleep restless with many dreams and frequent waking and again dozing*). There is another component to this fear of sleep: during sleep, the unconscious escapes all control mechanisms and can exact its compensating revenge in dreams.

Creation of an Alter Ego

The constriction of a typical school curriculum does not stimulate the *Lachesis* child with ASD. He needs the opportunity to act out his many imagined adventures in the right environment—for instance, that of a Waldorf school, where connection to nature is emphasized and a free-flowing curriculum is followed: this suits him well as his voice can always find a place to be heard. Otherwise, he is the first one to "check out" in class, where rigid rules and a lack of flexibility reign; he retires to his vast imaginary world. This world becomes an archetypal place where the teacher is a witch with monstrous power, thwarting any individual expression. Invariably, the teacher complains of the *Lachesis* child's lack of focus; he disturbs the class with sudden shouted descriptions of images originating from his vast arsenal of unconscious stored pictures, escaping the accusing eyes of the teacher fixed upon him. It is when these imaginary characters, personifications of his own emotions, continue to grow (while the hated outer reality tries to claim him and forces him to go underground) that this child runs the risk of creating an alter ego, one that can become stronger and stronger, with the ever-growing danger of dissociating and succumbing to a psychotic break. At first, this alter ego is used to justify any odd or violent behavior. This self-created personality has told him that he should do such things: the alter ego becomes the entity used to "kill" someone else by magic (often Mom or Dad or a teacher, someone who imposes harsh tasks on him). But the danger of infantile schizophrenia remains! For *Lachesis*, a great active imagination (*ideas, abundant*) is not without its dangers. Unlike dreams, which are self-limiting since we eventually wake up, active imagination resembles the seductive singing sirens, mesmerizing the person and pulling him so strongly toward the unconscious that the ego position may be endangered, leading to dissociation. This is particularly common in children with autism and with archaic egos.

Golden Tips from the Masters

- *Lachesis*, being a polychrest, is one of the most underprescribed remedies. How can that be? Because of its resemblance to other remedies like *Phos*, *Sulph*, *Staph*, and, of course, its twin brother, *Lyc* (the acute of *Lachesis*). In the absence of some very characteristic physical symptoms (especially cardiovascular issues, throat problems, intolerance to constricting clothing, and relief of symptoms through discharges), *Lachesis* is difficult to recognize on the mental plane.
- *Lachesis* is a major remedy for cardiovascular disease (strokes and heart attacks), and she often *experiences constrictive pain, oppressive chest pain and palpitations with numbness in arm, >by sitting up*. It is especially during those fits of jealousy that heart symptoms and fainting may appear: *after a jealous (hysteria) quarrel, she puts both hands on her chest and cried out, "Oh my heart!" Then fell down and was in an asphyctic state for 24 hours; no pulse could be felt, breathing hardly perceptible. Lachesis* prevents degeneration of the brain tissue in strokes and prevents recurrence of a stroke attack.
- *Lachesis* has bluish, dark, stagnant blood and purple discoloration and an anticoagulant action.
- Mystics or would-be mystics often require *Lachesis*
- *Lachesis* changes in character when pregnant! She becomes more like *Nat-m*, avoiding company, when pregnant. She can become depressive and sad.
- Often he can only sleep on his right side, NOT on the left (*sleep, position, right side, left impossible*)
- Palpitations common during pregnancy, <lying on left side
- One of the most important hints is hair loss **during** pregnancy (< > of normal)
- Frequent appearance of hemorrhoids during pregnancy; they can be big and even strangulating
- When *Lachesis* becomes manic, she goes on a shopping spree (during manic depression)
- Fear of suffocation (*Puls*); intolerance of tight clothes, especially at the neck, as anything touching causes suffocation; intolerance may extend to tight clothing around the abdomen or tight shoes
- Grief with a sense of revenge: "If I can't have him, no one will," often leading to murderous acts and stalking
- Palpitations, hot flashes, and hypertension: well-known **triad** in menopause
- #1 remedy in severe septic conditions of the throat

- Best remedy for rapidly maturing abscesses regardless of location (use a dose of 200C every two hours)
- Indicated in nosebleeds which are dark and generally accompanied by amenorrhea
- Strong incessant urging for stool with practically no result (black-type remedy)
- #1 remedy for asthma attacks in sleep which fail to wake

Lycopodium clavatum (Lyc). Club moss

The Cyber Delusion

The Cyber delusion in an excessive persona like that of *Lycopodium* is always deeply hidden in the unconscious. Being (shadow side) always contrasts with appearing (mask) in the *Lyc* person: he appears courageous, but in fact he is a coward, afraid of confrontation. Socially, he is a "strong" man, while in private life he often behaves like a mere child. His discipline in public goes miserably to pieces in private. His happiness in his work contrasts with bad moods and affects at home, so his family has a distinctly different view of him than does the rest of the world. The charming, extraverted man of honor in the world contrasts with one of tantrums and explosive moodiness at home, a man who terrifies his family. *Lycopodium's* overt behavior and persona are in drastic contrast to the reality of the force that motivates him, and his public persona is certainly different from his character. His behavior only partially reflects his being; it is mainly a mask that he wears for his own purpose: gaining power!

The real essence of *Lyc* is expressed in his Cyber delusion: that he *has done wrong, and everything will disappear*. First failures in life are usually as memorable as first successes, and many *Lycopodium* personalities are formed early in childhood and adolescence when the person suffers a deep humiliation (usually a remark about a part of the body with an unusual appearance like a big nose, or an unsuccessful first attempt at sexual intercourse), an event that damages the frail confidence of the young person terribly. *Lycopodium* (and everyone else!) has to realize that life is cyclical. Sometimes you are the windshield and sometimes you are the bug, through no fault of your own. True confidence comes from the gradual accumulation of self-efficacy over a long period of successes, as well as from the way one deals with failures. As *Lycopodium* has an early tendency to commit mistakes in writing, speaking, and spelling (*mistakes, using wrong words; misplacing words; giving wrong syllables; in writing, adds letters and omitting letters*), he is often held back a grade and may become, to his horror, a permanent member of what the other kids call the "dummy class." The punishment for his dyslexia, as well as cruelly being called a dummy, is exile to the shameful state of an outsider as his class moves forward and time goes on. Such an *ailment from mortification* permanently stigmatizes the young person and often paralyzes him with a preoccupation with failure, what other people might be thinking of him, and how he will be judged. Interestingly, dreams, the messengers of the unconscious, are typically corrective ones in the case of *Lycopodium*. A corrective dream can be instructive to the patient **if he is willing to listen to it.** Alas, as do so many people, most *Lycopodium* people think of dreams as nonsense; they throw away the precious advice of corrective dreams, which in fact provide warnings to the patient to change his conscious attitude as it will otherwise lead to calamity. *Lycopodium's* corrective dreams are clear enough: *that his boat will be foundering*, and *of people drowning*, the same theme that is expressed in the proving *fear of being unable to reach his destination*. In other words, it is a warning that he will fail in his undertakings despite the bravado he displays (the dream theme of failing examinations is often present). Other dreams also confirm the presence of *Lycopodium*'s excessive persona. The persona serves a useful function in that it mediates between the self (the naked ego) and society or the outer world, just as clothing is mediates between the naked body and society. Therefore, symbols of the persona appear in dreams as images of clothes, hats, dress, uniforms, armor, and masks. In dreams, the persona can be represented by a person who takes one jacket off when another one appears and so on. In other words, the "bare" selfhood cannot be reached; he does not dare to take his clothes off and be naked! I had a patient who, after one dose of 30C *Lycopodium*, had the following dream: he appeared as a man overdressed in an overly decorated, gaudy uniform that only covered the top of his body while the genitalia were naked. The dream was very amusing to my patient, but it was actually an important aspect of the totality of his symptoms that confirmed to me the indicated remedy, *Lycopodium*, so well-known for the excessive persona and the unbridled sexual desire for conquest. While he appears in his upper part to be a grandiose and impressive figure, the nakedness of the sexual sphere is shown in his dreams, when all inhibitory mechanisms have fallen away.

All this bravado cannot keep *Lycopodium* from forming delusions, usually at a later stage, pointing to the vulnerability and excessive fears that contrast so starkly with his excessive mask: *delusion, he was about to die*; *delusion, he is about to receive injury*; *delusion, he will be murdered*; *delusion, he is unfortunate* and *delusion, he is pursued by enemies*. As we will see, anticipation anxiety is written in capital letters in this individual. It is interesting to see that *Lycopodium* has the *delusion, he neglected his duty,* in spite of that excessive mask and over-preparedness in tasks (even in similar recurrent tasks with which he is familiar). Because of the oversized ego and misplaced haughtiness, his reproaches are mainly geared *towards others:* he plays the blaming game (*reproaching others*)! "I was hindered by so-and-so in my tasks, and that's why I failed." (This makes one think of *China,* which is similar to *Lycopodium* on the mental plane.) Do not expect introspection from this individual, despite the corrective dreams! The tendency to blame others distinguishes *Lyc* from *Aurum, Nat-m,* and *Carcinosin,* all of whom *reproach themselves* more than others. And then we have the super-ambitious *Nux-v,* who takes no prisoners (*ailments from deceived ambition*) and who reproaches himself and others in equal measure. It usually takes several doses of *Lycopodium* before the patient will show any introspection, finally dissolving these tormenting fixed ideas of his shadow side and bringing them into his consciousness; this, then, allows him to finally admit his "fears and vulnerability."

This fear of *doing wrong and everything will vanish* (fear of failure) and of being "unmasked" also produces some degree of competitiveness (*he employs every possible means to achieve his ambition*) and *suspicion* in *Lycopodium* (*Lyc* is the strongest black type remedy for suspicion in *Synthesis*), since he is driven by a love of power. As a result, the unbalanced *Lycopodium* man treats his wife and children horribly while praising those he can use to increase his social status; this is expressed by the proving *contemptuous, hard for subordinates and agreeable and pleasant to superiors or people he has to fear.* In fact, *Lyc* resembles *Nux-v* (with his CD *someone is in his bed*) in his fear for competition; this is expressed by *Lycopodium's* delusions: *the house is full of people; he is about to receive an injury* and *on entering the room he sees people at his bedside.* All these fixed ideas reflect his mistrust of others.

Causalities

Lycopodium is a prototype of the Thinking-Logos image-bound person, who resists with all his might the integration of his archaic female side, or anima, into conscious life. His will to control and take charge with a fighting spirit is the foundation of most of his causalities and compensations. Upholding his iron mask of power and success leads to many ailments from (A/F).

Literary and Scientific Failure

Lyc and its complementary remedy, *Lachesis*, as well as *Nux-v*, display competitiveness with a sharp edge. With *Lyc* and *Nux-v* (usually the father figure in the family), both of whom show dominance of the animus and are of the choleric temperamental type, life is all about business and the success of their enterprises. Both have *ailments from scientific and literary failure, from anger, business failure* and *from contradiction.* Lycopodium's anticipation anxiety increases at the sheer thought of failure, often paralyzing his mind: *internal anguish, and anxiety in the evening as things are half confused before her eyes; the head becomes benumbed, as if unconscious. She cannot grasp a thought because her head is occupied by an internal tension. He weeps and cries, at first about the past, then about the coming evils.* What she fears most, therefore, in spite of projecting the false image of a splendid helium-filled balloon, will indeed occur: a return to the Cyber delusion that she did wrong and that everything will fail and vanish: friends, career, money, power, and family!

As an adult or student, this can be a person who fails repeatedly in performance (exams, interviews for new jobs, etc.) in spite of an excellent mind and real ability. I have even seen this in families exerting no undue pressure and void of criticism of repeated failures. In fact, every effort may have been made to see that no inferiority complex was created as a result of any parental criticism (the opposite happens, unfortunately, all too often). Yet *Lyc* does fail, in spite of the fact that he is over-prepared and enters into his examinations with enthusiasm and optimism. But the moment he starts or has to start, his mind goes blank, and he has no idea why. A few hours after the examination, he remembers all of the information completely forgotten during the hours when he needed it and realizes where he made many blunders. The failures are not due to defective long-term or short-term memory, for his mind had remained engaged on other occasions when he was studying at his home. He can be a normal young man, but is obviously temporarily blocked by some force that he cannot recognize or control. This performance amnesia can lead to many *disappointments and mortifications,* two well-known A/F for *Lycopodium*. What a horror, what a humiliation for such a brilliant and able person!

Unfortunately, what one sees more often is the pressure from "high-society" parents who only "want the best" for their children. However, the family environment of perfectionism demands unrealistically high standards of children. Imagine the child returning home with a 95 on a test and being sternly asked, "How come you missed five points?" Sometimes all it takes is the raise of an eyebrow, a sigh, or a strategic silence from the perfectionist parent for the child to get the message that she has "failed," no matter how well he was doing. Perfectionism is only paralyzing in the presence of parental criticism and exacting expectations. It is one thing to strive for perfection (*Silicea, Carcinosin*, and *Lycopodium*), another to demand it. Overly demanding and critical parents feed the destructive idea that the child is not good enough and that, no matter what he does, he will be never good enough; the foundation is thereby put in place for the development of the under-confident *Lycopodium* person. We have now a child who doubts his ability to accomplish tasks and whose life turns into a punishing pursuit of perfectionism. So for the sake of social conformity with the masculine ideals of ambition, power, and success, parents with such high expectations teach their children to repress their subjective feminine sides, their affects, feelings, and needs. The child has been made to feel that love and approval are contingent on performance, making him believe that he is only as good as his achievements. As a result, this child wants to conceal his mistakes (*liar; cannot bear to be looked at, mental symptoms aggravate*), preventing him from getting crucial feedback, and he will not start anything until he is very sure of being perfect (*undertakes nothing lest he succeeds*). There is a great difference between excellence and perfection. Excellence involves enjoying what one does. Perfection means never being satisfied—no matter what. It undermines performance (*want of confidence*), creating potential future depression, anxiety, and even substance abuse! What such a child should learn is that success hinges less on getting everything right and more on how he handles getting things wrong. I remember a patient, a movie star from a highly ambitious family, who came to me with a diagnosis of "chronic fatigue," a catch-all phrase for mystery diseases. However, on looking at the trigger, I discovered that she had been nominated for an Oscar and that everyone, especially family and friends, had told her she was a "shoo-in" to win the Oscar; she herself had high hopes of being the winner. When this did not happen, the *disappointment* crashed her into the deepest abyss of despair, and for months she stayed in bed. She felt heartbroken and somewhat ashamed and humiliated. *Lycopodium* brought her a speedy return with an appreciation of the fact that being nominated was in itself a success!

Mortification and Disappointment

As has already been mentioned briefly, ailments from mortification and disappointment feature prominently in the formation of the *Lycopodium* personality, and no doubt *Lycopodium* should be added to ailments from *loss of position, loss of reputation* and *wounded honor* (presently not in these rubrics). *Lycopodium* is an intellectual, like *Sulphur* and *Lachesis*, but *Lyc* can't handle even the most insignificant failure as it exposes his fragile shadow side. Because of his intellectual prowess, much is expected from him, even as a child, just as is the case with *Aurum, Carcinosin,* and *Sulphur. Lycopodium,* however, succumbs to the weight of the expectations and the *scorn* (criticism) he receives (*ailments from scorn, being scorned*) when he experiences *scientific and literary failure.* In the case of one *Lyc* child in my practice, her father never posted her 100% results in the house, but if she earned anything less than 100% it was posted for everyone to see how she had "failed." *Sulphur* and *Aurum* have better tools to deal with imposed pressure, and they are more confident than *Lycopodium*; even *Carcinosin* has no lack of confidence in himself, though he usually suffers from great anticipation anxiety.

A *Lycopodium* dad, being the first representation of the animus, will instill in the young child the need to perform well academically. It is expected, even if left unsaid, that the child will be a high performer in school and society. This puts a tremendous strain on him to perform well in high school, where he often excels; the moment he enters college, though, the presence of many of his intellectual peers can pierce his balloon of pride; confronting the higher academic level and competition can create a sudden lack of confidence. More than one teenager is mortally wounded at such a moment, as his whole persona reflects timidity and a lack of clarity and authority (*lack of character*) confirmed by the use of a soft, cowering voice in the face of an authority figure. Such a persona causes what a *Lycopodium* person fears the most: lack of success in his jobs and enterprises, and the disappearance of "everything": his power, success, friends, and wealth.

Disappointment can be transferred to the unborn fetus as soon as intrauterine life starts on day one: there can be a lack of support or enthusiasm for the pregnancy, especially from the future father ("I am not ready to be a father," I have heard) and family; other mortifications may include interference from family members or wishing for a girl and discovering it is going to be a boy or vice versa (this happens more often than you might think). The emotions attached to these events are easily transferred through the psychogenic umbilical cord to the unborn fetus in what Jung called *participation mystique*, or mystical participation,[25] a

25. Jung, *Development of Personality*, 124.

term coined by the French anthropologist Lévy-Bruhl to refer to a child's perception of the conflicts between parents and beginning to suffer from those conflicts as if they were his own. Receiving feedback—or, worse, negative criticism—in marriage (and even more so in a state of pregnancy) can be an especially delicate affair. Unsolicited advice on driving, for example, might be received with gritted teeth—but though a husband's judgment of his wife's deficiencies might be "just" his opinion, in intimate relationships opinions are all that matter; they are received as complaints regarding the state of a relationship, and a pregnant woman is not always ready to listen to the feelings underneath criticism or demands for change (*offended easily*). An example from my practice shows clearly the A/F in the formation of a teenage *Lycopodium* patient suffering from depression and an apparent total lack of motivation. Three NWS seemed to have triggered her funk:

> First, a professor accused her of plagiarism when she presented a paper, although she had worked very hard on it and it was authentic. This shocked her to the core (*A/F wounded honor; A/F embarrassment; A/F mortification*) and made her very angry (*A/F anger*); after that incident, she did not dare to confront the professor with the falseness of his allegation when she saw him (*lack of character; cowardice; A/F suppressed anger*). The result was a failing grade (*A/F failure-literary, scientific*), and, again, she was too embarrassed to tell anyone (*A/F embarrassment*). She had anticipation anxiety about the future and felt guilty (*delusion, he has done wrong*) that she had not tried hard enough (*delusion, neglected her duty*). She then felt that she could not do anything right (*delusions, everything will fail*), that she was a complete failure (*confidence, want of*); she had no motivation to go back to school. In fact, she feared that she would fail any examination she might have to take, and she feared that her friends and parents would react to her as her professor had (*delusion, injury, is about to receive an*). An easier way out for her was to simply not go to school so she did not have to take examinations (*delusion, everything will vanish; fear of failure; in examinations*). Remarkably, she was much worse in general when a storm approached (*generals—weather—thunderstorm approaching* <). She also had very painful menses (*menses, painful*). *Lycopodium* turned things around for her!

Compensations

The Power Complex

To unite with other living beings, to relate to them, is a necessity on which man's very sanity depends. The way *Lycopodium* seeks this union with the world is by exercising power over others, by dominating them through loveless acts, and by making others a part of himself. But no amount of domination is enough to give a true sense of identity and union; knowing no other way to relate to others, more and more domination is sought by *Lycopodium*. But the ultimate result is defeat as, of course, such a goal can only destroy an individual's sense of integrity. Instead of pursuing his own course of individuation, *Lycopodium* is dependent on those whom he dominates. The straightforward, simple man, the simplest artist or poet, finds a fuller satisfaction in life than the power-seeker can ever know; this is because the latter must be perpetually engaged in some fresh manipulation if he is to avoid a sense of emptiness and failure. He confuses excitement and success in business with joy, and he mistakes the thrill of manipulation and success for a love of life. Yes, he will often win, because he has more than enough brute force and deception at his disposal (*abusive and insulting; anger from contradiction; anger at trifles; barking; liar*), and his shock of white hair evokes a certain respect. But he will not convince. For to convince he needs to persuade. And in order to persuade he needs what he lacks: honesty and care (*lack of character; deceitful*). He cares only for his business, not his family, which is only a burden (*flees his children; contemptuous, hard for subordinates, pleasant to superiors; aversion to responsibility; duty, aversion to domestic duty*).

For *Lycopodium*, interested only in obtaining power (*dictatorial, love of power*) and being right, innate vanity is accompanied by loquacity and speaking with a voice of command (*dictatorial, talking with an air of command*). In a discussion, he is likely to be the one with the most expansive posture, the loudest voice, the most amplified gestures and emotional displays. It is called "power posing," using voice and open postures to raise his testosterone levels, as he is convinced that this is the M.O. he needs in order to put down "revolt" (which is any dissenting opinion) before it can ever arise. It gives him a sense of action, the ability to pursue his goals without obstruction. He speaks before he thinks, and even though he may afterwards perceive that he is wrong and that what he asserts is false, he wants it to seem the contrary (*intolerant to contradiction; disposition to contradict*). When *Lycopodium* hears what he does not want to hear, he becomes angry and forceful (*anger from contradiction*). His interest in truth, which may be presumed to have been his only motive when he alleged his proposition to be true, now gives way to the interests of vanity and delusions of grandeur (*boaster, rich, wishes to be considered*): now, for the sake of vanity, what is true must seem false, and what is false must seem true (*haughty, stiff and pretentious; delusions, presumptuous*). Indeed, the desire for power and fame to bolster his persona is the last characteristic that *Lycopodium* shakes off. The thing about power and its kissing cousin, apparent confidence (which is fake in the case of *Lycopodium*), is that power and confidence influence others with or without their consent. What makes *Lycopodium* difficult is the coupling of his fierce demands with his inability to compromise. He is *contrary* and *intolerant to contradiction*. As a result, *Lycopodium* makes it a rule to attack a counter-argument, even though to all appearances it is true and forceful, in the belief that its truth is only superficial; moreover, he believes that the discussion may yield another case in which he may contradict that counter-argument (*disposition to contradict*) or succeed in confirming the truth of his original statement, evidence of the fact that he takes everything personally. The animus-driven *Lycopodium* does not fight for the truth but to win the battle for his proposition. As *Lycopodium* is skilled with words (making an excellent lawyer), he tries to win his verbal battles by making his opponent angry with repeated injustices, lying, or manipulating the facts, knowing well that when the opponent is angry he will be incapable of judging correctly and perceiving where his advantage lies (*ambition, employed every possible means; malicious*). Fair and thoughtful criticism is rarely welcomed by *Lycopodium*: every criticism is felt as a hostile attack against which he has to defend himself, as he cannot imagine that he can be wrong. Of course the real reason for this *easily offended* behavior is that he is afraid that people will find out about his narcissistic self-inflation, the only thing supporting and holding up his whole existence.

If there is one outstanding common characteristic among *Lycopodium* children (and adults), it is his great *fear for failure*. This child does not like what he is not good at, and he attempts to control his fear by avoiding any field of activity in which he does not believe he has a reasonable chance of success. He sticks to topics with which he feels safe and, in the case of the *Lycopodium* child with ASD, to his preferred activities. This, of course, will lead to much awkward and strange behavior. *Lycopodium* should remember what Thomas Edison said: “Success is ten percent inspiration and 90 percent perspiration.” Take the example, from my practice, of an intellectually gifted eight-year-old boy. He had the gift of the gab and was a natural performer, but he always longed for the applause of his peers; they, either out of envy or inability to understand him, shunned him at school. When the school day was over, his mother often found him sitting in a sandbox by himself, twirling little sticks in his hand, looking utterly lost. He was a brilliant boy, yet socially he was so awkward that his only good days at school were those days that he was asked to play the lead role in a play. How strange: he had no problem appearing in public, but once the applause died down, and his fifteen minutes of fame were over, it was painful to see him sitting in a corner, a shadow of the persona that had just shone so beautifully. *Lycopodium* was one of the remedies needed on his road to recovery.

Lycopodium is a person who does not want to feel inferior to others in any respect, especially in the intellectual sphere; she is always a victim of her own megalomania. No matter how great a person's gifts are, he is bound to be inferior to others in a multitude of ways. Of course, to *Lycopodium* this is unacceptable. *Lycopodium* thinks he is an expert on everything, and he is ever so susceptible to flattery (*flattery, gives everything, when flattered*)! Just as a cat purrs when it is stroked, one sees sweet rapture and delight in *Lycopodium's* face when he is praised—even when the praise consists of a palpable lie. As a *Lycopodium* child is often placed in classrooms of gifted children or those identified as having Asperger's syndrome, praising such a child for his smarts (which he likes) breeds the belief that things should come naturally—and when they don't, these kids think they are no longer bright. Or they choose unchallenging paths so as not to be exposed as "frauds" (*undertakes nothing lest he succeeds*). Being praised for being smart or for other innate abilities can lead to feelings of helplessness or self-doubt in the *Lycopodium* child when a setback occurs. Gallows appear on the horizon on which he should be hanged for perceived failure and incompetence. One should praise hard work while helping this child to think realistically about achieving goals. A parent must not fall into the trap of giving money as a reward for good performances: to the brain, receiving a sincere compliment is as much a reward as being given money!

Bossiness (*dictatorial; haughty, stiff and pretentious; impolite children; rudeness*) is *always* part of the *Lycopodium* child, and it is hard to teach him the art of empathy and respect for others. This bossiness is not a reflection of assertiveness, confidence, activity, or rambunctiousness, nor can it be called vivacious, courageous, or deserving of praise. It is rather aggressive, rude, disruptive behavior, and the *real* reason for it is the lack of confidence behind *Lycopodium's* mask. The *Lycopodium* child is too young to learn that a good leader is not bossy, and let's face it: many adults don't understand this either; they are blinded by their *love for power*. *Lycopodium's* failure to consider the feelings of others and tendency to push his agenda to the exclusion of all others constitutes an unfortunate, awful way to behave, and it can be corrected through correct use of the homeopathic remedy. A *Lycopodium* person is *intolerant to contradiction* and shouts incessantly that he is normal, but anyone who shouts incessantly that he is normal while behaving abnormally arouses the suspicion that he lacks insight into his illness.

Angel at School, Devil at Home

The parents of a young *Lycopodium* are often puzzled by the dichotomy in their child's behavior: as much as he is a dictator at home, he can be a follower outside of the home among his peers. Reports from school conflict with the family's experience at home. When an obviously honest teacher and an equally honest parent diverge widely in their estimation of the child ("an angel at school and devil at home"), one cannot dismiss the extreme variance as mere prejudice on either side. *Lycopodium* truly can be a man with two faces. An eight-year-old I once had as a patient was such a case. Though his younger sister adored him, he terrorized her, taking her security blanket away. When their mom gave it back to her, the boy would proceed to scream at the top of his lungs for a solid hour until his younger sister, worn down like the rest of the family, graciously gave him back the blanket. This was not an isolated incident of possessiveness and bossiness. When his mom tried to pass his first children's books on to his sister, he held on to them as though they were the most precious jewels, although up to that point he had had no interest in them at all. Unfortunately, Mom gave in and this boy won yet another battle, confirming that he was indeed the "alpha male" of the house. He "suggested" (read: ordered) that his younger sister play puppet theater and convinced her to say just what he suggested, and he threw a tantrum when she wanted to stop early before the brilliant script had been fully recited. Now, who is the head of the family? At school, though, he was the ideal student: meek, complying, and even rather timid in the classroom! What a split personality: certainly this is a child who possesses only two personas; a normal child, on the other hand, has an abundant and colorful set of personae to be used depending on the occasion (like having different clothes for different occasions)!

How fast a son learns from his unbalanced *Lycopodium* father! This can be easily seen in the *Lycopodium* child with special needs. No one has more of a split personality.

In school, terrified of the teacher's discipline and authority, he cowers, is submissive, and is most likely an "angel." Upon coming home, it is as though that child has been kidnapped and replaced by a demon. He throws off the chains of control and changes into a frenzied bully, ordering everyone around him to do exactly what he says. More than one parent has claimed that it seemed like his child was possessed: how else to come to grips with this grotesque transformation?

After talking to such a *Lycopodium* child for ten minutes, one pediatric neurologist declared to the boy's mother: "Your child is not autistic!" Never mind that this high-functioning *Lycopodium* child with Asperger's showed all the classic negative *Lycopodium* traits at home. Here, in front of an authority, he easily fools the specialist by being polite, curious, and yes, even *amative*! Another ten-year-old boy impressed his ophthalmologist by correctly naming all of the parts of the eye, showing off his knowledge, but again only to draw praise (*wants to be flattered*). He will ask a lot of questions, and when it comes to numbers, his delusions of grandeur are reflected by quoting the trillions and gazillions of dollars that he will earn! Money, after all, as he has learned from his father, is power!

Desire for What is Lacking

We are not surprised to see that what a person wants most is what he most lacks. *Lycopodium* wants power so much (*love for power*) simply because he knows he lacks it and needs it to really be the person he purports to be. Of course, the moment a situation demands responsibility and commitment (marriage [*the idea of marriage seems unendurable*], a new job, taking care of his children), his true colors come through as *he has fear of undertaking something* and *he flees from his children*; *forsakes his own children* and *has aversion to responsibility* and *has aversion to being kept in his house*. He will only love those children who are like him, those whom he succeeds in infecting with the same poisonous desire for conquests and power. He will project onto others in order to justify his own behavior (*reproaching others*; *reproachful delirium*), but in reality he runs away from the demands of life, demands that he accept his responsibilities and grow up. He always thinks about what is wrong with his partner, but never considers what is wrong within himself. What's wrong in *Lycopodium* is his incapacity to see another person objectively—as a real person, not merely as a meek subject. Sure, he falls in love with a woman who admires him terribly (*praised, loved to be*), but in the long run this is a bad mixture as her submissiveness becomes boring (though it was originally a big boost for his narcissism). Once boredom sets in, he needs a new subject to admire him, and the vicious circle goes on as he waltzes from one marriage to the next, not unsurprising, with the same "type" of woman, young, naive and pliable. Throughout his life, he will actively seek to "trade up" to someone with a higher score on his valuable characteristics list, not realizing that to trade up, to look for someone with "better" features, is incompatible with love. The energy spent in such a search would be better invested in improving his current union and, above all, in examining his shadow side. But he only loved a feature of his ex: her beauty, her flattery, or some other peripheral part of her or a delimited list of characteristics that will disappear or fail to remain exciting. Ultimately, though, he always fails to love her for the person she is, which one must do in order to be happy in love.

Animus in Control

Lycopodium fears life, and such a man always needs a mother figure who will help him in his struggle to deal with emotion-laden situations. In *Lachesis* (being of a sanguine temperament with the anima dominating), affairs of the heart take first place when it comes to competition. Well known is the cruel streak of the *Lachesis* woman undergoing menopause, and even before it, when she feels threatened by a younger rival: *jealousy with striking; impulse to poison others as she fears she is going to be sent to an insane asylum*, as she fears that the competing person will replace her (i.e. being insanely jealous of a sibling or friend who has a child while she struggles to get pregnant). *Lycopodium*, with a dominant animus, couldn't care less about affairs of the heart (he is the one breaking them, his wife's included), but he truly wants to be number one in the business world as he is *a boaster, who wishes to be considered rich*. Lycopodium does not hesitate to use the accomplishments of his parents, if they are successful, just to boast about his social status.

Unfortunately, an unbalanced *Lycopodium* father will often mold a *Lycopodium* son from the beginning, as the boy's perfect example is his "awesome" dad! A dominating *Lycopodium* father wants his child to be like him in temperament and character. *Lycopodium* has a choleric temperament and thus finds no sympathy with a phlegmatic earth type such as *Calcarea* or *Pulsatilla,* whom he considers weaklings. A *Lycopodium* father is only interested in seeing how much his child is like him, as any difference found in the son is considered a defect or at least an inferior characteristic. But if the child has a different dominant conscious function (feeling, for instance) from that of his thinking *Lycopodium* father, the child will only become a badly handicapped replica of his father, crippling his own growth as he tries to function according to a persona that becomes him like ill-fitting clothes.

The pseudo-*Lycopodium* child therefore has to cope with his parents' disappointments and accusations while constantly fearing that he will lose their love as well as the respect of society. There is no more effective method of weakening a child's will (*lack of confidence*) than arousing in him a sense of failure for not following in the footsteps of his elitist family. Without knowing it, such a child becomes a tool of others, crippling himself by disobeying the demands of his own conscience and by violating his dominant conscious function. The *Lycopodium* child therefore becomes aggressive with his or her mother and sister, the "weak" ones, the subordinates with the feeling dominant conscious function (*contemptuous, hard for subordinates and agreeable, pleasant to superiors or people he has to fear*), reflecting *Lycopodium*'s ultimate *aversion to women* and *aversion to family members*. This is, all the while, tolerated by the father—if it is not out-and-out encouraged! Therefore, the *Lycopodium* person jockeys for this first position from a young age, in the company of *Nux-v* and *Verat-a*, as he is *abusive and insulting towards his parents as well as disobedient, defiant* and *employing every possible means to fulfill his ambition*. He is one character that learns his lesson early.

There is also the delirium of social elevation in *Lycopodium*, and the sole purpose of these delusions is to emphasize the value of the personality (*pompous, important*). These delusions are frequently associated with aristocratic airs, literary and philosophical enthusiasms, boasting, extravagant and "original" views, and speeches. The only thing *Lycopodium* achieves with this is the creation of an iron mask that is glued onto his face, hindering any possible introspection later on.

Looking for the Old and Convenient: Routine

New environments and situations are scary for *Lycopodium*. To be suddenly placed in a new situation or a strange country, where the way of life is very different from his own, is at the first moment like stepping into cold water. *Lycopodium* is brought into sudden contact with a drastically different temperature, and he feels a powerful and superior influence from without which affects him uncomfortably. He finds himself in a situation in which he cannot move with ease and which threatens to rip off his mask. Anyone who performs the same task every day, who takes the same route to work every day, who eats an identical meal at the same time each day, can be disturbed by even a slight change in that routine, because his habit has become a property whose loss endangers his perceived security. As Mark Twain said, "There are several good protections against temptation, but the surest one is cowardice." And it is *cowardice* (and hypervigilance) that is behind *Lycopodium's* actions and thoughts. Courage entails that one be willing to face a present evil so as to prevent a greater evil in the future, while cowardice does the reverse.

The formation of habits can lead directly to failure! New situations and challenges evoke *Lycopodium's* true nature (which nature he does not acknowledge); they release him from his shadow side, and in those moments his superhero persona dissolves: he is *easily frightened and started; feels frightened at everything, even the ringing of the bell.* We see this also in the *Lycopodium* child with ASD when, for example, a toilet flushes unexpectedly (as toilets tend to do in airports) or a drinking fountain suddenly starts and stops! It is probably because this is happening unexpectedly, not giving him a chance to be prepared; such an event startles the man behind the mirror. Fear appears first, before anger, as it is the most primitive emotion—and yet it is the one which is most damaging to the stability of the ego (*frightened easily, at trifles*). There is *anxiety from anticipation of an event* as he is not able to predict all that can happen to blow his cover. It can even lead to *anthropophobia, especially for clowns or other masked figures.* It is interesting that a personality like *Lycopodium,* with such a big mask, is afraid of masked people. Perhaps *Lyc* is afraid to find out what is hiding behind the mask of a clown who expresses joy and laughter. He must instinctively know that such people are like him and that their emotions don't reflect the expressions on their faces. *Lyc* does suffer from a fear of confrontation, even when he must ask where one can find a certain item in a store. But at the same time, when on safe and known territory, he is not afraid to "bark" his opinion as it may help him to scare off his opponents (< > *Bar-c* and *Staph* who suffer from *cowardice, without courage to express their own opinion*).

Resistance to new things is a tricky thing in the life of a human being who is trying to grow up. *Lycopodium* and *Silica* fear all that is new, all that is different; they fear taking risks and have a strong tendency to recoil, to go back instead of going forward. Fear of what one is not accustomed to and fear of possible failure is expressed in resistance and, yes, even violent behavior when pushed. *Lycopodium* should heed Nietzsche's words: "What does not kill us makes us stronger." As resistance to new things can start out with low self-confidence as a child, it inevitably leads to a compensatory desire for power and social status in adulthood. Both *Lyc* and *Silica* are very well known for this, but of course we know that compensations are only self-deception. The question of how to avoid problems plagues both remedies. Both personalities are masters of compensating for their dark characteristics, which are usually well repressed in the shadow side. Their exterior appearances, or masks, often have little to do with what is transpiring underneath. Their compensations, therefore, will most likely just show the opposite of what takes place in conscious life; they will do anything (even as children) to convince you of the opposite of what is happening in the real, hidden self. This, obviously, creates a constant tension between a person's strengths and weaknesses.

Sexual Conquest

Lycopodium is mainly an extravert thinking type. With his posturing and excessive persona, he wants to portray a self-confident, influential, and powerful person. All his behavior is aimed at the object, not at the self, leading to a lack of introspection. As an adult, this extravert attitude can lead to *sexual excesses,* one of his NWS. But *Lycopodium* is the kind of man who believes that morals have nothing to do with his neurosis and that sinning intentionally is not sinning at all, because it can be intellectualized out of existence. He believes so much in the power of reason that he can even "unthink" a wrong he has committed. He is someone who believes too firmly in the power and dignity of intellect while violating the feeling value. He is blind to the archaic feeling function in himself and, therefore, finds himself rather isolated. To whom will he be sexually attracted? To a gentle, feminine woman who, because of an archaic thinking function, will find his ideas appealing mainly because they are his! She cannot make heads or tails of them, but she will listen beautifully with flattering attention and little interjections. *Lycopodium's* sense of self-worth is tied up in his relationships with women who admire him unconditionally and without limit (*flattery, gives everything when flattered*). Of course, if *Lycopodium* fails to obtain the admiration of the woman he has chosen, fear paralyses him temporarily—but fleeing the relationship becomes natural as such a failure threatens the basis for his narcissistic self-evaluation. When you praise a *Lycopodium*, a sweet expression of delight appears on his face. This is comforting for the *Lycopodium* man, as his partner's relative emptiness of intellectual ideas and her passive receptivity stimulates his superior thinking function as well as charming his *vanity*. Of course, he treats her as an inferior companion, parking her wherever he might choose and always expecting her to be waiting passively upon his return like a car in a parking lot. He is annoyed if she is not just where he left her, as though she herself does not exist. But *Lycopodium* is a commitment-phobe who fears that marriage is the end of his youth; he may also get itchy just at the thought of a long-term relationship (*idea of marriage is unendurable*).

When we examine *Lycopodium's* sexual behavior, it is of an asocial rather than a social nature, since *Lycopodium* flees from all relationship responsibilities. *Lycopodium* is the prototype of the obsessive-compulsive sexual neurotic who takes part in mechanical, soulless sex and who tends to reduce sex to a purely physical level at which his partner is turned into a mere object. Such a personality always has something major to overcome.

Anticipation anxiety is at the crux of his suffering, and it eventually, unavoidably, causes the unmasking of his personality in conjunction with the compulsive self-observation or "hyper-reflectiveness." This is also always accompanied by the attention he is compelled to pay to whether or not the intention towards his activities is effective. This is the same for any anticipation anxiety, be it anxiety about upcoming events, anxiety about failure, about sexual performance, about examinations, etc. His CD, *everything will vanish*, takes on a special meaning in his sexual relationships, where he is the king of one-night stands and uncommitted sex; this approach grows out of an expectation of immediate pleasure and gratification. Because of these sexual desires and thoughts, the married *Lyc* is the most prone to unfaithfulness in his relationship, being a sort of hunter like *Medorrhinum*. He walks starry-eyed, looking not into the eyes of his spouse or romantic partner, but over his partner's shoulder, in case there might be somebody better nearby. His love for power extends to sexual conquests, taking advantage of society's double standard by which married women with lovers are blamed more harshly for adultery than men. Also, *Lycopodium's* motto is "seize the opportunity," so he reasons that he can be only as faithful as his options allow him to be; in view of the status he seeks and often achieves, his options are numerous. Obviously, this is not the road to successful long-term relationships! *Lycopodium's* rather debauched sexual lifestyle eventually leads to sexual insecurity. *Lycopodium* is so self-absorbed and his powers of self-observation so acute ("Did I perform like a great conqueror? Am I the great lover?"), that he starts any conquest with the fear of not succeeding (*fear he will not reach his destination*). Eventually, sometimes sooner than later, this anticipation anxiety leads to the sexual performance failure for which *Lycopodium* is so well-known: *impotence, penis small and cold and relaxed; feeble erection, strong desire without being able to have an erection in old people; erections wanting after sexual excesses; erections wanting with his wife* (only remedy).

Lycopodium fixes his attention not on his partner but on the sexual act itself. And as much as he tries to "will it," and precisely because he is "willing it," the sexual act is bound to fail. It is a compulsion to engage in sexuality (based on his ego), and this has destroyed any spontaneity and naturalness in his sexual practices. It is not a spontaneous, natural consequence of intimacy, but a calculated power trip or conquest. Excessive intention, or hyper-intention, is easy to see in the sexual neurosis from which *Lyc* suffers: the more a man tries to demonstrate his sexual potency or a woman her ability to experience an orgasm, the more difficult it is to succeed. In such people, pleasure must remain a side effect and is destroyed when it is made the only goal. *Lycopodium* has the sex of a boy of fourteen without feeling. It is unrelated sex, a sort of auto-eroticism, a kind of masturbation on someone else, as Traditional Chinese Medicine (TCM) called it. *Lycopodium* remains an immature person; otherwise, he would only consider a sexual relationship in which sex was an expression of love. A monogamous approach is impossible for *Lycopodium* as his physical desire is never linked with a desire for psycho-spiritual union. Sex normally is, and should be, an expression of love; it is a vehicle of love, but love is not a side effect of sex.

As much as we see *Lycopodium* indicated in such cases of chronically faithless men, this remedy is equally indicated in poor sexual performance in "newcomers" or in those who are too excited in a new relationship. I have had patients who had been sexually impotent from the time of their first sexual encounter. As one told me, "I finally convinced my girlfriend to have sex with me and she consented to have sex at a safe, private place fourteen days from then. By the time those fourteen days were over, I was so agitated, so out of bounce with sleepless nights, excitement, and fantasy, that when it came to the real act, I couldn't perform." In the first place, this young man who doubted his virility had a normal reaction, not a pathological one. The patient had to realize that this was not a case of real impotence as he had feared; his fear created an anticipatory neurosis and thus became the starting point for a vicious cycle.

In the case of *Lyc*, the sexual performance and fear of failure (propelled by his CD) is only part of his total personality: *Lyc* has equal fears of failure in business, examinations, public appearances, meeting new people for the first time, and the like. No matter what mask he presents, we can assume that low self-confidence permeates his whole being and is not just focused on his sexual life. But the sexual aspect **is** a large part of his pathology when he consults the homeopath! Homeopathy, as with *Lycopodium*—just one of the anticipatory remedies we possess—is able to arrest the dangerous autosuggestion (CD) at the start, to nip it in the bud, so to speak, and keep it from developing.

Often *premature ejaculation* is another consequence that can be remedied by homeopathic *Lycopodium*. I have often read the stories of serial killers who were laughed at upon experiencing premature ejaculation for the first time. It creates in the syphilitic-predisposed person the desire to kill women as an act of revenge. The *Lycopodium* individual, with his love for power and domineering, often lacks the ability to lovingly devote himself to his partner, the prerequisite for the capacity to respond and perform sexually. Our therapy (and also psychotherapy) is aimed at eliminating the fixation upon the sexual act itself. Such a compulsion might originate from his own ego, from making a resolution to have sexual intercourse on a particular day, or to receive confirmation he is still loved, or to get confirmation that he is still a virile young man who is desired and can perform at will. In the psychology and pathology of men's sexual behavior, we see how misguided this striving for happiness is, how the desperate attempt to achieve happiness and pleasure is condemned to fail.

As one can observe from all of the above, sexuality for *Lycopodium* is initially a source of brief pleasure, but often, and sooner than he thinks, it becomes a source of protracted suffering. Normally, hunger, thirst, and the need for sexual satisfaction are physiological necessities; if they remain unsatisfied for any length of time, a painful tension is felt. Satisfaction comes from the Latin *satis facere*, "to make enough or sufficient." There is a distinct difference between the sexual desire of *Conium* and *Lycopodium*. In the absence of a partner, as is the case in *Conium* (due to death, conversion to religion or sect forbidding sex, spiritual conversion renouncing sex), it is not only physiological needs that go unmet: these needs are combined with psychological loss, the grief experienced at the sudden halt of these normal expressions from Nature, leading in *Conium* to hard cancers in the genitourinary system. *Lycopodium* has *irrational* desires when he uses the sexual act to prove himself that he is still virile as ever, that he is loved by his partner, and that he still is the one "in power," demanding what is owed to him in the marriage. Such an irrational sexual desire, born from his psychological needs, is insatiable, except at the brief moment of the encounter itself. Greed, as well as lust for power, is a bottomless pit, and the idea of the relief derived from the satisfaction of such is nothing more than a Fata Morgana.

The unbalanced and untreated *Lycopodium* person, incapable of loving himself and never able to love the other person for who she is rather than how she looks, is always stuck in the irrational desire that has become part of his life. TCM would call this an *ignoble misfortune*, one brought on by his own mistakes and attitude, while *Conium* suffers from a noble misfortune brought on by circumstances in life. An archetype that one is likely to meet among our *Lycopodium* patients is that of the eternal youth or *puer aeternus*. This is a person who remains too long in the adolescent psychological phase, as characteristics which considered normal in a youth are now carried over into adult life. Such a person seeks out experiences for their sheer excitement, choosing friends and women when he wants amusement but dropping them when they become in any sense a responsibility (*responsibility, aversion to*). Moving in and out of acquaintances is characteristic, and compulsive sexual activity, as mentioned before, is often the expression of this archetype. Childish *Lycopodium* indulges in casual and promiscuous relationships, only to drop each one when the first hint appears that some commitment may be required of him—or when he simply becomes bored.

Intellect

A crop of white hair (*early graying*) always commands reverence, much more so than the facial wrinkles of a *Nat-m*: one speaks of venerable white hair, and *Lycopodium*, who suffers from early graying, uses this as an asset to demand respect for his authority and wisdom. Of course he uses his intellect wherever he can: *he can properly speak about higher and even abstract things, but he gets confused in everyday matters*. This proving reflects the haughty persona he portrays while easily stumbling over everyday mundane things. Because of the hidden low self-confidence, his intellect has a sharp edge and urgency to it: he uses his education to *speak like a dictator with an air of command*, and *with a manner stiff and pretentious*, which serves him well when it comes to his profession as a teacher, priest, lawyer, broker, etc. Speaking with a voice of command has a purpose: he does not want to be contradicted! Intimidation helps! The intelligent *Lycopodium* never admits to any weaknesses but carefully conceals them; he is very sensitive to any allusion to them. The reason is that *Lycopodium's* whole world lies in the absence of faults and defects, so that every flaw that comes to light directly diminishes his overall existence as he wants to portray it.

Besides speaking with command, what helps *Lycopodium* to be admired by unsophisticated souls is his boasting. *Lycopodium*, the boaster, demonstrates an unpleasant increase of self-confidence and conceit. He is full of himself, knows everything, and imagines himself fully informed about world affairs but also about every detail of his presumed illness. As usual, such a one-sided conscious attitude of optimistic self-confidence conceals a profound sense of impotence, something that is very clear in the *Lycopodium* patient. The conscious optimism displayed by his excessive persona is nothing but an unsuccessful compensation, as shown in his dreams of a *boat capsizing* and the *fear that he will not reach his destination*, both expressions of his fear of failure in business, in school, or in sexual performance! The well-trained homeopath discovers certain traits of an anxious sense of inferiority and the *desire to be flattered by others* behind *Lycopodium's* haughtiness. The *Lycopodium* personality is puffed up; Jung called this "psychic inflation."[26] The motto of *Lyc* people is "L'état, c'est moi!" A perfect example is the often ostentatious behavior of politicians who act like reigning emperors; they are not subject to the common laws of their country (until they push their luck too far). There is a quest for high social position (also *Verat-a*). Such a person will not hesitate to hide behind his business or his titles, his social mask. Such attractions offer easy compensations for personal deficiencies.

As mentioned before, *Lycopodium* is the extraverted thinking type in Jung's typology. They are usually men who attempt to force everything into rational, intellectual formulations. In their frame of reference, everything can be planned and executed as reason and logic dictate. He has an answer for everything: "Is this clear to everyone?" he asks. "Who can doubt this course of action?" But *Lycopodium* is like the iceberg with an enormous block of introverted feeling and with his shadow side below the surface. *Lycopodium* is not aware

26. Carl G. Jung, *The Portable Jung*, ed. Joseph Campbell (New York: Penguin Books, 1976), 88.

that he has feelings, as any use of them is pure nonsense, hysterical and "womanish." But he has plenty of feelings that are expressed as vague needs and black moods that he promptly denies, rationalizes, and justifies. The situation, this person, the circumstances, left him no other choice, and *Lycopodium's* answer seems to come from the archetypal Old Wise Man resembling an absolute divine, compassionate, and intelligent character. The bitter truth is that such people are tyrants, not wise men, inconsiderate of those nearest them—of spouses and children especially, and then other relatives, friends, and subordinates—while seeking power among their superiors (*contemptuous, hard for subordinates, pleasant to superiors and people he has to fear*). The hidden part of the iceberg is made up of stubborn aggression, of dogmatic opinions (which he will passionately defend as they are the children of his animus) and resentment. *Lyc* fashions himself as the man who "knows" what is "right" and therefore becomes an individual who is dangerous to society in general.

While he can outshine most people in intellectual circumstances, he fails when the thinking mode, his dominant conscious function, must be set aside in favor of one of his auxiliary functions—let alone when he must rely on his subservient feeling function. He fears approaching such a situation without his strong side, his intellect (this reflects his CD, in which his intelligence now must vanish). At that point, *his thoughts stand still; his mind is awkward, and as it was, rigid, like numbness. He slips in words and syllables and chooses the wrong words. His thoughts become confused as he is unable to fix them. He uses wrong syllables, makes mistakes in writing and spells words wrong.* The stamp of ADD seems to fit him perfectly, and that stamp is, indeed, often affixed. In spite of his intelligence, he makes mistakes fueled by his hidden CD. It is a perfect example of how the unconscious guides the conscious. His reactions to all this make him hyperactive: *he can't sit still. He squirms in his chair, ready to escape! He can be excessively merry and laugh at the simplest things,* but when young *Lycopodium* experiences humiliation (mortification) at the hands of a parent, coach, teacher, or fellow student, *the child loses his cheerfulness and becomes quiet and dispirited, and is very much discouraged and tired* (*mainly at school*). The *Lycopodium* child can also successfully feign disease at the moment of examinations at school. He can convince his parents that he is not feeling well, and the parents, not knowing that there is a test that day, let him get away with it. It is here that not only the homeopath but also the parent must play Sherlock Holmes!

Obstinacy

Another positive compensation, at least an attempt to not be confronted by his Cyber delusion, is *Lycopodium*'s *trouble at concealing his internal obstinacy* (psora) *and vexation. He is self-willed, passionate and angry. He is obstinate, defiant and even looks for disputes.* It is like putting up a smoke screen! He needs to be obstinate and even scares people by looking for a fight to hide his sense of insecurity, which is shown in his strong reaction to disapproval: *he cannot bear the least contradiction and at once gets besides himself for vexation.* A child like *Lycopodium* (and *Silica*), born physically weak, will always compensate with mental prowess. Any challenge or disapproval of his opinion (which challenges his intellect or throws it into doubt) always meets with a flurry of abuse. So obstinacy regrettably also means that he *seeks disputes*! As has been stated here, *Lyc* will use his dictatorial manner to get away with this; the *Lyc* child becomes *disobedient, defiant, though not necessarily ill-humored.* This certainly reflects a certain degree of haughtiness and reproachful attitude (*reproaching others*).

Company

What else can *Lycopodium* rely on? If one dreads failing (his CD!), one often looks for support or company (psoric phase in which it resembles *Calc-c*, which it follows well), but only from close and trusted family members since *anxiety in others' company increases* and *there is even weariness of life, particularly in company. If people* (especially strangers) *come near her, she is immediately attacked with anxiety at the pit of her stomach, reflecting a deep feeling of distrust and suspicion.* The repertory shows this distrust in the rubrics *fear, approaching of others*; *looked at, cannot bear being*; *stomach, anxiety of people on approach* (only *Lyc*), reflecting a *deep feeling of distrust* and extreme *suspicion*. These provings reflect *Lycopodium*'s fear that people (outside of the family) will discover the real *Lyc*, the coward beneath the mask. The shadow side takes the lead in these circumstances. He worries: "Here comes somebody I don't know, and he will probably see through me immediately!" In contrast, *Lycopodium* knows his family members, as he has tested them from a young age on (*Sil*). As discussed before, a *Lycopodium* father creates a handicapped child, and the latter needs now support on the physical and mental-emotional plane, as expressed by the following provings: *child desires to be carried*; *dread of solitude*; *she is afraid of being alone, as she lacks confidence in her strength. Lycopodium* can be in the next room as long as he knows someone else is in another room (*fear of being alone, but desire to be alone, Lyc and Kali-c*). The child demands the presence of a parent when he is doing homework:

"I can't do it," he claims. All sorts of weird excuses start popping out. This assignment is only due tomorrow, so he tries to postpone it until the morning hours before breakfast. He wants to play a video game first; he needs to eat a little. *Lycopodium* is a true procrastinator, as there is always a gap between intention and action. This is not the same as laziness, which involves a lack of desire; with procrastination, the desire is there to start the project, but it consistently loses out to his appetite for delay. When Mom or Dad sits with *Lycopodium*, he has no difficulty successfully completing the school task; however, this is not enough to bolster his confidence for the next time. *Lyc* has also *timidity about going to bed,* reflecting his *fear of being alone* and his *fear of the dark.* This was evident in the behavior of a 14-year-old *Lycopodium* boy who complained every night that he could never fall asleep; but the moment he was allowed in Mom's bed, he always fell immediately asleep! Of course, the intelligent *Lycopodium* child will never say: "I am afraid." He will find more sophisticated expressions to help him reach his goal of joining Mom in bed.

Lycopodium children also drive their parents crazy as they never allow them to leave home in the evening to go shopping or see a movie, especially if a new babysitter is needed. They will become incensed when the parents leave, "punishing" them upon their return with temper tantrums and striking. And God forbid that Mom should leave him for a couple of days; he will show his anger in no uncertain terms, abusing her and trying to make her feel guilty. This has everything to do with the fear that someone else, someone not as close as his parents, will discover *Lycopodium's* timidity and will unmask his personality: *fear of being approached* can be taken literally but also figuratively. *Lyc* displays all his talents to others, and especially to the physician, in order to avoid intrusive personal questions (*Sil* too): as is true with a balloon, too much pressure can lead to a sudden, unpleasant noise (*Lyc* is *presumptuous),* and therefore makes a false impression on others.

Initially, the *Lycopodium* child receives support from family, as he can be very *amorous and amative,* still being in the psoric phase (part of the social mask). *They are so sensitive that they even cry when thanked.* This reflects how important others' opinions of him are to *Lycopodium* (*Lyc* has **concern**—not *despair—about social position,* like *Verat-a*): she likes her ego to be fortified and wants to be sure that others see her strong exterior side, not the insecure and cowardly inside picture (this makes us think of the fragile oyster in his shell, *Calc-c,* with which *Lyc* has a complementary relationship). *They can also be over-merry, with giddiness.* This behavior is really a mask hiding anxiety about being discovered (having fear of failure or dealing with suppressed anger). *Lycopodium's* excessive persona is again demonstrated in the following provings: *Lyc becomes sensitive, irritable, and peevish and cross on awaking. He is easily excited to anger.* These are frequently manifested around people *Lyc* knows, especially at home, but rarely outside of the home, where he is rather overcome by a *strong timidity about appearing in public.* Just like *Silica*'s, *Lycopodium's* anger is mostly directed at persons they can dominate and terrorize: a little sibling, the weaker parent, or an innocent animal: *makes ungrounded reproaches and beats the person whom she abuses.* Emotions in *Lycopodium* are often masked figures. With the homeopathic remedy, as well as love and understanding, the *Lycopodium* person can take off the mask and show himself in his real form. Anger then will reveal itself as fear. These fears, apparently meaningless and disproportionate, become related to his hidden sense of insecurity and low confidence.

Golden Tips from the Masters

- If *Lycopodium* does not work, think about *Kali-c, Nat-c, Chelidonium* and *China* as backups. They are complementary to *Lycopodium*.
- Primary action is on the liver and secondary action on the kidneys and genital system
- Dislikes math
- Quivering fibrillation of alae nasi
- The brain has developed at the expense of the body
- #1 remedy for erectile problems with performance anxiety
- An "angel in school, a devil at home."
- Non-descending right testicle
- Starts things, does not finish them (*postponing everything; undertakes many things, perseveres in nothing*)
- It is one of the greatest mental fatigue remedies and one of the greatest unrefreshed sleep remedies
- <from onions and beans; >after midnight (only remedy)
- Headaches when not eating on time; **hypoglycemia** when fasting or skipping a meal
- Increased and immediate fermentation of food when eating, with bloating below the navel and *fullness of stomach after eating ever so little*
- Dryness of vagina, severe enough to make intercourse impossible (vaginismus)
- Dry tickling cough at night
- Burning of the soles, sticks feet out from under the covers at night
- #1 remedy for uremic urinary lithiasis (increased uric acid)
- For back complaints where *Rhus-t* fails
- Major dyslexia remedy
- #1 remedy for varices in pregnancy, especially when located in the genitalia
- #1 remedy for intellectual sequelae of flu: unable to go back to work after a flu because of intellectual failures (memory, writing, misspelling, unable to read)

Lyssinum (Lyss). Hydrophobinum. Saliva of a rabid dog

The Cyber Delusion

If you have ever had a *Lyssin* case in your practice, you will never forget it. *Lyssin*'s purely primitive, animal behavior is puzzling and even disturbing: as if a sudden switch has been pulled, a well-functioning child transforms in a single moment into an aggressive, fearful, delirious, and biting individual who shocks all those around her. How can we try to look into the mind of this child and gain understanding? *Lyssin*'s Cyber delusion is ***something terrible is going to happen***. As we will note, many of *Lyssin*'s delusions express this same theme of fearful expectations. Hering describes in great detail the horrible feelings that overcome this person: *thoughts of something terrible going to happen come into his mind against his will; he could not get rid of the indescribable tormenting feeling that something terrible was going to happen to him; he feels as if he had heard unpleasant news, or would soon hear it; she felt as she was going to die; she feels impelled to do reckless things, such as throwing her child, which she carries in her arms, through the window and the like.*

Other delusions supporting the CD include *he defends himself against an imaginary attack and insults: they energetically defend themselves against attacks and insults, which in reality are product of their own fancy; she raved about the dog that had bitten her, imagined it to be near and fought as if to drive it away.* Then we have the delusion he *has suffered wrong: they believe that they are reduced to their wretched condition by the instrumentality of those about them (A/F; mortification).* Furthermore, this perceived persecution is expressed in similar fixed ideas: *delusion, being abused: they imagine that they are abused.* Also to point to the extreme intensity of the emotions, there is the *delusion, he suffers the torment of hell without being able to explain: declares amid violent sobs that he is suffering the torments of hell.* To round out the delusions supporting the essence of the CD, we also have *delusion, he is tormented* and *delusion, he is forsaken; after fainting spell, he wrote on paper: I am forsaken by all, even the birds of heaven, they do not look at me, they do not feed me if I am hungry; he wrote to his doctor: I am waiting with impatience that you give me and my young ones something to eat; he begged to pray for him and not to leave him alone.*

The above delusions all express the same agonizing feeling: a feeling of a perceived injury, of being perturbed or treated wrong by the person on whom one is dependent, leading to great anticipation anxiety and reducing the individual to his most primitive state where the instinct of survival is tested. The *Lyssin* person depends on someone (husband, family member, good friend) like a faithful dog depends on his master who gives him everything, from food and shelter to love and a daily walk (expressed by the secondary *delusion, feels forsaken* as mentioned above). In other words, *Lyssin* perceives himself to be abandoned and cruelly treated by another person, not all the time, but only in **episodes** and especially in those moments of the most common natural needs (*during the tranquil intervals he recognized correctly to questions put out to him, recognized those around him, and with a presentiment of impending death begged them to pray for him and not to leave him*). This is also especially felt in increased times of need, when there is more pressure in the patient's life, unlike *Hyoscyamus* or *Ignatia,* who have an insanely tortured "love, dependency, and loyalty" issue with the subject of their interest **all** the time.

When might *Lyssin's* periods of increased dependency and need for support occur? We will begin by discussing children. We know that until age five the child is linked by the psychological umbilical cord to the mother before beginning to wrestle for more independence and escape from the power of the collective unconscious; this is also an escape from the dream world of the Divine Mother, with all the responsibilities that come along with facing growing demands. It is then, at such moments of individuation or growing into an individual, that *Lyssin* moments could arise.

The child might feel increased need for support when entering a new school, when facing examinations, doing homework, when bullied in school (so much more prevalent now with the availability of social media like Facebook), when not fitting in well in school or being humiliated as the result of having a physical handicap, when suffering grief from the loss of a parent, grandparent, a pet, or a dear friend, and so on. One can have a good idea about such periods of increased needs of support when looking at remedies that ***follow*** *Lyssin* ***well,*** such as *Gels, Nat-c, Nat-m,* and the serpent poisonings, and what remedies *Lyssin* ***follows well:*** *Arg-n, Con, Gels, Hyos, Stram,* and *Lachesis.* One recognizes the forsaken, lonely feelings of the *Natrums,* the hearing bad news leading to the trembling *Gelsemium* person (*mental emotion or mortifying news always makes him worse,* *Lyssin* and *Gels*) as well as the grief and fright causalities of the snake venoms (*those who were afflicted with grief from any cause were much sooner* *affected with the disease – rabies*). For the adult, other instances of increased stress (*ailments from emotional excitement*) can be numerous and awaken the most primitive instincts.

I think that pregnancy (*strange notions and apprehensions during pregnancy*), during which, according to Kent, the woman changes into "a nervous race horse overcome by anticipation anxiety," is one of the most dangerous periods—not only to the expectant mother, but even more so for the fetus, in whom the seed of *Lyssin* can be planted. Much depends, no doubt, on the true constitution of the person. The sensitive *Phosphorus* and the vulnerable *Calcarea carbonicum* person, both filled with many fears and an inherent sense of compassion, care, and worry about family and friends, feel forsaken even when, in reality, they are not. So when these characters are confronted with the abovementioned challenges, it does not take much (if the other party does not deliver what they want) for them to feel insecure, needy, abandoned, frightened, and threatened, evoking the most violent and primitive emotions (*a sudden fright starts convulsions*). They indeed become nervous race horses excited by the slightest stress and by any sensory input via light or noise (*the sound of running water or pouring water aggravates all complaints*). The Old Masters had a special name for the extensive fears of such patients, who fear becoming mad: *Lyssophobia*: *feels as if he cannot physically endure his fears much longer, and shall be compelled to go to an insane asylum.*

Causalities

Emotional Excitement

To illustrate this causality, and the state of mind of a pregnant *Lyssin* woman who can unwittingly "infect" her child through **mystical participation,** I refer to a case from my practice. It is one of intrauterine transmission of apprehension in the case of a 12-year-old girl:

> She had come to me days before to consult for anticipation anxiety in relation to upcoming examinations. This all started when she was doing her Iowa advanced testing. Now, whenever examinations approached at school, she suffered from anxiety beginning days in advance. She was very intelligent when coming to consult and she led the whole conversation while both parents sat behind her. It was obvious to me that they adored their only child. I decided on giving LM1

> *Arg-n* and looked forward to good results. However, the next day, while I was having dinner with a friend, her parents tracked me down to inform me of some startling symptoms: their beautiful and intelligent young daughter growled like a wolf (sic) and bit the pillow on the sofa. She even nipped her mother when she tried to approach her! Then she started convulsing in her left leg. I knew immediately this was a case of *Lyssin* (*Lyssin* follows *Arg-n* well!). When I saw her the next day, I asked again about a potential intrauterine event which, when inquired about previously had not been divulged by the mother. Up to this time, nothing had ever indicated such bizarre behavior. She was a smart and perfect little girl. But as is so often the case, puberty wakes up many latent or dormant miasms! When I probed for an intrauterine event, the mother said to me that she was very dependent on her husband during that time, as she had no other family. And then he had to travel unexpectedly for months overseas. She had felt "forsaken and very lonely, utterly lost without the help of [her] husband." It had made her very anxious. Undoubtedly, I had found the "scene of the crime," as these feelings had clearly been transferred to the unborn fetus. As many keynotes of *Lyssin* appeared, and the young girl's fixed state reflected the Cyber delusion, I doubted neither my remedy nor my approach; but fate took this little patient away from me. A neurologist was consulted and she was put in a university hospital for observation and treatment. While she had no further seizures after my one dose of *Lyssin*, they discharged her anyway with two different anti-seizure medications. To increase the folly, a specialist in Lyme disease was consulted, who prescribed antibiotics based on a dubious positive nonspecific test. I never learned her fate, as the next month I moved away from my practice, but I am sure she was held on seizure meds for a long time. What a beautiful chance missed for homeopathy to work!

As seen in the previous history, the pregnant woman feels threatened when her partner leaves on a long trip, even to the point that she fears she will lose her reason (*fear of becoming mad*). *Lyssin* has even *complaints from abnormal sexual desire from abstinence*, like *Conium* and *Platina*! The husband leaving when she really needs him is now interpreted as a gesture of abandonment and felt as humiliation: "I was not worth staying for." And unfortunately for the patient, *it is very difficult for her to think, sometimes impossible*. It is for this reason that such humiliation/mortification occurs when the "protector" leaves: this could also be applied to a dog put in a kennel when his beloved master leaves and now becoming aggressive towards other dogs and people. Being left behind in circumstances which are perceived as dangerous leaves *Lyssin* with the urgent need to fend for himself and is perceived as "abuse": *imagine that they are abused, and energetically defend themselves against attacks and insults, which in reality are products of their own fancy.* Here again, a differential diagnosis with *Arg-n*, *fearful something will happen*, is necessary.

Mortification or Indignation and Anticipation Anxiety

A *Lyssin* state can be created in children who are put up for adoption, reflecting the state of mind of the pregnant mother who knows she needs to be there to feed and love this unborn child but is forced to give it up, especially when boyfriend/spouse or family insist on it (*feels as if something disagreeable will happen*). In other words, in this episode (pregnancy), she feels forsaken by those she is depending on: the essence of *Lyssin*. It might also be that the mother is not able to take care of the child because of drug or alcohol abuse. This reminds me of a case in which many *Pulsatilla* characteristics were visible in a girl who had been put up for adoption; apparently, though, *Pulsatilla* was only a simile as, upon having her first menses, this young lady showed typical hydrophobic symptoms: she showed immense fear whenever she heard the water running from the shower, further confirming the choice of *Lyssin* and giving us a glimpse of the natural birth mother's frame of mind while she was pregnant with this baby girl. I also had a memorable case of *Lyssin*, almost a proving picture, in a 28-year-old woman in foster care, mongoloid in nature. One will recognize the behavior of "a mad or fearful dog":

> This was not the common trisomy 21 child. A very experienced Down syndrome specialist said of her: "I have never seen anyone like her. Generally they are quiet but this one has never known inner peace." Noting her behavior in my office, this was an understatement! She scratched her face, banged her head, and had the IQ of a two-year-old. She bit, screamed, and wrestled. She did respond to persons she perceived as authorities and to those who had worked extensively with her, but not to others. She always remained in a special constructed zone, a play area that could be supervised from most rooms in the house. Without the security of this area and ongoing supervision, she would run away. In spite of

> her short stature, she was able to scale fences and block walls with surprising speed; she would also jump out of windows since she could not open doors which were locked. She enjoyed riding in the back seat of the family car. She attempted to grab food from others and would eat until food was taken away from her. When presented with a new situation or taken to a new place, like a doctor's office, she had to be sedated, as she often reacted with wild behavior like kicking, biting, and screaming. A common activity when not at a preferential task that did not challenge her was sitting with her back against the wall, her legs spread like a V and her hands flat on the floor between her legs, rocking rapidly and forcefully back and forth. Her behavior included self-stimulation through rocking, head-banging, grunting, and snorting. She refused to sleep in bed, preferring the floor. She ripped up stuffed furniture and ate the rubber. She was totally unaware of social conventions. She would remove her clothing outdoors whenever given a chance and touch her genitals. When she needed to urinate, no matter where she was, she pulled her pants down and would urinate within 30 seconds. She pinched others when upset and would kick or bite children who invaded her space. She had no interest in animals. She had a ravenous appetite: every time she saw food, she wanted it. She ate rocks, sand, dirt, feces, soap bars, etc. She once took a one-pound container of salt, tipped her head back and put as much as possible into her mouth. She would listen to commands if prompted by a loud "no" from a caretaker. She responded favorably to food rewards. She followed commands and would follow hand signals of "no," "sit," "stand," "come," "wait," etc. When frustrated she usually threw something. She could be affectionate and hold your hand, but then suddenly she would try to give you a head butt and then try to be affectionate again. She was partially deaf. She was very obstinate and she became wicked before her menses. She got a cold every time she had her period and played with the ropy discharge coming from her nose.

Her mother had been on drugs and alcohol while pregnant, and there was mental illness (schizophrenia) in the family; the father's history was unknown as he had abandoned the mother upon hearing about the pregnancy. It is clear that this unfortunate child had been "infected" with the syphilitic miasm. She reacted very well to *Lyssin*, becoming a lot less violent; it was not surprising to see *Hyoscyamus* following *Lyssin*. Remember that *Hyoscyamus* has the Cyber delusion *is going to be sold*. I wondered if that was the state of mind of the birth mother, abandoned by her family and in a frantic, dreadful state, already knowing that she was going to give up the child (going to be sold!) once she was born. The patient improved further on *Hyoscyamus* and was increasingly less violent, to the point where she could go to school (which she had not been allowed to do for a long time). Having the IQ of a two-year-old created a lot more delusions as this patient had few compensations available. It is amazing to see how many symptoms of *Lyssin* appeared in this case: she acted like an untrained puppy, with a minimum of understanding, and exhibited very impulsive, primitive reactions.

Compensations

Excitement Followed by Depression of the Mind

A perfect example of *Lyssinum's* effect on the nerves and spinal cord is seen through an alternation of symptoms: sudden outbursts of *violent destructive anger followed by quick repentance*. In the initial stage, the excitement seems to bring some unexpected benefits: *memory for single words is much improved; makes speeches in his delirium and thinks he is a man of great authority*. Hering states that, in this primary phase, *the mental faculties are in a superior state of excitement, shown by quick perception, amazing acuteness of understanding and rapidity with which they answer questions*. But soon after, a *certain confusion, unsteadiness and weakness of the mind occur and it becomes very difficult to think. School tasks, which before had been a pleasure to her had to be laid aside. The range of ideas is extremely limited and if left to himself, he is occupied with the same thing, bringing frequently forward same ideas within a short time space of time and always in the same manner. Then there is dullness and stupidity*. This kind of pathology became evident in the behavior and causality of the 12-year-old girl discussed earlier.

Impulsiveness and Biting

Given *Lyssin*'s syphilitic nature, we are not surprised to note a loss of control when the patient acts impulsively on insane ideas coming in his mind (here we see the close relationship to *Arg-n*, a phobic and very impulsive remedy). *Insane ideas enter her head; for instance to throw a glass of water, which she carries in her hand, into someone's face, or to stab his flesh with the knife he is holding. There is a strong and uncontrollable impulse to do certain acts, to spring at and bite any moving object that came within reach. She feels impelled to do reckless things such as throwing the child, which she carries in her arms through the window.* Due to its syphilitic characteristics, *Lyssin* starts with reckless and savage behavior: *inclination to be abusive and rude, to bite and strike; inclination to use insulting language, scold his friends, beat and abuse those near him; a kind of savageness in his temper.* These provings reflect a lot of impulsive, violent behavior, almost like a fixed response pattern dictated by *Lyssin*'s delusions.

This abrupt, unexpected, uncontrolled behavior, as if the person is under a sudden spell of mischief, is best exemplified by the biting seen in the previous examples. *Lyssin* is often called the biting remedy; as we will see, this is yet another compensation that the patient may use as a defense mechanism, as seen in the provings: *a strong and uncontrollable impulse to do certain acts, to spring and bite any moving object that came within reach; biting and snapping with convulsions; ordered her husband to go away, as she wanted to bite him, and joining the threat, she bit herself in arm; the child is continually tempted to bite her pillow at night.* *Lyssin* also has a *fear of being bitten.* It is interesting to see what allopathy proposes for biting children, as they have yet to find drugs to curb this behavior. This does not take away from the fact that many people, including teachers who work with such children, have found "solutions." Let's see how valid these solutions are!

I read the following: "My son too was a horrible biter. I read all the experts too who claim that kids bite out of anger, frustration, jealousy, fear and so on. But those explanations did not fit our boy. He bites for no reason at all.[27] He once walked past a child, bit the kid in the forehead and just kept on going. No amount of scolding or timeouts helped. We were told to bite him back, to have his dad lay down the law, to separate him from the group and a host of other punishing remedies. Nothing worked. He even bit the cat. Our pediatrician said, "Bribe him." At our next play date, I told him he could have ice cream if he did not bite anyone. It worked. Within two weeks he had stopped biting altogether."

What is wrong with this approach? This is someone who is introduced to the trade of bribing from a young age on. He knows he will always get his way, and I bet that this young man's syphilitic miasm will simply express itself in another way later on in life. He will remain

27. This really means that this child is very syphilitic in miasmatic terms!

self-indulgent and narcissistic! What will the parents bribe him with when he is 14 and his miasm flares up? A car? No matter what this bribing and biting means, it is putting the syphilitic miasm, which it clearly is, in latency—not dormancy. But it will inevitably turn this "good boy" into the unfeeling, manipulating syphilitic person he really is. He has learned an early lesson: "If I behave the way they want me to, I get what I want! I will pretend to be good until all my desires are fulfilled." How can one think that such an approach can continue to work into adulthood? It reminds me of incarcerated people who feign good behavior to get early release from prison. It is putting the accent on the "ME," inducing selfishness and uncaring behavior. We should remember that we are dealing here with the syphilitic miasm; people in this state can fool you remorselessly!

A teacher (syphilitic no doubt) had a better solution to cure the shark-like behavior of the children in his classroom: he had a bottle of water with vinegar in it on his desk. When a child would bite, he would explain that his or her mouth needed to be cleansed since biting can get dirt in the mouth. They did not like getting their tongues cleaned! So what about outside the classroom? All such "corrective" treatment will do is stir the presence of his syphilitic miasm, and the biting individual will most likely take revenge on some innocent child. And again, what other expression will take its place? The teacher shares no detail about that, and I doubt that a physician or parent would make the connection if the child were to demonstrate some new syphilitic behavior all of a sudden. Other parents take a hot pepper shaker and sprinkle this in the mouth of the biter. Someone else suggested that the biter, each time he bites, needs to bite a bar of soap. Other doctors advise dumping cold water on them. All of these methods are based on the Pavlov reflex, and they represent the best that allopathy can come up with. Biting is a syphilitic expression, but the causalities are of course different for each remedy. That *Lyssin* is not the only biting remedy is seen in our rubrics:

Remedies: Lyssin, Stram, Bell *are the three big biters.*

Biting in children: Bell, Op, Lachesis

Biting during delirium: (Bell, Stram)

Biting objects: Stram

Biting people: Bell, Stram, Op, Phos

We need to add here *Tuberculinum*, especially for biting children who show obstinate behavior and who bite when they are contradicted (*intolerance to contradiction*). Looking at these remedies, they have common issues or NWS: *abandonment* and especially *fright* are intertwined. The feeling of an imminent threat against one generates a need to be ready to defend himself; however, *Lyssin* does not accomplish this by running away, but rather with violence, possible biting, scratching, anything for defense! It is first fight, not flight, with *Lyssin* and the other biters!

Escaping and Restlessness

We already have seen in the delusions that *Lyssin* is seized with a strong feeling of apprehension (*thoughts of something terrible going to happen come into his mind against his will*). The word apprehension comes from the Latin *apprehendere*, meaning seize, gasp, cling to, take hold of, reflecting well the horrible and strong feeling of being held captive by these anticipation anxieties. This leads to a degree of intense restlessness, trying to escape the clutches of these strongholds expressed in the provings: *desperate efforts were made to break the chain; to break out of their stables furiously and run or jump over ditches and fences.* Although these last provings refer to a dog and a sheep respectively, one can see a similar desire to escape and run away in human cases (as seen before in the example of the adult woman with trisomy 21). Other provings describe this desperate restlessness: *driven incessantly about without any definite aim; restlessness driving him hither and thither, although weak enough to lie down; restlessness and anxiety at precordia, frequent change of posture and sighing*). This restlessness is also expressed at night: *she has been unable to sleep a wink for several nights; is driven from bed by indescribable anxiety; can but sit and walk or find momentary peace in prayer.* I also think about the *Lyssin* child who feels caged up in a school environment; he will show similar behavior. This restlessness inevitably leads to a dull mind and inattention: *strange sensation in head, with loss of memory; a certain confusion and weakness of mind; restlessness with great prostration; range of ideas extremely limited, if left to himself is occupied continuously with the same thing.* It is not hard to imagine, reading these provings, that such children would be classified under that ever-expanding umbrella of ADHD, OCD and ASD! On top of it all, the *Lyssin* victim suffers from *headaches while thinking and reading* and *is worse with writing* too (*like Calc-p*, *headaches from studying*)! It is easy to deduce that the person in such a prostrated, anxious, and restless state is very sensitive to *fright which can start convulsions and is susceptible to any outburst of passion or excesses of any kind.* There is also *hypersensitiveness of all senses* or overly acute senses: *when he hears water poured out, or if he hears it run, or he sees it, he becomes very irritable and nervous (hydrophobia); he has an exalted state of smell, taste and touch, with a feeling of anxiety and a fear of being alone.* There is also *hyperesthesia, a current of air, a bright light, a sight of any shining object, the slightest touch, and even a conversation in the vicinity of the patient, may throw him into a most violent agitation and bring on severe convulsions.* And I actually had the following proving in a case in my clinic: *cannot bear to hear others sing, or eat apples.* One can see in all these provings how strong *Lyssin*'s affinity is for the nerves and the spinal cord.

Golden Tips from the Masters

- *Lyssin* is also used for prevention of hydrophobia, in other words, prevention for rabies danger just like *Belladonna* and better than *Stramonium*
- Cannot bear the heat of the sun
- Resembles *Lachesis* in the bluish discoloration of wounds
- Ropy saliva like *Hydrastis*
- *Lyssin* feels forsaken with a sense of isolation and apprehension; *Stram* feels forsaken with a sense of isolation and terror.
- *Very strong craving for salt*!

Magnesia carbonica (Mag-c). Magnesium carbonate

The Cyber Delusion

Mag-carb's Cyber delusion of ***forsaken feeling, feels is not being beloved by his parents, wife and friends*** is reflective of a person born into a household which is simply and starkly inhospitable to him. He experiences coldness and emotional withdrawal all around him. I once had a patient whose mother had bluntly said to him, "I wish you had never been born." Such a person recoils and withdraws from an early age, rolling himself up in a ball, turning away from any eye contact, and retreating deeply into himself, dreaming deliriously of a "perfection" accessible only within himself. At best, such a child strives for perfect self-sufficiency. Often this child is secretly determined to reject intimate contact with the world. He is a stranger in the house of his parents, and his first thoughts were that he was a foundling, an orphan. Indeed, this "loveless" and solitary life has earned *Mag-c* the nickname of the orphan or the Oliver Twist of the materia medica; as Kent stated in his *Lectures on Homeopathic Materia Medica*, *Mag-c* also represents the illegitimate or clandestine child. This is a child who is not asked for his opinion, and who receives very little food, sleep, and attention. In this sense, *Mag-c* is different from related *Rheum*, another sour, greenish diarrhea remedy who *desires impatiently many things, but dislikes its favorite play things*. *Rheum* is the situation of a child who is only a part-time orphan, like latchkey kids who come home to an empty house and then become very demanding when their parents are at home!

So the central idea of *Mag-c*, *the lack of care, protection and nourishment* as a dependent infant or young child, is a different expression of its Cyber delusion. *Mag-carb's* parallel dreams confirm this notion: *dreams being lost in the forest* **and** *dreams being lost at home*. The latter dream brings home the intensity of the fixed idea: the world or the wilderness (forest being the relatively fixed symbol for danger, a place inhabited by ghosts and dangerous animals and the place where mysterious things happen like in fairy tales as well as being lost in the magical world of the unconscious, full of dangers and strange forces) might be a danger not only for *Mag-c*—it is also dangerous to *Mag-mur, Calc-c, Puls,* and *Stram,* but these other characters at least look for (and usually find) protection in the home, the relatively fixed symbol for love, nurturing, and sheltering. But *Mag-c* receives none of the love, nurture, or sheltering, putting him in a difficult and frightful position, so secondary delusions are formed: *delusion, he will be murdered, delusion, sees thieves* and *delusion, he has an incurable disease.* This is a person who continuously struggles to get a foothold in the conscious world before some of his fixed ideas bring him back to the unconscious (*delusions, about water and delusions, of dead people*), drawing him further into additional anxious delusions.

Causalities

Deceived Friendship and Grief

Mag-c suffers something even more fundamental in its nature than deceived friendship, as his isolation is produced by a total absence of emotional nourishment; the child needs to fend for himself from a young age. But what is more natural to a child than longing for a Divine Mother, which gives him certainty, protection, and love? For *Mag-c*, the mother remains a Fata Morgana for the rest of his life. *Mag-c* has not experienced this primary encounter with the mother (because the *mother is dead,* real, or absent) and so this soul mate anima will now appear in his dreams as a fascinating attraction, leaving him forever longing for that which has not yet been realized. Not having experienced the primary encounter with the mother, *Mag-carb's* unconscious can recreate the anima encounter in dreams; the object may appear in a nonhuman form, particularly as a horse, frog, or siren. His longing will drain his emotions and deprive him of his vitality, never allowing him to find peace within himself. Such a man will be seized by inexplicable moods: he may be elated one moment yet in the deepest depression the next, earning him the stigma of manic depressive or Bipolar Disease (BPD); these swings are a common feature of the *Mag-c* personality.

Children can be orphaned, but it is also possible for a child to be an orphan even in the presence of her parents. There are many situations that represent abandonment and grief. For example, children can be caught in middle of a divorce when parents are too busy with their own problems. Especially when the children are still very young—before the age of five, when their egos are still connected to the mother—they might get the impression that they don't belong anywhere or with anybody. This can certainly be the case if the divorcing parents are overwhelmed by their own negative feelings and there is no one else (like grandparents) to extend attention and love! Emotional orphans may grow out of circumstances in which children have to be invisible to escape punishment from cruel, controlling, violent parents. A state of a *Mag-c* can be created intra-utero when the child is unwanted and bonding with the fetus is avoided on purpose. I have seen cases of what can be called an accidental birth, a child coming along long after the others, ignored by older siblings and parents who are too exhausted for him and show resentment to this "intruder" in their lives. The child, for whatever "practical" reason, may be sent to a boarding school where now he feels abandoned by everyone, family included. I had a patient in Australia who had grown up on a farm with many animals and then, at age 11, was sent to a boarding school in a big town far away from home. He cried all year long. In this case *ailments from fright* play also a role: the new environment can seem threatening for a "nature" boy thrown into the vast wilderness of civilization, with all the noise and cacophony. I also think of a person who has only one good friend (usually *Calc-c* or *Nat-m*) and now is deprived of that sole source of emotional nourishment.

Compensations

Looking for a Safe Place

Support, especially from family, does not seem forthcoming. What to do? *Mag-c* is full of anxiety, even anguish, which will be only relieved when going to bed—the relatively fixed symbol, in dreams, of refuge, sex, and the place of origin, where the creation of the infant takes place: *anguish, ameliorates after going to bed; tremulous anxiety and fright, as if she apprehended some misfortune, disappearing in the evening in bed; very anxious, with perspiration, all day long, especially on moving about.* But even bed is not always a place free of anxiety: *for several nights was unable to fall asleep for a long time on account of anxiety; anxiety in warm bed, yet limbs cold if uncovered.* Mag-c is anxious all the time; he may say, "My brain is going all the time, I am constantly thinking, my thoughts jump from one thing to the next" (*Coffea*). He constantly thinks about going home (if he is at school or work), trying to find all kinds of excuses to go home (*homesickness*—in extended meaning, longing for a real home that gives protection) in order to get into that one safe place: bed.

This anxiety obviously comes from the fact that *Mag-c* is unprotected in a dangerous world: *delusion, he will be murdered; he is frightened easily* and he feels weak and sick (*delusion, he has an incurable disease*). In both of these delusions, we find the general fear of the *Carbon* person for physical harm and illness. His fears are very specific: *fears for accidents all day long and relieved when going to bed; fear for misfortune,* and *fear something will happen.* Of course he fears all this: he realizes he is on his own. He must be a practical survivor, and he walks around on eggshells; this always creates very *irritable children.*

Repressing Emotions

How does one survive perceived chaos and danger around him? By repressing his emotions—they are only a hindrance to actions or the thinking conscious function! His feeling part is secondary to the dominating thinking part, and feeling must remain totally in the background for him to remain protected. This is the extreme form of the imbalance between thinking and feeling: emotions are not even felt. *Mag-c* has to be practical in order to survive; he has to think clearly, so there is not much place for feelings. His feelings are his Achilles tendon, so suppressing them is also self-protection against the demons in his closet: releasing them would only lead to *great irritability* and *violent anger.* Neglecting and suppressing his feelings is a positive compensation for him as it helps him to deal with his Cyber delusion in order to survive. The adult and even child *Mag-c* discusses her case in a matter-of-fact manner. She is serious, *reserved,* and surprisingly unemotional when telling her homeopath her life story.

Being Proactive

A negative trait of *Mag-c* is his resemblance to a caged animal with a fiery impulsivity towards the slightest impression or stimulus. Being proactive is the best defense in a dangerous and unpredictable world. This is a defense mechanism for someone who needs to be on high alert. Unfortunately, because of *Mag-carb's* Cyber delusion, this impulsivity (loss of control) is released from his unconscious and comes crashing into his conscious life. But *Mag-c* cannot control or explain these reactions! He has sensitive antennae; they feel situations out and warn him of the slightest danger. He is driven by the unknown (calamities, feelings), so psychotherapy is often as useless as offering a tissue to cure viral pneumonia, and it requires much more skill (and, often, dream analysis) to find the key to *Mag-carb's* proactive behavior. No matter what his coping skills are, there are no sunny moments in *Mag-carb*'s life. No kind words from others, no personal accomplishments to boost his sense of self-worth, no superior goals to achieve through dedication and hard work, no exceptional command of language to attract others, no religion to support him. He is like a wounded animal (*chaotic confused behavior*) that needs all his energy and attention to cope with just about any ordinary circumstances, just to survive! That's why *Mag-c* is tough when he gets hurt: he knows he can only count on himself. And we should not be surprised that one of his chief complaints is chronic fatigue (*nervous worn-out,* except *industriousness before menses,* just like *Sepia*)! This worn-out state leads to isolation with *sadness and indisposition to talk; she is much <from talking and aversion to presence of others.* One can see that confusion with *Sepia* in the exhausted state can occur. Even *dipsomania* (to further dull his feelings) *and kleptomania are possible.* Worse, *Mag-c* is always on the defensive and shows it through very negative behavior: these are the *most irritable children, vexed, ill-humored, everything frets her; everything is disagreeable; everything that she looks at vexes her. She is so fretful that she does not know what she shall undertake. And she becomes completely out of sorts, which is increasing as time goes on.* Can you imagine such a schoolchild, such an adopted child, whom the caring teacher or the devoted adoptive mother wants to shower with love? All the caregiver gets is violent anger, changeable behavior, and irritability, which makes other people tiptoe around *Mag-c* on eggshells. Even the most resilient person often gives up, and this takes us back to the Cyber delusion, which is now once again confirmed in *Mag-carb*'s mind: *he is not loved by anyone*!

Dreams

We already have seen that *Mag-c* seeks refuge in the unconscious (bed) to escape the violent conscious world. His dreams reflect this; he dreams mainly *about water and floods,* the relatively fixed symbol of a subconscious in turmoil. In view of the intensity of his feelings in conscious life, parallel dreams keep torturing him, giving him no peace even in his sleep: *dreams he is lost in the forest and at home* (= orphan) and *dreams of going astray.* Of course, these are what Mag-c children would refer to as nightmares, but unfortunately they often forget the finer aspects of the dream. Besides parallel dreams, *Mag-c* can also have dreams which follow the principle of compensation: the more one-sided the conscious attitude and the more it deviates from recognizing the optimal possibilities of life, the greater the possibility that vivid dreams with a strong contrasting content will appear as an expression of the self-regulation of the psyche, establishing a psychological balance. For this reason, *pleasant, peaceful and quiet dreams* belong to *Mag-c* also.

Golden Tips from the Masters

- *Mag-c* is the Oliver Twist of the materia medica, the great "unloved" one, anxious, silent, insecure, thin, and unattractive. He longs for affection which he doesn't get
- *Mag-c* is to exhausted nerves what *China* is to loss of fluids
- The whole body gives off a sour smell (*Hep-s*)
- *Mag-c* is the chronic of *Chamomilla* and has its capriciousness
- Lax muscles, lack of tone
- Unrefreshing sleep, waking up around 2:30 a.m. feeling more tired than when they went to bed
- Sensitive to the least touch, like teeth touched by the tongue
- All secretions are sour (*Rheum*)
- Cravings for meat in children
- Green diarrhea, frothy like a frog pond or like chopped spinach
- Colicky babies who don't thrive because the milk passes undigested (< milk)
- Teething remedy and delayed dentition; canker sores appear when teething
- Main remedy for acute **left-**sided trigeminus neuralgia (*Mag-p* right-sided)
- Acute remedy for foot and leg cramps: *Calc-c* (chronic), *Cuprum* (acute in toes) and *Mag-c* (acute) take care of 90% of foot and leg cramps
- Coryza before every menstrual cycle

Medorrhinum (Med). Gonorrhea Nosode

The Cyber Delusion

Medorrhinum's Cyber delusion is ***someone walks behind him***. This fixed idea contrasts with the delusion *someone walks besides him.* In order to understand the meaning of *Medorrhinum's* CD, we need to look at his other delusions, but also at the remedies belonging to both rubrics. Let's start by looking at *Medorrhinum's* other delusions.

That someone is behind him is also indicated by the *delusion, his head is caressed on by someone; the delusion, he was pursued,* and the fixed idea that *someone is whispering him anything* and *he hears voices.* That these fixed ideas are not as benevolent as they might seem at first is evidenced by the confusion they create in the person to the point that he has the *delusion, he will become insane* and *everything seems unreal with exaggeration of time, passes too slowly.* Hering expresses these emotions also in the following ways: *sensation as if life was unreal, like a dream* and *she felt she must do something to rid her mind of this torture.* In *Medorrhinum*, all these delusions are sufficiently strong that they create a level of confusion leading to neurosis; there is a danger of progressing to psychosis if the tension lasts too long or if an additional trigger moves him closer to the danger line of dissociation. At this point, *Med* still has control over his ego, so he understands that his mind is overwhelmed with strange things and that, as a result, he is swinging from one emotion to another, from one extreme of the pendulum to the other. This excessive sycotic reaction creates instability in the person, and it never takes much for him to reach a breaking point expressed by a syphilitic compensation.

To get more information regarding the intentions of the person walking behind him, we examine *Med's* companions in the same rubric in our materia medica. We have in this rubric remedies like *Anacardium, Lachesis, Magnesium muriaticum, Silica,* and *Staphysagria.* All of these characters, except perhaps for *Silica,* who can be a terror at home, are under the influence of someone powerful, even to the point of being dominated and leading to a split personality like *Lachesis* and *Anacardium* (*two wills*). Even *Silica* seems to be a split personality, an angel at school and a devil at home. *Mag-m* and *Lachesis* are also in the rubric *orphans*. *Anacardium* and *Staphysagria* are dominated and violated by a sinister person in their life. *Med* is in ominous company with *Anac* and *Staph*, which indicates that the person walking behind him is not doing so in a benign manner; at the very least, his trailer evokes a paranoid and suspicious reaction (*suspicion, mistrustful*) in *Medorrhinum*, causing him to constantly look over his shoulder for any possible harm or danger (*thinks someone is behind her; hears whispering; sees faces that peer at her from behind bed and furniture*). Here we see even more clearly the contrast between *Medorrhinum*'s *someone walks **behind** him* and the rubric *someone is walking **besides** him*, in which we see remedies such as *Calcarea*, *Silica*, *Thuja*, and *Petroleum*. These four remedies all need someone to support them, either because they are fearful of dangers in the world (*Calc*), timid when appearing in public (*Silicea*), forgetful, lost, and confused (*Petroleum*), or convinced of their own exaggerated vulnerability (*body is made of glass*, *Thuja*). These characters are all in a somewhat symbiotic and dependent, welcoming relationship with someone benevolent. Having looked at all these delusions and rubrics, we now understand that *Medorrhinum* does not view people behind her as friends; rather, they are persons who arouse suspicion, or at least ruffle his feathers, creating instability in his daily emotions!

Causalities

Anticipation Anxiety

Anticipation anxiety can take numerous forms, but he who suffers from it (like *Medorrhinum*) is always dealing with events or situations that are not quite known to him. Unsure of himself and saddled with an *impulsive* makeup, he cannot call upon a strongly built ego to confidently look at and deal with the vicissitudes of life. *Anticipation from engagement* is especially present, be the engagement a job, an interview, a musical performance, an examination, or a visit to parents-in-law. What is the reason? It is precisely his **dual** nature: at any time of the day, *Medorrhinum* can be at two opposite ends of the spectrum, whether compassionate and empathetic, or vicious, malicious, and hurting people and animals. He has no control over who shows up, so he is at the mercy of his conflicting emotions. In good moments, he certainly can feel guilty and remorseful (*anxiety of conscience as if guilty of a crime*), but when the dark side shows up, he can also exhibit *cruelty and inhumanity*. *Medorrhinum* never finds a balance and is subjected to an inner force that overshoots a healthy center. How can such a person ever approach social situations confidently? (It must be said, though, that *Medorrhinum* is usually unaware of this abnormality and thinks everyone is just like him.)

The anticipation anxiety is especially visible when *Medorrhinum* is walking, as he is very afraid that someone is following him, that someone will harm him (*fear, someone is behind him*), especially *in the dark*, so he starts walking faster and faster as if an uncontrollable inner force is at work, looking behind him to see if someone is there. Even if no one is, the fixed idea does not disappear. There is also *anxiety when time is set*, when he has an appointment or needs to take a train, airplane, or bus: a feeling of unrest takes over, forcing him to feel nervous and unsettled. Often there is *a constant state of anguish, always a feeling of impending danger and evil, but knows not what*. In view of his changeable and unstable behavior, it is not surprising to see that *Medorrhinum* has a great *fear for misfortune*. Of course, *Medorrhinum* is the last one to take the blame for it (*lack of responsibility*), although he can torment himself by reflecting on the ways that he could have avoided these misfortunes (*thinking of complaints aggravate*).

Compensations

Libertinism or Debauched Lifestyle: "Seize the day!"

I refer to *Medorrhinum* as being mainly a male person because numerous studies show that women are generally far less interested in casual sex and relationships than men are. It is *Medorrhinum* who will write the *Casanova Field Guide* or "How to Sweep Women Off Their Feet and then Drop Them Fast." *Medorrhinum* is a person who welcomes the rapture of losing himself in irrationality, in pure emotion, in the drunkenness of passion and the abandonment of the ego sense. Thinking he is God's gift to women, he wants to be "made mad with [so-called] love" and has no apparent need for knowledge or reason. Drinking alcohol with abandon, experiencing fleeting infatuations with as many women as possible, abstaining from sleep, and, above all, staying "on the move (*unusually active, going as if on wings*)," *Medorrhinum* resembles a person in a permanent state of *mania*. It takes gregariousness, a lack of inhibition, a desire for unrestrained liberty, impulsiveness and absence of deliberation, a highly developed sensibility to beauty and refinement and an appreciation for fine things to produce such a lively personality (*strange exhilaration of spirits*). A modus operandi for novelty and earthly pleasures makes him an outgoing risk-taker, a modern satyr (*libertinism*).He has a sweet tooth for every woman and indulges freely in his vice (*idea of marriage seemed unendurable*). In his eyes, every gorgeous woman is equally devoted to having sex, cooking and washing his car! The less he knows about a woman, the more alluring she is at first and the more driven *Medorrhinum* is to interact with her. Other people have to provide his pleasure, but a bond based on such intemperate self-satisfaction, unfortunately, is as volatile as the emotions that underlie it and as hollow and fragile as the hedonic sense of happiness it causes. *Med* thinks of himself as a James Bond, knocking out the bad guys (his competition in sexual conquests), jumping in his Aston Martin (always on the move, impossible to be caught as he is an extraverted dervish with an exhausting aversion to downtime), staying at the Ritz (luxury), and having beautiful women throwing themselves into his arms (thinking about sex every five minutes). Of course the other side of the coin, besides driving around Monte Carlo in his snazzy sports car, is that he will have to deal with the health consequences of all that drinking, smoking, carousing and insatiable casual sex—but that confrontation is for later and does not stop him now from seizing the day! Only later will he find out that his inner vacuity, this craze for society, diversion, amusement, and luxury of every kind leads to misery. Too late in life, if ever, *Medorrhinum* finds out that the early bird gets the worm, instead of "*Medorrhinum* always gets the worm." And maybe, just maybe, he who considered himself a free spirit, when the light shines on him and exposes him, will realize that he has, in fact, been an irresponsible person in every facet of life (*lack of responsibility*). He is an escape artist, forever slipping out of the responsibilities he resents having to fulfill. But without the dissolution of this strong sycotic inheritance, he may remain a highly *impulsive* person, steeped in his daydreams of irrational scenarios where obligations disappear into thin air (*desire to procrastinate*); just like the flighty Scarlett O'Hara, he will use her favorite line: "I'll think about that tomorrow (*postponing everything to the next day*)."

Because of his inner emptiness of soul, *Medorrhinum* is a person who confuses excitement with joy and thrill with love of life. He is without joy in the midst of abundance. He is poor in spite of all kinds of gadgets because he *has* much but *is* little. As if taken up by a tornado, *carpe diem* is his daily motto. In his turbulent, undisciplined life, he goes from one person to another, from one event to another, and always seeks the thrill in everybody and everything. He really thinks that life is 90% fun and 10% responsibility (*aversion to responsibility; libertinism*), the opposite of what life really is. He never does anything to find meaning in his life or to direct his life toward a worthwhile goal. There is no more mistaken path to real happiness than this kind of high living, for *Medorrhinum's* whole object is to transform his secretly miserable existence into a succession of delights, pleasures, and amusement of every kind: a process which can only result in excess and debauchery, disappointment and further delusions. This is a person who always feels a tremendous sense of vigor; he is willing to take unbelievable risks, in everything from drag racing and hitchhiking in dangerous places to ingesting unsafe street drugs. *Medorrhinum* resembles Icarus, son of the architect of Crete who was imprisoned with his father in the labyrinth he had designed. Carefully collecting feathers from birds, Icarus used candle wax to fashion wings and escaped; but, deluded and overcome with this wonderful sense of power, he ignored all common sense as he soared delightedly up and up—where the sun melted the wax, resulting in his death. Playing with fire is indeed part of *Medorrhinum's* makeup. Such warning dreams of flying and falling are not uncommon to this type.

Medorrhinum is gonorrhea. It is a product connected with sexual instinct and drive (sex, drugs, and rock and roll!). Who gets gonorrhea? Usually not someone who is moderate in his sexual activity, but someone who is immoderate and driven by his sexual desire to such a degree that he is not afraid of catching a venereal disease. Reckless sexual behavior is part of his excessive thrill-seeking behavior. But the danger is half of the excitement and he often feels like a snake-charmer must feel when he lures the cobra from the reed basket that holds it. *Medorrhinum's* sexual desire is so pliable that it is aroused and mobilized by any kind of uncontrolled desire—lust, conquering, possessing, power, narcissism, feeling invincible and irresistible, and many more—everything, in fact, except love! *Medorrhinum* shows remarkable unconsciousness in his behavior. He is the lover who is motivated only by his need to conquer and to satisfy erotic appetites while failing to see human dignity in, and to accord individuality to, the object of his desires. For *Medorrhinum*, the world carries a permanent banner which reads: "Welcome to the Meet Market." He is the hunter who is hooked on the hunt and, armed with irresistible charm and charisma, only thinks about conquests; he leaves each conquest days later after breaking hearts and wrecking marriages. He proclaims to each new conquest, "You are the love of my life." What this innocent swept-away woman does not know is that *Medorrhinum* has more lives than a cat. So his love life is compartmental and short-living, and there is plenty of place for many new "loves of his life." *Medorrhinum's* neediness stems from falling in love at first sight as he agonizes more over how to get a woman than how to **keep** her. And for those women he leaves, being a "bad boy" and not being too available makes him even more desirable and mysterious! He enjoys "a meaningful overnight relationship" or a one-night pass that can be renewed indefinitely and at will; his weapons are high self-regard and a sense of attractiveness and entitlement. His victims croon for wit, curiosity, excitement, and passion, and *Medorrhinum* knows he can deliver all of it as he has honed his behavior over the years to aid and abet a reproductive payoff. To woo the desired woman, *Medorrhinum* will grossly exaggerate his income, his status (heir to such and so, inventor to this or that, physician at a prestigious institute), commitment ("you are the one"), and affection for cuddly creatures ("I would love to have a dog together," avoiding the topic of kids), always a plus point for the momentarily stunned sucker. A warm glance from this charmer seizes everyone within range; when *he* is attracted to someone, his whole body switches on. It is like hearing the first bars of his favorite song. Alas, his billboard of top hits is endless! Once the goal (the overnight relationship) is attained, his interest evaporates for lack of true love, and then it will be someone else's turn! Women should be warned that if the physical aspect of the relationship overwhelms the bulk of your time together, you are at risk of being with someone who won't be good for you in the long run. Indeed, *Medorrhinum's* instinctual, most often unconscious attitude is "*love* her and *leave* her"—in other words, he takes flight after he gets what he wants, discounting his victim as a true person. The lack of appreciation of the other as a separate and distinct person with different needs prevents genuine relatedness.

Medorrhinum's subjects of love are at first mesmerized by his extraverted, charming mesmerizing behavior and his carloads of seductive tricks: "He immediately gave me his home number, he asked about my family, he mentioned children in the future and the desire to settle down and he alluded to a concert next week. It is clear that he is really into me." It is as though she has struck romantic gold! With *Medorrhinum*, though, a relationship is doomed beyond all repair when the "tear-your-clothes-off" period of sexual and emotional excitement ends. For him, there is no greater ecstasy than that of getting the woman in bed. It is like unwrapping a present. The real and only thrill is to see how fast he can get to this point. If he gets the feeling that she isn't likely to go home with him on the first date, he will often cut the date short to save time and money. Time lost is time for *Medorrhinum* when he has not lived a life full of thrills, sexual enjoyment, riches and abandon to all the fun the world has to offer. Unfortunately, time is not the Corrector where his judgment errs! With his roving eye he scans women on parties, family gatherings, and business retreats; then he scores and moves on. *Medorrhinum* is utterly blind to what he is doing, which is anything but advantageous to himself and his victims. Sex is never a vehicle of love for *Medorrhinum;* on the contrary, his sex act in Traditional Chinese Medicine (TCM) would be called "masturbation on someone else." We are dealing here with a person whose sexual desires are strong and uncontrolled. *Medorrhinum* is the prototype of a man with poor impulse control, and he is overwhelmingly represented in diagnoses of *impulse control disorders*—predilections that lead to alcohol and drug abuse, sexual excesses, sudden and unexpected violent outbursts, and problems holding a job. *Medorrhinum* is ruled by his emotions: there is passion and infatuation in abundance. "I give everything in my relationships," he says, seduced by the power of his own words. He is a smooth and fast talker, generating a symphonic burst of desire in his victims. But upon closer examination, the passion has less to do with the partner than with simple satisfaction of his deep sexual drive and desire for conquest—Atilla the Hun on the move! *Medorrhinum* is not concerned about his partner, only about the fulfillment of his passion. The attention he showers on his partner is, again, a means of getting what he wants, an expression of malignant narcissism: to satisfy himself. At parties, he is sizing up women with only sex in his mind, showering them with a lot of attention and compliments (*thoughts, sexual thoughts at every woman he sees,* only *Medorrhinum!*). He actually wants more than just sex (*Lyc*); he wants a passionate relationship more than anything else, to the point where his feelings overwhelm him (*cannot speak without crying*). Of course, the burning fire never lasts for long. And *Medorrhinum,* in the quest for the next passionate encounter, is never willing or prepared to stay around long enough to experience the full range of feelings that makes us human.

While this debauched lifestyle can be part of the hard, unfeeling *Medorrhinum* type, who is just a selfish conqueror of women, there is also the opposite type: the extremely sensitive *Medorrhinum* type whose desire for sex is equally intense, and whose flame of passion burns just as hot, but in whom sex finds a different expression. This rather timid, non-aggressive, and sensitive type has a tendency to homosexuality. Such men are endowed with much anima (inflation of the anima) or have feeling as a predominant conscious function, so they love nature, flowers, and animals (*animals, love for; love for her pet in children*), the contrary of the macho, unfeeling, and cruel *Medorrhinum* type.

Swinging from Exhilaration to Depression

Medorrhinum is a person with unstable vitality (cyclothymiacs) and periodic drops in mood and energy. The mood alternations are easily seen in his emotional makeup. At one moment he is extraverted, lively, charming, charismatic, and seductive, the life of the party (*strange exhilaration of spirits*). He looks like the kind of man that parents would be pleased for their daughter to bring home. But then, unexpectedly, he can transform into the opposite persona, into a character that is very gloomy and depressed, and on the brink of committing suicide (*alternation of happiness and gloominess*): *spirits in the depths, weighted down with heavy, solid gloom by torrents of tears. She wakes at an early hour with a frightened sensation, as if something dreadful had happened* (*fear of misfortune, and fear on waking*); *could not rest in bed; felt as if she must do something to rid her mind of this torture. He has a tendency to suicide, gets up at night and takes his pistol but his wife prevents him* (*suicidal from sadness; and by shooting*). He is like Dr. Jekyll and Mr. Hyde! He is obviously not the easiest person to live with, and certainly for the homeopath he is a client who (just like *Nitric acid*) can be impossible to please: *he cannot see any improvement, even when it is pointed out*!

Inner Restlessness

Drastically swinging from one extreme to the other, with mental and emotional symptoms, is not a sign of stability or inner peace. *He is always in a great hurry; when doing something is in such hurry that he gets fatigued. He is hurried always, but accomplishes nothing. There is a constant state of anguish and an always feeling of impending doom but knows not what. A wild and desperate feeling, as of incipient insanity. There is impatience, excitement and wild feeling* (*wild feeling in the head*). Of course this restless mind leads to the typical confusion we see in a *Medorrhinum* person. *We find a dazed condition from the loss of the thread of thought which annoys and causes a dread of saying the wrong thing, and a difficulty in stating symptoms. He forgets entirely what he has read, even the previous line. He cannot remember names* (*memory, weakness for proper names, and cannot spell right; he wonders how the word "how" is spelled. He loses constantly the thread of his talk.* Medorrhinum starts a sentence automatically, but then he starts thinking about other things and must pause, realizing that he has lost his train of thought (*memory, weakness for what he was about to say; vanishing of thoughts, while speaking,* Thuja also). He is also a great *biter of fingers; he bites his nails till they bleed,* and the *Med* child *desires to play at night*. The reason for this changeability? Even though Casanova types like *Medorrhinum* seem the life of the party, they are very insecure about their lovability.

Medorrhinum learns very late, and sometimes never, that warmth and support from a fellow human easily prevail over the titillation of the hunt.

Narcissism

There is no better myth to describe the persona and shadow of *Medorrhinum* than the one of Narcissus and Ameinius. Just substitute Narcissus with *Medorrhinum*. Renowned for his beauty and charisma, Narcissus was the object of affection and admiration of all who saw him. His disinterest and selfishness often led to the ultimate destruction of his admirers, most notably Ameinius. In his desire for Ameinius to prove his love, Narcissus sent him a sword upon which he was meant to fall. (In our times these are the women who kill for their *Medorrhinum* paramours, as seen in the TV series *Wicked Women*.) Before taking his own life for the love of Narcissus, Ameinius asked the gods to punish his vain paramour. Upon seeing his reflection in the water of a spring (the real person behind the mask), the cursed Narcissus fell in love with his own image. Although he tried to touch his reflection, possession was impossible. After he realized that he was the image in the spring, Narcissus took his own life, dying with the agony of unrequited love experienced by those who had loved him.

The charm of a *Medorrhinum* person is that he is charismatic, entertaining, and exciting; he is also assertive and manipulative: the prototype of the irresistible "bad boy," which makes him quite attractive and compelling to many women in the real world. The appeal of this bad boy is so great that sparks fly on first encounters; even the most intelligent women fall under his spell. In homeopathic language we call it, "intelligent but naïve" (*Nat-m)* as indeed attraction can make enemies of the brain and the heart! Like the peacock's tail, excitement and cockiness coupled with a certain swagger and stride are irresistible to the opposite sex. The rock stars and the dudes with the smoldering eyes at the bar make women weak in the knees, signaling to them, "Here is your alpha male!" *Medorrhinum* is a compulsively fun-loving rogue, in love with his own social power. Of course there is nothing reasonable or objective about a *Medorrhinum*. Usually *Medorrhinum* possesses high self-esteem, self-focus, and self-importance (*egotism, self-esteem*). He likes his own body, his eloquence, and there is nothing about him that brings him even the slightest dissatisfaction. The only things that are real and important are those directly affecting him, just today and not tomorrow! Whatever is going on in the outside world is without importance and hardly exists at all (*great selfishness*).

Having good self-confidence and being an extraverted is one thing, but with *Medorrhinum* we have a game of vanity, entitlement, and exploitation on display. *Medorrhinum* dazzles and seduces others without suffering the consequences of a bad reputation. At first glance, *Medorrhinum* is irresistible: well dressed and well groomed, full of humor and exuberance, and often more sculpted than the average person, he stands out in a crowd. Just like *Sulphur*, he likes the sound of his own voice and does not hesitate to use highly charged sexual talk. Promiscuity is a key strategy for *Medorrhinum* to maintain control and reign in the dating world. For a woman, indeed it is attractive to see all the apparent options Mr. *Medorrhinum* has, and yet (for the moment as long as it lasts, four months being the maximum) she feels he continues to choose her, which is mesmerizing to this naïve victim. Days after meeting her, he sends flowers to her office; the unsuspecting, overwhelmed victim, relishes the surprise deliveries and the admiring notice of colleagues. *Medorrhinum* is not a psychopath; he is more of a fun-loving individual, a gentle star with "charismatic airs" and a widespread social network, a vast source to tap for further conquests. *Medorrhinum* is more appealing than appalling. Having a "bad reputation" is not a setback for him: as long as there are still many women out there who think he is irresistible and beautiful, he does not mind being called a jerk by those he has left hurt and baffled. But tell him that he is forgettable, and he is crushed (*despair after light critique*). Even women who are caretakers and/or have set out on a mission to alter his negative traits (*Nat-m* comes to mind) are no match for the restless *Medorrhinum*. *Medorrhinum* likes drama, but not that kind of drama!

Religious Fanaticism

It is not uncommon that, as *Medorrhinum* gets older and finally settles down (if this is at all possible) that he looks at his excessive and extreme youth filled with alcohol and drug abuse and feels guilt (*anxiety as if guilty of a crime*). (This holds true only for some, not all!) These guilty feelings can lead to a religious fanaticism (*religious affections*)—and in the extreme, *because of his restless, uneasy and unbalanced nerves*: *he has feeling as if he had committed the unpardonable sin and was going to hell.* We also find some *Medorrhinum* types who exhibit their instability through this paradoxical connection with religion. All too often, U.S. history has shown charismatic and passionate preachers who visited prostitutes at night. Their magnetism can be so strong that they are able to "cure" people in front of their followers—because their religious power sometimes creates a miracle amidst the frenzy of religious fervor.

A typical *Medorrhinum* case:

At the time of consultation, a 50-year-old man presents with the following:

- Poor sleep: going to bed at 11 p.m. and then tossing and turning due to sinus congestion (nostrils blocked)
- Delays going to bed because it is unpleasant: he wakes throughout the night with the feeling that people are in his room and touching his head. He feels that this is due to doing a lot of traveling; he used to barricade the door when traveling and staying in hotels. Now it is just the thought that "someone in his room is caressing his head." Med has A/F *anticipation and foreboding, delusion, sees faces, and head is caressed on by someone, and seeing people. Woke up with a frightening sensation as if something dreadful had happened, could not rest in bed, feeling of impending danger* (H.C. Allen)
- Right ring finger (interesting observation in regards to being married) very sore, rheumatic, can't bend without pain. All symptoms are right-sided
- Diarrhea, hemorrhoids, and polyp in rectum. Since undergoing earlier hemorrhoid surgery he has had sharp attacks of diarrhea. Stools are always urgent, watery, and debilitating
- Hypertension for years, not improved with meds
- Right shoulder pains and lower back pains (rheumatism)
- Frequent nosebleeds for the past two years

First dose: *Medorrhinum* 30C, ½ tsp from 4 oz up.

Result: Sleeping really well. No more nosebleeds. No more attacks of diarrhea. No more shoulder pain. BP now always normal! Return of old symptoms (itchy palms of hands with scratching, psora instead of sycosis). Polyps feel smaller, no bleeding with hemorrhoids. Back pain is gone. No new symptoms.

Golden Tips from the Masters

- *Medorrhinum* is either cruel to animals (*kicks animals*) and hunts them or shows a pathological attachment to animals.
- Children are often hyperactive, violent, with frequent temper tantrums and allergies
- Amelioration from discharges and at the seaside and from lying on the stomach
- Strong craving for citrus, oranges, sour green apples, and fats, with aversion to eggplant; cravings often present during pregnancy, the hallmark of sycosis!
- There is a fear of losing control like that of *Calcarea*
- Keynote: rocks the head from side to side
- Marked tenderness of soles and heels, can't stand tickling, and hot soles, sticking them out from under the blanket (*Sulph, Puls, Calc-p, Carc*)
- Chronic rheumatism ameliorated by humid weather and alternating pain, going from left to right to left (*Lac-can*) and with a history of gonorrhea (*extremities, pain rheumatic, gonorrhea, after suppressed*)
- Great remedy for chronic recurring sinusitis, especially if *Hydrastis* and *Kali-bich* do not hold
- Great remedy for obstinate vaginitis and dead *fish like odor* of discharge (leucorrhea). First give 200C *Medorrhinum* followed by *Thuja* 30C (5th edition).
- Great remedy for pelvic inflammatory disease (PID), prostatic infections and endometriosis
- Great remedy for genital herpes if sexually active; *Nat-m* if the etiology is grief
- #1 remedy for Reiter syndrome (arthritis, conjunctivitis, and urethritis)
- Good remedy for cases of AIDS
- For rhinitis from birth on with green discharge (typical sycotic discharge)
- One of the best asthma remedies in children, typically with relief from lying on knees and elbows and marked amelioration at the seaside. <2 a.m.
- Think of *Medorrhinum* when there is only swelling of the ankles, regardless of the etiology (R.A., heart disease)
- Condylomata around the anus
- Unruly eyebrows and too-wiry hair suggest *Medorrhinum*
- Great indication for left-sided sciatica (Burnett). Burnett stated that his own prepared version, which he called *Glinicum*, "wiped out half of the sciatica cases that came [his] way."
- Most useful remedy in vomiting during pregnancy (C.M. Boger)

- Cures many cases of severe asthma, the results of suppressed gonorrhea (Kent)
- Thick, long hair on the extremities, from the elbows and knees down (hirsutism)
- For intractable cases of rheumatism (*Syphilinum* too)
- Has clairvoyance for misfortune: gets the feeling something will happen; anticipates and feels matters before they occur, and many times correctly
- Breasts cold, especially the nipples, the rest of the body is warm
- Mental symptoms worse at night (Kent)

Mercurius solubilis (Merc). Mercury. Quicksilver

The Cyber Delusion

Mercury has the Cyber delusion ***that he is surrounded by enemies, everyone is an enemy***. Or, as Hering states, ***there is constant suspicion; he considers everybody his enemy***. *Mercury* is convinced of the ancient Roman saying *Homo homini lupus est*, or "Man is wolf to man." There is a great degree of suspicion and paranoia in this individual, as we see in the provings: *morose and mistrustful, treated his associates almost insultingly; looked upon everyone as his worst enemy*. "Everyone hates me! Everyone wishes me ill and wishes I were dead! Everyone is out to get me one way or the other, even my friends (*delusion, he is about to receive an injury*)!"

There are many *Mercurius* despots that come to mind. Stalin is one example, and history is filled with others: Hitler, Caligula, Julius Caesar, Napoleon, Ivan the Terrible and others who have obtained absolute power in their lives and whose reign was characterized by mass torturing, unprovoked violence and towering inhumanity. In reading about Stalin, I have always been struck by the description of the immense suspicion that he fostered, even towards his closest and most cruel collaborators, to the point that almost none of them escaped eventual death at his hands (*kill, desire to kill beloved ones*) after being arrested on trumped-up charges by Stalin himself, who viewed himself as a god (*dictatorial, despotic*) sitting in ultimate judgment as to who should live or die, who should eat or starve—a god limited only by illness, age, and eventually death, although as long as his collaborators were not sure of his death, even when he was exhaling his last breath, they did not dare to utter a bad word about him, so strong was their fear of him. It is not at all uncommon for such despots to project the contents of their own shadow or dark side on others, as this is by far the easiest way of avoiding dealing with their own demons. Stalin was fond of saying, "It is your fault entirely; you should have changed; you should have been a better party member and a pure ideologist. I, Stalin, being the anointed judge, must therefore punish you." The underlying message is: "Unless you agree with me and go along, you'll regret it" (*malicious; intolerant of contradiction.*). If he does not have enough enemies, *Mercury* produces them so he can justify his actions propagated by his CD: everyone is an enemy! Intimidation is *Mercury's* natural behavior, and he displays unpredictable acts that are random and seemingly out of the blue. The dictator *Mercury* keeps his subordinates guessing and scared (*mood, alternating; want of moral feeling; disposition to become a criminal without remorse*)! Such erratic behavior is a powerful weapon because it defies accurate prediction; flying into a rage or staring someone down and dismissing him summarily (a favorite tactic of Stalin) are common strategies to create an atmosphere of terror. *Mercury's* meanest motive (control to gain absolute power, *dictatorial*), his lowest appetite (*sexual excesses; love for sexual perversity*), and his most common passion (*anger from contradiction; anger so he could have stabbed someone*) become to him laws by which the lives of others are to be guided, and to which, if necessary (out of paranoia), they are simply to be sacrificed. Stalin was the Mercury prototype!

The more the *Mercury* person tries to be a god, the more he isolates himself from the human race: Stalin, feeling lonely and bored (*company, desire for, while alone aggravates; ennui, tedium*), pleaded (read: "ordered") with some close friends to visit him at his dacha at odd hours of the night, but many of them were so scared that they found any excuse not to be thrown into his orgies or long nights of boozing, drinking, and womanizing (*gluttony*). There was no limit to the lust and ruthlessness of this powerful dictator and narcissist; it bordered on madness. Of course, many tried to kill or overthrow him: this CD, expressing a pathological degree of suspicion (*delusion, he is about to receive an injury*), is generally based on a nucleus of reality and prevents *Mercury*, as was the case with Stalin, from descending into the hell of full psychosis or true madness, although a few under pressure might dissociate in any case (*delusion, she will become insane*).

Deep down, the *Mercury* person is possessed of the delusion, *it seemed as though he had committed a crime* and *delusion, he has done wrong* and *is a criminal.* The latter delusion also explains why he considers everyone else an enemy. *Mercury* is a person who has almost no freedom to choose good over bad and evil, because the balance of psychic forces in his character (the king of Syphilis) leaves him no choice. Having the fixed idea that he is a criminal and capable of violent acts, he projects this sentiment on everyone else around him: "No one is to be trusted! Everyone is probably like me: a criminal!" But *Mercury's* lack of insight and degree of perceived suffering are reflected by that other fixed idea: *delusion, he is in hell, suffering the torments without being able to explain*. The Cyber delusion is also supported by other fixed ideas expressing the same message: *delusion, about criminals; animals are jumping on her; he was about to die; he will be murdered; he is persecuted; he is pursued by enemies* and *he sees thieves in the house*. Possessed by such fixed ideas, *Mercury* shows great paranoia: hypervigilance and suspicion run high through this remedy; however, this individual does not become paralyzed without doing anything. When cornered in almost any adverse situation, his best defense is the offense (*delusion, tries to shoot with a cane*), eradicating his enemies!

Inundated by such a strong Cyber delusion and secondary delusions, *Mercury's* essence is, unsurprisingly, instability, according to the triggers he is subjected to—almost like *Pulsatilla* or *Medorrhinum* changeability—and this on the mental, emotional and physical level as seen in further proving symptoms (*anxiety and apprehension with a feeling that he had no control over his senses*).

Causalities

Allopathic Medical Suppression

There are various ailments from (A/F), ranging from the apparently "innocent" ones to the more common emotional causalities. I use the word "innocent" with my allopathic medical hat on, considering the many allopathic therapeutic aggravations of applications. The last thing my allopathic colleagues would expect is for the "wonder drug" cortisone to play havoc with the patient's inner structures, as cortisone cream is "only" for local use in eruptions. This has become such a popular approach, facilitated by the over-the-counter availability, that there are very few doctors or patients in this world who have not at least seen once in their lives the "miracle of disappearing symptoms" which later turn out to be a disappointing Fata Morgana. Besides cortisone, modern man seems to find pleasure also in suppressing perspiration, wrongly reacting as if this expression (which in reality is an exteriorization) is synonymous with "uncleanliness," just like all eruptions. The latest popular allopathic suppression is the suppression of menses for the "convenience" of patients (from the Latin words *con*, or "with," and *venire*, or "to come"). But this convenience "comes with" something, indeed: the destruction of a natural process, a crime against Nature for which humans will pay!

As Hahnemann explains exteriorization in A201-202, miracles of disappearance of disease and their symptoms don't take place; rather, **transference of disease** occurs, moving from the interior to the exterior when the therapeutic intervention is curative. Unfortunately, in the case of suppression, the seeming disappearance of diseases and their symptoms are in reality contrary to the observations of healing, as the internal disease is being increased (though general allopathic practices deem it cured by dint of the disappearance of the localized symptom). Despite the warnings of some of our greatest past homeopaths, (of which I consider Compton Burnett one of the most brilliant in terms of demonstrating the evils of suppression—well documented in the book *The Best of Burnett*), this transference takes place in *Mercury*, as described here by Hering in his *Guiding Symptoms*: *after suppressing of foot sweat, whenever he sees an open window or a cutting instrument* (*knives*!) *he breaks out in a sweat with great heat of the head, and is seized with an almost uncontrollable desire to commit suicide.* So deep is the action of suppression that it leads to acts of destruction and self-destruction! Destructive acts, including suicide, have resulted from such suppression; to the detriment of society, though, suppression and its dangers are either misunderstood or ignored by the medical authorities.

Deceived Ambition

One of the fixed ideas of *Mercury*, even in a *Mercury* child, is that he will be "the greatest, the invincible, and the reigning and uncontested emperor." While many children with autism flee into a world of fantasy, the *Mercury* child's only goal is to flee into a world with imaginary friends who are all fighting on his side, helping him conquer the world so that everyone will obey his orders and wishes. He is more the *revolutionary anarchist*, the freedom fighter who actually is more a despot than a liberator (*dictatorial, domineering and dogmatic*). When a child is imprinted with such a dictator's mindset, it is not uncommon and not incomprehensible for him to clash with his parents and siblings in response to the slightest contradiction (*ailments from discords between chiefs {parent} and subordinates {children}; he has a disposition to contradict*). And as the dictator and revolutionary fighter, he feels justified in his behavior and experiences no guilt at all (*want of moral feeling; disposition to become a criminal without remorse*). One can see that *Mercury* will have a difficult life as a person who remains *discontented with everything and everybody, reproaching others* for the obstructions put in the way as he attempts to live out his misdirected ambitions.

Egotism

Egotism reflects *Mercury's* need to stay on top no matter what. And such an ego is easily insulted and humiliated. This egotism is certainly the causality of other A/F: *ailments from disappointment, from deceived ambition* and *discords between chiefs and subordinates; discords between one's parents;* and *discords between one's friends and between one's servants.* These latter provings confirm the Cyber delusion that no one is to be trusted and that fights and wars are necessary to establish *Mercury's* power position! Certainly the *Mercury* person is not the only individual suffering from such causalities, but one can hardly expect compassion or understanding from such an extreme carrier of the destructive syphilitic miasm (*lack of remorse and hatred for those who have offended*). This person does not forget an "insult" and is bent on revenge. *As he is offended easily and takes everything in bad part,* revenge is swift; many despots throughout history have demonstrated this. *Contradiction* of such a person raises the most intense negative feelings, even *a desire to kill the person that contradicts him.* The *ailments from mortification* and *insults,* also due to *deception causing grief and mortification,* seem to give the *Mercury* individual enough justification to start down the destructive path: he believes in "an eye for an eye" rather than the proverbial turning of the other cheek. *Mercury* is the wolf in sheep's clothing; through his ruthless nature—a nature that is predisposed to destroy—he fulfills what is dominant in his syphilitic miasm, as the use of force and violence is rooted in him. Frighteningly, that mass of sheep can be easily persuaded to act like wolves, contrary to their nature, as witnessed in the history of war, past and present. Such is the power of the wolf *Mercury.*

Compensations

Impulsiveness and Destruction

To establish his perceived birthright of dictatorship, an impulsive *Mercury* child with ASD becomes the bully in school, initiating fights, inciting others to start problems and intimidating everyone around him. He does not hesitate to wield a stick or bat to instill fear in others (*anger so he could have stabbed anyone*). He often intimidates other children into forming a "band of brothers" with him. In addition to the stamp of ADHD and ASD, this behavior earns him the stamp of the allopathic oppositional disorder (O.D.). This child shows a *chaotic and confused behavior: he can be cheerful and alternating this behavior with lack of sympathy. Considering everyone an enemy* leads also to *strong disobedience even to his loving parents* (*aversion to family members*) and to intolerance of any authority. *He can be impolite and impulsive and can suddenly kill with a knife for a slight offense.* He does not hide his rudeness, often exhibiting *a peevishness and ill humor and takes everything in bad part.* When not getting his way, the child *can spit in the face of people.* And no matter how many times he is admonished, the *Mercury* child *is impelled to touch everything,* at home, in stores, and in school, and he *tears things* belonging to others (*he has a feeling that he had no control over his senses*). If some other child wrongs him, whether intentionally or otherwise, his thwarted *sense of injustice* prompts him to plan as how to get back at this "offender" (*malicious and vindictive*). Everything has to go his way, but he often neglects to do what he promises (*he is unreliable in his promises*). This can lead to being expelled from school, as he refuses to do homework and even cuts school with great frequency. Of course, *Mercury* never considers (and is indeed blind to) the consequences of his behavior or its effects on others. Confusion can be observed in other emotions: *he weeps alternating with laughter,* also reflecting his stunted emotional growth. Destruction on the physical plane is seen in *frequent temporary loss of vision; ulcers of cornea and destructive iritis. His teeth are loose and drop out; they become denuded of the gums and turn black and his gums recede from teeth.* One of the most common places to establish the physical process of syphilitic breakdown is indeed the mouth, where *gums recede, causing loosing of the teeth, with bleeding gums and formation of pus pockets* (*pyorrhea*) *exuding a very offensive mouth odor.*

The instability in *Mercury* is also expressed in destructive impulsive behavior towards himself and others: *desire to kill the person contradicting her and great desire to commit murder or suicide, particularly during the menstrual cycle; something urges her to kill her husband of whom she is very fond, and she implores him to hide his razor.* This impulsiveness is easily seen in children with ASD and ADD but is far more controlled in the *Mercury* adult, who feels the same urges but is initially able to control them. The adult *Mercury* person hides behind an excessive mask and tries to keep the beast locked up in the unconscious, in his shadow side. This is quite a fragile control mechanism, as the primitive suppressed beast will unleash all its ferocity in reaction to a simple misunderstood word, a small event, or a bad memory, particularly during the menstrual cycle. The internal conflict, the fight between his impulses (*fight, wants to; anger, so that he could have stabbed anyone; pulls one's nose in the street*) and the desire to control these murderous impulses and keep up the excessive social persona, takes a lot of energy from *Mercury*. This also means that these bad deeds are done only on an impulse, as if to release accumulated internal tension. The messengers of the unconscious, dreams, are often the first to let the cat out of the bag as the syphilitic dreams escape the tight inhibitory control of the conscious: *frightful dreams at night*, often pursuing others with knives or dreams of *thieves, animals and shooting*. Often, under the influence of homeopathic *Mercury*, the change from syphilitic to sycotic and psoric dreams is a first sign that the patient is moving in the direction of a cure, even before any other symptom has changed!

The impulsive destructive nature is also seen in the rubric *ennui*, black type for *Mercury*. It is not just boredom, weariness, tiredness, or dissatisfaction that defines *Mercury's* tedium. The word "ennui" is derived from the Latin *inodiare*, "to make loathsome or hateful." *Mercury's* quest for power and superfluity leads not only to restlessness (*great restlessness as if he had committed a great crime; no rest in any place, constantly anxious* and *almost uncontrollable desire to travel far away*) but also *to foolish, disgusting actions*, suspicion (*morose and mistrustful; treats his associates almost insultingly*), and of course hatred (*desire to kill the person contracting him*). As mentioned above, Stalin was an example of this persona, feared by friend and foe. Not being able to call his intellectual powers into play (*obtuseness of mental operations; muddledness of head*) or finding resources within himself to engage in some fruitful activity (*believes he is losing his reason with illusions of fantasy*), this boredom becomes a burden leading to paralysis and melancholia. As much as unbearable pains torture *Mercury* at night, boredom is his form of torture during the day.

Foolishness and Hyperactivity

In his quest to be accepted as the popular, or rather feared, leader, the *Mercury* child possesses still other tools. He is *audacious*, has no sense of danger and *is a boaster*, and loves to engage in dangerous, thrill-seeking activities that require energy and speed (jumping from walls, car roofs, roller skating, ice hockey, roller hockey, American football, etc.). He is constantly moving around—unfortunately, also at night, which makes for *sleepless nights* for him and his parents (*restless at night, in bed driving him from one bed to another and restless after the least exertion*). He has *convulsive gestures, puts everything in his mouth and shows strange and ridiculous motions of the hands* (*fidgety with fingers*). He can use *nonsensical speech, with difficult articulation amounting to stammering and laughs silly, making strange faces*. Foolish behavior takes even such extreme forms as *licking up his feces, mud and his own saliva from the floor*. This child is hard to control at school, and it is difficult for him to engage in activities as he is so restless that *he cannot remain sitting for one moment in the same posture; he is forced to change from one seat to another; there is no rest in any place*, and *he is constantly anxious.* When this child grows up, he might be able to hide some of this foolish behavior, but at heart he remains the same person and will use psychology to hurt others in business or in his personal life.

Withdrawal and Depression

Behind the foolish behavior of a clown, the spectrum of darkness and depression is always hiding. Because of his asocial attitude, *Mercury* is isolated (the contrary of what he desires—an empire!) and has an *aversion to family; feels estranged and ignores his family,* often annoying them through his *disobedient and willful behavior. He loathes life* and complains about everything as if the whole world has made a pact against him and is conspiring to make his life difficult (*complaining about relations and surroundings*). He even *has a narrow tolerance to temperature* (he does not want it too hot or cold); *Mercury* is called the "living thermometer" as he suffers quickly from cold, seeks warmth, and then suffers immediately from the heat. Excessive perspiration all over the body, *staining the linen yellow* upon the slightest stimulus, also aggravates the *Mercury* person. *He is suspicious and sulky,* and approaching this child or adult is always difficult as *consolation aggravates* and *he is averse to being touched.* When not finding an audience to dominate, he is *indisposed to talk and shows aversion to play with others.*

The *Mercury* person constantly struggles with a desire to kill himself (*he fears to injure himself when left alone*). He can't remember things (*vanishing of thoughts*), *can't concentrate while calculating and studying and reading,* and gets lost while returning home from school or work (*confusion, loses his way in well-known streets*). When he does not answer a question, it is simply because he does not understand the question: *there is obtuseness of mental operations with great inclination to sleep and muddledness of the head. He shows every mark of imbecility with foolish, mischievous and disgusting actions.* He is dyslectic and makes *mistakes in calculating, spelling, reading and speaking.*

Interesting in this person is that he becomes sad when the sun is out (*sadness in sunshine*). The sun, a symbol of happiness and light, is shunned by him: it does not resonate with his inner being. He prefers dressing in black, the relatively fixed symbol of withdrawal, sin, the hidden, rebirth in seclusion and the personal unconscious; *Mercury* children tend to draw pictures of knights, swords, and dead people. When the *adventurous* *Mercury* person has an *almost uncontrollable desire to travel far away* and *wants to go abroad,* it is not about socializing and connecting as it is with the *Phosphorus* child; rather, it represents an attempt to escape from his world full of enemies: *desire to flee with nightly anxieties and apprehension*. *Mercury*'s thinking, his extraverted and excessive persona, and his choleric temperament relate better to the Genghis Khan's way of traveling ("conquering and ruling"), even in his own environment. Hormonal changes seem an additional stress to the *Mercury* person, throwing her directly into the black depths of unrest: she has a *great desire to murder or commit suicide, particularly during menstrual period*. Almost contradictorily, the best place for *Mercury* is his bed, but the worst time is the night! So you see a person who feels better lying in bed the whole day long (*bed, desire to remain in bed*), often suffering from chronic fatigue and immune deficiency syndrome and with increased thirst and perspiration but who, when trying to fall asleep at night, is plagued by an aggravation of all existing symptoms: *head pain at night; fear of insanity at night; extremities, pain, night, bed, drives out of; pain, bones, night; extreme restlessness at night, beginning around 8 pm and lasting till morning and an inexpressible pain of soul and body* (we could call it anguish) *with anxious restlessness as if some evil impended*.

Sexual Excesses

Sexuality will be used as an outlet for the *Mercury* person to exert (in his mind) total control over another person. The syphilitic miasm stands for loss of control, so sex will be uncontrolled and rather destructive in nature: *nymphomania*. This is a person who never evolves beyond the most superficial level in love—the sexual attitude—, consciously disregarding his partner's inner personality in order to obtain what he wants. *Mercury* is more likely than any other personality to engage in abnormal sex, be it incestuous or sadomasochistic. For *Mercury*, the idea of sexuality is purely mechanical and un-psychological as his partner is viewed as "a piece of meat," an object that he can bite, hurt, and then throw away.

Golden Tips from the Masters

- Heavy, foul sweating at night does not ameliorate (the Chinese called night sweats "rob sweats" as they rob the person of precious Yin Qi)
- Headaches at night with the sensation a being in a constricting band
- General offensiveness (fetid) of all excretions
- *Mercury* people catch cold easily because of a lack of defense mechanisms. They have a sudden loss of energy with the slightest change of temperature
- Keynotes: metallic taste in the mouth and excessive salivation, making the pillow wet
- Intense thirst in spite of a moist mouth
- **Geographic tongue** with imprints of teeth on the sides
- #1 remedy for swimmer's ear
- Great remedy in Parkinson's disease (tremors, salivation, stuttering, general weakness)
- Great remedy in AIDS patients with swollen glands and recurring fevers
- Use 30C *Mercury* to limit withdrawal symptoms when mercury fillings are removed
- In cases of colitis ulcerosa (DD with *Merc-cor*) with the classic tenesmus and diarrhea filled with blood and mucus because of ulcerations
- Great remedy for acute mononucleosis: extreme debility, swelling of neck glands, fever, and loss of saliva in sleep
- *Hepar-sulph* is the peacemaker between *Mercury* and *Silica*. So if *Silica* is indicated after you have given *Mercury* (for instance, with abscesses), first give a dose of *Hepar-sulph* and you will never have a problem!
- In low potencies it hastens suppuration; in high potencies it aborts suppuration (*Nash*)
- *Mercury* is <by heat of bed and >by rest in bed; *Ars* is >for heat in bed and <for rest in bed (H.C. Allen)

Natrum carbonicum (Nat-c). Sodium carbonate

The Cyber Delusion

Nat-carb's Cyber delusion is ***there is a division between himself and others***, which is also expressed by the delusion ***he is forsaken and deserted***. There is a kind of abyss in front of *Nat-c*, or some intangible barrier preventing her from reaching others (this is the opposite of *Kali-c*, who has an abyss *behind* her). *Nat-c* sees the distance that is created between herself and others and can't figure out how to overcome this wall or abyss that divides and separates her from society. The resulting isolation is neither welcomed nor desired as *Nat-c* has a *fear of being alone, yet is averse to company*. This sounds like a contradiction, but *Nat-c* is indeed torn between two opposite emotions which she tries to overcome through other delusions or fixed ideas which are, in fact, wishes to escape the strangulating hold of her CD. The *delusion, the body has become heavy and thick* supports the difficulty this person experiences just in trying to move forward, to connect. Then there is the conviction that *she cannot succeed, she does everything wrong, and does nothing right,* undermining her self-confidence (*want of confidence*), not a good characteristic for one who might want to undertake any journey, let alone socialize, leaving the fairy tale world of the collective unconscious with its protective and loving Divine Mother archetype.

Nat-c people, adults and children alike, are stubborn, with a primitive, little-differentiated, archaic ego. The attention is still mainly aimed at the self (but not 100% so, as it is with pure *Carbon*) and, together with the stubbornness, leaves little place for others to verbalize their wills or opinions (we see this readily in *intolerant to contradiction*). The child usually expresses this sentiment by saying: "I want to do this! Don't help me!" It looks like this is a very independent child. The reality is very different. Independence, in the case of *Nat-c*, is easily confused with and translated as loneliness. It is easy to see, too, why these children might be categorized as having ASD; they have difficulties connecting to others, even with intimate friends or family: *aversion to family members and to society* and *estranged from family and friends.* And one must add to this *company, aversion to, of intimate friends.* This is puzzling, given that the *Natrum* element is so desirous of connection to others, but the Cyber delusion will lead us to greater insight.

Driven by her CD, *Nat-carb's* flight into fantasy will be the primary compensation (*delusion, of fancy illusions*). These are children who create stories by themselves in which they are the heroines, the controlling forces over what happens in their own little fantasy world. Such children are seemingly totally engrossed in their actions, playing with toy cars or trains while listening with headphones to fairy-tale music that encourages this kind of fanciful, imaginative retreat from reality. Other delusions allude to this fantasy world: *delusion, he is on a journey,* as they are seemingly totally disconnected from their environment. Then we have the *delusion, of a wedding* and *delusion, he hears music,* showing again in extended meaning the desire to connect to a pleasant world and to feel a sense of belonging somewhere (to a family), which in real life they seem incapable of achieving. Because these children are still young, they create a world of smallness in order to fit in that world, in order to be part of it: *delusions, things appear small.* Creating such a miniature world (like carrying small toys around everywhere) is comforting to them: the child is large in comparison with the little toys/stuffed animals he plays with.

The difficulty for *Nat-c* is entering the adult world, or even the limited world of the child's reality, to connect to others. I remember a former patient, a child who would go so far as to invite her friends to her home, but when they arrived, she would go off to play by herself, leaving her mom and her friends stunned and puzzled. For such an intense, compulsive force to be present in such young child, a child who has hardly begun to live, it must go back to the intrauterine life; these same feelings must have been found in the pregnant mother! But for what reason? It can only be that the mother felt isolated and estranged from friends and family during pregnancy, causing this fixed idea.

Causalities

Anger with Silent Grief and Anxiety

This NWS recalls cases of the young woman who might be excited to be pregnant for the first time but whose joy is tempered because of neglect, indifference, or even anger from a husband or partner who is not ready to have a family or fears that this baby will get all the attention. Maybe she feels, rightly or not, forsaken by her family because they did not show enough enthusiasm about her pregnancy. Or maybe the pregnant mother was hoping that this child would be the peacemaker between her and her estranged parents and this has not been the case! Maybe her husband has to travel frequently for his work and her family lives far away. It certainly would explain her anger and grief and her isolation from family. Sometimes, as is evidenced in the next example, the secret story is unbelievable—but then again, society is often quick to judge others without knowing the facts.

A woman who thought she was infertile adopted a child. When two months later she found out that she was pregnant, she could not tell anyone out of fear that she would be labeled a fraud and that the adopted child would be taken away. Only her parents and spouse knew. The pregnant woman said, "I wanted to protect my nest and my reputation." She wanted to communicate her joy about her pregnancy, but she was frightened to do so, which created that communication gap between her and others (the rest of the world). It is interesting how the *Nat-c* child created by this event taunted her adopted sister by saying, "I came out of mommy's belly, not you" (*malicious and spiteful*). This might well have been to boost her standing in the family: "I, but not you, belong somewhere!" In reality, she was referring to *her* real trouble: she did not know where *she* belonged!

Another possible causality of anger with grief can be found when expectant parents are not married, which in a conservative family might lead to all kinds of rejection: maybe an abortion is advocated, strongly against the mother's wishes, leading to estrangement from "well-meaning" friends and family who exclaim: "You are both too young. You are immature. You cannot afford this." Or there can be a secret story of rape or incest. Is there any more horrible reason for being subdued about being pregnant? How can the pregnant mother express her joy to the world? And it does not have to be rape. There are enough *Lycopodium* and *Medorrhinum* men out there who abandon the pregnant mother right away when they hear the news of pregnancy (*lack of responsibility*), yet the mother is committed to the unborn child. *Lycopodium*, *Medorrhinum* and *Fl-acid* are people who confuse excitement with joy, thrill with love of life. Besides leading to ailments from *anger with fright* ("What am I going to do now with no help; who is going to help me raise this child?") to *anger with silent grief* (they are too embarrassed to tell anyone they have been dumped), it all leads to *ailments from anticipation anxiety* and *emotional excitement* (stress), two other NWS for *Nat-c*.

One *Nat-c* child I saw (diagnosed with high-functioning autism), was constantly on the lookout for clocks that might chime; he got upset at birthday parties because there was always singing, and he was startled and scared at the sound of fountains. One can deduce from this that *Nat-c monitors his environment in order to avoid things that will distress him*. This creates, of course, *anticipation anxiety*! The mother's story of this child also reflected *Nat-carb's* CD of *division between herself and others*. Here is another story from my practice:

During her pregnancy, a woman's attorney husband became well known for a case he handled and fell in love with his own grandiose persona. He was not interested in how his wife was feeling during the pregnancy; he only told her, "Make sure to record me on this or that TV show and collect the articles in the newspapers." As her family was unavailable, it led to total isolation, and she kept numb until the end of her pregnancy, not even caring anymore if the father would be there for the delivery! Busy with his trial case, he was unaware of his own crime!

Sometimes *anxiety with silent grief* is created in the *Nat-c* child by a stern mother, one who is strict and dominating in her actions. Such a mother might always insist on doing the next thing right away: time to wash your hands now, to leave for an errand now, to put things away because it is time for dinner...***now!*** I remember such cases from my practice. Regardless of what the child might be doing at a particular moment, it was time *now* to brush her teeth and go to bed. Her mother's supercharged and nervous voice became immensely disturbing to the point of creating anxiety and grief in the child whenever the mother approached her. She knew that when Mom came around, her peaceful entertainment would be over, broken up with an irritating persistency. In this particular case it created fright, anger, and grief as well as an aversion to her mother (*aversion to certain persons,* and *aversion to family members*). Her mother's behavior was in sharp contrast to that of her father, who always came gently in ahead of time to say, "We will have to go to bed in fifteen minutes. Or we will have to leave in half an hour." She adored her father, but her mother made this girl high-strung and angry (*ailments from emotional excitement*), leading to Tourette's-like behavior with *swearing* and creating a rift with her mother that continued into her adulthood. Even when, as in this case, the father supplies the child with enough emotional nourishment, a single relationship should not carry the weight of having to assume double significance—especially for a girl, for whom the formation of her natural anima comes largely from the mother.

Mental Work

Mental work is not a positive tool for *Nat-c*. When we see in the provings *occupation ameliorates* and *attention to details*, these traits are connected not to schoolwork but rather to the creation of a fantasy world, steering this child away from the adult world. Where *Nat-m* and even *Nat-p* in their initial phases have *desire for mental work*, *Nat-c* has outspoken, *mental work is impossible or fatigues*! This child needs a break after spending barely 30 minutes on homework or after a single class—something impossible in the structured setting of mainstream school but better dealt with, and certainly more quickly found out, with home schooling. *Nat-c* easily reaches the point of *confusion of the mind from mental exertion* and *concentration difficult while studying and reading*. No wonder these children, *absorbed and buried in thought* (in their fantasy worlds), have been labeled with every name in the manual of psychiatry: from OCD to ASD to ADHD!

Compensations

Desire to be Magnetized

The combination of loneliness, stubbornness, and an immature ego coupled with shyness does not help *Nat-c* overcome her sense of isolation. And indeed life is a struggle for this child. The lack of intimacy she experiences also results in a *desire to be magnetized* and *mesmerizing ameliorates*. In other words, there is a desire to be supported, to be "carried" by someone. This mesmerizing has more to do with the fantasy visions that *Nat-c* creates than with realities in life, as she has a tendency to *aversion to mankind and society, anthropophobia, misanthropy* and *especially fear for men*. There is a continuous effort to try to make contact, but at the same time, *Nat-c* flees before any serious contact is made as the obstacles seem too steep to overcome.

Music

Music is the other magnetizing force. We can't expect that *Nat-c* will listen to fast rock-and-roll music like *Tarentula* does: this does not fit her mood at all, and even *piano music creates anxiety; she is affected by playing on a piano, a short time, with painful anxiety of the chest, trembling of the body and weariness*. The most helpful music for such a child is classical music or film music (like that from "Beauty and the Beast"), another dream world into which she can escape. The *Natrum* element certainly refers to the seriousness of the child (*serious, earnest*), which is reflected in the kind of music she listens to. So this music is a positive reinforcement, as it resonates with *Nat-carb's* special world. But we should remember that a serious child is met with seriousness; people respond to a happy and outgoing child with laughter and play. From the beginning, this child unconsciously blocks the avenues by which the outside world would reach out to her.

Conscientiousness About Trifles

Another positive tool to connect to "a world" (not ***the*** world) is her strong *conscientiousness about trifles*. Unfortunately, this can lead to *monomania* and OCD, again mentioned in the spectrum of ASD: children play for hours lining up their little cars and get mad when someone interferes; or they get attached to one or more objects, like a certain toy or doll that they always carry around with them, playing the role of the protector. *Nat-carb's* interest in detail is indeed a positive tool for the child as she uses it to enrich a comprehensive fantasy world, but this characteristic can also be a positive indicator of ASD. As is the case with *Silica*, attention to trifles is sapping her mental strength, leading to indecisiveness (*irresolution*) and *irritability from trifles. Conscientiousness about trifles,* as seen in *Arsenicum*, *Lyc*, *Staphysagria*, and *Sepia*, often leads to OCD and also to *undertaking many things but not persevering in anything* for many of these characters. In *Nat-c* it only leads to *weakness of memory for mental labor* and *an inability to perform any mental labor as her head is stupefied if she tries to exert herself.*

Loquacity

All the positive compensations of *Nat-c* are really means to reinforce a permanent world in which *Nat-c* is able to live and thrive. If we see *loquacity* in *Nat-c* (the most loquacious of the *Natrums*), it is not because she wants to connect to others; she wishes to connect to companions in her created fantasy world (to which she talks all the time) (*occupation ameliorates*). This lining up of toys and talking to the figurines and little soldiers makes one think of *Calc-c*, but the difference is that *Calc-c* is, initially, not yet ready to go out into the world (sometimes he never is, even as an adult) and connect to others beyond parents or other immediate family. *Calc-c* has only just discovered himself and feels content in the safe environment of the home, where he has no difficulties engaging with others. Through stubbornness and temper tantrums, in fact, he can get all the attention he wants so much. *Nat-c* has gotten lost somewhere, and family does not (or never has) represented that safe haven as it does for *Calc-c*.

Nat-carb's conversation goes on *ad nauseam* about the same topic (*loquacity until exhausted; loquacity vivacious; loquacity cheerful and exuberant*), even *talking in her sleep*: one of the favorite things is observing and talking about small animals like ladybugs or little goldfish, for which they show great concern (*sympathy, compassion*). Therefore, this remedy should be in the rubric *talking, of nothing but one subject,* where we find remedies like *Arg-n, Lyc, Med,* and *Stram*. Of course, the talking of one subject is very different in these remedies. *Med* and *Lyc* talk not about ladybugs but about ladies (their sexual conquests); *Arg-n* talks about all the calamities that could occur when she goes out from home, the "what if" situations, and *Stramonium* talks only about the dangers he faces in this world.

Poetry

Once the *Nat-c* child knows how to read and write, her loquacity takes on another form, and her fantasy world expands with another positive tool: writing! *She talks in verses and writes stories*. These first stirrings of poetry reflect the aching feelings of homesickness, so weaving poetic fancies are a compensation for what is lacking: connection to the warmth of the family. You see the refinement of the *Natrum* element again in this trait, as writing is for *Nat-c* a form of "communicating" with the outside world, a world that seems too difficult to reach and explore. However, this compensation only appears to be a positive one for the child: it will increasingly cut *Nat-c* off from the real world, as that world finds *Nat-c* too serious and eccentric.

Creation of Imaginary Companions

What can we do to survive if we are not able to connect to anyone in this world? Create our own imaginary world! When we come up against an obstacle and no adaptation is possible, then introversion with increased fantasy activity takes place—with the sole aim of removing the obstacle, even if it is just in fantasy. Because of a psychological need dictated by her CD and the proving *fear of being alone yet averse to company,* a fairy-tale life is called into existence (*delusion, of fancy illusions*). This child feels her relationships with others to be lacking, as mentioned in the causalities above. Often, the fantasy self or dual personality is projected onto some small animals (like the ladybugs in the previous story) or onto some toy or collection of dolls. In her play, the *Nat-c* child assigns varying personalities to her dolls, singling some out as the

Golden Tips from the Masters

- *Nat-c* is a combination of *Lycopodium* physically and *Nat-mur* emotionally!
- Is close to *Sepia* and easily confused with it (also has the sensation of downward pressure in the pelvis among other symptoms)
- Fear of spraining the ankles (very weak ankles) because of lack of tone
- #1 remedy for NWS sunstroke (single or recurrent) with headaches, hypertension, and fatigue
- Aggravates from the least change in weather (headaches!). Has narrow range of temperature tolerance like *Mercury* with especially cold limbs in the winter and headaches in the summer heat.
- A "new-age" remedy for people who are very idealistic, sympathetic, and always working on themselves spiritually as well as sacrificing themselves for others
- A great remedy resembling *Nat-mur* (gloomy and heavy) but nice, selfless, and sweet, avoiding confrontation and sensitive to other people's feelings
- Complementary remedy to *Kali-sulph* and *Sepia*
- Obstinate cases of infertility
- Unusual aggravation from food around 5 a.m. and 11 p.m.
- Indicated for "old dyspeptics" with constant eructations, sour stomach, and rheumatism (Kent)
- Sadness, depression, and melancholy are worse after a meal but diminish as digestion advances
- Urine is characterized by sour odor
- The herpes family (herpes labialis, zona) is very related to *Nat-c*!

Natrum muriaticum (Nat-m). Common salt. Sodium chloride.

The Cyber Delusion

Nat-mur's Cyber delusion is ***his mother is dead.*** Recalling that the CD is the driving force behind every effort, plan, thought, and action, guiding the consciousness of the individual, we know that this same thought will be discovered throughout *Nat-mur's* story; it reflects the impetus behind his expressions in every phase. In order to gain far-reaching insight into dreams, the other half of human existence, the homeopath must be experienced in the matter of relatively fixed symbols. Such insights have great diagnostic and prognostic value. We call these symbols "relatively" because, when they occur in dreams, we are uncertain as to whether they might have variant or additional meanings. There are many such symbols, and they might differ in individual cases with subtle shifts of meaning. One must study mythology, folklore, religion, and language in order to determine their meaning in a scientific way. As a relatively fixed symbol, *mother* stands for a life-giving vessel, the hollow form (uterus) that carries and nourishes, and it thus stands for the foundations of unconsciousness. The symbol of the mother is equal to love, protection, homemaking, and a sheltering attitude. There is also the Divine Mother, the archetype of the collective unconscious. Mother is food; she is love, she is warmth, she is earth. To be loved by her means to be rooted, to be at home (*Nat-m* has *homesickness*). The negative aspect of this Mother archetype, the "witch," is over-protectiveness, possessiveness, and unnecessary meddling; of course, the archetypal mother may also be absent because of cruelty, dominance, or alcohol or drug use. In *Nat-mur* we see a person who has known only the forbidding, life-destroying aspect of the mother, not the natural nourishing and protecting attributes. Now the reader understands that, more than any other remedy, *Nat-m* reflects the intrauterine crime of lack of emotional nourishment, creating a child that from day one seems *too serious, too lonely and out of sorts.* Such experience can be embedded in the fetus through mystical participation when the crime of abandonment or lack of nourishing is perpetrated on the mother while she is pregnant.

This "not belonging," a sensation of isolation and estrangement, and "looking for a mother," is the main feeling and true essence of *Nat-m* from the beginning of its story until the end. The drive to bond lies deep in our DNA. Disappointment when we fail to connect or when the connection is broken is virtually guaranteed. That's why the ultimate rejection—the departure of a loved one—is among the most stressful of all experiences. In *Nat-m*, this state of isolation and loneliness is accentuated by the fact that sympathy and communication with others is longed for, yet an inner command—one stronger than the desire to connect—forbids the acceptance of help and urges the *Nat-m* person to look for strength within herself, especially in later stages of adulthood. Initially, such person may not be clinically depressed, but she suffers from what psychologists call dysthymia, a mild, low-level, pervasive depression that saps life of its beauty, even as one continues to fully function. This is a state involving the absence of *joie de vivre*, or "joy of life," and life will move forward without its victim. One can only shudder upon reflecting that so many people born in a *Nat-m* state are going down an all too well travelled road due entirely to what TCM calls a noble misfortune. Jung and Hahnemann both expressed this misfortune as a *mistunement*, a deviation of the intended constitution through psychic trauma. We must remember that much childhood material (and of course the intrauterine trauma even more) remains indisposed of and unprocessed in the psyche because of the rapid flow of the years and the overwhelming rush of the newly discovered world. Early childhood memories are diagnostically important for adults: the very fact of something being remembered from a period most of which is forgotten marks it as a signpost pointing to a traumatic or highly feeling-toned complex (NWS). The maternal role can be taken over by someone else, saving the person from entering the *Nat-m* state: it can be another family member (grandmother, older sister), but it can also be a teacher, physician, neighbor, or anyone who extends sympathy and love to this lonely person.

The mother can be dead even when she is alive! Everything depends on whether the mother fulfilled her role as a source of emotional support when needed. I had a patient who discovered, upon coming home from school, that his mom had given the dog away because the dog was too rambunctious and annoying; another patient's mother put the piano obtained with her daughter's hard-earned money in the cellar. When asked why, this mother simply said that she was redecorating the house. In each instance, the mother demonstrated that nothing about the child mattered; she had her own agenda and followed it. In these cases, the one place where a child should be able to get unconditional encouragement and love was fraught with indifference and self-interest on the part of the mother. Let's take another example: I met a patient who, as an adolescent, was afflicted with a number of anxieties: *anxiety in a crowd* (agoraphobia), *for flying, for tunnels, for small spaces, for robbers* and *even people.* Looking back in her life, from age three on, she recalled that her father and mother had done nothing but fight, and that her mother, rather than giving emotional nourishment, had pushed her own needs on the child. This situation was an example of *ailments from too early responsibility*: a child of three should not bear the cross of emotional turmoil between the parents and feel that she needs to be the nourishing mother of her own mom. Although the mother was alive, she was not "alive" in the sense of giving support and protection to her child, who was carried away in the whirlwind of marital disarray. This child could only express her mother's needs and lived all her life with her mother's needs in mind, not her own. There was no room for personal needs, so this person was not seen and took on the identity (including the desires) of her mother (*delusions, of errors of personal identity* and *delusion, her head belongs to someone else*). With her identity erased, such a *Nat-m* child is not seen or heard while someone else's existence is practically grafted onto her. This sets up a dangerous precedent for the *Nat-m* child, as it often translates into the future life and relationship choice of a certain kind of partner: one that keeps the *Nat-m* person in a cycle of not expressing her own needs, though she continues to have those needs and yearns to be heard.

An example from my practice:

> A man had a chief complaint (CC) of dull pains in his lower extremities. This condition had started after a contentious divorce that had lasted for about five years. He had moved to his native country to be close to his family for support. However, once he arrived there, his mother and sister did nothing but harass him with their small problems and criticize him constantly while at no time giving him much-needed emotional support. In other words, two female figures that could have provided an opportunity for him to restore his wounded anima failed at that time to give him any emotional support; worse, they represented the negative side of the mother, the critical and opinionated side! They never

> asked him, "How are you?" or "How are you dealing with your grief?" This was, for him, the proverbial straw that broke the camel's back; it exacerbated his CC. The *betrayal* had such a painful impact on him that he again left his native country to start a career elsewhere. But the memory of that negative experience remained with him, always present in the unconscious and also manifesting itself and torturing him in his conscious life.

Let's investigate *Nat-mur's* other delusions. There is a sense of disconnection, of not standing with both feet on the ground. *Delusion, of floating in the air*: is this the start of a disintegration of the person, or is it symbolic of her naivety? Or both? Is *Nat-m* on cloud nine all the time? What is the reason? What kind of person is *Nat-m* according to Jung's conscious functions? She is dominant Eros (feeling) and archaic Logos (thinking). This is the opposite of *Sepia*, who from the beginning of life suppresses her female attitude, a "masculine protest." This means, at least in the beginning psoric phase to which this delusion belongs, that *Nat-m* is somewhat naïve, as some provings indicate: She *could have laughed and sung all day long*. Always **smiling** no matter what! In further provings, we see *lively, good-humored and cheerful; remarkable inclination to laugh, constant laughing; she laughed so immoderately at something not ludicrous, that she could not be quieted and tears came into her eyes, so that she looked as though she had been weeping*. This does not sound like a *Nat-mur*, but it is! She will do anything, including exhibiting peculiar behavior (like laughing when attending a funeral—*laughing about serious matters*), to get into the relationship that she seeks. The primitive thinking function is easily overtaken by the dominant feeling function, so a "reasonable" approach for *Nat-m* is to speak through her feelings (*although evidently a well-educated and intelligent woman, her mind seemed hopeless and confused*). At this point, *Nat-m* thinks it is possible to find a human being whose every quirk, habit, and preference aligns perfectly with hers, fitting like two perfect pieces of a puzzle. Other provings expressing this dominant feeling function are *excitable, capriciousness, cheerfulness, passionate at every trifle*, and *hysteria with fainting*. The word "hysteria" shows how she can lose ground in her excitability. This psoric first phase and first theme, in which *Nat-m* tries to connect to others, is related to the overwhelming desire to belong, to seek the eternal Divine Mother, the connection with the collective unconscious that has been missing since she was a youngster. Apparently unlimited possibilities and partners breed the illusion in *Nat-m* that the perfect person, the long-awaited prince, is out there and has only to be found. Floating in the air also represents, therefore, a disconnection from the earth (consciousness) and a regression into the unconscious, where her

Eros and feminine qualities (her Yin side) can flourish. Women naturally have an easier time connecting to the unconscious than men do; women most often have feeling as a dominant conscious function, while *Sepia's* dominant thinking function in women, according to Jung, "is a regrettable accident."

Purposely taking on someone else's identity (yielding) leads to constant praise of the paramour. This is usually not difficult in this psoric phase as the archaic *Nat-m* animus connects automatically (called projection) to the dominant out-of-balance animus of a man: one falls in love with the opposite, which is good only if both want to learn from it. *Nat-m* adapts to a relationship/marriage more quickly than her partner: sadly, as she lowers her expectations, she adjusts all too readily to the partner's baggage, which often merely leads to an increase in that baggage. *Nat-m,* at the apex of the rebuff-sensitivity scale (*easily offended; sensitive to criticism; delusion, she is criticized*), pays a particularly steep price just for wanting to belong. In this initial naïve stage, *Nat-m* falls "in love with love," convinced that the Prince Charming she has met on a first date is THE one! All week long, after the initial date, she builds up an ironclad case to prove that he is perfect for her, marveling at how their interests coincided (*intelligent but naïve*). Her friends are going to be so impressed! Then she gets an email, and the message is an unaffectionate business-wise request to reschedule! What horror! What pain! She expected reality to conform to her fantasy, always a formula for disappointment. Such sudden dose of rejection, often from peers, family and especially romantic partners, precipitates a deep-seated sensitivity to rejection in *Nat-m* as well as increased longing to finally belong, to connect to someone, anyone! Being in love with love, called infatuation, is an intense state that displays familiar features: almost always thinking of that other person; waiting constantly to touch or holding on to that person, to hear from that person every five minutes and to be together; excitement at the other's presence and to feel lost without him, not knowing what to do; not being able to fall asleep and feeling that without that person, only for a short separation, life is not worth living. The story of romance becomes the predominant foreground event in her life, in fact the only event worth thinking of. In other words, a person can (and *Nat-m,* at this point, always does) enable her partner, child, or friend to live his delusion, which eventually leads not to more intimacy and closeness, but, to *Nat-mur's* dismay and surprise, to more distance and separation. She is too eager to curry the favor and admiration of the lover, bending over backwards to accommodate all his requests. She gives the impression of offering: "May I be your puppet on a string?" She is a people-pleaser, committed to bolstering the well-being of that desired person even at the expense of her own (*delusion, head belongs to another*). *Nat-m* may say to herself later, "I was so good; I did everything he wanted, and now look what has happened. We are more separated than ever! And now I am losing him!" This is a cruel reality in which *Nat-m* cherishes the illusion that she has married a hero, unperturbed by her own low self-worth and looking for validation from others, losing control over her own life. But it really points to the impatience and naivety of *Nat-m* in this stage; she must exercise and appeal to her archaic thinking conscious function before she falls prey to her impulsive behavior, wishing to connect to someone at all costs. She does this more out of despair than out of true love. And off *Nat-m* goes in search of the next relationship!

Of course, there is also another reason for the *Nat-m* patient to dissolve her early relationships in a hurry. She resembles a tiger that wants to leap over things rather than emulating a tree that stands still and takes root, eventually overcoming many adjustment problems in her relationships. So she runs away as she is unable to form a decent relationship with her partner, forgetting that to bear fruit, a tree needs time. Many things fail, as is often the case in Nature, but man must have the courage to undertake and to cultivate.

Further delusions will be found in her various compensations as *Nat-m* tries to rectify her hopeless situation with the creation of additional fixed ideas, most of them not leading to any real solution—as can be expected from any delusion, whether benign or malignant in character.

Causalities

Unresolved Grief and Disappointed Love; Deception and Betrayal

We are wired for attachment in a world of impermanence. This does not bode well for a *Nat-m* person; early loss poisons *Nat-mur's* ability to trust, feel safe, and give herself fully in subsequent relationships. Grief and disappointed love are unfortunately all too common in our lives. But, as mentioned before, *Nat-m* is not inclined to express this grief and get help from others. On the contrary! *Nat-m* suffers grief in silence and does not even *cry except when pitied* (*ailments from silent grief*). The non-expression of grief suffered during pregnancy will lead to delayed and *late learning to speak* in the *Nat-mur* child, as "speaking up" to ask for and receive consolation is not an option for a *Nat-m* person. There is truly a longing to belong (*homesickness*), to be loved and connect to a kindred soul. However, such a serious and insecure person is bound to be lonely. Seriousness is not as appealing to others as an open, friendly character: seriousness is met by seriousness, while joy instills joy in others! The *Nat-m* child's inner life is like a house in which the curtains are always drawn to block the sun, impeding the entrance of joy. Such a child *dislikes being in the sun* and will, for instance, as I have seen in my practice, walk in the shade all the way home from school. Because of this psychological barricade, the disappointment continues (*prolonged grief; ailments from disappointed love*) and the *Nat-m* person seems to be trapped in a never-ending spiral of *bad news, old disappointments,* and *suppressed anger*.

As devastating experiences go, few events (and alas how often do they happen in this world) can match the emotional havoc following the discovery that one's partner is having an affair. Heartbreak sparks a common scenario: hibernating (*aversion to company* and *fond of solitude*), thinking the world has ended (*delusion, being doomed*), and keeping Kleenex in business (*weeping when looked at; weeping when alone* and *weeping when spoken to; whenever alone she wished to cry and she did not know why*), for starters. It can feel like a part of your body has been ripped off or like you have been socked in the chest (*tightness and feeling of tension and pressure in the chest*). When falling out of love, *Nat-m* remembers the steep fall, never the initial love. Above a suddenly shattered world hover pain and rejection, doubts about one's worth (*delusion, she looks wretched when looking in the mirror*), and above all, the rupture of trust (*deception causes grief and mortification*). Such an event fractures time, oversimplifying it into the periods before and after the going of separate ways. Sudden breakup and deception leave *Nat-m* socially paralyzed. It has become easier to break up using social media such as Twitter and Facebook and avoiding doing it face to face, which is particularly difficult for the sufferer. When communicating the bad news face to face, there is at least a degree of courage required and some built-in consolation, so that the injured party is capable of weathering the inevitable pain and sadness helped by *Ignatia* (*Nat-mur's* acute). Often, the *Nat-m* victim is deeply traumatized and emotionally distraught by the betrayal and desperately tries to piece together what has happened; such a rejection has the potential to shatter her sense of self. The result is an ongoing self-criticism of *Nat-mur's* personal life, like a continual readout of her emotional heart rate. Adultery resulting in the shattering of faith—the faith in love, loyalty, friendship, trust, and honesty—is a key factor in the development of a *Nat-m* person. It is *ailments from bad news* and *deception causing grief and mortification* that engage her deepest vulnerability: the fear that she is unlovable.

This deception is also felt as *a loss of honor,* and for a *Nat-m* person loss of honor brings a shame greater and more threatening than any other kind. The loss of face, the overwhelming shame, and the derision of others are like daggers in her heart. There is no statute of limitations on the hurt and anger that follows a partner's affair. Because of these *old disappointments,* the *Nat-m* person is extremely sensitive to the slightest perceived grievance (*easily offended, takes everything in bad part, and ailments from being scorned*). Note the mention here of *old disappointments*: this sets the tone for *Nat-m*. As salt preserves everything, the *Nat-m* person seems to preserve all her feelings too (*thoughts persistent, haunted by unpleasant subject* and *tormenting thoughts*). *Nat-m* has a permanent relationship with the grudges she holds. As much as she is depressed and aggravated by the many slights and deceptions that befall her, she remains reluctant to bury her pain and move on (*disagreeable thoughts; dwells, recalls disagreeable memories*). She is a champion at itemizing every real or perceived unfair knock she ever suffered, known as "grievance collecting." *Nat-m* can slip into rumination—a spiral of morbid self-involvement that is extremely difficult to shake (*thoughts persistent, haunted by unpleasant subjects*). One can call this "the cultivating of depression," the mental habit of taking wretched feelings too seriously and burrowing into them. Sad thoughts and sorrow become familiar demons that now arrive as welcome visitors (*tries to recollect past disagreeable occurrences, for the purpose of thinking of them and indulging the grief which it causes*). *Nat-m* is not haunted by the past; she herself haunts her own past. How often this is seen in marriages in which one or both partners fall into the process of transference, the tendency to perceive another person as a character from one's early childhood, as the father or mother. They might initially fall (the word is appropriate here!) genuinely in love with each other. However, they discover later (or sooner) that they have fallen in love with a phantom, with a transference object, with the projection of their archaic anima or animus, with qualities possessed by their mothers or fathers but that are, on closer view, absent in the partner (opposites attract!). Frequently, such partners end up hating each other as a result of disappointment in this ghost figure! As one woman expressed to me: "We couldn't take out the garbage without a Geneva Accord!"

Discord Between Parents

It is evident, and generally accepted by modern scientists, that one of the most important tenets of normal early development in a child is the creation of a world in which a sense of security comes from the parents' love, courage, and honesty in facing the problems of daily life; it is crucial to offer an environment in which the child can grow normally, with his psyche firmly rooted in a loving spirit. Carl Jung used the term *participation mystique*, or mystical participation, a term coined by the French anthropologist Lévy-Bruhl, to describe a situation "in which the child feels the conflicts between parents and to suffer from them as if he owned them."[28] Jung stresses the fact that children are so deeply affected by the psychological atmosphere of the home that many children's problems can be traced to ongoing parental problems. Even when parents take great care not to discuss their difficulties in front of a child, it is not at all certain that the child remains unaware of them. "I always make sure my child does not witness any discord between me and my husband," a mother may reassure herself. But, as Jung stated, "Secret and unresolved issues can and will influence the child's health profoundly and taking the easy road, avoiding painful discussions, is not a solution. It is like a poisonous vapor that seeps slowly into the child's soul."[29] Jung stressed the fact that the child sees much more than the parent ever suspects. The child intuits the harsh things in life that parents don't want to face or have repressed. This is true for any child, but for the child with autism and a stagnant ego, such an "infection" is even more harmful if not treated successfully.

Up until age five, the ego of this child is still too unformed to be able to set up barriers against the invasion of forces moving in the unconscious world of the adult to whom he is still bound by the psychic umbilical cord. When the physical umbilical cord is cut, of course, a child becomes a separate physical entity; according to Jung and later psychologists such as William Emerson, though, the all-important psychological cord remains. A real psychological separation from the mother does not occur until much later, until about the seventh year. This is not to say that the child is a psychological duplicate of the parent, as the child has his own constitution and personality, but each child remains affected in his development by the attitudes of the parents and those in the close vicinity of the home. As everyone who has children knows, an infant reacts instantaneously, or even simultaneously, to every emotional change in the mother and in the environment—regardless of whether the mother is aware of her own state. Human infants exhibit the capacity for emotional contagion from the age of about six months, and in the beginning, the contagion is so complete that the individual is unable to distinguish between emotions that originate from one's own situation and emotions

28. Jung, *Development of Personality*, 124.

29. Ibid., 125.

originating in another person. In the first phase of ego evolution, the child's psyche seems to operate as a relatively undifferentiated unity, with no subject-object separation; additionally, there is no early differentiation between psyche and soma or between subject and environment.

Anger and Perceived Humiliation

What kind of anger does *Nat-m* experience? Anger that is *suppressed and with silent grief.* Here we see the nervous temperament of *Nat-m*, not the choleric or sanguine temperament, because most of the pain is held in. Anger is, of course, a cover for fear, which is much more damaging to the ego; therefore, the displacement is ideal when confronted with the *fear for men* or the fear of what men can do to her (*deception causing grief and mortification*). *Nat-m* is an introvert feeling type, but, as we see, it brews a storm for which the offending party will pay with damnation (*hatred to those who have offended; hatred and revenge*). It does not help that the offending party steels himself to apologize; even if he was fully justified in his original behavior, *Nat-m* will hear nothing of an apology! "Hate is, the eternal negation. Considered from the context of the emotions, it is a form of atrophy and kills everything but itself."[30] Hatred that is one-sided and not expressed can lead to destructive violence (*violent and vehement at trifles*) as well as unhappy love (*love, disappointed, from sadness with silent grief*), unsatisfied neediness, and a sense of rejection (*offended easily; takes everything in bad part*). The anger is not as strong as the grief, so a reaction can come later (depending on the dominant miasmatic state and true constitution of the person); if the anger remains unexpressed, though, *Nat-mur's* wrath does nothing but grow!

There is nothing that drains blood from the heart more than relationship problems, whether with family or with lovers and friends. Such problems affect the heart directly and disturb the distribution and the circulation of blood; this is part of the reason for which *Nat-m* withdraws into her shell for quite some time after a heartbreak. However, the male part of her (or sword side, or animus) will inevitably appear, taking revenge for any perceived humiliation when the archaic thinking function overcomes the usually dominant conscious feeling function: it is the making of a perfect storm in which *Nat-m* finally asserts that she is coming into her own, that her life will now take an entirely different course!

---

30. Oscar Wilde, *De Profundis, The Complete Works of Oscar Wilde,* (New York: HarperCollins Publishers, 1958), 897.

Nat-m can be the victim of bullying from a young age, being called "weird," a "freak" and whatever else children can come up with (*ailments from mortification; ailments from anger with indignation*). But it is during this delicate period of childhood that one learns resentment (*hatred to those who have offended*). Repressed feelings contained for a long time are bound to break into consciousness—either through an event, word, or gesture referring to that painful old complex in the shadow side, or by appropriate treatment with homeopathic *Nat-m*. At that moment, pent-up feelings of anger and hostility burst forth with unimaginable strength. It is like a copious bowel movement after a long period of constipation or, to use Freud's terminology, a catharsis—which is not always welcomed at that moment by the family of the patient or even by the patient herself. It seems more convenient for everyone involved to let sleeping dogs lie, but doing so results in a freeze in the patient's individuation process. It is much wiser to proceed cautiously with well-determined, judiciously applied homeopathic *Nat-m* doses. Only with the right key (the homeopathic simillimum) to open the door of the guarded vault of the unconscious, together with the judicious management, dose, and potency (and not withdrawing more than what the vital force allows) can the process be considered safe, leading to a successful outcome for the patient!

Compensations and Consequences

Naivety in the First Stage

Often, as a child, in the solitude of unexpressed bitterness toward the mother, *Nat-mur* has populated her adventures and inner world of fantasy with nature and animals (*animals, love for; love for horses*). They were the trusted ones and never rejected her. Equally trusted are her imaginary friends and lovers in the illusionary world. The escape into *delusion, of fancy illusions* entails the creation of an ideal fantasy world and a disconnection from the real world. If we want to know the meaning of this, we need look no further than *Nat-mur's* acute: *Ignatia*, with her CD of *being married and pregnant*. Even *Nat-c* flees into such a dream world, since she has a similar preoccupation: belonging to the *Natrums*, she is looking for a mother and all that accompanies her. *Nat-c* has *delusions, about a wedding* and *hearing music*, although she is unable to connect to the outside world; she remains so throughout her life if untreated—fixed in that *Carbon* state of inertia and immobility, unable to move forward. *Nat-m* is more like *Nat-c* in this first stage: often born with that sense of loneliness, she will look at any person as a source, a nourishing vessel, foolishly falling in love and not understanding why it turns out so badly time after time. But there is no point of return; she persists, as she is overcome by the desire to connect to others. ("There must be someone out who fits me!") At this point, everyone out there in the world is a potential mother! A friendly word, a compassionate gesture, an unselfish deed: all are sure signs that she is loved by the person. So the fancy world that the immature young *Nat-m* has created for herself is a world of the birds, the bees, the flowers and eternal love! What other delusions belong to this group? *Delusion, delirium with conversing*: driven by her CD, there is frantic behavior (delirium) even in her conversation, because she will do anything to secure the relationship. This delirious talk is certainly noted by the target of her attention.

Before withdrawing into her cocoon like a wounded animal, *Nat-m* in this first phase tries to be *yielding* to the source of love; this is expressed by the *delusion, head belongs to another, delusion of being double,* and *delusion, errors of personal identity*. These fixed ideas are most often created in people who are dominated (*Alum, Anac, Nit-ac, Viol-tricolor, Hura Braziliensis,* etc.), with the danger of leading to a dissociation or psychotic break. But is this the case here? *Nat-m* does not realize that to be part of a couple in a loving relationship does not mean that she must give up her identity as an individual. Alas, at this point, *Natrum* **wants** to give her identity away; as she is being voluntarily dominated, this is **not** a sacrifice, although this is not the way *Nat-m* will see it. *Nat-m*, in this psoric stage, does not love herself enough to cultivate her own true persona and ego. She will do anything to secure that relationship, even if she has to give up most of her personality and her own wishes, because she has no greater wish than to get to know and to belong to that other person, and then to become one with the essence of the desired person! At this point, *Nat-m* has a vacuum in her ego consciousness: despite all the stimuli that come to her from the outside, only one obsessive thought persists, creating mental poverty (*thoughts persistent*). She is possessed by the thought of that other person, breeding the illusion that the perfect person is out there, just around the corner, waiting to be found. She is *absorbed, buried in thought, as to what would become of her* and *forgetful of purchases, goes off and leaves them.*

It is easy to see that she suffers from an error of personal identity, but is she double? Two personalities? Has she come to the point of having *two wills*, which would really indicate the presence of a split personality? To determine the answer, we must consider the other dominant remedies in this rubric and determine whether a certain theme can be observed: *Anac, Bapt, Gels, Nux-m, Petroleum, and Stramonium* are all in this rubric. We think also of further remedies such as *Anhalonium* and *Alumina*. All of these remedies show remarkable poverty on the mental level as well as loss of independence, just like *Nat-m* in this phase. All of these remedies are double in the sense that **most of the personality is subsumed into that of the other person**; depending on the remedy and how much the person must give away in order to receive the needed support and reciprocity, a small percentage of individuality remains intact. In this way, *Nat-m* invites others to come into her world and to dictate what they want her to be: submissive, resigned, and complying (*Nat-m* is *yielding*). It makes us think of *Carcinosin* and, of course, *Staphysagria*, with which *Nat-m* is often confused. These secondary delusions are reflected and exposed by her infantile behavior, which reflects an archaic ego and plain foolishness. She will do anything to attract the attention of others, but she is not aware of her often inappropriate and primitive behavior.

It is also easy for *Nat-m* in the psoric phase to let other people do the talking for her: *she is distracted while talking and does not know what she ought to say*; *she is awkward in talking and easily makes mistakes*. By trying to forget who you are, you reduce your substance! Not being your natural self also leads you to feel jealousy and hatred towards others who are more successful in securing a relationship (*hatred and revenge*). It certainly invites domination, insensitivity, and rudeness, all of which are triggers that deepen *Nat-mur's* isolated state. *Nat-m* in this phase makes me think of a song from the 1960s called "Puppet on a String" ("If you say you love me madly, I'll gladly be there like a puppet on a string"); there is no doubt as to **who** pulls the strings: not *Nat-m*! Typical *Nat-mur* expressions at this stage include "I am so into him," confirming that she has given up her own identity! She wants to **be** the other person, thinking it will secure the relationship while in fact setting herself up for failure after failure in her relationships (*ailments from disappointed love*).

Loss of Self-Esteem and Further Isolation

In the second phase, when relentless attacks on her heart have reduced *Nat-m* to a shadow of herself, we see many secondary delusions appearing as a form of protection and compensation. There is the delusion *she is pitied on account of her misfortune and she wept*: there is a lot of self-pity and weeping. She starts ruminating excessively about her failures to succeed in a trusting relationship (*sad thoughts, persistent*), and she therefore becomes a prisoner of her past. She begins to dwell on the fact that her partner left her; her brain runs a file search and pulls up thousand possible reasons for which he might have abandoned her. What follows is melancholy, low self esteem, obsessive wondering about what went wrong, fantasies about its being set right, lingering in strategic places (restaurants, work place) to catch a glimpse of the person, making telephone calls to hear the other's voice on the answering machine; no other activities hold interest for her (*indifference to everything; indifference to pleasure*). Occasionally, *suicidal thoughts* may arise. Does all this lead to any substantial of introspection at this point? Although Eros/feeling is her dominant conscious function, meaning that connection with the unconscious should be favored, this is clearly not the case at this point. In the sycotic phase, *Nat-m* will exaggerate her efforts; she will continue to try to connect, often to a person who is as lost as she is (an alcoholic, a drug user, or a fellow sufferer). But *Nat-m* is determined to form a new entity with that particular person, to create a unit that allows her to use the word "we," convinced that the person she has found is the right one and desperately wanting the other to feel the same way about her. *Nat-m*, when she feels that a relationship is troubled, rather than fleeing the hornet's nest, she is gripped by a grim determination to make it work no matter what (*loyal in relationships*). It often leads to getting married to the wrong guy to rescue him, even becoming involved with a married guy (*love with the wring person, a married man,* only *Nat-m*)! But *Nat-m*, believing that she needs to make a relationship work at all costs, is on an exhausting and corrosive path—one that rarely works! Great sadness is present, and although we know *Nat-m* to be a silent weeper (*sadness, cannot weep*), it is not the case in this phase. Tears actually come rather easily when she is pitied by friends, therapist, or homeopath about her misfortune (whether ignoble or noble, as her situation is as often as much her fault as it is others'). This is expressed in several provings: *she is very much inclined to weep with disinclination to work; he rejoiced over something but his joy speedily passed off; sad and weeping without cause; attacks of complete hopelessness and internal despair, that deprived him of all power. Whenever alone she wished to cry and she did not know why. Consolation aggravates and fluttering of the heart follows.* There is even *lachrymose depression,* which is < *being spoken to with concern for the future.* Recurrent deceptions and betrayals lead all too easily to further fixed ideas: *there is delusion, sees thieves*—her heart is stolen, not her possessions. She wanted to give everything away, heart included, but this precious gift has been taken for granted. As a consequence, she starts looking in the mirror with a sense of antagonism and horror: *delusion, wretched, when she is looking in a mirror* and *delusion, of being emaciated.* There is self-loathing and hatred eating away at her confidence that she will meet the right person. The emotional trauma has begun to take a toll on *Nat-m* in this phase as her body changes under the pressure of grief and deception and lack of confidence. Water retention appears throughout the body: *edema in the face, especially around the eyes* (Apis, Nat-m), *edematous swelling of the feet* and cellulite in thighs, causing her body to assume a pear-shaped form. Most of her sadness is reflected in her face, and she is horrified to see her suffering etched there: *face waxy; face wrinkled; face bloated; lips chapped and cracked, corners of mouth cracked, circles around the eyes; face pale* and *herpetic eruptions,* making her look like a much older woman (*delusion, of being emaciated*).

She now takes on the delusion, *she is doomed.* She is stuck in this phase, and it is hard for her to imagine finding a solution; this is not only because of a lack of self-confidence but also because of repeating the same questions: "Did I do everything I could? Where did I go wrong?"—a rather misplaced sentiment, as *she reproaches herself. She is continually haunted with thoughts that something unpleasant will happen* and *she is gloomy and foreboding* (we see the anticipation anxiety, the apprehension, and the stress from which a *Nat-m* patient suffers). Because of the rather bleak situation she is in, *she suffers from despair* and *has a hopeless feeling about the future.* This delusion leads to many fears: *of dogs, of evil, of losing her reason,* which can actually lead to the delusion, *fear of people, of robbers* as well as *sees thieves.* All these emotions express a sense of forsakenness and stifling solitude. In order to regain some sense of power, self-control, and superiority to undo the horror of deception and rejection, as well as the feeling that she is unattractive to the outside world (*delusion, wretched when looking in the mirror*), *Nat-m* can fall into the trap of starving herself (*anorexia nervosa*); now, the power to keep on defeating hunger feels like true triumph, something that eludes her in everyday life. But *Nat-m* does not consider the dire consequences of this self-destructive behavior, which include *amenorrhea, infertility,* and brittle bones breaking; and yes, she now correctly sees a corpse sticking out of a fancy dress when she looks in the mirror, transforming her delusion into reality (*delusion, wretched when looking in the mirror*). The anorexia starts dictating everything she does and is, from going to bed when other people get up, from avoiding intimate and pleasurable gatherings (*indifference to pleasure*), to the absolutely necessary isolated run in the park. Such an illusion of control, a Pyrrhus victory, extends into everything else in her life: how she behaves at work (withdrawing as not to fall into the seductions of food and drink), how much money she spends, and how often she sees family (who might deter her from her chosen path). But along with coldness, tiredness, oversleeping, *sleeplessness from grief,-weakness of memory for mental labor,* trouble concentrating (*on attempting to concentrate has a vacant feeling*), self-hatred, *self reproach* and hunger comes excruciating loneliness: social contact dwindles quickly, because it can't be separated from food and drink.

At this point, it is not uncommon for *Nat-m* to resort to the bottle, which sometimes restores her appetite: *food is again relished and appetite returns after drinking wine several times.* She can even become addicted to alcohol, as such an addiction represents the search for a sense of security, a sense of being loved, and, in *Nat-mur's* case, a sense of control over her life. Eventually, though, *Nat-m* will learn that alcohol does not console her or fill up her psychological emptiness. Drinking and anorexia both blunt the bleakness of her existence while making things worse. Gratification through alcohol is temporary and illusory, and drinking results only in greater self-disgust (*delusion, she looks wretched when looking in the mirror*; *reproaches herself*), reduced bodily control (*awkward and drops things from nervous weakness*), and poorer coping ability (*hypochondriacal anxiety*).

The opposite reaction is also possible: comfort eating, a common form of self-sabotage (*sadness with canine hunger*, *Ignatia* too). It is, of course, paradoxical that *Nat-m* tries to help herself with hurtful behaviors. There is a lot of *self-reproach, guilt and homesickness* (the latter with the extended meaning of "longing for the good old times"). One thing is sure: the feeling of guilt and self-accusation creates sadness, self-loathing, and loathing of life (*suicidal ideation*), a mix of very unpleasant emotions to which *Nat-m* succumbs.

In despair, and unable to chase the bitterness from her heart, she asks herself at times if she is becoming insane: *delusion, she becomes insane.* This does not mean that she has already progressed to dissociation; all of us have had moments in which we have asked ourselves the same question. But certainly the first cracks in the walls are showing, which is not surprising as we know that *Nat-m* is a dominant feeling person prone to hysterical outbursts. Although her ego is still in control of her conscious, *Nat-m knows* in her more lucid moments that she is losing control; her weakness at this point is on the physical level, not the emotional—like *Phosphoricum acidum*, for instance, as evidenced in the *Nat-m* expressions of *cold sores, numbness in the face* (*os zygomaticus, multiple sclerosis* (MS), *infertility, vaginismus* [*painful coition*] and so on.

To make matters worse, a touch of paranoia sets in: *delusion, she is persecuted.* She is convinced that someone (or society, or fate) is deliberately obstructing her path (*China, Aurum*).

Of course, she fails to see that the regressive infantile mode of her persona makes her a perfect victim, which will only continue the vicious cycle of connecting and failing. As she feels she has been injured in the past, she is *now easily offended* by innocent remarks. It is as though she is convinced that everyone knows about her suffering and that people are out to hurt her. Such paranoia leads, again, to isolation—which only exacerbates her suffering and her incapability to reach out to others.

All these delusions show *Nat-mur's* anguish about her situation. The cave to which she wants to withdraw is called despair; and the ground is paved with the gravestones of abandoned hope: *despair about the future, despair with the pains* (emotional) and *despair, thinks everything is lost* (*Ignatia*!). *Nat-m* removes herself from humanity and real life at this point, forgetting that there is no prison into which love cannot find an entrance. She forgets that when we grief we don't have to turn into cold marble or trees. The most terrible thing about a broken heart is not that one's heart can be broken—hearts are made to be broken—but that in *Nat-mur's* case, grief and deception turns her heart to stone.

Intellect and Introspection

In a later phase, when heartbreaks have become part of her past, *Nat-m* often develops into a very serious young woman, prone to thinking herself unattractive (*delusion, wretched when looking in the mirror*) and to withdrawal on account of it (*disheartened all day, without definite cause*); she remains, however, an excellent student who stays near the top of her class. There is hope for *Nat-m*. If she can become introspective, gaining insight into what is unique and authentic in her and in her suffering, she can transform herself and infuse her life with new meaning.

Revenge and Hatred

Looking at *Nat-mur's* causalities, it is easy to see how she can justify seeking revenge in her life. As a result of suffering so many emotional injustices, *Nat-m* burns with a thirst for revenge (*hatred and revenge to those who have offended*); it is often said that revenge is sweet. This is confirmed by the many sacrifices *Nat-m* makes simply in order to take revenge and without any real intention of gaining recompense. But one must remember that *Nat-m* suffers nothing as painful as the *deception and betrayal* of others. Suffering inflicted by the will of others includes a bitter and painful addition to the injury itself: namely, the recognition of someone else's control together with that of one's own impotence. By returning the injury, *Nat-m* imposes her will upon the offender, which, at least in her mind, cancels out his dominance over her.

Having been rejected through, perhaps, a casual text message—after always being there for her "soul mate," showering attentions on him by phone and in person, and shopping for the perfect cute cards to send him (hello, Mr. *Medorrhinum*!)—*Nat-m* often executes well-planned acts of revenge that are perfectly proportional to the original injury in every way. After reading over the break-up message "way too many times," *Nat-m* might use his own words and post them on Facebook, asking friends, even strangers and acquaintances to comment; this, of course, always evokes a flood of anger towards Mr. Casual by other equal hurt parties. *Nat-m* defeats his overinflated ego by sending him these responses, which make him look like the adolescent and jerk he is. He has stolen *Nat-mur's* sense of self-worth, and revenge for *Nat-m* means getting it back by stealing his! This tell-all is a classic (and, in *Nat-mur's* mind, classy) act of revenge made possible in an instant, by the push of a button through social media.

Nat-mur thus acquires the satisfaction she sought, magically undoing what has been done to her in reality. However, "an eye for an eye" is a rather primitive reaction of the crippled and out-of-control *Nat-m* person, and it is only a fleeting delusion. Instead of looking in her shadow side, *Nat-mur* keeps sowing thorns in the garden of her heart. The pleasure she hoped to experience is annihilated by the fact that exacting this revenge subsequently breaks someone else's heart; her motivation is now gone, but the proof of her wickedness remains visibly etched on her face (*delusion, wretched when looking in the mirror; malicious, spiteful and vindictive; face, cracked, lips; cracked corners of the mouth*). *Nat-m* is walking through a desert of existence which she has created; while she is traveling, no sun protecting tree is found, every rock loses its shadow, and every oasis dries up. Solitude, suffering, and sadness are her fate! *Nat-m* should consider what the famous Persian poet Hafiz (1320-1389) revealed in one of his stunning verses: "The heart is a thousand-stringed instrument that can only be tuned with love."

Not all *Nat-m* persons react vengefully, as some prefer to live productively; they may join support groups or become psychotherapists or crusaders, therefore proving that the desire to turn tragedy into a positive force can be stronger than the desire for revenge. The most destructive consequence for the betrayed *Nat-m* person is that her disappointment can lead to a hatred of life (*indifference to pleasure; to everything*), with increasingly cynical behavior and a growing aversion to mankind (*censorious, critical; aversion to opposite sex* and *family members*). Life itself does not progress and seems to circle around one center of pain; suffering becomes one long moment, creating a paralyzing immobility. At this point, *Nat-m* has forgotten the four pillars of a life of well-being: positive emotions (**not** hatred, revenge, and loathing of life), engagement with what one is doing, a sense of accomplishment, and, above all, a good relationship.

Living in the Past: Living in a Cocoon in the Final Stage

Finally, *Nat-m* crashes into the third or syphilitic phase. *Nat-m* can present, at this point, two separate types: the **passive** one, remembering the "good old times" as well as dwelling on her past sad times, or the **active** one, playing the role of a crusader.

Let's look at the passive type. It is a mistake for this *Nat-m* to think (as she often does) that she has moved on, that she has dealt with her past issues, that she has freed herself from suppressed material. In reality, she has only removed herself from it; in most cases, it remains in the unconscious, which is the mother of conscious and will therefore directly influence her conscious actions and thoughts. In spite of all this, most people who need *Nat-m* are the first ones to try to convince you that they have moved on and that they now live a normal and productive life. Often, in an attempt to reduce emotional volatility, well-meaning friends or therapists have rushed *Nat-m* into moving on. This is not the best course of action, which is shown by the rubric *persistent sad thoughts* and the proving that *Nat-m*, unlike *Sepia*, likes to think and reminisce about sad episodes caused by others (*tries to recollect past disagreeable occurrences for the purpose of thinking on them and indulging the grief which it causes; gloomy thoughts, recalls insults long since suffered. Always in his thoughts he seemed to seek for past unpleasant occurrences, in order to think them over, making herself morbid. He tormented himself, he seemed to prefer disagreeable thoughts, which prostrated him very much*). So the disagreeable occurrences have basically become part of her life, of her baggage. We humans can get used to carrying such a suitcase—even if it never gets emptied. As stated in A38, new events **postpone and suspend** but do **not** cure the old events! This is evident when some slight word or gesture, or a birthday or holiday, releases the suppressed material from the unconscious. It is all the result of burying distrust and resentment that continue to worsen, sometimes for decades, forever precluding the possibility of future closeness. The first qualities to disappear are openness, insightfulness, cooperativeness, empathy, and trust in future relationships—so the next person *Nat-m* meets has to suffer for the sins of a stranger! Establishing closeness with future partners becomes very difficult. She wears gloom as a king wears purple; she often swears never to smile again. Yes, hearts are made to be broken, and *Nat-m* is proof of this, but hearts are not made to turn to stone! *Nat-m* must forgive her enemies for her own sake.

Even more, these suppressed (not repressed, which are deeper and entirely forgotten) memory fragments remain in their primitive and childhood state; as such, they are still strong and immediate. Only when they are reintegrated into the adult consciousness (through therapy or homeopathy) can they shed their infantile and primitive aspect and be corrected. These infantile memories are like an avalanche, surprising *Nat-m* and those around him with their crude, violent nature. New delusions are now formed: *delusion, talking with dead people*; *hears distant voices* and *voices of dead people*; *sees faces when stooping*. "Dead people" symbolize a regression to the unconscious: remaining in and withdrawing to the unconscious. The world of the living is left behind (*anthropophobia*; *avoids company*). Part of life is striving for a relationship, but that part is now dead; relationships do take another form, one of nourishing *Nat-m's* soul through connection with a narrower segment of the world: her fellow sufferers, motivated not by injustice, but more by *grief causing hatred*. *Nat-m* has now retreated into a cave, close to the Eternal Mother. Both the cave and the Divine Mother are symbols in dreams of the collective unconscious; this is the return to safety and protection, the womb. The person has become a caveman again, shunning the light or consciousness and lowering herself, hauling herself into that protective hole (*delusion, sees faces when stooping*). "Stooping" is getting closer to the lower parts of the Self, or, more precisely, the personal unconscious, and trying to immerse oneself in it. This type of *Nat-m* experiences profound discordance because she is in the company of others but she never truly connects to them. In a world abound with anonymous faces, burning the candle at both ends, eating and sleeping amid people who remain distant and aloof, *Nat-m* is at risk of slipping into detachment, isolation, and possible dissociation. *Nat-m* measures time by throbs of pain, deceits and betrayals, and the recall of bitter moments (*dwells over past on past disagreeable events and recalls disagreeable memories*). The remembrance of her suffering is necessary to *Nat-m* as evidence of her continued existence. There is only a small light in the cave (there is always Yang in the Yin), and that small light is the symbol for the remaining connection she has: her kinship with those who have suffered similar fates. Society has no more place for her and has none to offer. Her tears made clefts in the rocks of her unconscious where she finds a place to hide, a secret valley in whose silence she can weep undisturbed.

The second psoric type, the **active** one, takes another road; still, though, she is unconsciously attached to a past event. The active *Nat-mur* person has found solace in volunteering or in becoming an activist. She volunteers for political campaigns, libraries, hospitals, or the like, and may be involved in a group supporting victims of some sort. Loneliness is still part of her life, but the blow is softened by other interests that keep her busy: a profession (psychotherapy, perhaps), a recreation (attending concerts of classical music or baking for her church), or a relationship with God. She even makes a great business out of her "crusader's plans," expressing her views and suffering on websites and blogs, which is ideal as she now lives only for that purpose (I think of the crime fighters and MADD [Mothers Against Drunk Driving]). Even if there is still a husband at home, and he is the cause of her continued grief, the person in a *Nat-m* state can now simply accept this; she pays little, if any, attention to him. Often a beloved dog or cat takes the place of the husband/friend to fill the void. Together with the crusader business, the animal leads her to think that her life is "fulfilled"; little unhappiness is expressed, as it is relegated to her unconscious. For this *Nat-m* type, the ugly dress that makes sorrow grotesque to look at, the separation, the deceit, the silence, the solitude, the shame, each and all of these things, *Nat-m* has transformed into spiritual experiences.

For the crusader *Nat-m*, there are two sources of emotional nourishment and spiritual enlightment: she has her crusader's goal and the memory of her loved one who met an unfortunate death, to whom she talks. "I am doing this for you, dear, so your death will not have been in vain." The quality of such communication (*delusion, talking with dead people and ghosts*) is entirely different from that of a conversation with a living person. When we are in the company of others, there exists an interpersonal energy: all of us have felt it as we experience in person the uplifting and the depressive powers of others. Interpersonal energy has, of course, a changing character, but even the worst moments make us feel alive as we struggle against the tide's ebb and flow. Communicating with dead people, though, leads to further isolation, indicating that *Nat-m* does not believe there to be anyone out there worth communicating with. Such a person truly lives in the past; there is no thought of present or future. It is healthy for the past to serve as a guide for the future, but remaining in the past is like dying minute by minute, as if one is attending one's own slowly evolving funeral.

Of the two types of *Nat-m*, the crusader is clearly compensating in the more favorable way: she has at least found a positive solution, yet it is sometimes she who fares the worst. Why? Granted, **both** types are stuck, motivated by sad memories, and neither of the two continues her path of individuation (although both, especially the crusader, are convinced they are indeed doing so). But the crusader suppresses her feelings of grief; "forgetting" is not equivalent to freeing oneself from the past. On the contrary, the situation becomes worse: by refusing to face her demons, she allows them to attack her from behind—where she is unaware and defenseless. Certain situations, gestures, or innocent words can be enough to raise the beast (the delegation of unresolved issues) from the unconscious and provoke "normal insanity" (temporary upheaval) when her deeply buried emotions are aroused. The *Nat-m* person gets in a rage about the past incident as though it has happened quite recently rather than (for instance) thirty years ago (*quarrelsome, gets into a passion about trifles*). It only leads to *Nat-mur's* opinionated and even harsh judgments about others (where her animus is dominating—*censorious; contemptuous; consolation, kind words aggravate*), as she feels entitled to cite her "noble misfortunes." However, it is not uncommon that the *Nat-m* patient will try to convince the homeopath that she is over this grief: she claims that she does not wish to talk about past offenses as she wants to move on. For *Nat-m*, it becomes "us against the others" (*Nit-ac*): either you share her opinions, drive, and interests or you are to be ignored (if not hated for resembling the antagonists in her life story). Frequently, this leads to great turmoil in her own family as the driven and centered *Nat-m*, consumed with her crusade, isolates herself from relatives; divorce is often a sad consequence, fueling even further the fire of grief, injustice, and betrayal.

The first *Nat-m* type (the passive one) knows her enemy: she **knows** she is stuck, she **wants** to be stuck in the past, and she **accepts** it as her fate. She appears to be more selfish than the crusading *Nat-m*, but this one at least knows her enemy. She does not suppress her feelings; she **wallows** in them! Most *Nat-m* people of this type are still unforgiving of the perpetrator of the perceived or real injustice (*hatred of people who had insulted him-delusion*), which leads to further—but now accepted and somewhat comfortable—isolation. But in one sense, it is certainly also detrimental to such an individual: life becomes meaningless for people who prefer to close their eyes and live in the past, and they suffer now from a **spiritual** disease. Compared with the crusader *Nat-m*, this passive kind of *Nat-m* simply ignores the challenge to attain some last meaning and greatness in her suffering. The crusader at least sees an opportunity in her grief and tries to turn her life into an inner triumph, throwing herself wholeheartedly into her sole cause as it gives her inner strength and points to a goal to which she can aspire. I think that, in the end, both types are in need of homeopathic *Nat-m* to rescue them from the stagnation that overtakes their lives. Only then will the rejection-fearing *Nat-m* feel more secure, which will pave the way for a happier existence and the possibility of future relationships with human fellows. An empty email inbox will be no longer a sign of impending doom (*delusion, being doomed*) and harsh reproach; it will be, rather, just an empty inbox and not a rebuff.

All these third-phase syphilitic delusions point to self-imposed exile and loneliness, either to communicate with dead relatives (often in dreams) or to protect oneself with an impenetrable wall from the world, which is viewed as an enemy territory. *Nat-m* hides the depth of her wound not only from other people, but even from herself. It looks like she has made a marvelous adjustment, but if anyone comes too close, she retreats to her tower of safety and takes up the drawbridge, convinced that her isolation has been forced upon her by other people, unfortunate circumstances, or noble misfortunes.

Nat-m patients, often dominated by the introverted feeling conscious function, are still waters that run deep and are usually women. Their emotions are contained within, which tends to separate them from other people. Because their feeling function is held so intensely within, in their final stage, they come across as being as cold as the wastes of the North Pole, remote and difficult to approach. *Nat-mur's* only safety is to build a wall around herself (living in a cocoon) so that nobody can get near her, shielding herself from outside contact and never trusting anyone with her real thoughts and feelings. *Nat-mur* people seem shy and inarticulate, and they find communication difficult. At times this makes them appear paranoid and hysterical. Only homeopathic doses of *Nat-m* can break through the illusory wall that hems such a patient in; few from the outside world will ever be able to find the key to the quasi-invisible door to her world or to reach the precious little oasis of reality in the desert of her soul. But the walls of her sheltered, tight circle of security crumble when

Nat-m can finally open her soul to the psychotherapist—whom, incidentally, she at first did not consider to be "a real person," but more a fixture there to listen to her, to unload on as she ridded herself of her garbage and the skeletons in her closet. Upon leaving the office, though, she goes back to her prison cell of self-isolation, which is now dutifully restored with mortar and pestle to hide the temporary opening; at the end stage, her heart is closed as a fist, at least towards most people (*company, aversion to presence of other people* and *desire for solitude*). In addition to engaging with a psychotherapist, *Nat-m* needs to talk to the offending party (often the husband or ex-lover) about what happened, but the other party can't bear or has no desire to talk about it. They have become two persons unable to communicate, one speaking Greek, the other German. As such, *Nat-m* finds relief only with her trusted psychotherapist and, occasionally, with a good friend with whom she can discuss her deep mistrust of society. However, *Nat-m* and her therapist must beware: scrutinizing the patient's past, and trying to understand every bit of it before trying to move on, can become a kind of addiction that keeps the focus on the past and not on the present or the future. At this point *Nat-m* might avoid intimacy altogether—averting stormy relationships but losing out on the chance to find acceptance and support. This, of course, puts her at risk for loneliness and depression.

The Awakening

Both *Nat-m* types are somewhat resigned to their fate. They come to terms with their lack of a relationship; they accept the loneliness. ("I don't think there is anyone out there who would be right for me. I never want to get married again. I am happy the way I am now.") Of course, when homeopathic *Nat-m* is administered, those suppressed feelings of forsakenness, betrayal, and deception might come up—something the patient may not initially appreciate, as it rocks the core of her soul like a boat caught in an unanticipated storm! "My life was serene until I took your remedy!" she cries out. What she does not realize is that, when the unconscious is totally discarded, as much as half of her conscious life may be as good as dead! Reducing her life to a fraction of its potential deprives *Nat-m* and others of many possible pleasures and certainly hinders her individuation process, the psychological process that makes us into individuals and keeps us from living ghostlike existences like those of many *Nat-mur* people! Once such a person rises from the ashes of her former existence, she is the first one to recognize the value of admitting her mistake and moving forward.

"Promise me one thing," one of my patients said to her best friend: "never suppress your feelings for as long as I did!"

Nat-m has the tendency to suppress the truth about her emotions, and doing so creates unconscious knowledge. Few humans are aware of such well-guarded knowledge, and *Nat-m* suppresses the truth because if it were made conscious it would make her life (and others) too difficult and too dangerous. There is resistance when the painful truth threatens to come to the surface; such repugnance for her suppressed emotions is clearly demonstrated in slips of the tongue and in many other telltale symptoms: crying, not answering questions, looking away, awkward expressions, or even saying the very opposite of what one claims to believe and then seemingly forgetting it a moment later. *Nat-m* and other characters (*Lycopodium* and *Veratrum-a,* to name two) use a great deal of their energy to hide their own knowledge from themselves—and, of course, homeopathic *Nat-m* unseals the cave where all this knowledge has been stashed away: the homeopath must administer properly adjusted doses with timely repetition in order to ensure that this healing process does not become a tsunami, crashing into consciousness, as it can when the healing process goes too fast!

A child is no different from an adult in the repression of feelings. Having fewer tools to deal with painful issues such as loneliness and abandonment, the child needs to repress these feelings for fear of losing the love of her family forever. Flight into a dream world is necessary. One child's dream world was created by reading the adventures of the noble native American chief Winnetou, who in children's books was always there for the underdog, protecting the weak. However, this particular child was led to hang on to this ideal world even at a later age; as a result, whenever she set foot in the real world, "it was not at all so nice" as in her dream world. Having such shocking experiences every time she ventured out into the real world led eventually to physical symptoms in which she felt thrusts and shocks coming from her stomach and rising to her throat, keeping her awake at night. And before she could leave home, she had to encourage herself for hours to go, fearing the painful shock stemming from the dichotomy between the unconscious desired, imaginary dream world and the "cruel," real, conscious world. Such a child, unfortunately, grows up to an adult who is conflict-avoidant, not addressing things that are bothering her or asking for what she needs, hoping that difficulties will go away magically without having to disclose her wants and needs.

Always Looking for the Mother

It should be evident to the reader by now that *Nat-mur's* CD is present throughout her story, though it assumes slightly different forms. In the psoric phase, anyone can be the mother for the insecure, yielding *Nat-m*. In the second, sycotic stage, after having had multiple partners, the imaginary mother will be personified by a single source: her boyfriend, spouse, or a close friend. At this phase, *Nat-m* has settled down, has become a different individual (alas, not necessarily more mature, although possibly successful in business) and is now betrayed in her mind by the single maternal figure she counted on. In the third, or syphilitic, phase, the search for the mother has become symbolic: looking in herself, and withdrawing, she is on a quest for the Divine Mother of the collective unconscious, which can take the form of an animal, a recreation, or a crusade.

Golden Tips from the Masters

- The physical complaints are related to three issues: **1**. Reduced assimilation with tissue breakdown and underactivity of all glands: anorexia nervosa, >from fasting, face wrinkled, face cracked, face pale, dry lips, dry hair, emaciation of the face (from above downward), recurrent fevers, vaginismus, and hypothyroidism. **2.** Derangement of blood: anemia and disturbed regulation of body warmth (desire for open air, aversion to sun). **3**. Derangement of elimination: constipation, hay fever, urticaria, oily skin, herpes, retention of water
- Aggravation at the seashore: What does aggravation at seashore mean? It cannot be the salt air that aggravates, as salt is often craved by this person; it represents, symbolically, the border between the conscious and the unconscious and might reflect the urge to free oneself from all the suppressed material in the unconscious (sea).
- *Ignatia*, *Bryonia*, and *Apis* are acutes of *Nat-m*
- A combination of grief/guilt and deep resentment; cautious and skeptical individual with sharp tongue
- Fear of robbers and being attacked, fear for bodily harm
- These patients always ask for a bit of extra attention because they feel they have been neglected. *Nat-m* is a person who nice to know but not always nice to live with!
- Bursting, hammering headaches responsive to *Bryonia*. Never give *Nat-m* during such a headache as it would cause aggravation.
- #1 remedy for blocked eye ducts and Sjögren's disease!
- Strong dislike of oysters and fats
- #1 remedy for herpes labialis: these attacks are associated with emotions and stress.
- #1 remedy for psoriasis: Use *Nat-m* 6x! (also *Ars-iod*)
- Good sequence of remedies: *Sepia—Nat-m—Thuja*
- Indicated in cases of infertility (major remedy), MS, and Hodgkin's disease.
- No remedy on our materia medica is so often indicated in severe cases of malaria, whether acute or chronic
- Malaria prophylactic: take a 30C potency once a week for 6 weeks prior to exposure. Cures malaria from overuse of quinine
- #1 remedy for anorexia nervosa and bulimia (fear of rejection)
- *Nat-m* stands for the **S's: S**adness, **S**ensitive, **S**olitude, **S**ingle, **St**uck, **St**unted thoughts, **S**ilent, and **S**uppressed emotions

- Hard chill around 11 a.m. with great thirst and most violent headaches, the latter relieved by perspiration
- *Nat-m* is a warm-blooded individual (< > of *Nat-c*); both *Nat-m* and *Nat-c* are disturbed by being in a room full of people and suffer extreme weakness in summer heat
- Important remedies in early arthritis: #1: *Nat-m*; #2: *Sulphur*; #3: *Rhus-t* (Elizabeth Hubbard)
- Emaciation from above downward, especially of the neck: *Nat-m*, *Lyc*, *Sanicula*. From below moving upwards, especially emaciation of the legs: *Abrotanum*
- Approach of fever heralded by excessive thirst before the chill and during the chill, but no thirst during the fever when the hammering headache starts

Nitricum acidum (Nit-ac). Nitric Acid

The Cyber Delusion

In *Nit-ac* there are two main groups of delusions with a common denominator: the sense that there is danger everywhere in the world, a feeling which can lead to isolation and hypervigilance. It is more than the sense of danger of *Calc-c*, who is afraid of suffering and calamities everywhere (*talks about nothing but murder, fire and rats*). *Nit-acid's* first group of fixed ideas refers to the conviction that everyone seems to be out to harm him. The second group indicates *Nit-ac's* hypochondriasis: he is convinced that his health is poor and that few people can be trusted to help him in his quest for well-being (*delusion, he has an incurable disease, delusion being sick* and *delusion he is about to die*). No amount of reassurance can help him. His brain is so powerful that it really can convince itself of illness. He knows something is wrong because he believes what he is thinking, and what he is thinking is what he perceives himself to be feeling. These delusions tend to reduce the *Nit-ac* to a restless and fretful but combative individual. His nightstand is always topped with a cornucopia of pill bottles, and his hands routinely tremble as if his fingers housed jumping beans. His Cyber delusion is expressed by the ***delusion, he is engaged in lawsuits*** (***anxiety as he was engaged in a lawsuit or dispute, causing uneasiness***). This "engaging in lawsuits" means that life, as mentioned before, is a constant struggle for *Nit-ac*, and not merely a metaphorical one against want of health, but also an actual struggle against other people. *Nit-ac* discovers adversaries everywhere, lives in continual conflict, and dies with the sword in his hand. His CD is supported by the *delusion, about criminals.*

Everyone, or almost everyone, is considered an enemy (*Mercury*). The government, newspapers, and TV newscasters are engaged in a conspiracy against him, scheming against his welfare and that of his family. Doctors are not to be trusted, as they are in cohorts with pharmaceutical companies; the Internet and blogs are God-given resources to bolster his lawyer-like arguments (*disposition to contradict; intolerant of contradiction; contemptuous and cynical;*

irritable when spoken to). These lawyerly thoughts disappear and reappear constantly in his mind (*thoughts, disagreeable and tormenting*). He will argue with any authority; entering the army is **not** a good option for *Nit-ac*! In fact, he does not trust any authority; the lawsuits refer also to the fight for the preservation of his health: he feels he needs to be his own protector, his own doctor, his own attorney, and his own scientist. Intoxicated by what he feels is a life full of magnificent actions, *Nit-ac* identifies himself equally with ancient conquerors and saviors of society (*excitable during debate*). *Nit-ac* seems to resemble *Causticum*; however, *Causticum* always acts alone or in small groups, with a mind that is focused, determined, and cunning. Everything is well thought through and justified in *Causticum* (*cannot support injustice*), while *Nit-ac* is *impetuous* (*impulsive*) and overcome with *raging and raving delirium* as well as *cursing and swearing*. The question is: does *Nit-ac* have the tools to find a more peaceful solution to his problems? How many lawsuits does he win or lose? Before we explore this, we must, however, ask: how did he get into this anxious situation in the first place?

Causalities

Discords between Chief and Subordinates

The main NWS or ailments from (A/F) come from *discords between the chief* (of the family) *and subordinates*. Since the chief of the family has traditionally been the father, *Nit-acid's* Cyber delusion often stems from the intense control and domination exerted on him during childhood by a dominant father figure. The motherly principle is that of unconditional love; the mother loves her children not because they please her, but simply because they **are** her children. Fatherly love, on the contrary, is often conditional: it depends on the achievements and good behavior of the child. A father most loves the child who is most like him. Having failed to fulfill his father's criteria for success, *Nit-ac* has become a combatant and insurgent because of the strict authority and expectations of the father. This continuous struggle will mark the *Nit-acid* personality: he will aggravate when admonished (*admonition aggravates*; *intolerant of contradiction*), and he *swears and curses*. In other words, he is a volcano ready to erupt; at the same time, though, he is a nervous wreck continuously worrying about his health and *sensitive to all external impressions, especially to noise, and splashing of water*, and *easily startled from fright*. Even Nature's wrath and violence seems to unsettle *Nit-ac* (*mind symptoms aggravate during thunderstorm*). This main NWS of discords leads to some other NWS: *ailments from hurry, fright, grief and emotional* *excitement*. The latter NWS are all very understandable, thinking about the tight-fisted father who wants the youngster to follow his rules exactly. One thinks of *Lycopodium* fathers, who are quite abusive and domineering towards their families while yielding to superiors at work. The one-dimensional *Lycopodium* person, thinking only on a single plane, will do the most damage to those youngsters (teenagers) whose dominant conscious function is different (for instance, feeling). The betrayal of the youngster's dominant conscious function will lead to strong neuroses. In the case of *Nit-ac*, neurosis has everything to do with health and resistance to authority. Later on, any small unkindness, or even a well-intentioned remark, might drive him to absolute rage (*anger, violent*; *excitable with violent palpitations*), confirming for him that, indeed, it all comes down to "me against the rest of the world." *Nit-ac* is incapable of gaining insight about his real motivations through introspection, and he therefore projects everything (his unconscious) onto others. It is always the case that someone else has put him in a situation and should be blamed (*excitable during debate*; *irritable when spoken to*).

Compensations

Irrationality and Hypervigilance

There is one thing that *Nit-ac* seems unable to achieve: the confidence to approach his health issues with calmness and common sense (*despair with rage, cursing and imprecations*; *delusion, talking insane*; *delusion, talking irrationally*; *suicidal disposition with fear of death*). When he was younger, his ego was not allowed to develop; it was always challenged by the critical father figure, so now rebelling against others' opinions has become an automatic reflex—even later in life and even if opinions are given with the best intentions. This has caused the birth of secondary delusions about his health: "I am really sick and fear for my life" is his motto, and the *Nit-ac* person thinks that no one can be trusted to take the initiative to guard his health. The doctor had better be of his opinion and follow his advice as to what tests to perform—or he will look for another physician who will acquiesce! *Nit-acid*, therefore, approaches his health issues with an enormous amount of anxiety and fixed ideas of demise: *he has anxiety about his disease, with fear of death*; *morbid fear of the cholera*. This last idea reflects his fear of an incurable disease—in our time, fear of cancer.

Nit-ac has *anxiety from night watching* and is *sympathetic*, which makes us think of *Cocculus* with his proving symptom *little concerned as to his own health, but is very anxious about others' sickness.*

Upon closer inspection, *Nit-acid's* sympathy and concern do not go that far as he is *estranged from his family*. In the first place, the night watching is about his own health (*he is often anxious about his illness and constantly thinks about his past troubles; anxiety during sleep; sleep is anxious with sobbing, restless and unrefreshing and difficulties of going to sleep*). If *Nit-ac* devotes himself to night watching for someone else, it is for a friend who is always there to sympathize with him when he complains about his ailments (*lamenting, wailing; hysteria*) or for someone who shares his opinions. *Nit-acid* knows only two classes of people: those who are against him and those who are with him. It is this latter class, always a minority, that he is afraid to lose for the selfish reason that he needs their support (*after continued loss of sleep, long lasting anxiety, over exertion of the mind and body from nursing the sick, great anguish of mind from loss of dearest friend*). This is somewhat analogous to *Bar-c*! Towards his few friends, *Nit-ac* often has a guilty conscience, fearing that he might have offended them, something he cannot afford to do as it might lead to losing that crutch he counts on—just like *Arsenicum*, as we see in the *delusion, he has offended people*. Due to an uncontrolled temper (*fits of rages with curses and maledictions*), *Nit-ac* counts few people as friends, and everyone else out there is at best a stranger in his eyes, if not an enemy (*delusion, he is surrounded by strangers*). For *Nit-ac*, there are two ways to look at a problem: "my way and the wrong way." He cannot recognize the validity of others' views as potentially offering a more holistic approach to a given situation. He is incapable of learning from the other person, of learning to increase his ability to respond in a variety of ways. And being "for" *Nit-ac* and of his opinion means doing everything *Nit-ac* wants; it is a very selfish stance. If *Nit-ac* has a partner, she must give up her life to help achieve *Nit-acid's* goals, which, with his undeveloped ego, are rather limited.

Looking for Support

Nit-ac is driven by his fixed idea that death is near and yet no one has diagnosed his mysterious illness (*delusion, he has an incurable disease; fancies he will die soon, yet he is not physically ill*). What *Nit-ac* calls optimism is really mere persistence: he never gives up, as he keeps looking for the "genius" healer who will finally find **his** disease (no doubt a special one). *Nit-ac* is driven from physician to physician, anguished by his tormenting illness, real or perceived (*at once she is taken with a peculiar anguish, runs to her physician, but he is not at home, hires a carriage to drive to the home where she expects to find him; during her ride all her anguish is gone; arrived at home she feels as bad as ever, and feels herself thus forced to drive about the whole day; driving ameliorates the mental symptoms*).

He is convinced that no physician has ever diagnosed him correctly, as he must be suffering from an incurable disease (*anxiety about his disease, with fear of death; morbid fear of cholera*) or *from an impending disease* which surely will lead to his death (*fear for death; hopeless despair*). So this is, in a sense, a positive compensation: as long as he is on the road, thinking he will find a trusted physician who will solve the riddle of his illness, he feels better. That also means that the homeopath will have a hard time getting him out of the office at the end of a 30-minute follow-up visit! His talk is only about his disease, but at the same time he is very pessimistic and sucks the energy and patience out of his physician as he is convinced that "nothing will help." While optimists bask in the sunshine of the world's approbation (*Phosphorus* comes to mind), the pessimist mopes in the shadows. While the energizing force of optimism can convince a person to overcome any health issue, *Nit-ac's* pessimism about the outcome of a health issue mobilizes him to act with alacrity. There is nothing like a looming disaster (real or perceived) to make him get things done. *Nit-ac* believes he is a marked man, destined to suffer the torments of hell, roaming the earth in search of a little bit of relief that can only be found with a single trusted friend—who may be his always-empathetic homeopath. That trusted person is the raft he clings to, to clear the skies and escape the stormy seas. That is, until the homeopath or physician finds out he is composed of the letter **P**: **P**issed, a **P**est, **P**essimistic, and never **P**leased! Hahnemann calls it, in his *Chronic Diseases*, "a crabbed humor."

Hatred and Vindictiveness

Nit-ac is in the company of *Nat-m* when it comes to these feelings. Being a narcissist in the sense that he feels he belongs to an elite segment of the population that is always right—and that he sees himself as a targeted victim of the authorities—his honor can only be restored by revenge, which is based on his wounded narcissism. In order to "cure" his injury, *Nit-ac* must disobey the offender if not annihilate him. His motto is: "I get even and I move on with my life." Here is an example from the practice:

> While walking the dog in my neighborhood I got to know a 40-year-old man whose main topic of conversation consisted of complaints about anyone in his life: his co-workers, family, children, the drivers on the road, and especially the police (*lamenting, bemoaning, and wailing*). He often became beet red when telling of his altercations. He described one incident in which the police, when

> driving by his house, were concerned with the terrible abusive language (*cursing, swearing*) they heard coming from his house. It turned out that the ruckus was due to the fact that he had spilled a pan of hot water on himself. The arrival of the police only aggravated the outburst, and he turned the verbal abuse toward them (*cursing; rage with cursing*). He also recounted having gotten into an argument with his brother while doing errands in another town and deciding to walk home in the pouring rain. Obviously, his chief complaint was anger and irritability. I knew there had to be something else at the root of his problem. He also related to me that his brother, who was five years older, was killed when he was in the seventh grade. His brother had been very popular and very protective of him, and had always walked him to school. It turned out that his brother had been killed in a motorcycle accident just after having an argument with him, and he was the one who found his body (*ailments from grief; ailments from fright; anguish from loss of his friend*). He waited there until the police came. The worst part of the whole event, he said, was that after the police arrived, they put him in the police van and would not let him out. He viewed this as an act of cruelty, became hysterical, and smashed the interior of the van (*ailments from anger; ailments from anger with indignation; violent anger; anger from contradiction*). His brother's death was the beginning of the family breakup. The father became very abusive, physically and emotionally, and had numerous affairs (*ailments from discords between chief and subordinates*). My dog-walking companion said that, after all this, he could never fit in society and could not hold down a job because of altercations with co-workers (*quarrelsome; intolerant of contradiction; contrary*). He only had one close friend in life (*aversion to company*) and harbored an intense hatred toward police and anyone with authority (*hatred, unmoved by apologies; hatred of persons who had offended; irritability when spoken to*).

No one can convince a *Nit-ac* to accept an apology; you might as well swallow your tongue: *long-continued rancor, insensible to apology and excuses; he is unmoved by apologies, obstinate.* In fact, to justify his own behavior, he constantly thinks of people who have offended him, a little like *Nat-m*, who reminisces about sad events with joy and only cries when she feels she is pitied (*she falls to thinking of an occurrence long past, and cannot rid herself of it; he is always absorbed by these ideas, without being able, in spite of strenuous efforts, of thinking of anything else*).

Meltdown

Since he is surrounded by "enemies" and constantly engaged in lawsuits, the vigilant *Nit-ac* can never let down his guard. Like anyone else who remains chronically hyperalert, this state finally wears him down, so that even the most insignificant unexpected event may shake him profoundly: *very easily startled and frightened; starting up from fright and falling asleep; great weariness and indolence, as if completely exhausted and bruised.* The *Nit-ac* personality edges easily toward a nervous breakdown: *discontentment with himself, even if he makes a trifling mistake. He cannot get rid of his sad thoughts; he has an easily excited annoyance and impatience.* This *hopeless and boundless despair,* coupled with *attacks of rage with curses,* hardly helps him escape his Cyber delusion (that he is always engaged in lawsuits). Here is another case from my practice demonstrating the onset and course of a *Nit-acid's* life:

> This was a 30-year-old man with CC "I have a short temper (*anger, violent*); I am ticked off at trivialities (*anger at trifles*). Can't anything go my way?" He reported: "Since I was a young child, I would throw things out of the window and hit the wall (*striking the wall*); I was always fighting and liked to manipulate others to be the hero (*malicious*). My father split up with my mom when I was six. I was the first of four children. Mom stopped taking care of me when I was 9 (*ailments from early responsibility*), and I have not seen her in 15 years (*estranged from family*). From age 13-15, I was bullied for being an outsider; I always was the new kid on the block and was always picked on. I was a loner but I would stand up for myself; in fact, I loved the conflict. I had a sharp tongue and liked to insult people (*contemptuous; cynical*). I liked provoking people. From age 14-21, I was always looking for the next fight (*delusion, he is engaged in lawsuits*). At age 19 I went into the army, which is filled with idiots, for two and a half years. I was injured and ostracized by the army because I never followed the rules. I had been involved in a car accident with back and head injuries; I tried to return to my work for the army too early and couldn't do it, but my superiors called me a malingerer (*ailments from discords between chief and subordinates*). I decided to be my own lawyer and challenged the military authority, which made things worse for me (*delusion, engaged in lawsuits*). The military psychological abuse (*ailments from rudeness of others; ailments from discords between chief and subordinates*) became

> very personal, but I pushed back; finally, though, I had to admit defeat, which caused a severe depression (*sadness from anger; sadness indisposed to talk; indifference to pleasure*). I wanted to kill someone (*rage with cursing; violent, rage leading to deeds of violence*); I was like a robot (*unconsciousness, stupor*). I can't forget those abusive people in the army, and I wish I could do something to them (*hatred towards people who have offended; hatred for persons abusing him*). Whenever anything goes wrong, I take it personally, even when I'm walking the dog (*anger about his mistakes; discontented with himself*). Nothing goes my way! I curse a lot when things don't go well (*cursing; rage with cursing*).

One can see from this example how the *impetuous* (impulsive, volatile) *Nit-ac* is subjected to many real and imagined injustices, prompting him to react even if he can't win or if he is exposing himself to retaliation. Only judiciously applied doses of *Nit-ac* can avoid a meltdown and release him from the chains of his Cyber delusion.

Golden Tips from the Masters

- *Nit-ac* wakes up irritated and dissatisfied and hates drafts; is always on edge
- Better when riding in a car (< > of *Cocculus*); nausea >with motion
- Sensation of having a "bone" in the throat: prickly pains everywhere
- Is the most pessimistic remedy of the materia medica (< > of *Phosphorus,* most optimistic one)
- Alternating with *Thuja* to resolve the roots of sycosis
- Bad-smelling urine, like horse's urine
- #1 remedy for ailments due to overuse of antibiotics (diarrhea)
- Remedy for ingrown toenails (*South pole of magnet* too)
- Easily bleeding warts (*Sabina, Thuja*)
- Anal fissures (*Ratanhia*)
- *Painful scars acting up* (*Graphites, Staphysagria*)
- *Nit-ac* exhibits a singular power over the rectum and anus: it has cured prolapses, fistulas, and even fissures (C. Burnett)

Nux vomica (Nux-v). Poison-nut-Strychnos

The Cyber Delusion

Nux-v is a person who will become one with his mask (identification with his persona), exercising only one facet of his ego as he has not completed a process of individuation: his world is driven by ambition and work! The other two persona classes, the excessive and the inadequate personae, in contrast to the situation of identification with the persona, know that there is another person behind the mask, respectively a coward or one that is dominated. *Nux-v* becomes an obstructed personality, as he demonstrates psychic arrest or a lack of individuation. Persona is a product of the ego that serves to make an impression on others while concealing the true nature of the individual. *Nux vomica* identifies with a mask or persona with only one facet, as it is entirely formed by the one thing that is important in his life: ruthless ambition! This limited mask is the whole ego; there is nothing behind the mask. The person **is** the mask! This attitude sets the tone for *Nux vomica's* approach to the world, which is driven by his Cyber delusion. *Nux-v* has many delusions (44 of them!), but the central idea is expressed by different delusions with the same meaning (one of the criteria for calling it a Cyber delusion). We can therefore accept that the ***delusion, someone is in bed with him*** is the prime motivation for his limited attitude toward the world. This is not like *Pulsatilla's delusion a naked man is in her bed.* The latter indicates the desperate need of *Pulsatilla* for attention, as well as her need for procreation to sustain her exaggerated maternal instincts. She wants someone in bed with her; without such a person she feels *all alone in the world. Nux-v*, though, would love to be all alone in the world; then, there would be no one threatening his growing empire (*company, aversion to presence of other people; desire for solitude*). Indeed, with *Nux-v*, it is all about professional competition or *increased ambition* (not the romantic **and** professional competition of *Lachesis*). This is also expressed by the *delusion, someone gets into bed with him in the evening, and he has no room in it* and the *delusion, his bed is sold.* He hates to see someone competing for his bed (business)!

One sees immediately from these delusions the fierce competitive spirit of *Nux-v*: he wants to be the only business in town, and he is therefore very suspicious of everyone (*delusion, he is about to receive an injury*). Other delusions of *Nux-v* expressing the same sentiment are *delusion, he sees vermin crawl about and creeping of worms* and *he is pursued by enemies and his house is full of people*. Everyone is an enemy of his business; no one is to be trusted, as in his mind, they are all maggots eating his flesh and leeches drinking his blood; he is convinced that *someone is always ready to sell his bed* (*delusion he is poor*). Wealth is desired for the importance it brings, as well the things it buys. It does not escape *Nux-v* that, especially in Western society, a wealthy person is generally treated as important and successful. For this reason, he (and others like *Lycopodium* who *wants to be considered rich*), believes riches to be the currency of importance.

For *Nux-v*, wisdom does not always accompany age. In his case, age sometimes shows up all by itself. Unlike Socrates, who when viewing articles of luxury exclaimed, "How much there is in the world that I do not want," *Nux-v* is seized by an inner libido to want it all. "Citizens of Athens," Socrates asked, "aren't you ashamed to care so much about making all the money you can and advancing your reputation and prestige, while for truth and wisdom and the improvement of your souls you have no thought or care?" He might well have been addressing the *Nux vomica* people of this word! *Nux-v* might well be wise about business matters, but he is not a wise person. *Nux-v* does not understand that possessions can do little for his happiness as he is without true mental culture, so his fate is to be driven further and further from inner peace (*mental activity restless; anxiety about business; exaggerated anxiety*) until, perhaps, a warning dream of falling from a mountain ominously predicts his demise. Indeed, for *Nux-v*, riches become like sea water: the more he drinks, the thirstier he becomes! The pursuit of goods has become an end in itself, and in such a person, tending to his livelihood overshadows his life; when he deals with business, he knows how to get ahead, how to manipulate others. But when it comes to the question of living, he is weak and even less than half awake! The more he focuses on a materialistic pathway to happiness, the less happy he tends to be and the less happy he makes others. Certainly, some aspects of life improve with wealth: one does not have to wonder if food will be available each day as I have witnessed in Third World countries, and there is the temporary satisfaction of buying something one doesn't strictly need, as I witness every day in modern society. But happiness, fulfillment, and contentment cannot be bought. He forgets the age-old adage that money does not buy happiness or love but often corrupts both. *Nux-v* damages his ability to form personal bonds, treating others as objects to be manipulated rather than as unique individuals with their own desires. You cannot expect such a person to look in the mirror and see the man he is, realizing mournfully what he might have been. He is convinced to his dying day that his way is **the** way to live! He fights a constant battle to climb the social ladder, but his constant fear of failure creates a permanent state of anxiety and stress, bringing to light the Pyrrhic victories which lead him to lose the war on life (*anxiety about business*; *anxiety about the future*).

Nux-v has his own malicious streak, the hallmark of egoistic conduct (*malicious, spiteful and vindictive*). Don't confuse a good ego with a bad ego. A good ego, like a balanced *Aurum*, is one that expands while following the path to individuation, while a person tries to become an individual through service to humankind. *Nux-v* is really a true egoist, a man who fails to individuate. He takes direct delight in the failure of others and is always conniving and scheming to obtain even a small personal advantage from a situation (*competitive ambition increased*). *Nux-v* should be added to the rubric *employs every possible means to increase his ambition* (*Veratrum*). Between him and the others in the world, there is a mighty fixed abyss of indifference: "*Après moi le déluge*," he says (in other words, the world may perish for all I care, as long as I have gotten all I want and am not here anymore). Egoism indeed contracts the heart, whereas doing disinterested deeds for others enlarges the heart. Egoism leads to anxiety and worry as it entails too much self-interest (*delusion, he is dying*; *delusion, everything will fail*; *delusion, happened, of having anything*; *discontented and displeased*), whereas a reduced interest in our own selves leads to calm and confident serenity. *Nux-v* is not preoccupied with the afterlife but only with what can be reaped in his present life. "Death," *Nux-v* says, "does not concern me." When we are, death is not, and when death is, we are not. It is materialism that is his God, not spiritualism, although he would proclaim to be spiritual if it were to clinch him the next deal.

Even in a *Nux-v* child, a materialistic and ambitious attitude (it is all about *possessing, not being*) is already ingrained. For that child, anxiety about business is usually seen in a need to have the most toys and goods. A guarded person who demands and receives the undivided attention of his parents, he strives to be the leader in class, the king of business, the CEO, the one who has the most ambition to make money in the first place! He will be ever the eager entrepreneur from the moment he pitches his first lemonade stand; he will outsell everyone else because of his zealous pursuit of success in business. He is fiercely independent, driven by his *desire to be considered rich*. We can immediately see the suspicion, even paranoia, of the

Nux-v person. He is neither a light-hearted person who can take a joke at his expense nor a joking person (*delusions, that people are beside him, carrying all sorts of pranks with him,* and *delusion, he is being mocked and laughed at, even persecuted*). He might appear to be an extravert, but that is only in the sense of having his focus on what objects he can own, devoid of introspection, which reflects his search for hedonic pleasures. His "being," how important he is in his eyes and others,' his "happiness," is based on what and how much he **has**. But anyone who seeks happiness in acquisitions is doomed to disappointment (*ailments from disappointment; anxiety about business*) as hedonic pleasures have a limited staying power. *Nux-v* indeed has the delusion that he realizes an authentic life, but in order to truly be authentic, *Nux-v* must learn to set aside pleasure-seeking well-being—the kind of shallow, short-lived pleasure he gets from acquiring things—in favor of a deeper, more meaningful state in which gratification is not usually immediate. This way, he will not blame others or get defensive when he meets with less success then he had hoped (*anger about his mistakes; anger so he could have stabbed someone; being beside himself; reproaches others; rudeness*).

Nux-v has a fixed idea *that he is on a journey*, and the young *Nux-v* is purely goal-oriented. He seeks the unrestricted satisfaction of all his desires; this does not lead to happiness and independence, as the child will learn later, but the *Nux-v* person is on a mission to accomplish (*delusion, he is on a journey*). The journey of *Nux-v* is not of a spiritual nature but consists of a trip towards wealth and fame; *Nux-v* takes a purely materialistic path because having nothing is equal to being nothing for this person. We will see that materialism is the driving force behind *Nux vomica's* life, and that nothing and no one should get in the way of reaching his goals. Following the law of compensation in dreams, such a one-sided attitude always is compensated through opposite dreams, warning dreams of failure causing *fear of terrible dreams*: *Nux-v* has *dreams that teeth are falling out and dreams that the filling of teeth is falling out.* In the book *The Interpretation of Dreams (Oneirocritica)*,[31] the mouth represents the house and the teeth the inhabitants of the house. If all the teeth fall out together and the person is a "merchant or businessman" (*Nux-v* is!), then this dream predicts lingering illness and wasting away, but without resultant death. Such a dream is a **warning** for *Nux-v* to change his lifestyle as he is burning the candle at both ends (= wasting away)! Another common *Nux-v* warning dream is

31. Artemidorus, *The Interpretation of Dreams (Oneirocritica)*, trans. Robert J. White (Torrance, California: Original Books, 1975), 44-46.

climbing a high mountain and then falling from the peak of the mountain. Usually the dreamer wakes up before he is on the ground in the dream. Other warning dreams for the worn-out businessman are dreaming that he drives a car which is out of control, usually a symbol that he is not living with due awareness or care. Sometimes in dreams, a *Nux-v* person cannot find a parking place for his car. A parking place is a socially accepted place to rest or to make some sort of change. Not finding a parking spot in a dream when you are looking for it refers to the dreamer's difficulty relaxing, getting away from the demands of the "traffic" of his life, certainly something that applies to a *Nux-v* mentality!

Causalities

Ailments from Deceived Ambition

There is open to man alone a source of pleasure, and of pain as well, a source that can give him all kinds of trouble. In the case of *Nux-v*, I refer to ambition and the feeling of honor and embarrassment or shame, or in plain words, what he thinks other people's opinion of him is (it should be added to the rubric *longing for the good opinion of others*). *Nux-v* is in the rubric *A/F lost honor*, and indeed, honor is dearer than life itself to this person; the important thing is what others think of him, the enhancement of position that he so assiduously seeks throughout his life. The main goal of the *Nux-v* person, from youth on, is to become "someone in business," as his relationship to the world is one of possessing and owning property. This includes not only houses and businesses; he also "possesses" people: wife, children, servants, employees, friends... he wants to be famous for having his name in big letters on a building (the *Sulphur* child too), to retire by the age of thirty as a millionaire, and to be known as being in a powerful position, the undisputed "king," often in the financial (Wall Street) or political world. But a person is bound to go through many disappointments if, even from childhood, he has only the goal of acquiring as many gadgets, toys, and goods and as much power as possible. Keeping up with the Joneses is always a losing battle! This trait can be seen in a youngster where ruthless competition results from his wish to win every game, even if by cheating, because he is fixated on worldly goods and their value, and yes, winning! When the world does not bend to all his wishes and things don't always go his way, it will provoke his *anger and disappointment*, and *ailments from deceived ambition and business failure* are a major trigger for illness. Losing a game, for a *Nux-v* child, is a "business failure" (*sadness for reversal of fortune*; *sadness after loss of place*). Of course it becomes even more serious when he is older (*he has not slept for a fortnight, brooding at night long over a lawsuit, by which he may gain or lose a million*). It will provoke his *jealousy* (towards those who are more successful: *ailments from disappointment*) and a *feeling of wounded honor*. And who is ultimately responsible for failure in his business? Not Mr. *Nux-v*! People working for him are just loafers collecting their paychecks, he claims! But angry confrontations tend to alienate people and provoke self-protective responses and actions. *Nux vomica's* anger will drive a wedge between him and his listeners, regardless of his words or intentions. If one is so determined to get the most toys in his life, he tries to succeed until he becomes the prisoner of his Cyber delusion—with a very high price: an inevitable physical breakdown and illness. *Nux-v* does not realize that the abundance of goods he strives for is nothing but superfluity that often turns out to be fatal excess.

Mental Work

Continued mental work aggravates him, and he is indisposed to it, particularly to that form, which involves elaboration and connection of subjective ideas independently of external objects. In other words, the *Nux-v* person simply acquires knowledge that he writes down and memorizes, but he does not come to life spontaneously in response to what he has heard; he will not produce a new idea and is incapable of critical thinking, but he follows the lesson to the T as a guide to having more and being more successful. Mental exertion occurs day and night and often causes a headache in the morning; this will eventually, much later in his life, lead to *laziness and aversion to work* (*man, worn out, averse to business*). It is part of a *debauched* lifestyle: "work hard and play hard" is his motto, which includes (thanks to his money and toys such as a yacht or airplane) sexual conquests (*ailments from sexual excesses*). These are selfish as he never has interest in truly knowing people, but only in adding them to his collection of beautiful **things**; in this way, he creates quite a few enemies during his life journey, both cheated business partners and jilted lovers. But *Nux-v* remains blissfully blind to such issues: after all, winning is everything, even if it involves trampling on someone else's honor or heart. Too late in life, *Nux-v* learns what he must do to be healthy: avoid excessive violent and unpleasant emotions (*anger with red face; exaggerated anxiety*), avoid mental overstrain, and take daily exercise in the open air (*business man, worn out*). Without proper daily exercise, no one can remain healthy. Aristotle said aptly, "Life begins in movement," as this assures the ceaseless motion of each individual part in man: the heart, the lungs, the intestines, all the glands, the arteries and capillaries are all moved by our Vital Force to keep us healthy and alive and prevent internal tumult; internal motion is supported by the external motion. Burnout—emotional exhaustion, physical fatigue, and cognitive weariness—will set in if one's job is too stressful or intense or, in the case of *Nux-v*, when he has been doing it for too long and excessively. The destructive power of burnout is unforgiving. It leads to stomach ulcers, recurrent myocardial infarction and apoplexy, increase of coronary atherosclerosis, and yes, death. Sleep deprivation and physical exhaustion are at the root of his demise! *Nux vomica's* fate and punishment is also to be easily *angered from contradiction*; he suffers a gloomy, hypochondriacal existence and a life wrecked by overuse of stimulants, tranquilizers, and purgatives which he uses to deal with a *deficient appetite, ineffectual stool, poor digestion, nightly back pain and insomnia*. What a price to pay for that heap of gold! What a folly to sacrifice his health for some gain, profit, or promotion, not to mention for fleeting sensual pleasures. It does not help *Nux vomica's* health that he is prone to angry outbursts directed at his wife, children, and subordinates (*ailments from discords between chief and subordinates*). When angry, he can behave like a little kid, with a face reddened from excessive anger, stomping his feet on the ground (*anger with red face*; *anger from contradiction*). Real happiness is never found, as much of our happiness depends upon health alone and *Nux-v* is far too busy with his pursuit of possessions to realize it—except when sickness and death knock on his door. How much does he want to exchange his belongings then for the treasure called health! As is so easily seen in people condemned to a sedentary lifestyle, there is a glaring disproportion between outward inactivity and inner tumult (*exaggerated anxiety*; *violent anger when obliged to answer*; *concentration difficult when reading or studying*). If he is fortunate, *Nux-v* will begin to see that material ambitions are silly, that the pleasures of friends and family are paramount, and that he should reorganize his life with new priorities in mind.

Compensations

Industriousness, Fastidiousness, and Competitiveness

Nux-v is a person who lives entirely by will power and rational control, devoting his whole life to success and to providing for his family **and his ego**! *Nux-v*, who identifies with his persona, is a person who also suffers from "weekend neurosis." He is an invincible (at least in his mind) workhorse who feels empty and adrift except when working. He has misused the persona appropriate to work and fails to cultivate a wider sense of identity. He is a true workaholic! He is as industrious as an ant, ceaselessly occupied from morning until evening in an endeavor to increase his heap of gold. The "weekend neurosis" creates a kind of depression which afflicts people who become suddenly aware of the lack of meaning and content in their lives and who, when not busy, feel the void within themselves quite painfully (*sadness without weeping and sadness with sighing*). Boredom in *Nux-v* becomes a real scourge. It is quite common in the unbalanced *Nux-v*, a miserable wretch who is always concerned with filling his purse but never his head, and for whom his wealth now becomes a punishment: it either pushes him into a never-ending race to **have** more rather than **be** more, or it delivers him into the hands of tormenting boredom. *Nux-v* never learns until it is too late that a life driven by love is preferable to a life driven by greed. He might become outwardly rich, but he surely remains inwardly poor. *Nux-v* never learns the hard lesson that happiness has nothing to do with an obscene accumulation of unshared wealth and that true moments of happiness lie in simple things like walking down the beach, the wind blowing in your hair, and your dog greeting you with an enthusiasm that is hard for a human to match. Acquiring never-ending personal amounts of property hinders his individuation path at every step. *Nux-v* forgets to walk out the door, allowing his mind to be strengthened and invigorated by a clear sky and plenty of fresh air. Minds must relax, as they rise better and keener after a rest. Just as one must not force fertile farmland, as uninterrupted productivity will soon exhaust it, so does constant effort sap one's mental vigor; a short period of rest and relaxation always restores one's powers. No doubt the real cause of happiness that lies within us is greater than anything that can come from objects, but *Nux-v* remains blind to this until the end of his miserable existence.

One of the greatest regrets people have when they are dying is that they did not take time to stop and enjoy the little things, and that they did not follow their passions and go along with their instincts! Only sudden death from exhaustion, as *Nux-v* rushes in all directions and travels here, there, and everywhere looking for new investments and deals—a death forewarned by dreams of falling from a cliff or a mountain—can relieve his miserable life. Aggressive and acquisitive, he expects every situation and every person to heed his driving will, and he insists on having his way in everything (*anger from contradiction*; *intolerant to contradiction, and contrary*). Materialism, greed, egotism, and the dogged perseverance so characteristic of *Nux-v* can all be traced back to his habits of excretion. No wonder, then, that *Nux-v* is such a well-known remedy for constipation (*constipation, with ineffectual and frequent urging to stool*), the type of constipation that reflects his tense and always unsatisfying business transactions and achievements in life. If *Nux-v* is successful in nine out of ten undertakings, he is not pleased but annoyed and irritated that one has miscarried; furthermore, he is likely to blame one of his employees for these failures (*reproaching others*). Each failure in business (*ailments from deceived ambition*) increases his nervous tension, and each increase of nervous tension increases the probability of failure; it becomes a vicious cycle. This increase in tension can lead to many physical complaints: *oppressive headaches, impaired vision, and trigeminal neuralgia; want of appetite, burning in the pylorus area of the stomach and extreme gastric irritability and sexual impotence.* If Nux-v could only listen to his forewarning dreams... but to expect this from such a materialistic, foolish person without treatment is in itself just a dream!

Restless Mind

Another positive tool, although it is (like everything else) abused and misused by the *Nux-v* person, is his *restless mind.* He is always creating some new plan, always busy with some activity that will lead to gaining more goods (which he guards carefully once they are acquired). His sleep can be restless as even at night his mind cannot relax: *ideas are abundant and clearness of mind in bed* (his bed is part of conducting business, of new plans for the next days and reviewing the success or failures of the previous day). He often *wakes at 3 a.m.*, and this leads to *unrefreshed sleep.* Nux-v *is zealous and industrious while being conscientious about trifles.* There is no time to waste for *Nux-v*; *time goes too slow and he is always in haste.* In order to be successful, he wants to keep order in his things (*very fastidious*) and loves to order others around to do exactly what he wants as "he knows better" (*intolerant of contradiction and contrary*). It is his way or the highway, and no one can put restrictions on his wishes (he does not like tight clothes either, as they "restrict" him) and ambitions (*contrary and disposition to contradict; obstinate and resists wishes of others and impatience when spoken to*)!

From childhood, *Nux-v* has a good chance of growing up with **addictions**: to fast food, coffee, drugs (he is inclined to be a heavy recreational drug user), and alcohol (*desire for alcohol yet aggravates from it*). *He is zealous and industrious while being conscientious for trifles.* Of course all these efforts are one-dimensional, not promoting a healthy lifestyle. He easily falls prey to *dipsomania* in an attempt to maintain his drive as it increases his thinking and scheming *-(mental strength increases, more intelligent during drunkenness,* Sulph and *Nux*). Eventually, though, this leads him into a destructive syphilitic cycle as it will yield *confusion of the mind after carousal, and from* *spirituous liquors, and suspicion,* setting him up to return to his Cyber delusion. The clearest ideas and strongest ambitions will eventually be drowned in these excesses. They turn out to be the "help" that harms—in other words, *Nux-v* shoots himself in the foot and puts obstacles in his own chosen path. This self-defeating behavior is like a false friend: it seems helpful at the time to achieve what he wants now, but in the long run it is very harmful, especially when repeated. That dipsomania plays a huge role in the *Nux-v* character, as seen in the multiple rubrics indicating *Nux-v* and dipsomania: he *must get up at night to drink* (and not milk!); *alcoholism with hypochondriasis; alcoholism from idleness* (the weekend neurosis); *alcoholism with irritability,* **only** *Nux-v*; and *alcoholism during or after pregnancy, Nux-v* **only**!

Extraversion and Boasting

Nux-v appears to be very *social* and an extraverted, but this is only a mask: a mask that has become his entire self. He is *amorous* as he understands that syrup catches a lot of flies, *cheerful, gay and mirthful.* We also see a little of *Lycopodium, Fl-ac* and *Platina* in *Nux-v*: *being kind with strangers but not with his family and entourage.* As usual, we have to ask the "why and for what purpose" of this behavior to see the difference among these remedies: *Fl-ac* because he *is always ogling women on the street* and uses his charm to get a sex interest in bed; *Lycopodium* because *he has love for power* and wants to be recognized by his peers; *Platina* because she can only have respect and awe for someone more intelligent and famous than she is; and *Nux-v* because he might need that person to further his career or business! This characteristic of *Nux-v* is also expressed by further provings: *avarice as regards his family but generous too much towards strangers.* The saying about a friend in need is apropos here, but for *Nux-v* it works in the opposite direction: no sooner are you his "friend" than **he** becomes a friend in need, asking you for a favor or for a loan/investment for one of his sure-to-be-successful schemes. He increases his chances of appearing to be a prosperous businessman through his *boasting behavior and squandering through ostentation* (also *Verat-a*, to gain coveted social standing!). *Nux-v* has the plush office, the big car, the three-piece suit, the remodeled kitchen with high-end flooring and energy-efficient appliances. All this is not cheap, and he knows that others know that (*fear of rags; wishes to be considered rich; delusion he is poor; avarice but squandering on himself*). Who could doubt that he is the talk of the town and the king of business? Who would not want to invest their money with this sure winner?

Jealousy

While successful in business, *Nux-v* is impoverished in feeling, in interpersonal relationships, and especially in any desire to seek a higher meaning in life. The force of emotion represents an energy that he should not disregard. If he ignores it, his prevailing egoism and the libido of rational functioning can destroy him; this is often foreseen in warning *dreams of falling*. What *Nux-v* does not know is this: he is poor, in spite of all his wealth, because he **has** much but he **is** little. Since the *Nux-v* person's goal and preoccupation is always that nobody should have more than he has, he is prone to feel envious toward anyone who has even an ounce more of anything. His mental greed has no saturation point, since possessing more things does not repair the inner emptiness, boredom, loneliness, and depression it is meant to overcome. In addition, since what he has can be taken away in one form or another, he always must have more in order to fortify his existence against such danger. He asks himself: "How much in the world is there that I still want? What is there that I don't have yet?" He fears his neighbor's aggressive intention to take away what he has (*delusion, someone sleeps in his bed*). To prevent such an attack, *Nux-v* becomes preventively aggressive himself (*irritability with anxiety*; *mania with rage*; *passionate*); *Nux-v* always looks the part, ready to act in any role in order to sell himself in the world: what kind of person is playing that role is of no importance, as long as playing the role fulfills his ambition and helps him get what he wants. *Nux-v* roams the earth for profit, a person who buys cheap and sells dear, ruthlessly pursuing wealth—the sole driving force of his life. All it leads to in the end is a depersonalization and meaninglessness of life as anything acquired is never enough. To still his growing dissatisfaction, *Nux-v* does not hesitate to put his own health at risk by means of increasingly unrealistic "get-rich-quick" schemes that most often do not work.

Even the *Nux-v* child feels bitter envy toward those who have more. It leads to *boasting*: "I have more than you, I am stronger than you, I am smarter than you…" Interestingly enough, as he is very frugal with his belongings and toys, the *Nux-v* child does not hesitate to bribe new friends he thinks he can use; he shows a generosity that surprises his family (*avarice in regards to family, and generosity towards strangers*; *generous too much for strangers*). Of course, it is just because a bigger prize is in view: that new friend has something he can use. He might be smarter, more popular, or physically stronger. Always good to have someone like that in your camp! *Nux-v* wants to give the impression that he is the most successful, translated in his mind as having many toys: he is a *boaster, and squanders through ostentation on himself*. He has the latest and most fashionable clothes, shoes, and electronic gadgets to impress everyone around him. Of course, they don't call these "con games" for nothing. How else can one explain *Nux vomica's* ability to influence others to the point of wheedling money out of them, which attests to his near-magical social power? The boasting is often accompanied by fault-finding in others: *censorious, critical; he is inclined to find fault and scold and violently approach others for their faults* and jealousy often creates *quarrels and scolding. He can get angry without any provocation and he quarrels, reproaches, scolds, insults from jealousy, mingled with unchaste expressions and has a fiery, excited temperament*! But as much as *Nux-v* wants to be high on the social ladder (*ambition increased; anxiety about business; fear of misfortune; fear of poverty; steals money without necessity*), he lacks the substance, compassion, and trustworthy judgment to climb high in others' estimation.

Anger to Reinforce his Persona

If you have a *Nux-v* child, you have an angry child! Impatience, jealousy, mortification, noise, and failed ambition all provoke anger. It is often *violent anger, when contradicted or interrupted in his favorite task, and angry outbursts even about his own mistakes* (perfectionism) or when stuck on *trifles*. Family members, especially younger siblings, are frequent targets of his rages, in which he shows *a red face, is beside himself with cursing,* and can have a *sudden impulse to kill for a slight offense*. Of course, in *Nux-v*, anger resembling madness is a mere mask to hide weakness. The *Nux-v child is being kind with strangers* (he wants to impress them with his big plans) *but not with his family. He is easily offended* and does not hesitate to *strike while talk of others aggravates*: "Leave me alone," he says; "Be quiet!" This is not the time for a discussion! Unfortunately, this child can be a bully at school; he loves to fight those he considers weaker.

The Slippery Slope: Debauched Lifestyle

As he feels he is losing control somewhat, *Nux-v* (or "Mr. Know-it-all") thinks the best positive tool is to be *obstinate and resisting the wishes of others*. Without knowing it, he **is** losing control as he is *passionate* in the sense of being *angry and intolerant to any contradiction. He is impetuous and impatient when spoken to* and bullies his way through the day with foul language and cursing. As Hering expresses it, *Nux-v suits the very particular, careful, zealous person, inclined to get angry or excited, or of a spiteful, malicious disposition*. A perfect example of the choleric temperament! He will lose control faster than the other ambitious character, *Aurum* (*delusion he is not* *appreciated*), who begins by showing silent resentment, only later *trembling with anger because he is not appreciated* (*Pall*).

Health indeed outweighs all other blessings to the point that one may really say that a healthy beggar is happier than an ailing king. But the "wannabe" king, *Nux-v*, is compromising his health every step of the way. In the end, alcohol, lack of sleep (because of a restless mind), a debauched lifestyle, and a focus on trifles all lead him further and further away from potentially positive paths. Only *hypochondriasis and irritability and suspicion are left. He has a passion for reading medical books* (not to help others but to offset the many physical ailments caused by his debauched lifestyle and to find drugs to support it) and *has loquacity about his health* (only remedy). *Nux-v* should be added under the rubric *loquacity about business,* where we see *Bryonia and Hyos. Bryonia* is driven by the fear of poverty, and *Hyoscyamus* aims to conquer the subject of his adulation before he is sold! Nevertheless, *Nux-v* is now like a racecar out of control: the once fast-thinking individual *chooses now expressions which are not suitable with a slow train of thought; he cannot read or calculate for the loss of connection of ideas*; he suffers greatly from an overtaxed mind (pronounced *ailments from mental work/exertion*). *He is inclined to find fault in everything and is very much inclined to violently reproach others for their faults.* We can easily see how this behavior only reinforces *Nux vomica*'s Cyber delusion that everyone is out to kill his business and livelihood! However, unlike *Aurum*, *Nat-s*, and *Sulphur*, at this point he might also *think of suicide, but he lacks the courage; he talks about it but does not commit suicide.* He resorts to *restless wandering,* thinking about how the world has mistreated him (*melancholic in consequence of losing his position*); this is reflected in the rubric *sadness for reversal of fortune* (*Lachesis, Sulph, Sep*), the last two remedies being the chronics of *Nux-v*.

Golden Tips from the Masters

- *Nux-v* stands for spasms, sensitivity (to light, noise, music and voices, all black type remedies), effects from over-drugging and overuse of coffee and tobacco, and chilliness
- Disciplined and efficient workers
- Sensation as if a weight is in the stomach 1-2 hours after eating
- First half of the tongue is clear, a heavy fur covers the posterior part (location on tongue of the excretion organs in TCM)
- Spasmodic sneezing, especially after lots of spicy food
- Headaches and migraines in sedentary persons
- Clears the field and neutralizes the effects of too many medications or wrong remedies
- In case of being struck by lightning, a person should be put into a freshly made opening in the ground, in a half-sitting, half-lying position, with the face toward the sun, and be covered with fresh ground. As soon as he begins to move his eyes, give *Nux-v* internally every half hour. The complaints which frequently follow restoration may generally be removed by *Sulphur* and *Nux-v*. For blindness, use *Phosphorus*
- If *Nux* fails in digestive illness, think about *Carbo-veg*
- For constipation, *Hydrastis* is far superior to *Nux-v* (Hughes)
- #1 remedy for a hangover
- <in dry and windy weather
- Coryza during the day, nose stopped at night
- *Nux-v* is the chilliest remedy in our materia medica (also serious ailments from cold are removed by it)

Petroleum (Petr). Crude Oil

The Cyber Delusion

Nowadays we are in the midst of a brain failure epidemic. Yet allopathy has not figured out the story of human memory—why it exists, how it works, how it fails. Worse, the care of dementia patients often means coping by doping these poor patients with excessive doses of strong psychotropic medications, causing severe side effects and often rendering patients' conditions worse than they were originally. This practice is especially alarming in nursing homes, where powerful antipsychotic drugs are used to quiet disruptive people with dementia; it is easier and cheaper than taking staff time to fix the problem. These dangerous drugs are prescribed for about 30% of all nursing home residents, whether they are psychotic or not. This does not come as a surprise to me: older people are often overmedicated, and individuals in nursing homes are especially vulnerable. It is in nursing homes that *Petroleum* will become a major polychrest together with other forgetful remedies.

When beginning to lose one's memory bit by bit, one realizes that memory is what makes our lives. Life without memory is no life at all. Memories are an integral part of our reason and the basis for our actions as they often create fixed ideas (CD). And death is nothing but the final amnesia, the one that erases one's entire life; one indulges in good memories and, alas, also in sad memories (as in *Nat-mur's* case). In *Petroleum*, part of the patient's life is erased—and with it his past and his moorings in time. Let's investigate his Cyber delusion.

Petroleum's Cyber delusion is ***body is divided***. Just as in *Silica* (*delusion, left half does not belong to his right*), it reflects a sense of confusion, a sense of duality and a certain split personality; but *Petroleum* is very different in nature from *Silica*. *Silica* is literally a split personality with an excessive persona, a mask that he takes off at home when he feels secure, even terrorizing his household. *Petroleum* is a personality with an inadequate persona due to a great degree of confusion caused by severe memory loss; he therefore lacks the tools to rectify the situation, as we will discover. *Petroleum* is helpless **everywhere**, while *Silica* is helpless once he sets foot outside of the home. *Petroleum's* CD is supported by other delusions: *delusion, he is divided in two parts; has three legs; he is three persons; of being double; body is divided and scattered about, tossed about.* This last delusion reflects the scattered brain of the individual; it is natural, then, that many *Petroleum* people become victims of forgetfulness and Alzheimer disease. The confusion is so pronounced that *Petroleum's* identity is erased (*delusion, errors of personal identity and confusion of mind, sense of duality*); he therefore needs someone for support (*delusion, someone walks besides him*). Looking at the other remedies in this rubric, we find *Calc-c, Sil,* and *Thuja*. For *Calc-c,* it is when he leaves his safe home and faces the dangerous world that he needs support (*delusion, he is about to fall into annihilation*); *Sil* needs a family member because now the mask has fallen off and *Sil* does not feel at all confident he can survive on the outside (CD, *left side does not belong to her*). *Thuja* is another individual who always needs support, especially in the outside world, because he has a fixed idea of vulnerability and needs reinforcement from others (CD, *body is from glass; body is brittle*).

Petroleum, on the other hand, needs someone to literally guide him (a "shadow," as we call it in the ASD world) because his mental capacity is diminished. So it is a benevolent person walking next to him, unlike the case of *Staphysagria,* who has someone walking **behind** him (controlling). That *Petroleum* is very confused is confirmed by still other delusions: *everything is strange; familiar things are strange.* Even in the most private place, his bed, he has the fixed idea that *his bed is occupied by another person,* a reflection of the dissociation that can take place in such a state. This has nothing to do with a spirit of competitiveness as it does in *Nux-v,* who has the same fixed idea; rather, this delusion expresses that the confusion for *Petroleum* extends to every place in his life, not just the outside world (*feeling of helplessness*). These delusions fit the patient with Alzheimer's perfectly, since such a person does not recognize family members and gets lost in his own neighborhood (*confusion, loses his way in well-known streets; mistakes in localities; forgetful on which side of the street his house was*).

These delusions of duality and loss of identity point to a depersonalization and make up more than half of *Petroleum's* fixed ideas. *Petroleum* never seems to be able to integrate his whole personality (*confusion as to his identity, with sense of duality*); there is always the feeling of having someone in bed with him or walking next to him. It makes one think of other split personalities like *Anhalonium, Thuja, Anac,* and *Lachesis;* one wonders if *Petroleum,* in its further evolution, will also be doomed to flee into a different world (*delusion, of fancy illusions*) or will dissociate into schizophrenia. I have also wondered if *Petroleum's* pathology would lead to cases of true insanity, or at least bring a fear of insanity in *Petroleum's* mind. Or would the quick destruction of his mind spare him this awful fear? These questions can only be answered, of course, once we understand how a *Petroleum* state is created.

Causalities

Suppression of Skin Lesions

Petroleum has many expressions in common with *Glonoin,* another forgetful remedy, but its etiology is entirely different. In *Petroleum's* case, suppression of a skin lesion is a major cause of forgetfulness (*eruption suppressed*). Compton Burnett describes several cases of skin suppressions in *The Best of Burnett;* in his descriptions, cases of angina pectoris, ossification of the heart, asthma, hydrocephalus, cataract, and even death occur after suppressing skin eruptions. During Burnett's lifetime, besides *Petroleum,* zinc ointments were (and still are) popular. When I was a doctor in the army, zinc ointment was used for just about any kind of skin rash, especially for buttock rashes in children. To our horror, we see that *Zinc* is a black type remedy for suppressed eruptions, and again, Burnett gives us countless cases of such suppression with zinc. Allopathy is unfortunately quite blind to the dangers to patients that stem from suppressive treatments. TCM, however, understands the relationship between *Skin* and *Lungs,* in which the progression of suppressed eczema to active asthma often comes about as a result of cortisone application. When the forgetfulness is corrected with *Petroleum,* the previous rash, which is a combination of *Sulphur, Graphites,* and *Silica,* will return. It is indicated in eczema with deeply cracked palms and bleeding eruptions; the patient can't wash her hands as they keep on chapping; the eczema is <during the winter (often manifesting itself as painful cracks in the fingertips) and well in the summer, which is a great guiding symptom. Patients with eczema or psoriasis using cortisone creams in the long term can become confused and forgetful. As long as the patient is using cortisone cream, a cure is impossible. The longer the skin symptoms have been suppressed, the more violently they will come back, which often prompts the patient to revert to cortisone use again if he is unwilling to go through such suffering. More than ever, in these cases the

advanced Hahnemannian methods are a must: low potency 6C in 5th edition, in judicious careful repeated doses to minimize the exteriorization and aggravation!

Motion Sickness

A second A/F, one not found in *Synthesis* under "Ailments from," is *ailments from riding in a car or motion sickness* (Cocc). We do find *Petroleum* under *vertigo, riding aggravate* (Petroleum); *riding in a boat aggravates* (Cocc), *and riding in a carriage* (car). Characteristically, there is *vertigo on rising and on stooping, in occiput as if intoxicated, like seasickness,* for which *Petroleum* is a great remedy.

Sexual Excesses and Fright

I have put these two seemingly unrelated causalities together as they have both an impact on the Kidney Qi or Essence, a well-known connection in Traditional Chinese Medicine. *A/F fright* is the most prominent trigger. When we look at TCM, fright and fear relate to the *Water* or Kidney element, and severe fright damages the Kidney Yin, responsible for **short-term** memory (the Heart or Fire Element is responsible for long-term memory). It is, therefore, unsurprising that short-term memory should be affected first; its close relationship with the Heart organ, through the controlling cycle, will lead in time to total memory loss, even in familiar surroundings and including memory of long-ago events. When we talk about the Kidney Qi, another A/F will make sense: *A/F sexual excesses.* Any ejaculation (the Chinese called too-frequent sexual intercourse "unregulated affairs of the bedroom") will lead to a decrease in K Yin Qi and will contribute to *Petroleum's* confusion. Although TCM knew about such triggers 5,000 years ago, allopathy remains blind to them and prefers to analyze the brain with technical tools (scans, MRIs, etc.), failing to recognize that these identify only advanced pathology and leave physicians unable to establish a true cause for the deformations identified. The other causality of decreased K Qi is also present here: *anticipation anxiety* directly connected to the K organ.

Compensations

Petroleum, when suffering such unfortunate events as severe loss of memory, becomes a confused personality with an almost erased identity. One thing stands out in *Petroleum*: he seems to be a rather weak person without much self-confidence (*lack of confidence; dipsomania from weakness of character, cowardice, without courage of own opinion, weakness of will* and *feeling of helplessness*). As we turn to positive compensations, we see that this does not bode well.

Conscientiousness about Trifles

Comparing to *Sil* again, *conscientious about trifles* turns quickly from a positive tool to a negative one with *Petroleum* as it is a factor contributing to getting stuck in the thought process (*thoughts persistent, haunted by unpleasant thoughts*) and not going forward; this happens even faster than in *Silica*, for which "conscientious about trifles" is a black type remedy. Because *Petroleum*'s mind is not sharp (*imbecility*) and is rather weak (*deficiency of ideas*), we find another *A/F*: *aggravates from mental exertion.*

Alcohol Use and Loquacity

Petroleum needs alcohol to feel relaxed; otherwise, *he has aversion to answer and shows anxiety in crowds and when in company.* Alcohol is an escape and, alas, a negative tool with which he hides his confusion: he shows *loquacity during drunkenness; dipsomania from weak character, and talking foolish during drunkenness, with disposition to slander. He is inapt to talk in public and desires to be silent* (except when drunk!). Part of the reason for aggravation is that *Petroleum* does not tolerate alcohol that well: *a little wine taken at dinner goes to his head and makes him stupid.* There is even *delirious loquacity with delirium about the same subject all the time.* A proving says also, *talks of nothing but one subject.* When the patient has Alzheimer disease, no doubt the subject is the distant past which he remembers as if it were yesterday; he can go on for days repeating such stories. *And he is complaining constantly.* This last proving makes us think of *Calc-c*, who *talks about nothing but rats, mice and fire,* expressing *Calc-carb*'s fears of the outside world. Talking constantly about one topic in *Petroleum* has also to do with his sickness (*delusion, being sick*), linked again to his confusion since he now *worries and cares causeless. Petroleum* also feels causeless worry about his family: *towards evening anxiety and apprehension about his family, which he left behind going on a short journey; the anxiety increases until he becomes inconsolable.* Unfortunately, but not unexpectedly in view of the alcohol addiction, *Petroleum* even has *disposition to slander and maliciousness with anger, with swearing and malicious rage.* He is not an easy customer to deal with, but such character changes must draw our attention to *Petroleum* if they are accompanied by pronounced short-term memory loss.

Looking for Solitude

Although *Petroleum* needs an aide in order to function, he actually has an *aversion to company and a desire for solitude. Presence of other people aggravates his symptoms* and it is even worse with strangers: there is *an aversion to the presence of strangers.* There is *anxiety when in company, fear of others approaching him,* and *presence of strangers aggravates.* Hahnemann talks about *great timidity and lack of determination.* This is very much related to confusion and *loss of will and weakness of will.* The approach of strangers and of almost anyone else represents for *Petroleum* some kind of danger (*fear of evil; delusion sees thieves; delusion sees frightful images in the dark*). So *Petroleum* prefers quiet and isolation: *reserved; quiet disposition; indisposed to talk, desire to be silent;* even *talk of others aggravates* and there is *inaptitude to talk in public. Petroleum's* confusion leads also to great *timidity, a bashful timidity.* Company is certainly not drawn to such a quiet, confused, and shy individual, and *Petroleum's* oversensitive character is not helpful either: *offended easily, takes everything in bad part; quarrelsome, violent anger, violent and irritable, offended at trifles and morose.* There is also *sadness and despondency with inclination to weep.*

Indolence

There is *exertion from mental work and deficiency of ideas, apathy with ennui* and *although very intelligent, aversion to work, indolence.* Hering states that *Petroleum* is *always quiet, turned to himself and no ambition to work. Weakness of memory* does not help such an introverted person either. The threatening disintegration of *Petroleum's* personality (reflecting the CD) is really the crux of this introversion and indolence and all the other negative consequences. Memory loss takes a severe form and is a great cause of the mind's confusion and sense of duality.

Breakdown

Petroleum's real theme seems to be destruction on every level: mental, emotional, and physical. On the **mental** level, *Petroleum's* memory is the greatest victim, sharing many feature of Alzheimer's, especially the disintegration of the ego. In the final phase, *Petroleum's* mind is so utterly destroyed that *he has an aversion to think, is unobserving,* and his personality borders on *imbecility.* His thinking is rapidly reduced to a great fog: *sluggishness, difficulty of thinking and comprehending, as if he was enveloped in a fog. He is unconscious as in a dream, and he does not know where he is.* Hahnemann states: *the whole day he is only half conscious, as if only half alive; he lacks* *strength to think.* No wonder *Petroleum* is a very *indecisive person who undertakes many things but perseveres in nothing.* Even the dinner table is an enemy: *after eating a little, the head seems befogged, dizzy and confused.* The end result is often that he suffers from unfounded and irrational fears, such as *fears for evil and others approaching him and he imagines that little time is left to him to make his will.* Being certainly a sycotic-syphilitic remedy on the whole, this mental defect will explain his erratic emotions as he loses control over his ego; these emotions are mainly syphilitic in nature: *violent anger, cursing, dipsomania, frightened easily, melancholic insanity, and desire to kill. He takes everything in bad part so that he is very quarrelsome, offended at trifles, even more when he is intoxicated with a malicious fury and disposition to slander. He vexes himself about everything, even the least trifle and despite great efforts, he could not cheer up.* *Petroleum* becomes wild and unmanageable. As his senses are further destroyed, further deterioration sets in: *he sits still, he is in a dream, not knowing where he is and shows a weeping tearful mood, especially after drinking. He is always quiet, turned to himself and no ambition to work.* At this point, he seems to be totally disconnected from the world and his loved ones. *There is eccentricity alternating with sadness,* or as Hahnemann says, *frolicsomeness and extravagance then sadness and discouragement,* showing him to be only a shell of the human being he once was and pointing back to his CD: his divided spirit and body.

Golden Tips from the Masters

- It is especially known for a horrible eczema resembling *Sulphur*, but it is more a combination of *Sulphur*, *Silica*, and *Graphites*: *painful, unhealthy skin, with even slight wounds suppurating easily with splitting of the skin, especially in the winter when hands crack and burn and itch intolerably. Especially cracking of fingertips.* Think about it for people who work a lot with petroleum products or car mechanics who wash their hands with petroleum and can therefore prove it. It is hard for them to clean their hands because of these cracks. This eczema is only helped with Vaseline, which contains petroleum!
- *Sepia* is a complementary remedy to *Petroleum*.
- #2 remedy for genital herpes (*Nat-m* #1)
- *Petroleum* and *Rhus-t* are great for eruptions on the genitalia, male or female, but *Petrol* produces small vesicles, *Rhus-t* large blebs (Kent)
- It is a remedy of single parts in sweating, eruptions, and coldness (Kent)

Phosphoricum acidum (Ph-ac). Phosphoric Acid

The Cyber Delusion

This is the exhausted form of *Phosphorus,* the eternal traveler and communicator who ends up in the *acidum* state—this is not surprising in view of *Phosphorus's* low physical and mental stamina. Every *acidum* remedy consists of two different stages: first, a sycotic one with exaggerated efforts leading inevitably to a syphilitic one including total exhaustion, paralysis, indolence, and withdrawal. And where *Phosphorus* has the CD, *all alone on an island, Ph-acidum's* Cyber delusion is ***sees ciphers***. A cipher is a non-person, a nullity, zero, nothing, an emptiness. This CD is confirmed by other delusions: *sees dead persons, has visions, sees figures,* and *delusions, of fancy illusions.* Such rubrics reflect a disintegration of the person, a disconnection from reality, as *Ph-ac* either flees into an isolated, desired world of her creation or suffers from visual hallucinations and remains in a dark world (unconscious) as a direct result of her exhausted state. In addition to visual hallucinations, she has auditory hallucinations: *delusion she hears invisible things move, she hears rain, noises, hears a clock strike, and the ringing of a bell,* all a result of brain fag. All these hallucinations seem to take an unfriendly tone: as part of the disintegration she exhibits the *delusion being laughed at, being mocked.*

Causalities

Prolonged Grief

Ph-ac is one of the most forgetful remedies of the materia medica, with a central theme of exhaustion on all planes; especially, and in the first place, *Ph-ac* has a **great weakness on the emotional plane**. Where *Picric-ac* starts with exhaustion on the mental plane and *Muriatic-ac* on the physical plane, *Ph-ac* can become sick through intense *prolonged grief,* and will, depending on the family miasmatic traits, progress rapidly to weakness on both the physical and mental planes. With *Picric-ac* it will be in the first place from ailments from (A/F) mental exertion; just like *Calc-p, Picric-ac* gets headaches with the slightest mental effort. With *Ph-ac,* it has everything to do with disillusions in love and friendship, others' rudeness, recurrent emotional shocks, and loss of communication that can occur with friends (*ailments from deceived friendship*), lovers, and family. The grief can be prolonged or may be a major sudden one that abruptly breaks down the person's VF. There is also grief about an *abortion, miscarriage,* or *after a long time illness,* such as chronic fatigue and fibromyalgia. But common causalities are certainly ailments from *disappointment, mortification* and *disappointed love,* which seem to abolish all feelings and emotions: "I don't want to see anyone," they say. "I don't feel anything anymore; I am like a stone." Other grief causalities are *death of a child* (which can include a miscarriage), *bad news,* such as hearing she has cancer or another serious disease, or the sudden and unexpected death of a loved one.

The crux of *Ph-acidum's* suffering is a serious grief similar to that of *Nat-m*: the breaking of her heart (*deception causes grief and mortification, in which she dwells over disappointments and shows hatred and revenge*), or successive smaller situations causing grief; these lead in the end to her dissociating from the real world and seeking refuge in a fantasy world (*as if in a dream*) or, more often, withdrawing from any activity in real life: a burnt-out or frozen state to be compared with the final *Sepia* stage (with *indifference to everything*) or to the hermit *Sulphur* (*averse to amusement; aversion to all persons; desire for solitude,* which should be added to the *Ph-acid* portrait). *Ph-acid,* therefore, should also be added to *silent grief,* as the person in such a state is inclined to cut off all contact with the outside world, disconnecting telephone and internet, closing the blinds, and lying in bed staring at the wall. This paralytic grief leads to *drowsiness, night sweats towards the morning, sweat and flushing of the face and crushing weight on the vertex.*

Extended and severe grief takes also the form of *ailments from homesickness.* There is no better remedy than *Ph-ac* for the adolescent who leaves home and familiar surroundings to enroll in college, often far away from family and close friends (*homesickness, with silent ill humor*). Only *Capsicum* is better than *Ph-ac* for homesickness: *Capsicum* has *homesickness with sleeplessness and with heat in the throat and red cheeks.* Many tragedies like suicide and severe depression could be avoided with doses of *Ph-acid.* In all these causalities we see an initial exhaustion on the emotional level: patients understand mentally what is happening to them, but they are overwhelmed by the emotions (< > of *Ignatia*).

Emotional Excitement

With her *Phosphorus* traits, such as *sympathy* (*amativeness, amorous*) and excitability, she also suffers from *ailments from care, ailments from emotional excitement, fright, and ailments from unhappy love,* especially at the end of a love affair that was particularly involved sexually. It is basically the *Phosphorus* person running out of energy after many exaggerated efforts to connect, or remain connected, to loved ones and multitudes of other friends. She exerts herself on numerous trips, posts on YouTube and Facebook, and exhausts the minutes on her cell phone, all to relieve the feeling of isolation—one of her biggest fears. "Stay connected" is *Phosphorus*'s motto, but unfortunately this leads to being disconnected in the *Ph-ac* state. *Ph-ac,* however, is not solely a remedy of pleasure, travel, and love. One must also take her business connections into account: *ailments from cares and worries* and *business failure.* Not surprisingly, the business fails: not only because of exhaustion, but also because of easy dissatisfaction with it and changeability of interests due to her tubercular character. *Ph-ac* is a good beginner, but a bad finisher.

Sexual Excesses

Excessive sexual activity is modestly referred to in TCM as "unregulated affairs of the bedroom." Excessive sexual activity weakens the Kidney energy, which harbors what the Chinese call the Ancestral (or miasmatic) Qi and the Essence, a precious substance inherited from the parents and partly replenished by the Qi extracted from food. The inherited Essence nourishes the fetus, and after birth, it controls growth, sexual maturation, fertility, and human development. Insufficient Essence may be a cause of infertility, impotence, and mental and physical underdevelopment in children, as well as declines in short-term memory. "Excessive" sexual activity entails ejaculation for men and orgasm for women, and it can also include excessive masturbation. Thousands of years after the development of TCM, homeopathy continues to recognize the same causalities of disease in the ailments from masturbation and loss of fluids for which *Ph-ac* is such a highly rated remedy. We mentioned ailments from *sexual excesses through masturbation*: this refers to the rather shameless and *lascivious Phosphorus* behavior (*naked, wants to be naked; nymphomania before menses*) and the *libertinism* of any *Phosphorus,* male or female. *Ph-ac* is *distressed by culpability after masturbation,* an expression of her *conscience as if guilty of a crime.* A differential diagnosis with *Staphysagria* and *Picric-acid* is necessary in this case. *Staphysagria* has frequent sexual dreams and, driven by her platonic love for her love objects, she feels good after masturbation. *Picric-acid* masturbates a lot to relief his mental tension during exams, but the more he masturbates, the worse his mind works, leading to exhaustion, short-term memory, and failure in exams (*almost complete loss of memory of the occurrence of the day*).

Loss of fluids can come not only from *excessive masturbation*, but also from *loss of blood, excessive perspiration* and *increased urination during menses* and *during perspiration* as well *as loss of sperm (pollution) during stool* (all proving symptoms of *Ph*-ac). We also have *ailments from fright*, the emotion linked to a decrease of the same Kidney Qi.

Compensations

Short-term Excitability

For a very short time, the homeopath can expect *Ph-ac* to use her *Phosphorus* characteristics to retain a glimmer of hope of connecting to others. This sounds like a psoric compensation, but there is nothing moderate in *Ph-acidum's* character; her behavior expresses all the exaggerated sycotic efforts of the first phase of an acidum: *she is amative, a nymphomaniac and excitable*, but this lasts only for a short time. In fact, *excitement aggravates her* easily. And the lasciviousness (sycosis) takes on the form of masturbation, but the only consequence is *sadness from masturbation, exhaustion, prostration of the mind; prostration of the mind after masturbation; hysteria after sexual excesses; hypochondriasis from sexual excesses, forgetfulness after sexual excesses, and distress by culpability*, all *from masturbation*. As mentioned before, it will also lead eventually to a decrease of energy on the mental and physical level: *long lasting effects of seminal emission, whether occurring during sleep or when awake, with every effort at stool or urination or from excessive venery. The whole system seemed weakened.*

Homesickness

Initially, *Ph-ac* still longs for her home (*homesickness with inclination to weep*) in that she yearns for that time in her life when she was happy, loved, and successful, having many friends because of her outgoing, lucky, happy attitude. Homesickness can be especially connected to a lost love: the *Phosphorus* aspect tries very hard to reconnect with and communicate again with the one she has lost, and she would do anything to have her soul mate back; *Ph-ac* returns to the subject of love and asks repeatedly to start over again (< > *Ignatia*, who has more hatred and hardness and reacts more with hysterical behavior, even on the physical plane with *globus hystericus and convulsions*). *Ignatia* has more of a weakness on the physical plane, while *Ph-ac* is weakened by the slightest grief on the emotional level. Both being exhausted in the final syphilitic stage, *Ph-ac* also contrasts with *Sepia* in that *Sepia has aversion to loved ones* rather than longing. And when you insist on talking to a *Sepia* person in her last phase, you will only arouse her ire, while a *Ph-ac* in its end stage lacks any strength to react at all, as if stimuli are not even received (*unconsciousness after emotions; mental insensibility*).

Aversion to Company

Ph-acidum's first negative reaction—as long as she still has some energy left—is *irritability towards anything but especially on awaking and when questioned*! Don't ask her, "How do you feel this morning?" At this point, a DD with *Sepia* can be difficult! (This is similar to *Nux-v*, the acute of *Sepia*). Irritability is a defense mechanism to protect her weak, emotional soul from slipping into the horrible depressive phase. As a result, if you treat a *Ph-ac* patient and the patient goes from indifference and apathy to irritability, this is the **right** direction of cure and no other remedy but *Ph-ac* is needed. Usually, like *Sepia*, feeling depleted, *Ph-ac* wants to be left alone and has a very hard time engaging in any conversation. *Ph-acidum's* negative compensations reflect, especially, the aversion to communication: *aversion to answer*, and *desire to be taciturn* is the usual reaction. One can expect no more than *monosyllable answers, reflecting long before she answers, answering incoherently, and unintelligible, while stupor returns quickly after answering*, as conversation taxes her very limited energy. *Ph-ac speaks unwillingly and talking is irksome*. For *Ph-acidum's* mind, everything goes too fast, so the whole action and thought process needs to be slowed down. *She is also averse being spoken to*. Any conversation is hampered by *forgetfulness while speaking; she has to hunt for words; she is unable to think long and there is dullness of the mind while reading. Her memory is weak for expressing herself and for remembering occurrences of the day*. So even if a question finally registers in *Ph-acidum's* mind, the patient's face looks vacant as she cannot find the right word (differential diagnosis with *Helleborus* necessary). *There is chaotic and confused behavior and aversion to thinking*, comparable *to Sepia*.

Depression and Withdrawal

Following initial irritability and withdrawal from conversations, *Ph-acid's* situation only becomes worse if the situation is not remedied; irritability is now replaced by emotions of a destructive syphilitic nature, especially a kind of depression that imitates that of other remedies: *her sadness increases even when walking in open air, and the longer she walks the worse it gets* (< >Aur, Puls). *She has the inclination to sit still* (compare *Puls*, and *Pic-ac*) and *has even aversion to the slightest thinking process* (any attempt to complete a whole idea is met with resistance as it is too tiresome). (Note: *Ph-ac* should be added in the repertory of *sits still.*) *She has dread of the future and sits there brooding over her condition* (compare with *Aurum*, but unlike *Aurum*, *Ph-ac* stops working, is averse to business, and exacerbates from music). *Ph-ac* understands what is happening to her (*brooding over one's condition*), but her weakness is on the emotional level, which leaves her with little desire to act or react. For a long time there is no true insanity but merely a deep lack of interest due to exhaustion (< >*Ignatia*, a feeling person, who is more hysterical and does not understand what is happening and *Pulsatilla*, who sits still in complete insane apathy and stares at an object as though she were a statue with her stillness). As mentioned before, if after administering *Ph-ac* the irritability comes back, this confirms Hering's *Observations of Cure* and no other remedy is needed (a mistake here would be giving *Nux-v*; continue with *Ph-ac*!).

Without intervention, *Ph-ac* in this phase of stillness spirals down into a world of loneliness and apathy, mirroring a severe form of depression. Her depression takes on a grave form as *she refuses to eat; she becomes indifferent to everything; she has indolence and aversion to work, and becomes weary of life. She becomes very weak and indifferent to affairs of life.* There is *indifference to those things that used to interest her most.* Life becomes useless, and there is no more meaning to it: "I don't want to live anymore; what is the point?" "My emotions are frozen." Especially after disappointed love, she disconnects her phone (*quiet disposition*), does not open her mail or read newspapers, and only *fruits and fruit juice are desired. There is a total loss of appetite from grief. There is a feeling of drowsiness and inclination to lie down.* We can see the connection and return to her CD as she feels dead and feels that around her is dead and non-existent: *even pinching is not noticed.* The patient seems, and in fact is, incapable of any response; she has sunk into total apathy and a burnt-out state. It is only at this point that there is danger of disintegration of the personality with insanity: *everything is as in a dream*, and *melancholic insanity can occur in which she picks at bed clothes, and makes gestures, grasping and reaching at something. There is semi-unconsciousness, in which she answers correctly when spoken to, but delirium and unconsciousness return at once.*

Golden Tips from the Masters

- *Ph-ac* is a chronic fatigue syndrome remedy when etiology fits
- Most prominent remedy for unrefreshed sleep
- *Ph-ac* loves sodas and carbonated drinks; desire for fruits or juicy things after loss of fluids i.e. post-operative or after a miscarriage
- Important diabetes remedy after grief, with dry mouth, dry eyes, and much thirst for juicy refreshing drinks. Together with *Phosphorus*, it is the most important remedy for diabetes.
- On the physical plane, we see *hair fall on the head from grief* (*only remedy*) and the presentation of *night sweats*. This hair fall is sudden and quite extensive and can also be seen in *falling of the hair from the genitals* (*Nat-m*, *Phos*), but it is the only remedy under the rubric *genitalia, female, hair falling after grief*. Sometimes the emotional shock turns the hair gray or white (*Nat-m*, *Phos*), but again, it is the only remedy of *hair turning grey after grief*.
- Grief causes also occipital headaches. Also interesting is the *frequent desire for stool* (diarrhea for months), *which is passed involuntarily while passing flatus* (*Aloe*), but there is no pain or any marked debility or exhaustion with this diarrhea. Diarrhea sets also in from catching a cold on a hot summer day with a cool evening.
- Tinnitus ameliorates by lying down
- Frequent urination during menses and during perspiration

Phosphorus (Phos). Elemental phosphorus

The Cyber Delusion

The Cyber delusion of *Phosphorus* is ***that she is on a distant island***. Her central idea is one of *disconnection*, which is also found in other fixed ideas such as *her body is scattered about the bed, delusion of being double, delusion of floating in air, delusion of errors of personal identity and that she is some other person* as well in the fixed idea that *familiar things seems strange*. This disconnection in *Phosphorus* people is an example of what are known as out-of-body and past life experiences, events common in *Phosphorus*. The whole psychic force or libido of the *Phosphorus* person, then, is aimed at connecting to others—to as many people as possible, including not only those in her neighborhood, but also anyone in the world in general. How envious to many people is *Phosphorus's* easy way of enjoying life, her independent persona, her radiant outlook. For a *Phosphorus* person, close ties with family and friends and the cultivation of strong social connections in general are not only important to living a fulfilling life: they are vital to *Phosphorus's* healthy life. The CD reflects a sense of isolation and being fenced in—being removed from everyone. We can indeed find *Phosphorus* under the rubric *forsaken*. However, the forsaken feeling of *Phosphorus* is quite different from that of other remedies (*Aurum*, *Pulsatilla*, *Nat-m*, etc.) in this rubric. *Phosphorus's* first goal is to connect to others as she is driven by this incomprehensible feeling of isolation. This is understandable to most people in view of *Phosphorus's* positive tools, including her beauty, sympathy, and loquacity. So there is definitely a difference in *Phosphorus's* approach to people ("How many friends can I find in the world?") and that of its inimical remedy, *Causticum* ("How many enemies are out there?"). It looks as though *Phosphorus* is more geared towards pleasure and *Causticum* towards serious issues in the world. While *Phosphorus* writes an ode to the one she loves, *Causticum* is busy composing a manifesto about the injustice in this world.

Phosphorus is a *compassionate* person, which means that she does not make a distinction between her own ego and others'. For *Phosphorus*, the suffering she sees in others touches her almost as closely as does her own. Her act of compassion is not oriented to each situation individually, but to the world in its entirety as she has boundless compassion for all living beings, humans, animals, and all of Nature's beauty. She is mindful, which makes her more connected to other people—an empathetic feeling of being "at one with the universe." This provides an explanation for another theme of *Phosphorus*: *delusions, seeing accidents.* There is always fear about something: that *something bad will happen* to her or to those close to her. Such a fixed idea is always an intrusion on the patient's life as all possibilities are anticipated with fear. There is panic regarding the idea of imminent danger and death, especially when she is alone; she experiences the same apprehension for her children and husband when they are away from home.

Another theme is *Phosphorus's* delusional fears and distortions: *delusions, fingers are thumbs, sees something coming out of corners, sees frightful images; hears voices; sees dead persons; is about to be choked,* as well as *delusion, will be murdered and delusions of fire, sees frightful phantoms, sees thieves and is pursued by the police.* It should be apparent by now that *Phosphorus's* outings in the world will somewhat be inhibited by the magnitude of her fears of bodily harm as they are created by her intuitive feeling side. Then again, her CD (that is why it is the CD!), reflecting her *Wanderlust* with a dominant anima, surpasses everything—even her greatest fears. *Phosphorus's* fears are also related to Nature (*fear for thunderstorms*), fears of *impending disease,* fear of lack of company (*fears of being alone*), *and fear of death.* As one can see, loneliness stemming from a lack of communication is a dominant emotion.

It is not surprising, in view of her persona, that *Phosphorus* demonstrates some delusions of **grandeur**. She believes that she *is a great person* and projects herself as such! Her delusions of grandeur do not have much to do with achievements, although she has the *delusion, she is doing business* and the *delusion, she is hard at work.* While the flamboyant *Phosphorus* can be very successful in business—as long as business relates to beauty, acting, and decoration—she is not eager to engage in the business of thinking because it exhausts her too much (*great indisposition to mental or physical exertion; brain fag from mental overwork and constant strain of eyes*). While she is not on the same level of haughtiness as *Platina*—for one thing, she is much warmer and more charming than the white-gold queen—*Phosphorus* feels she is *rich and noble,* which probably helps her to connect to just about anyone in the world from the poorest to the richest (delusion, *as if she is rich and delusion of wealth; delusion, she is a person of rank; delusion, she* *is distinguished; delusion her chair is rising up and delusion, she is the incorporeal light*). These last two provings express her elevated standing, in her eyes, among the general public; this is generally and gladly acknowledged by the recipients of her warm radiating presence, "a ray of light" that falls upon the darkness of their existence, but this quality is also envied by others who are entangled in the negativity of their own beings.

Causalities

Fright and Anticipation

The sensitive *Phosphorus* person is full of fears, especially those related to her own body and her family's well-being. Her *sympathetic* nature explains the fixed idea *of accidents of her relatives*. This mirrors the extreme concern *Phosphorus* shows for anyone in her wide circle of friends and family, so when Mom and Dad leave on an outing, there often arises in the young child *fear something will happen*—not out of the selfishness seen in the *Arsenicum* person, but from genuine concern and love (*anxiety about others*). Her own fears are easily projected on others, such as her *fears for impending disease, robbers, and death*. Need for protection and connection leads logically to fears *for being alone*, as *Phosphorus* loves and needs company, warmth, and communication. As much as a *Phosphorus* child remains close to the collective unconscious and its language of fairy tales and archetypes, she remains *afraid of ghosts, death, and visions* once the unconscious takes over (*fear of the dark in the evening in bed*). This child loves homeopaths: they seem to be genuinely interested in her fantasy stories, and homeopaths neither draw blood (during which she usually faints like the *Calcarea* child) nor undress her for a physical examination, which creates much anxiety (*anticipation before going to the dentist and physician*).

Grief

Grief in the *Phosphorus* child's life is mainly related to disconnection from people and animals that are important to her. Divorces are traumatic (for the *Calcarea* child too); moving away from friends is always injurious to her soul; the death of a beloved pet, which is another family member, has the same detrimental effect as losing a sibling; the sickness and suffering of a family member are made her own; and losing even one friend at school causes immense grief in her life in spite of the fact that she makes friends very easily. The *Phosphorus* child, unfortunately, gets attached all too easily and far too soon to humans and animals alike. It is therefore not uncommon that this child reacts to these grief events with serious diseases such as juvenile rheumatoid arthritis (JRA, an autoimmune disease) or anorexia nervosa and bulimia. For *Phosphorus*, losing support is seen as *deception causing grief and mortification*. And, in general for the *Phosphorus* child, *headache is caused by grief and undermines her constitution*, taking the wind out of her sails.

What are the differences between *Phosphorus*'s grief and that of its inimical remedy, *Causticum*? *Causticum's* grief is long-lasting (similar to that of *Nat-m*) and so is hard to overcome. *Phosphorus*, as we will see, has more tools to help her overcome the grief. While the death of a child, parent, or friend surely affects *Phosphorus* deeply, it is his reaction to such an event that sets him apart. Every emotion in *Causticum* is influenced by a sense of justice. Therefore, grief over the death of a parent, child, or friend (which includes people anywhere in the world who suffer injustice) is strongly expressed by protestations against the injustice. With a *Phosphorus* person, such a death is also more connected to her own fears, especially her fear of death; she asks herself: "Am I next?" In *Causticum*, the grief is deeply felt, and it is expressed differently than it is in *Phosphorus*: *Causticum weeps from sympathy with others*. Surprisingly, *Causticum's quiet disposition* leads to more weeping than in *Phosphorus*. We see *Causticum weeping at trifles, weeping easily, and weeping after drinking* and being *sentimental during drunkenness*. Weeping in *Phosphorus* does not seem to persist (*hysterical alternations of laughter and weeping*) as she looks for the beauty and intimacy in this world rather than the injustice. We find *weeping, alternating with laughing, weeping spasmodic and weeping after anxiety*. This has much to do with the fact that *Causticum* looks for places where unrest reigns, while *Phosphorus* looks for a world full of like-minded people; she is focused on friendship, laughter, and sharing experiences and values. Their *ailments from*: *cares and worries, hearing bad news* (*horrible things and sad stories affect her profoundly*), and *emotional excitement* can be viewed in the same light. *Causticum* and *Phosphorus* both care, but their motivations are different. For *Causticum*, everything is related to serious events both in her world and in the rest of the world. *Phosphorus* is equally moved and excited by beauty, friendship, travel, and the like. So the bad news that *Phosphorus* might hear is that she has to cancel her adventure trip! And emotional excitement can be about all the friends she is going to party with, unlike *Causticum*—who gets worked up about war, dictators, and meddlers in people's lives!

Sexual Excesses

One of *Phosphorus's* NWS is definitely different from *Causticum's*: sexual excesses. Indeed, *Phosphorus* does not shy away from a powerful positive tool: her beauty! She can resort to some extravagant moves if necessary: *shamelessness; lascivious; uncovers herself and wishes to go naked.* Causticum is *sentimental, sympathetic and serious,* **not sexual**! *Phosphorus* does not hesitate to flaunt her beauty in a flirtatious way, especially when younger. *Phosphorus* is attracted to the intellectual and successful type, one who excels in the thinking conscious function as it complements for her extreme feeling conscious function. Flirting is second nature for *Phosphorus*, and it belongs to her persona, but she is a warmer person than *Lycopodium* and *Medorrhinum*, who disregard the partner's inner personality consciously as they really don't want to know their partners. *Phosphorus* has also *ailments from celibacy* and *fear for celibacy.* Celibacy does not mean being literally unmarried. In its extended meaning, it can also suggest not being connected to anyone: having no friends or others caring for *Phosphorus*!

Compensations and Consequences

Creativity and the Arts

Conveying the contents of the *Phosphorus* soul is not only done through talking (*loquacity*), but is commonly expressed through a love for drawing, sculpting, theater, dancing, clay model making, crafts, painting, and writing in verse as *Phosphorus* is not only intelligent (*active concentration and easy comprehension*) but also interested in all kinds of extracurricular activities (*desire for numerous various things*). These are all forms of communication, which is the major compensation of the *Phosphorus* child and adult, and when such communication is lost because of moving, the loss of a friend, or the death of a family member, the ensuing grief easily sends this child into her own dream world, reflecting autistic characteristics. This is the child that is very verbal from a young age, charming everyone, a popular grade schooler with friends clamoring for her attention. She is the best artist in the class and the best dancer in junior high, often the first violinist in the all-city orchestra. She is often the homecoming queen, edits the high school paper, wins creative writing awards, and is usually voted most likely to succeed. She is inclined to be fascinated with crafts, painting, and art from a young age. She learns to sew in order to have all the pretty clothes she wants. While this child can excel in sports, especially swimming and running, she often runs out of energy (*great indisposition to mental or physical exertion*). Even on the mental plane, this is a child who needs to take numerous breaks from mental work, (*dullness and unable to think long; no capacity for mental work; brain fag from mental overwork*); otherwise, she will *understand a question only after repeating and becomes detached and sleepy.*

Vessels of Light

Some lucky souls are born with brighter outlooks than others; they simply see beauty and opportunity where others hone in on flaws and dangers. *Phosphorus* belongs to the first category. *Phosphorus* is derived from the Greek words *pher* or *phoreo,* meaning "to carry, bear" and *phos* or "light," which defines this person perfectly. In her pure state, *Phosphorus* possesses genuine personal advantages that mold her personality in the broadest sense. She **is** the way of lightness, playfulness, charm, attraction, and sensuality. She is wholly awake and fully alive. She is attuned to beauty, pleasure, and enjoyment, the play of love and life. She is the radiant vision, appearing an angel of beauty and love. Life looks worthy and bright. She gives lightness and poetic inspiration, enjoys and grieves easily, loves and rejects often, connects and repels even more. She dances and plays with a life that for her is simply a game and an illusion. Happiness, for *Phosphorus,* comes from within as well from without: she avails herself of the manifold blessings which surround her and has a personality that allows her to appreciate them. She feels that life is indeed a glorious inheritance to be enjoyed! She is a person who, when in balance, loves life to the fullest; she is capable of wandering, always ready for an adventure and to see something new rather than being tied to the security of finding confirmation in the old. For *Phosphorus,* life seems full of fortuitous circumstances as she is fearless (in spite of the many fears she has) when it comes to trying something new. If an opportunity appears, *Phosphorus* will usually take it, as it allows her to live in a sort of never-ending fantasy world. Instead of giving in to worry about what could go wrong, she says to herself, "Isn't that interesting? I'd like to give it a try." Variety in life increases her day-to-day happiness. She maximizes her chances of good luck by maintaining a large network of friends and acquaintances. Serendipity smiles on *Phosphorus* and her relaxed approach to life. If our world is shaped by our perceptions, then the world of *Phosphorus* is interesting and full of beauty and meaning, an exciting adventure; *Calc-c* might see the same lifestyle as shallow and superficial, because *Calc-c* wants a steady home and security, not adventure!

When cheerfulness knocks on her door, *Phosphorus* throws the door wide open, never missing the opportunity to increase her happiness. We all might experience similar external events, but *Phosphorus* always manages uniquely to make it a life of wonderment, a life to be gazed at with bright, open eyes. Being of a sanguine nature, she sees a scene of conflict as a way to connect more deeply with the other person, extending her far-reaching compassion. In contrast, a choleric temperament such as *Nux-v* will explode in anger, throwing his whole being against the barrier of conflict to destroy it rather than trying to resolve it; a nervous temperament such as that of *Nat-m* immediately resorts to a protective mode, walling herself off to avoid further injury.

We all could learn something from a *Phosphorus* person about how to enjoy life and all its manifestations as she is driven by a love for all things: she has an uncanny ability to simply recognize the beauty of a cloud formation while listening to her friends the birds serenading her in thanks for the gourmet food she has provided. (This does not necessarily mean she is used to cooking gourmet meals for her husband. After all, there is more to do in life than spend time working in the kitchen!) Thank goodness, a love of life can be contagious—and *Phosphorus* is its permanent messenger!

Travel and Distraction

As D. H. Lawrence once said, "The great home of the soul is the open road." This can be said of any *Phosphorus* person! *Phosphorus* is characterized by a tubercular dissatisfaction, fidgety character, and quickness in shifting interests; therefore, a need to change physically (restless traveling from one city to another) as well as mentally (changing study topics or interest all the time) and emotionally (easy connection to others but very often tires of and dispatches them) is not uncommon. Travel (the world is her home) is therefore the ideal solution: there are millions of people out there to be met and, if so desired, to be left, although she loves to stay in touch with many people around the world. (This is uncomplicated now thanks to the internet, which is the greatest invention for the *Phosphorus* person.) *Phosphorus* also likes to read adventure and travel stories as well as animal stories.

Dissatisfaction will be the driving force for her restless nature as she moves from one city to another, from one continent to another—if not literally on her numerous travels, figuratively in her dreams or thoughts. She will light a candle of Moroccan scent; a carpet has to be imported from an exotic country; books of travel to dangerous destinations are absorbed in a dreamlike state, while the furniture and other gadgets in her house are a keen reminder of previous trips (*excited imagination*). *Phosphorus* is keenly sensitive to the value of beautiful surroundings, and never wearies of describing the various items (treasures) in the rooms in which she lives and even those in which she would have liked to live (like the temples or houses of ancient times). Often blessed with a *Carcinosin* eye for harmony, with true accordance of all real beautiful things irrespective of age or place of origin, she decorates a room not for show, but a room for her to live in and recall the wonderful moments of her many journeys. Carpets, paintings, frames, books, chairs, and hanging mosque lamps are fondly viewed not only because of their place of origin but especially of the way they were purchased: "That one I bought from an old man, who told me that it had been kept in the family for a long time." "This one I procured after having a delightful conversation over mint tea with a lady who told me the story of the love of her life." (Touching her heartstrings certainly helped clinch the sale). Every acquisition comes with a story that is as tenderly remembered as the item itself. One can fancy her lying on the Persian sofa on the pillow purchased in Malaysia, in the midst of books, engravings, and carpets, her mind wandering and traveling along the four corners of the Earth. Her love for travel will distract her mind. She is the eternal seeker for truth and enlightenment, but often forgets to find it within herself. This is most easily observed when death must be faced; she has great fear of death, or, as one female acquaintance said to me (while continuously traveling all over the world), "When the money is gone, I'll die the next day." Her life's purpose meets its end when she loses the financial means to maintain this lifestyle. At this point she suffers from a spiritual disease. She then asks herself: "But what if I am dying? What if I am suffering from a terminal disease that stops me from doing things that give meaning to my life?" In the context of the end of life, the last opportunity to give meaning to her existence and enrich others' lives, it is interesting to note that the word *despair*, coming from the Latin *asper* or "rough" and *are* or "to be," or being in a rough place or spot, a syphilitic expression can be also translated as suffering without meaning. And such a syphilitic expression is, again, a spiritual distress. A person can still give meaning to life, providing an example to others, by coping with such a situation, with his fate, his fears, and his distress. It will take great patience and courage, not always common characteristics of the restless and excitable *Phosphorus*. But she should remember that people who face death and pain without flinching have earned and received the greatest gift granted to humankind: showing others that there is meaning in life until the very end.

Phosphorus is also the housewife who changes furniture and wallpaper constantly, the businessman who changes job frequently, and the student who chooses another major every year. Being extraverted intuitive types, they are the great beginners but rarely the finishers. They can be skillful politicians and diplomats, but often the irresponsible adventurers and excitable fashionistas. Their nemesis lies in the opposite conscious function, which is the introverted sensation; this means that they tend to misjudge and overlook concrete conditions and limitations and often put themselves at risk in spite of their numerous fears.

Company and Intimacy

There is a theme of **diffusion** in *Phosphorus*. She wants to spread outward into the environment. She finds joy in being friendly, being warm, in considering and respecting another person and making him or her happy. She organizes her life around goals such as fostering community, connecting to family, and engaging creatively. *Phosphorus* is a person who experiences falling in love as exhilarating and intense. As it loses the desired intensity quickly, love ends in the wish for never-ending conquests, always with the illusion that the new love will be better than the previous ones, and will result in finding *Phosphorus's* soul mate. In this conquest, the tubercular person is greatly helped by her beautiful physique: the *fine eyelashes, tall figure,* beautiful eyebrows and angelic face. Lucky women like *Phosphorus* have big, beautiful eyes, while other constitutions just seem to have big eyes thanks to the clever application of eye shadow. Trying to explain *Phosphorus's* appeal is very much like attempting to justify one's fascination with a beautiful song. The melody haunts and the lyrics tantalize. There is no one portion of the tune that stands out, no single compelling line among the lyrics which will go down in history. Each note and word is part of the whole, and the whole mesmerizes and is unforgettable. So it is with *Phosphorus*! The chest is usually unremarkable and even boyish (although she is the first one to correct this minor mishap of Nature by having breast implants); the arms are slender and the neck photogenically firm. The chin is determined. The mouth is enchanting, small and drawn, turning up at the corners only slightly, almost royally, when she smiles. The eyes are captivating and seductive; the voice can be soft or enthusiastic, but its tone is always comforting. Nothing can exceed the grace of her movements and the charm of her manner, both of which give her the delightful distinction of being different from others. Her heartfelt laughter brings sunrays on a drairy day. Her speech is both "with it" and educated. When young, she is often a shopaholic and a rather compulsive one: she sees something she likes and buys it because she wants to look pretty. The internet, of course, has become a fertile shopping ground for the spontaneous *Phosphorus* woman. When smarter and more mature, she limits herself to looking, buying less, as even a *Phosphorus* person can only have so much. On entering a room, she draws awed gazes, and men who have gotten to know her are willing to travel many miles to cherish her company. Of course she is spoiled. All charming people are; it is the secret of their attraction. *Phosphorus* never wants for company. She is like a chameleon, a woman of a thousand faces. Her beauty is such that it seems to realize every form of fancy, to embody each dream of the creative imagination. She can be reserved and professional in business. At social functions she fits in beautifully, even stands out, both at formal charity fundraisers and on more casual occasions; she is welcomed and fêted at elegant gatherings, but neither is she ill at ease guzzling beers in the back of a pickup with bare feet hanging out over the open tailgate. Her grades at school and university are good, but could be better with a less active social life.

Phosphorus is little impressed by fame and only slightly more by fortune. Her abundant beauty and inviting charm easily capture the imaginations of *Sulphur* and *Lycopodium* men; they are carried away and wish to support her honorably in some form or another for the rest of her life. Beauty is indeed like an open letter of recommendation, predisposing the hearts of others to favor the person who presents it. But *Phosphorus* is sensitive to those around her and to the suffering of others. *Phosphorus* is a person with a strong feeling function: she can look into the face of someone and realize what that person is experiencing—pain or pleasure, hurt or anger. She genuinely cares (*sympathy, desire for*) for the underdog and those who encounter mishaps in life. Despite modern stress, competition, and struggle, it is natural to *Phosphorus* to rejoice upon a friend's success, simply because sympathy with joy intensifies the sum of joy in *Phosphorus* herself. She desires to give and receive love. Besides a strong feeling function, the conscious function of intuition is always strongly developed in a *Phosphorus* person, either as the dominant primary function (in which she approaches everything in the world with this function) or as the auxiliary function, subordinate to the primary function. Feeling tells her that she likes someone; that she also has empathy and intuition provides her with the uncanny ability to know what **may be**: smelling a rat, having a hunch. With this intuitive function, *Phosphorus* sees things in a broad context. For instance, in viewing a lovely landscape, where the sensation type like *Calc-c* will note every detail of the flowers, trees, and the color of the sky, the intuitive *Phosphorus* imagines where it all came from and speculates about its future: "What will happen to the Nature that I see with all the destruction and pollution that exist?"

Phosphorus becomes easily animated, and also attracts attention with her appearance, speaking style, and evident warmth. Behind this is the feeling that she is not getting enough attention, love, or care for herself. Because of this insecurity, she wants more friends and company. *Phosphorus* makes friends easily, and she likes to stay out of the house. The house is a source of sorrow for her. If she did not get love at home as a child, she seeks it outside by having numerous friends; however, most of the friends are superficial, since close friends are hard to make in general.

Connection (even via the phone or computer) can mean security for the *Phosphorus* person; it is like being part of a big "family." Such a quest also reflects the fiery or sanguine temperament of this person: *very excitable, cheerful, and vivacious,* and these emotions must find an outlet in exchanges with many people. One of her dictums is "If no news, send rumors!" She can go from small talk—conversational hors d'oeuvres with each topic sampled and savored—to deeper topics such as the suffering of people caught in wars. But there is another side to the coin: *Phosphorus* is often *clairvoyant,* sees auras around people, and also *hears voices, sees something coming out of the corner of her eyes and can have horrible visions at night.* This is due to a great *sensitivity to all external impressions*: the *Phosphorus* person is very *impressionable, easily mesmerized and magnetized by others,* but also sensitive to *thunderstorms,* of which *she is very afraid.* There is also sensitivity to *noise, and light,* from which she wants to shield herself. This leads to two opposite forces at work in *Phosphorus*: on one hand, he wants to connect but on the other hand, because of his great sensitivity and impressionability, she is often stuck because of fears, especially of *ghosts, devils, phantoms and hearing invisible things move,* which in turn makes her fear *losing her reason.* To overcome these fears, to be able to explore the world—which is the driving force of this *precocious being*—connection to others is a desire and a necessity, providing protection for her well-being.

This attractive, *sentimental,* and extraverted person (with a great growth spur at puberty, often causing growing pains-*Calc-p*) loves to be massaged, held, and kissed. This child *accepts and craves for affection* and, when it is received, *easily returns affection.* Because of her *sympathetic and affectionate character,* she is also *sensitive to the crying of children.* This bleeding-heart mentality is also expressed by a great tendency to bleeding on the physical plane, especially *nose bleeding.*

She equally *desires sympathy and compassion,* and lack of love (whether real or incorrectly perceived) is a major reason for which this child may show autistic characteristics like *difficulty in concentration* and *learning with difficulty,* withdrawing on her own (*refusing to answer, reflecting long before answering*), quite a contrast to her normal, bubbly personality; she resorts to *great fancies and daydreaming, desire to bite, confused behavior, excitability preventing sleep,* and *automatic gestures* (spinning, flapping, and strange and funny gestures), especially *during sleep.*

Homesickness

As much as she loves to explore the world, *Phosphorus* is very much tied to the family; when going away to school or moving away from home at a later age, homesickness can set in. The internet and the mobile phone (texting) are her great friends. There is no better remedy for homesickness than *Phosphoric acidum*, the exhaustive state of *Phosphorus*. It is not uncommon, when moving away from her beloved neighborhood, for a *Phosphorus* child to be afflicted by an autoimmune disease such as juvenile diabetes or JRA. The grief and forsaken feeling that homesickness creates is apparently enough to turn the body against itself, as expressed in these destructive diseases.

Depression

Grief and cut-off communication are the main causalities of the extreme form of depression that can be found in the *Phosphorus* person; this is called a *Phosphoricum acidum* state. In this state, she *will refuse to eat (anorexia nervosa), sits there as if in a dream, brooding over her condition, her hair falls out; she becomes indifferent to everything, has indolence to work, and shows a weak memory for expressing herself* (the opposite of her normal loquacity) as she is *forgetful for words while speaking.* Although she is better with consolation, when in the grips of such a depression *she is irritable when questioned and desires solitude as she suffers from silent grief.* She even thinks that *others are mocking her,* which makes her become even more withdrawn. Children at this point may *masturbate,* but this only *increases their sadness and lack of energy. Phosphorus* will develop a total *aversion to thinking* with *disconnected thoughts and complete aversion to mental work.* Such a dark and dramatic change from her usual lightness, stemming from the abovementioned causalities, should catch the attention of every parent of a *Phosphorus* child. *In her apathy, Phosphorus is indifferent even to her own children, answers no questions or replies wrong.*

Golden Tips from the Masters

- *Phosphorus* and *Causticum* are inimical remedies and should never be given following each other without first cancelling the previous remedy with an antidote!
- When aggravation after doses of *Phosphorus*, give *Psorinum*!
- #1 remedy for NWS lightning (with *Nux-v*) with brain damage (loss of memory, confusion, and loss of energy)
- #1 remedy for fatty degeneration of the liver
- String amelioration with short nap (< >*Lachesis*); headaches disappear after a short nap (*Sepia*)
- Rare and peculiar symptom: the anus may stand wide open; diarrhea and feces oozing from a wide-open anus; stool as soon as anything enters the rectum
- In pregnancy, cold water intake relieves only until the water becomes warm in the stomach, then symptoms of morning nausea return. Also: pregnant woman has nausea and vomits when putting her hands in warm water
- Antidote of MSG
- Bright red bleeding without clotting
- In pneumonia *Phosphorus* does NOT want to lie on the affected side (< >*Bryonia*)
- #1 remedy for diabetes and hypoglycemia
- NWS general anesthesia
- NWS pneumonia
- #1 remedy for rheumatic stiffness with morning aggravation
- Environmental illness: sensitive to noise, odors and people's energy and electrical magnetic fields
- *Phosphorus* has an aggravation 36 hours after it is taken. No matter what potency it is, if it is the right remedy there will be an aggravation (Dr. Case)
- Is one of the persons who love massage!

Platina (Plat). Platinum

The Cyber Delusion

Platina is a very self-assured, even cocky individual who puts herself above every mortal (*haughty*). While she is indeed called white gold, *Platina* is far from perfect; it will become apparent that her state is not one that we should strive for. Life is *Platina's* personal express lane; although there are seven billion people in the world, it is all about her! Vanity is her name! There is nothing shy about *Platina*, who, rather, demonstrates hardness to others and shows respect only for those few whom she considers better than herself (*contemptuous, hard for subordinates and agreeable and pleasant to superiors or people she has to fear*). *Platina's* beliefs and delusions keep these unpleasant elements behind bars in her unconscious, and it is for this reason that she is unable to evolve into a completely free spirit with a balanced ego. *Platina* is unaware that the course she has chosen in life is a wrong one (*delusion she is doomed*) until she becomes a prisoner on the physical plane (paralytic destructive consequences; *paralytic weakness; great numbness in face around os zygomaticus*). Paralysis, MS, and numbness of the face reflect the stagnation of Qi/Vital Force on more planes than simply the physical; it is the physical expressions, though, that make *Platina* realize that her path of individuation—however glamorous her life may seem to be to her—is an inferior and incomplete one. Her only possible rescue: for someone to allow her to entertain and cultivate her Cyber delusion, which in turn averts pathology as long as she can maintain that CD. This brings us, now, back to the beginning of our story. Let's investigate *Platina's* driving force: her Cyber delusion.

Platina's Cyber delusion is ***the delusion of humility and lowness of others while she is great***. Without any doubt, *Platina* is the haughtiest remedy of our materia medica. She feels an urgency to grab the spotlight, instead of making a serious effort toward becoming a contributing member of a group. Driven by her CD, she is not at all concerned with how others are evaluating her. If her family is affluent, accomplished, and famous, *Platina* believes that her ancestors' achievements are transgenerational and feels entitled to pride in recessive traits and titles she apparently possesses but does not exhibit. It should come as no surprise that most of her delusions confirm the Cyber delusion as *Platina's* life reflects the life of a self-perceived queen, the Cleopatra of our materia medica. *Platina* fails to see that genuine humility in life is a sign of inner strength and that modesty involves self-awareness joined with a belief in the intrinsic equality of people. *Platina* is unaware of Aristotle's statement that virtue resides in the golden mean between extremes—a balancing act between acknowledging one's accomplishments and virtues and hiding them from view. No remedy has more delusions of grandeur than *Platina*, and this reflects the essence of her CD: *delusion, everything in the room is diminished while she is tall and elevated; delusion, she does not belong to her own family; delusion being noble; delusion, she is a proud person; delusion, on entering the house after a walk, people seem mentally and physically inferior; delusion of superiority; delusion, as if he is rich; delusion, things appear small; delusion, he is swollen; delusion, she is very tall; delusion, of wealth; delusion as to the greatness of her body and delusion she is a great person*. In Hering, we read: *pride and overestimation of oneself; looking down with haughtiness on others*. Although the word "pride" is used in the provings, vanity is a better word for the true *Platina* state. Pride is the firm conviction of one's worth, self-esteem that comes from **within**. Vanity, on the other hand, is the desire to awaken a conviction of one's worth in others; it is this attempt to arrive at such esteem from **without** that is characteristic of *Platina*. Pride is earned through merit; vanity is the secret hope of acquiring self-esteem based on delusional and deceiving behavior. *Platina* has a blind and exaggerated vanity, which makes her despise her home and treat her family like Philistines (*delusion does not belong to her family*).

Platina, considering herself a person of rank and position, always behaves disdainfully towards people who (in her warped opinion) are in a lower position than she is. Vain as she is, she can be talkative as well as taciturn *(indisposed to talk, alternating with jesting)*. *Platina* might spend hours in front of the mirror attending to her makeup and hair as the beauty of her body is the only existing reality she knows. Vanity, for *Platina*, is false pride: she tries to arouse certainty of her worthiness in others, but her translucent pseudo-ego deceives only the feeblest of minds. Vanity has barred up the windows of her house, and the name of the warder is contempt (*pompous; contemptuous to everything; casting off people against her will*)! *Platina* is unable to let go of the feeling that she is always right; she is smug and superior with others in order to cultivate an impression of extraordinariness. Her self-righteousness, *increased ambition*, and self-satisfaction are simply fun for her. Indulging in these feelings and thoughts not only provides her with a sense of power over others, but also gives her the false comfort of thinking that she doesn't really need to change—because she is so much better than others!

Snobbery can be a symptom of narcissistic personality disorder, a condition marked by grandiosity, an inflated sense of one's own importance, a deep need for the admiration of others and recognition of superiority, and a preoccupation with power and prestige while exhibiting little regard for other people's feelings. *Platina's* troubles, though, go beyond snobbery: her relationships are impaired because she is unable to enter anyone else's world. When *Platina* has the delusion that *she is alone in the world and she feels deserted*, it is unlike the neediness of a *Pulsatilla* who has this delusion as her Cyber delusion; *Platina* feels all alone in the world because she is the queen, and apparently there are few other queens whom she considers to be of her standing. Unlike *Pulsatilla*'s, hers is an accepted and even welcomed position of isolation (*delusion she has no place in the world*), a position of honor, of not belonging to the class of commoners, which suits her well. Far from being insecure, with her high self-esteem, she exhibits an orientation towards extreme social dominance: she believes that some people, like her, are innately superior to others and therefore deserve more esteem in society. As with the other remedy associated with pride, *Lachesis*, she believes she is in contact with superhuman beings (*delusion, is under super human control*) who are guiding her life. But as with *Lachesis*, this will result in a 'life unlived.' Selfishness and egotism are hallmarks of *Platina*. For her, the world is a non-ego; it does not belong to her (*delusion, she does not belong to her own family; she is all alone in the world*); her relationship to the world is a hostile one to the extent that she feels *contempt* for it rather than hatred. It is as if *Platina* is rocketed off to a distant planet.

Although we find in *Platina* the rubric *marriage, excited sexual girls are obsessed with the idea of marriage*, once she grows up it is all about the opportunity to have sex and not to have children. Children are unwanted (*aversion to her own children*) and maternal duties seem unbearable (see clinical example further); the mundane demands of marital life are responded to with impatience, irritation, and even indignation! In *Platina* we find a resistance to the mother complex: "I want to be anything but my mother" is her motto! This resistance to the mother complex always leads to menstrual disturbances (*menses clotted; menses, absent; menses intermittent after abortion, only Platina; menses painful*), *vaginismus*, failure to conceive (*complaints of vaginal genitalia; sterility*), and problems in labor (*childbed, mental symptoms during*).

It is evident from her behavior that *Platina* suffers from a kind of mania (*mania with violence; delusion being at war*). Existing in a perpetual state of mania is living dangerously. One exhibits vast energy levels, elevated moods, intensified mind, and amplified senses; these begin as assets, but they end only in delusions of grandeur or megalomania; mania often creates an insidious mechanism to self-destruct as well as danger of dissociation (*delusion, she will become insane; delusion, divided or cut into two parts; delusion, she was about to die; mania with deeds of violence*). This is the fate of many *Platinas*. It is astonishing to see *Platina's* annoyance in response to the slightest disdain, disrespect, or slight: all the while, *Platina's* life passes by her like a dream—an annoying source of illusions, heartbreaks, bereavements, embarrassments, disappointments, disbelief, and irritations, all due to the fact that she cannot bring herself to look at her ever-growing shadow side. Thus, she remains a prisoner to her mighty delusions.

Causalities

If we consider *Platina* as a being with excessive needs looking for balance, then these NWS will make sense.

Sheltered Family Upbringing

This is a causality that you can't find in any repertory, but it is, nonetheless, a very real A/F that leads to the creation of a *Platina* person. The formation of the excessive persona usually starts in childhood and causes much confusion in adult life, since the persona has been unconsciously accepted in early childhood:

> I remember such a patient from my practice; she complained to me that she found the demands of life with her children too hard. Resentment, bitterness, and jealousy were apparent; what was notable about these resentments was that many of them were aroused by the everyday, ordinary experiences of life. The sacrifices she made for her children and her husband (who did not earn enough in her viewpoint to supply her with a nanny and a maid) were those which most people make, but she felt like life had singled her out to struggle with these common situations. She worked herself up over the ordinary difficulties

> of marriage, although she usually failed to see her own part in creating her marital problems. "Other men's sins are before our eyes; our own are behind our backs," said the Roman philosopher Seneca. While this is true for many people, it is an inherent part of *Platina's* makeup. She was an only child, born in a wealthy and important family, and at school she was treated differently because of her well-known, politically well-connected family. She was called "Princess" by her parents, and she readily identified herself with the corresponding fantasy figure. The princess could do no wrong, and in her ego adaptation she **was** the princess. This did not change when she married a powerful Wall Street broker; she could accompany him to banquets and on outings, and she was treated with the reverence she expected. But everything changed when her children were born. As she could no longer accompany her husband, in her own words, she became a commoner: the ego adaptation only worked as long as the environment remained undisturbed. But now, even with her own limited qualifications, she wanted to put the genie back in the bottle; she still expected to be treated as a princess whereas, to others, she was now an ordinary woman with no special abilities.

Reflecting the CD of *Platina,* people who were not recognized in societal circles were unacceptable to her as equals; she expected life to arrange a new setting of superior privileges for her, even in her now-ordinary life. The persona formed in childhood had become so much a part of herself that it was almost impossible for her to see herself as part of common humanity. When she took up tennis, she refused to play with the beginners (where she belonged) but insisted on playing with the advanced players! In essence, she was in danger of identifying with this consciously chosen nobility persona. So her princess persona smiled, was courteous and gently condescending, all with a consciousness of the charm of this image. But the egotism, the resentments, and the emotions which would eventually destroy her were invisibly harbored in her shadow side. Her ego had not only accepted but welcomed all the influences that had played their parts in building up this persona, and so the ego had become identified with the image. She developed numbness in the face, which is a typical symptom motivating *Platina* to seek medical treatment, at the os zygomaticus (*face, numbness right side, and numbness zygoma*); this alternated with the periods of depression that are common for *Platina*. When the numbness was present, the depression was absent, and vice versa (*mental symptoms alternating with physical ones; the body suffers when the mind is cheerful and the body feels well when the mind is affected*). Developing such a neurosis was her way of regaining importance: what physician would not pay attention to this serious physical symptom of the central nervous system?

A common dream for a *Platina*, appearing often after initial treatment, features her nakedness. In such a dream, she accepts herself as she really is, not as society wants her to be. One must be able to strip herself of all self-deception, to see herself naked in her own eyes before she can come to terms with the elements of her own unconscious and know who she really is in order to change it. She appears naked and unashamed and has the courage to begin investigating her shadow side. At this point, the persona worn before the world can cease to be a concealment of inner reality.

Decompensation in Pregnancy/Delivery: Mental Shock

Other causalities and delusions leading to a *Platina* state are illustrated by means of the following clinical example:

> During pregnancy, I feared that I was going to miscarry (*A/F fright*) when I was spotting at around eight weeks. Thankfully, it lasted only two weeks, but during that time I had much sadness (*A/F grief/anticipation*) because I wanted the baby more than anything. I also found out that the umbilical cord was near the rim of the cervix, which proposed risks of rupturing during delivery—so a C-section was the only option. The C-section turned out to be frightening (*A/F fright*) about midway through, because the umbilical cord did in fact rupture and the panic in the room was palpable. There was much blood loss during this event. I thought I might die (*death, presentiment of; death, thoughts of*), but instead of being scared I felt at peace knowing that the baby was safe in my husband's arms and that if I died it would be OK because they had each other. I was passing out (*faintness, after loss of fluids; from hemorrhages after delivery—proving: profuse hemorrhage; from pain*) so they gave me a shot of methadone; I immediately felt pain in my heart and felt that I could not breathe. I was frightened but did not want the baby to feel it, so I meditated (*meditation*) on something pleasant.

I did not sleep the first night as I wanted to stay awake so that nothing would happen to me (*anxiety with fear*). I had many strange thoughts; I was fiercely protective of the baby and told my husband not to leave him for a second (*fear something will happen; mental symptoms during child bed*). I had the baby sleep in my room because I did not want to be separated from him. The second day, I experienced such terrible gas pain that I thought I was going to die (*thoughts of death; delusion, die, he was about to*). I could not even sit still because I felt my insides would explode from the pressure. I cried a lot and felt I needed to leave the hospital. I was so frightened. I finally was released after two days. I started to feel fearful at home that something would happen to the baby (*fear, happen, something*). I was afraid that the night nurse we had hired would hurt the baby (*fear of people*), so I begged my husband to send her away. I also thought that my family was evil and did not want them near my baby (*delusion, all persons are devils*). As time went by, I became increasingly frightened and thought that there were evil spirits in the house (*delusion, devils are present; delusion, specters, ghosts, spirits, is pursued by; delusion, devil is after her*). I made my husband take the baby outside while I cleansed the house with sage and yelled at the evil spirits to get out (*delusion, specters, ghosts, is conversing with; delusion, being at war*). The next day, I told my husband I needed help, so we went to the hospital; it was a nightmare, because there I became even more afraid and also claustrophobic (*fear for narrow places; fear for crowds*). The doctor and nurses wanted to examine me, but I clung to my husband, not wanting them to touch me (*fear of people; anthropophobia*). I left and took one Prozac that they had given to me. The next day, I could not get out of bed, and I thought my husband was the enemy (*delusion, everyone is an enemy*). On the way to the hospital again, I felt that I could not breathe; it was like an elephant was sitting on my chest. I felt like I was losing it. I felt that I had somehow caused the end of the world (*delusion, he is possessed by the devil; delusion, he is evil*), that now everyone hated me, and that people were waiting outside for me with torture devices. I had visual disturbances in which I saw three eyes, and they were Satan's eyes (*delusion, has visions; delusion, everything seems horrible*). I believed I was going to experience eternal torture and wanted to scream (*delusion, scream, obliging to*). I was admitted to the hospital and stayed

> for three weeks, not wanting to see anyone but my husband. I felt that spirits were on me and that my body was not my own (*delusion, being possessed*). An old person had taken over my body. I was so scared at the hospital; I thought they were all vampires wanting my pure blood. Evil spirits would come and kill everyone that I loved (*delusion, pursued by ghosts*). All the while, I prayed (*delusion, religious*) to be a good mother and wife. When people coughed, I thought they were drinking my blood. I was very wary of all people… I thought I would be the only one left in Hell (*anxiety about salvation of hell; despair, about religious salvation*) and would be raped and tortured; I was the most horrible person on earth and needed to be punished for sins I had never committed **[which is symbolic: she pays for the sins of her forefathers]** (*delusion, she is disgraced*). I had a terrible fear of vampires.

This beautiful woman was saved by successive doses of *Platina* and restored to health. She returned to a loving relationship with her husband and cared tenderly for her child.

Loss of Position

Platina only tolerates a selective group of people for company. She often finds her hero in a man who has accomplished deeds of significance and has attained power in the world. Her hidden motive is ambition, and if she succeeds in acquiring her hero, *Platina* will live in complete identification with his achievements. Her husband's position is her position; his accomplishments are hers. She is the one who says, "I feel so exhilarated! **We** just have been made CEO of a Fortune 500 company!" It is quite intolerable to see with what haughty disdain *Platina* usually speaks to women who are beneath her (almost all of them, not just her servants!). In *Platina's* case, there is only one decisive consideration in determining status: which man she has succeeded in ensnaring in order to sustain her Cyber delusion. It is only when circumstances in her life change, causing *Platina's* narcissism to be severely wounded, that she can no longer maintain her CD; as a result, her ego collapses. Her true pathology, then, only appears when the CD is no longer supported. This can occur when, for example, her husband loses his job and position; when the company goes bankrupt; or even, as in the example given above, when children might interfere with her special image in the eyes of others. This reflects *Platina's* *ailments from deceived ambition, delusion, she is disgraced, ailments from* *embarrassment and mortification and delusion, she is doomed* and *she is about to die. Platina* does not produce anything; rather, the object of her narcissism is something she *has*—her body, her looks, her wealth, her fame (inherited), all things that further inflate her ego but have nothing to do with real achievement, which requires effort and work. But after the disgrace of losing what is so dear to her, *Platina* is now *easily offended,* and *trifling things produce profound vexation; she remains a long time sulking* and there is *crying after being mildly reproached.*

Compensations

Narcissism

Platina can exemplify true narcissism. Her personality is mysterious and exciting as well as aggressive and out of reach to the common individual, which makes her very compelling and desirable. No doubt, at first sight, she is rated as more attractive and alluring than others, as she is always impeccably groomed. *Platina* is enraged when told that she is not beautiful, special, or smart—but she is not much affected if told that she is a turn-off or a witch (*boaster, squanders through ostentation; want of moral feeling* and *unfeeling, hard hearted*). While some of her narcissistic traits are commendable, such as exuding confidence and self-sufficiency, she unfortunately also exhibits the toxic levels of haughtiness and entitlement found at the other extreme end of the spectrum. *Platina* thrives in entertainment-related fields (film, music) and in leadership situations (often those of her husband) in which she can dazzle and dress provocatively while showing contempt for the rest of the world; here, she must neither cooperate nor suffer the consequences of acquiring a bad reputation, which is a ticket to ill-earned, but welcomed fame. *Platina* does not give a damn what you think of her, because she has no doubt that what she thinks of herself represents reality—and that every word she says and everything she does is just wonderful and earnest.

Platina often loves the sound of her own voice *(Sulphur)*, although it does not always sound pretty to others. Conversation is used to maintain power in an interaction; she can brag, refocus the topic of conversation, and show lack of interest by glazing over when others speak (*arrogant, reserved; cold and haughty in the company of friends, too well satisfied with one's self; mania with great pride and fault finding; clings obstinately to her ideas, without however growing angry about it*). The result of such narcissism is a distortion of objective judgment; *Platina* is typified by the following attitude: that which is mine is great and good, and that which is not mine is inferior and bad. Another consequence is the **lack of love** and lack of empathy from which she suffers: obviously, she cannot love anyone else if she is only concerned with herself. This will lead to many delusions and distorted fixed ideas, but *Platina* is either blissfully unaware of them or simply does not care. It is much easier to project everything on others or suppress in the shadow side; *Platina* may conclude that the others are jealous or just not smart enough to realize how inferior they really are.

When *Platina* is younger, much of her haughtiness lies dormant behind the mask; she can be charming. Because of her self-centeredness, though, in reality, she dislikes others. Of course, her initial excitement and charm is hard to resist (*attacks of cheerfulness; very lively mood, so that she could have danced, half an hour after weeping; involuntary inclination to sing and whistle*). Just like *Aurum*, from a young age, *Platina* knows she is different—from another cast, so to speak (*delusion does not belong to her own family*)—but there is a marked need for attention in *Platina*, and her passion serves her well in her search for a soul mate. We see in the provings *inclination to embrace everybody; attacks of cheerfulness and amativeness, and kisses everyone*: something we would immediately link not with *Platina* but rather with *Pulsatilla*. Seeking admiration is like a drug for *Platina*. She certainly is *affectionate* at this time, but where to find an ideal partner? There are enough highly sexual partners available (*Sulphur, Medorrhinum, Fluoric acid*), but they generally lack the spirituality she demands. Therefore, just like *Nat-m*, she will have a slew of heartbreaks in her first stage, leading to *ailments from grief*. In the second stage; a differential diagnosis with *Nat-m* will be necessary and often difficult! Whereas *Nat-m* (the introvert feeling type in this second stage) will tend to wall off her emotions, even becoming ill-humored and vindictive, *Platina* reacts differently because of her increased sense of ego. At this point, she is capable of hiding her emotions, especially her haughtiness, behind an excessive mask. This suppression of her emotions is helped by a high degree of intellectualization (*easy comprehension*) and spirituality. *Platina* has no difficulty maintaining her Cyber delusion as pride and overestimation of herself surface: *she employs every possible means to fulfill her ambition*. At this moment, she says, "Of course it is not easy to find a soul mate for a perfect, beautiful being like me." She has no trouble being *dictatorial and contemptuous, looking down upon people usually venerated, with a kind of casting them off*. This might lead, already at this point, to a sense of isolation: *she thinks she is left entirely to herself and stands alone in the world; delusion, she has no place in this world* and *everything familiar seems strange* and even *the delusion, she does not belong to her own family*. But there is no danger of severe pathology (dissociation) yet; she can still compensate with autoeroticism, narcissism, and self-love. After all, she still revels in the delusion, *she is a great person*, so her superiority complex keeps her in a certain balance—although, unbeknownst to her, it is a rather frail one.

Remarkably, we can't find *Platina* under the rubric *hatred*. She actually has no feeling but **contempt**, which is worse than hatred. Hatred is a thing of the heart; contempt is a thing of the head. In fact, hatred and contempt are mutually exclusive. Genuine contempt stays hidden away in secret and lets no one suspect its existence. The contempt that *Platina* feels is the unsurpassed conviction of the worthlessness of another human being. The opposite of love is not hate but indifference, which is more painful than hate. Even in its most destructive form, hatred springs from frustrated emotional involvement—but *Platina* never reaches a state of emotional involvement with anyone! If something goes wrong, if someone leaves them, they think that they have been misunderstood and that their gift—the white gold that they are among human beings—is not appreciated. You can do or say almost anything to *Platina* without raising an outward expression of ire, but if you pierce her narcissism there will be a great show of rage and a desire for revenge—almost as though you have tried to kill her. *Platina* has an intense interest and attachment only for self, which is a huge, overt compensation for her true spiritual poverty and lack of introspection. But she often looks like the motionless and emotionless figure of a department store mannequin. As she is skating on thin ice, the ultimate curse and punishment for this kind of self-love is an extreme form of self-destruction associated with CNS diseases such as paralysis and multiple sclerosis.

Religion versus Sex

Inevitably, when heartbreaks occur, *Platina* starts slowly falling out of the balance she maintained in the psoric phase, and a sycotic phase commences in which she demonstrates a *very restless disposition so that she could not remain anywhere*. In this second stage, she realizes that the ideal partner, one who will match her ambition, will not be easy to find. The two intense, opposing desires—the sexual and the spiritual—cause an inner conflict; a balance between the two is no longer possible. In fact, it was never possible except in the mind of *Platina*. There is an **alternation between religion and sex**, and depending on the person's upbringing and background, one focus will be accentuated. If she has grown up in a family in which sexual expressions were permitted, her sexual nature will become more pronounced and out of control, even leading to *nymphomania and erotic insanity*. In this stage she might exhibit lesbian/homosexual tendencies (*love, lovesick, with one of their own sex*) when her quest for a male soul mate does not succeed. If she has grown up in a strictly religious family, the balance will fall to passion in religion: she can become a nun or a pastor, or follow a guru who forbids sex (*haughty, religious haughtiness*).

Before *Platina* chooses, there are days that she follows one path and days that she follows the other. We see in the provings *religious affectations, altered with sexual excitement*. It is reflected in preaching from the pulpit during the day and visiting prostitutes at night. Alternations of mood are also present, which is another expression of slowly losing control: *sad and sullen one morning, the next one extremely happy so that she felt like embracing everyone and could have laughed over the saddest thing; she could have danced half an hour after the weeping*. Suppressing all sexual feelings can lead to a negative cycle, resulting in brooding and depression: *sits alone, sad and morose, without talking; weeping mood >in open air* (Puls); *she often weeps involuntarily which relieves her* (Graph). There might even be a murderous desire—*killing her loved ones and her own child*, like *Sepia, Nux-v*, and *Mercury*—but she will rarely act upon this emotion.

In a further stage, *Platina* is bound to fall into either extreme sexuality or excessive idealism leading to egotism. Promiscuity is a key strategy for *Platina* to maintain control over the delusion that she is an exceptional person. Obliterating all other emotions, sex becomes number one: it is an *aggressive erotic insanity*, like that of *Tarentula, Apis, Bar-m, and Verat-a*. At this point, *Platina* does not hesitate to approach strangers with sexual propositions—with the only goal of satisfying herself. There is also excessive masturbation throughout her life, often starting at a young age (like *Origanum*): *sexual desire premature* (Plat, Origanum) and *sexual desire in virgins* (Plat and Con, only two remedies in this rubric). Usually *Origanum* starts at an earlier age (3-7), while *Platina* starts frequently around puberty. Sexual and lascivious dreams appear. We find *Platina* under *sexual thoughts intrude and crowd around each other; sexual desire insatiable* and *sexual violent desire with involuntary orgasms*, which can occur when she undergoes a gynecological exam. She detests condoms as they decrease her sexual satisfaction, and abortion is the solution to her pregnancy; no one has a stronger aversion to children (*dislikes her children, calls them too little*). Of course, she blames society for this aversion in herself: she does not want to bring up a child in a decadent society. If she has a husband at this time, she does not want him to leave home or go on a trip—because she fears he will meet with an accident and she will lose a good sexual partner (*fear, happen, something will, and that her husband would never return*). And if he does go on a trip, *Platina* has a back-up, a "Plan B" partner, waiting in the wings to offer protection and resources and to fulfill her needs when the regular guy is not around.

Excessive Idealism Concealing Arrogance

If the sexual outlet is suppressed, the only other outlet is excessive idealism. In this case, *Platina* allows her ego to grow enormously; she might become an advocate of sexual abstention like *Lyc* or *Lachesis*. Now she becomes *arrogant and reserved.* I even knew a *Platina* in South Africa who could play the perfect role of an empress: she had a big throne in her home and many servants. Such surroundings will feed her *delusion, she is great* and close the vicious cycle. *Platina* is ill-humored at this point, reacting to slight vexations as though she cannot be bothered with the everyday events of a commoner's life. *She only talks when she is obliged to and she is only agreeable to superiors or people she has to fear, while being contemptuous and hard to inferiors.* This arrogance leads often to being scorned and to situations of failure and injured pride, once again closing the inevitable vicious circle. The suppression of sexual feelings often leads to pathology on the deepest physical level, starting with *numbness in the face,* especially the *right side,* and with a feeling of coldness. Numbness is also present around *the mouth, on the lips and the os zygomaticus (Nat-m).* There can be also *formication* in the lower jaw, the anus, and the vagina—leading to *vaginismus* and making intercourse impossible (*Nat-m*).

Golden Tips from the Masters

- Pathology on the physical plane starts rather late for *Platina*, but when it starts it involves deep pathology of the central nervous system. We see cases of MS and paralysis
- Looks like *Ignatia* and *Thuja*
- Violent sexual desire with early masturbation, going from one partner to another
- Hysterical numbness and paralysis (*Ign*)
- Best remedy for alternation between psychic disorders and physical disorders
- Great sensitivity of the vagina: examination is very painful; can't be touched (*vaginismus*)
- Multiple personality disorder (*Anac*)
- Constipation of travelers (*Nux-v*)
- *Platina* ameliorates from walking in open air and sunshine, the opposite of *Nat-m*

Plumbum metallicum (Plb). Lead

The Cyber Delusion

People such as *Plumbum*, with an excessive personality—even progressing sometimes to identification with their persona—have built up a massive protective mask. Rather than a balanced, ever-growing ego, *Plumbum* builds up a pseudo-ego, a very rigid and dogmatic yet brittle and fragile one. Being subjected to constant pressure from within to maintain his image leads easily to paranoid delusions or delusions of persecution; he always thinks that others are conspiring against him. This results in inflexibility, overly critical behavior, and a lack of genuine responsiveness. Frequently, paranoid delusional ideas are a mixture of wish-fulfillment and a sense of being injured or persecuted, a feeling sometimes compensated with megalomania but more often with very violent reactive fears. The idea of persecution usually stems from a relationship infected with mistrust. When *Plb* meets with a mishap, during the first moment of terrifying fear, he immediately jumps to the conclusion that he has been injured or insulted deliberately, called delusions of reference (*delusion, there are conspiracies against her*). Prejudices of this kind, if they establish themselves, inevitably lead to delusions of *strange machinations*, as we will discover in *Plumbum's* provings.

The simplest form of schizophrenia is paranoia, the classic persecution mania. It consists of a simple doubling of the personality. The patient strikes us at first as completely normal; he may be a very respectable person, a great professional—nothing is suspicious. We converse normally with him, and at some point we let fall a word that hits his highly feeling-toned complex (for instance, a situation related to jealousy and suspicion). Suddenly the jovial face before us changes and the eyes are imbued with a piercing look full of abysmal mistrust and inhuman fanaticism. He is totally transformed and has now become the hunted, dangerous animal surrounded by invisible enemies. The other ego has risen to the surface. *China* and *Plumbum* are perfect examples of doubling personalities with their persecution delusions. This persecuted subject has completely replaced the healthy ego and has in fact suspended it according to A38 (the stronger of two dissimilar states postpones or suspends the weaker one).

This pathological idea of persecution is created by a psychogenic event, rarely an organic disturbance of the brain (as seen in head trauma or brain tumor which changes the character of the patient). This psychological event must usually be something out of the ordinary, else it would not have such a profound, even dangerous effect. The highly feeling-toned complex or NWS (creating a Cyber delusion) is deposited in—and remains in—the unconscious or shadow side. In this shadow world, the ego is somewhat dark: if we explore it, we can always discover something new about ourselves. As with delusions, this feeling-toned memory complex, hiding and invisible in the unconscious, can still lead to certain actions as if it were present in the conscious mind, when it is called up through minor gestures, incidents, acts, or words. We have to remember that the greater part of all of our psychic elements (the real person versus the mask) resides in the unconscious, cast away from our conscious so as not to disturb our frail balance (and, in children, as a way to protect them—to offer a degree of safety). Let's investigate the fixed ideas and, above all, the Cyber delusion.

An inquiry into the history of the provings reveals that *Plumbum* has many delusions of paranoia and persecution. I therefore chose as the Cyber delusion, *everyone around him is a murderer* (*delusion, he is about to be murdered*). Hering expresses this as *he thought his life was in danger from assassination or poison and that everyone about him was a murderer*. Not only does it reflect *Plumbum's* essence very well, confirmed, as we will see, by other fixed ideas, but it is also italic for this rubric and the only remedy in this rubric. In other words, enough criteria are present to accept this delusion as the mother or primary, archaic delusion. This is slightly different from *Mercury's* CD, *everyone is an enemy*. *Mercury* is the dictator, and in order to rule and avoid assassination, he must distrust everyone. It is *divide et impera*—divide and rule. *Mercury* plays a very active role in the attainment of his goal: to become the despot feared by everyone. Realizing as he does how temporary and fragile such a position can be, he targets and eliminates his enemies (that is, those with dissenting opinions). He is convinced that he needs to be proactive in killing his enemies before they kill him. *Plumbum's* message, though, is more one of receiving, not inflicting an injury (like the snake venoms)—his role is more of a passive one as he feels he is the target (*delusion, he will be murdered; delusion, his life is in danger).*

Plumbum's CD and passive role as a perceived victim are supported by numerous other fixed ideas which, taken together, create a huge vacuum in his ego: *all persons are devils; people conspire to murder him* (*Ars, Tub*); *he is about to be poisoned* (*Lachesis, Hyosc, Kali-br*) and *he is pursued by enemies*. There is always a dark cloud of possible assassination hanging over his head. Both *Kali-br* and *Lachesis* seem to be remedies closely related to *Plumbum* when it comes to the formation of these fixed ideas.

Additionally, *Plumbum* suffers from another set of delusions. *Plumbum* is a paralytic state of past glory lost, and now in a later state (possible retirement) he suffers the fate of so many who once basked in the limelight with power, materialism, position, and glory and who now are forced to spend their time on what they consider to be simple tasks. But only those who have not followed their path to individuation and Self-realization, will look at this afternoon stage of life as a loss and degradation; *Plb* is unfortunately one of them, suffering from retirement as do *Aurum* and *Arg-n*: *delusion, they are pursuing an ordinary business; he is engaged in some ordinary occupation*; and *he is working on a machine*. This can be compared to *Cuprum's* delusions of *gathering herbs, selling green vegetables and repairing old chairs*. These are the ordinary jobs in which he has become the master, and he basks in the limelight of being considered the best shoemaker, car mechanic, or hairdresser. Fueled by the delusions *he is a general and a great person*, *Cuprum* can still have a fulfilling life as long as he stays healthy. He still has a big pseudo-ego bolstered by self-proclaimed glory, and he slowly transforms himself into a cramped and frantic individual. In contrast to *Cuprum*, *Plumbum* is past his peak, and the ordinary business is now all that is left, a setback and a far cry from the glorious past as expressed by *Plumbum's* *homesickness*—in the extended meaning: longing for the precious good old times. *Plb* resorts to daydreaming and creating a fantasy world: with the *delusion, of fancy delusions* and an *exaltation of fancies*, he can still reign as the undisputed king; he thus pretends to be someone else and holds on to his excessive persona: *delusion, errors of personal identity; delusion, of being double* and *delusion, he is some other person*. All characters with delusions of fancy illusions are in danger of dissociating at some point, but *Plb* (just like *Platina*) will exhibit severe central nervous system pathology before dissociating under emotional pressure.

Causalities

One clue about triggers appears clearly in Hering's statement about *Plb*: that *his affections or diseases are more of the emotions than the intellect.* Kent expresses the same idea: "*Plb* is intensely emotional (full of melancholia, sadness and a feeling as if something terrible would happen, that he has committed the unpardonable sin) while the intellect is slowed down."[32]

Anticipation

As is to be expected in view of the paranoia produced by his Cyber delusion, *Plumbum's* main A/F seem to represent constant preoccupation with what can happen to him: *ailments from anticipation and presentiment; anxiety with restlessness and yawning.* This is fueled by his suspicion towards others, who he thinks are conspiring to kill him, as we have seen before. Murdering him, in an extended context, means obstructing him in his ambitions, as seen also in *China*—another personality that embraces the *delusion, he is persecuted. China* is an intellectually artistic but rather naïve person who perceives others as preventing him from reaching his desired goals. *China* even has the fixed idea that *others are tormenting him and that he is hindered at work and pursued by enemies.* For *Plumbum*, extreme anxiety leads to *anguish,* its destructive equivalent, rather a bleak and foreboding sign when it comes to possible compensations.

Sexual Excesses

There is only one other NWS: *A/F sexual excesses.* It is only a moderate one, and *Plb* is not classed in the hypersexual group of *Lycopodium, Fl-ac, Plat, Med, Lil-t,* etc. *Plumbum's* provings clarify this rather unusual aspect. It is not uncommon for a man subjected to great anxiety, fear, and anticipation to resort to relief from masturbation, as seen also in *Picric acid.* This seems to be the case with *Plumbum*, leading, as is well known, to a loss of strength or Qi with the loss of fluids and contributing to a slowly developing paralytic state. As masturbation always involves a sense of guilt and often self-contempt, as with drunkenness, the long-term practice of masturbation can become a serious pathology, moving toward depression and further delusions in *Plb* in spite of only being a normal-type

32. Kent, *Lectures*, 786-787.

remedy in the proving. Hering states: *mental disturbance of eight to ten years' duration in a man addicted to masturbation; has several times attempted suicide; greatest despair and dejection; and hears voices and sees shadows of demons.*

Compensations

Company

Looking first at the psoric compensations, we see that *Plumbum* initially likes company, probably to relieve his anxiety about his paranoia: *desires the company of a friend* (specifically a friend: **not** anyone else!), *aggravates while alone*. But there are several *Plumbum* traits that will make it difficult for him to find company or to engender sympathy for his position. For starters, *Plumbum* cannot talk about his problems with truthfulness: she *exaggerates her symptoms* (DD *Calc-c*) and has *loquacity*. However, there is *babbling, prattling, incoherence and wandering in her speech*, which is obviously not conducive to a good, rational conversation evoking sympathy and understanding. Additional difficulty in making contact with others (aside from friends) stems from *Plumbum's* pronounced *timidity about appearing in public*. I wondered if this last proving had to do with the fear of his mask being ripped off, as is true with *Silica*, *Gels*, and *Lycopodium*! When *Plb* exhibits a psoric trait (*timidity, desiring company*), it turns out to be an obstruction rather than a help in getting through day-to-day activities. *Plumbum's* Cyber delusion of everyone around him being a murderer limits his reaching out to others, the main reason for his timidity in public, and can stealthily lead to the sycotic trait of *suspicion and mistrust*. In a further state, *Plb* loses his ability to walk, experiencing *paralysis and violent neuralgic pains in the extremities, even fainting in a room full of company*. Then this *paralysis can be preceded by mental derangement and shooting, darting pains in tracks of larger nerves*. Obviously, looking for company will be limited at this point.

Industriousness

Industriousness, although a proving, is not pronounced in *Plumbum*: *talks of business* and, most likely, as we have seen before, *Plb* will exaggerate in doing so. Though not every job is glamorous or exciting, we know from his delusions he nonetheless keeps on talking—probably about his old business, and not his current ordinary job. *Plumbum* is not *fruitlessly busy* like

Verat-a and *Lil-t*, who give the impression that what they are doing is important (*delusion, they are pursuing ordinary business*); *Plb* does not possess the boundless and frantic energy of these two remedies. *Verat-a* is busy fruitless to alleviate his despair about his social position; *Lil-t* must keep busy to ward off those incessant sexual thoughts (*has a conflict between religious ideals and sexuality*, only remedy, *too occupied with religion*; *and, busy, fruitless, to repress sexual desire*, only remedy). *Plb* is simply prattling and babbling about business, and makes a halfhearted effort without much result!

Religion

It is important to investigate what comfort and support religion may provide for *Plb*. Does it give meaning to his life? Examples of a psoric religious compensation would be *wants to read the Bible all day* (Calc-c) and *metaphysical concerns* (Calc-c). With *Plb* it is nothing like that. Here we have a sycotic expression: *religious mania, and religious melancholy*. *Plb* is even found in the rubric *religious fanaticism*, in the company of *Sulph*, *Veratrum*, and *Puls*, although there is *anxiety about religious salvation*. Contrary to *Kali-br* and *Lachesis*, who derive positive strength and feedback from religion, *Plb* is a tortured individual who tries to turn to religion to regain peace of mind: *delusion, she is lost for salvation* and *anxiety about salvation*. In Hering we find: *fixed idea that Plb could only obtain peace and safety through absolution from a priest of the Papal Church, although she had been a zealous Protestant; and after being permitted to visit a priest and converse with him ceased to talk and think of the Church*. Being saved by religion, for *Plb*, is a remote possibility, while *Lachesis* is convinced he has been chosen to have direct contact with a superior being (even talking to God when in a dissociated state); *Kali-br* and *Veratrum* often take a religious message from door to door or preach the end of the world as God's messenger.

Sex

Plb is *amorous* (*Nux-v, Plat, Verat-a, Causticum*), but again, as with religion, presents it immediately in a sycotic fashion: *nymphomania and lascivious* and *slight provocations produce erections and emissions* (compare with *Conium*). The loss of spermatic Qi (part of the Essence in TCM) in this fashion is one aspect of A/F sexual excesses; it is not, however, the only one, as we will discover. Religion and sex often go hand in hand and can alternate: suppression of one leads to excess of the other, as seen also in *Platina*.

Emotions of Contrast to Hide Fears

The homeopath can see that *Plb* does not really have psoric compensations; he falls almost immediately into the excessive sycotic phase. Speech (*loquacity and exaggeration of the facts*), religion, sex, and other sycotic expressions are frequently present. As *Plb* suffers greatly from anticipation anxiety, the homeopath should not be surprised that fears are easily incited. These fears reflect his Cyber delusion, as we see in *fears of being touched and fear of being approached*; *fears of being poisoned, something will happen, and of being murdered.* Fears of touch and of being approached will certainly be evident from *Plumbum's* attitude in the homeopath's office: probing questions will be looked upon as personal attacks and an invasion of privacy (*Lyc, Sil, Nat-m*), and the patient will be fearful of having his mask ripped off; it is essential for the homeopath to act in the *Plumbum* patient's dominant conscious function (in this case, feeling). The *fear for water* needs always to be taken in its extended meaning too: water is a relatively fixed symbol for the unconscious, and *Plb* is afraid or unable to explore his unconscious; he has, rather, a *desire for light* (compare with *Stram*), the relatively fixed symbol forconsciousness. Before *Plb* plunges into the depths of the syphilitic miasmatic stage, he tries to hide his worries through his excessive persona with what Jung called emotions of contrast (usually a sycotic trait). *Plb* indeed plays the clown to cover up his tortured soul to the world: *foolish behavior, hysteria, makes gestures*; *he assumes strange attitudes and positions.*

Plumbum's final stage, which leads him to the homeopath, is best expressed by paresis or arteriosclerosis on every level. All symptoms and diseases seem to develop very slowly, but, alas, they also do so insidiously. It is as though the Trojan horse has invaded the body: the enemy is already within the city's walls, but the victim has no clue! Because of this, sometimes it is too late to recognize *Plumbum*'s symptom picture when he seeks help; it may also be that the disease is too far advanced to be cured (compare with *Conium*). The final pathology on the physical level is very specific: degeneration of the brain through CVAs (cardiovascular accident) and arteriosclerosis. Indeed, *Plumbum's* triad is CVA + paralysis + forgetfulness. After a CVA, we often see *trembling of the hands on holding objects* (*Mercury*, besides the trembling, has abundant night salivation and bad breath). *Plumbum*, parallel to the state of arteriosclerosis it represents, is a slowly progressing state, built step by step, but it will eventually lead to paresis and atrophy on all levels.

In cases of Alzheimer disease with the ensuing characteristics on the mental level, one recognizes many expressions of AD: *the memory becomes weak for expressing oneself, weakness of finding words and for occurrences of the day. Plb* becomes anxious when talking, but she always tries to start a conversation and then stops because she can't find the proper word (*babbling, prattling*). These patients are also slow to receive impressions in chronic cases (*Mercury, Ph-ac*). It is parallel to what we see in neurology: the patient reacts slowly to a pinprick (compare with *Cocc, Alumina*, and *Ph-ac*). We have the rubrics *answers slowly; stupor returns quickly after answers; answers monosyllable and unable to answer. Plumbum's* mind is sluggish, but the patient makes great efforts to answer your questions. *Plumbum's* paresis on the mental plane is further expressed by *unobserving behavior* and *confusion as to his identity and losing his way in well-known streets,* which are also expressions of AD. Initially, it is not as extreme as in *Glonoin* and *Petroleum*, but eventually *Plumbum* turns into *extreme dullness of mind, slowly growing apathy, idiocy, imbecility, in which he does not recognize his relatives* (compare with *Glonoin*) *and sheer insanity,* during which *Plb* shows *increased strength* (*Tarent, Stram, Plat*), an additional challenge for the families of such patients. *Plb* is also indicated in ALS (compare with *Lathyrus sativa*) and paralysis of intestines (DD with *Alum*). *Weakness and painful lameness of arms. Numbness and want of power, wrist drop and foot drop. Plb drops things from the hand. There is wasting away of muscles* (atrophy) *and diminished sensibility on whole R side of body. Lame feelings in legs as if feet were made of wood* in case of extremely long-lasting sciatica. The *extensors are most affected. Paralyzed parts may swell after the emaciation and painfully contract. Hemiplegia is often accompanied by hyperesthesia of opposite side).*

Golden Tips from the Masters

- Hyperesthesia in acute cases with loss of power is a great indication for *Plumbum* (Nash)
- Keep in mind that *Rhus-t* is the acute of *Plb*. *Plumbum* represents a spastic paralysis affecting the upper extremities while *Alumina* (*A/F domination*) is a flaccid paralysis affecting the lower extremities and leading to diseases such as MS
- Complete paralysis of urinary organs because of spinal degeneration. Unable to urinate due to the lack of physical sensation of the need to do so (neurogenic bladder), the will to urinate is not sufficient to make it possible; inability as if from paralysis. Everything tastes sweet. Immense thirst is a big keynote!
- Claudicatio: feeling of a tight band tied around the leg = a marked *Plb* symptom!
- Paralysis and atrophy of muscles: think of *Plb* and *Causticum*!

Pulsatilla pratensis (Puls). Wind Flower

The Cyber Delusion

Pulsatilla's CD, ***he is all alone in the world,*** refers to the fixed idea that *Pulsatilla* always feels alone no matter how much attention is given to her or how many people are present. There is a great need for constant attention; without it, *Pulsatilla* feels abandoned by the beloved protector, which can be just about anyone who gives her the care she craves: mom, dad, friend, teacher, anyone! So the worst action parents can take with a *Pulsatilla* child is to tell them that they are going to get rid of her—the "attention-seeker"—or put her out on the street if she doesn't behave. Talk about confirming a fixed idea! All too often, I have heard mothers' stories about how a specialist advised them to let the child cry for months in his crib in order not to spoil the child. I treated one mother who suffered a mental breakdown as a result of following such injurious advice. Additionally, when one considers the remedy for many such children, *Pulsatilla,* and its corresponding fixed idea—I am all alone in the world—then one can only imagine that by doing such a thing the mother, the nourishing source, is unconsciously doing exactly what the child already feared in the first place: increasing his fixed idea of isolation. The result is a worsening of the child's state, as it originated with an expression of the child's desperate attempt to feel the intimate bond with his mother, to protect herself from the dangers outside of the home.

Making friends for *Pulsatilla* is not the same as it is for *Phosphorus,* another restless tubercular remedy whose home is the entire world. *Pulsatilla* is a member of the *Carbon* family, and she is therefore more attached and interested in family and close friends than in the world's suffering; friendship for her, then, is a means to assure continued attention and security. The homeopath recognizes the *Carbon* element in *homesickness and obstinacy* while *horrible things affect her profoundly.* Love from family is security; just like *Phosphorus,* though, *Pulsatilla* welcomes attention from anyone, focusing especially on those in her immediate neighborhood. Attention directed toward her is translated as love, no matter what the source is. If it is not a person, it might be a pet, preferably an affectionate dog. A differential diagnosis with *Phosphorus* will be necessary—but the difference is clear when the homeopath contrasts the fiery, passionate, and fast spirit of *Phosphorus* with *Pulsatilla's* slow, phlegmatic temperament, tendency to irresolution, and slow movements (among other characteristics).

This central fixed idea or CD is supported by other fixed ideas in the person, whether adult or child: she has *the delusion, of being deserted and feels doomed and being away from home* (the protective environment). *She is always alone and does not belong to anyone; she is not appreciated and she is surrounded by strangers, and familiar things seem strange* are other fixed ideas that can roam around in the unconscious of the *Pulsatilla* person. *Pulsatilla* often ends up not knowing what to do with her life; she is like a traveler in the desert without a map. What a lonely place to be! No wonder the Cyber delusion needs to be satisfied: *Pulsatilla* wants to be emotionally close to someone who can pay attention to her and spend time with her. And because of the CD, *Pulsatilla* strives to keep the ideal of an infant's happiness: to always be fed on time, to be held when needing comfort (all the time), to be heard when voicing the smallest request (perpetually), and to be entertained with the full attention of the mother or loving source (uninterrupted). The world is viewed as a dangerous place, and it cannot be faced without the support of close family or friends (*delusion, pursued by enemies*; *delusion, about criminals*; *delusion, sees devils and will be taken by the devil*). Such people remain obstructed personalities as this fear can hinder the path towards *Pulsatilla's* individuation while also becoming overbearing to others. *Pulsatilla* doesn't want to grow up. Throughout her life, there will be an intense search (sometimes successful, sometimes not) for that supportive person or entity; this desire will not go away unless resolved by the homeopathic remedy. Significantly, *Pulsatilla* is a black type remedy for *dreams about cats,* the cat being one of the symbols of anima or female characteristics such as love, protection, cleanness, nourishment, and shielding the person from danger in the world. There is always a way out for such a sensitive, demanding person: escape into her dream world, which is filled with imaginary people and animals created according to her most fanciful wishes. Unfortunately, though, her retreat into this dream world reinforces the CD and creates a wide gap between her whimsical wishes and the stark reality of the adult world (*delusion, of fancy illusions*; *delusion, she hears music*).

The birth of *Pulasatilla's* CD is linked to an exaggeration or hypertrophy of the maternal instinct in this person. An exaggeration of this feminine side is above all an intensification of the maternal instincts. I once had a patient, a 37-year-old unmarried woman, whose maternal instinct was triggered when her neighbor had a new baby; as a compensation, my patient had immediately bought a puppy as an outlet to transfer the maternal feelings that had been triggered by the birth of her neighbor's child. *Pulsatilla* unconsciously lives in complete identification with all the subjects and objects in her care. First she gives birth to her children, and from then on she clings to them and dotes on them to the point of suffocation—for without them, she feels her existence to be utterly empty. Therefore, she will always suffer from empty nest syndrome when her children leave home. Her mind is not cultivated for its own sake; it is, rather, stuck in an infantile and primitive state. For this reason, *Pulsatilla* is prone to remain stuck in her CD. At the slightest negative remark or criticism she falls apart; additionally, we see such susceptibilities as: *easily offended*; *sensitive children*; *sensitive to reprimands*; and *is sensitive to opinion of others* (also *Sil*, chronic of *Puls*). Love, linked to the mother complex, means shelter and safety—and we see that all delusions in *Pulsatilla* are linked to this theme. *Pulsatilla's* delusion, *a naked man is in her bed* not only indicates the desperate need of *Pulsatilla* for attention but also reflects a need for procreation to sustain her exaggerated maternal instincts.

Causalities

Grief and Disappointment

We must not forget the tremendous influence of the intrauterine trauma in cases where an increased need for protection is an appropriate reaction of the pregnant mother. Many children who undergo such trauma suffer obstruction of the personality from birth, and the accurate and diplomatic questioning of the mother regarding emotional traumas during pregnancy is a must. In *Pulsatilla's* case, the decisive event must have involved both grief and a feeling of forsakenness on the part of the pregnant mother. The grief can be anything such as the death of a beloved dog or, in certain cultures in which the future grandmother customarily stays with her pregnant daughter to offer support for a time, her failure to do so. And even when her mother does come, each day the pregnant and postnatal woman fears the moment that her mother will leave, and this is always in the back of her mind. She might always say to her husband in the evening when he comes back from work: "Pay attention to me now. Forget work. It is my turn." This clearly reflects the needy *Pulsatilla* state that is being transferred to her child. Whether real or perceived, lack of attention is considered deception by a *Pulsatilla* person (*deception causes grief and mortification*).

Because of her *yielding character*, *Pulsatilla* can also succumb to another kind of grief. Many families prohibit expressions of grief and anger and teach their children to suppress these emotions. A child, especially one like *Pulsatilla*, learns quickly from the lack of affective display within a family what will be tolerated and what will not. Wanting above all to please her parents, but feeling devalued with no means of expression any kind of emotion, this child often sinks into deep depression in adulthood. Freed from the family shackles, she has now become a *Pulsatilla* person in full bloom: a person for whom small setbacks and difficulties regularly turn into huge catastrophes that take over her life. And now she will cry constantly, for just about any reason. However, we must not assume that this grief always leads to a desire for consolation. In the final syphilitic phase, *Pulsatilla* descends in the depth of a paralyzing depression (*sits still, wrapped in deep sad thoughts and notices nothing; silent grief; answers, aversion to answer or answers monosyllable; indisposed to talk, desire to be taciturn; indifference to joy and suffering*).

Jealousy

When a new child is added to a family in which a volatile *Pulsatilla* is the first-born, the familial unit can become a tinderbox. A *Pulsatilla* child always wants parents to pay more attention to her than they do to her brothers and sisters (*affection, craving for affection in children; desire, full of infinite desire*); it is for this reason that a *Pulsatilla* person elevates whining to a Homeric art form (*moaning, whining in children, while being carried*). No wonder, then, that an emotion like jealousy, which propels this child, can turn vicious and *malicious*. When someone punches you in the face, you know for sure that it is aggression. But *Pulsatilla* is smarter than that! She is passive-aggressive, engaging in very sneaky behavior that she can easily hide and deny (*deceitful; mischievous*). With an innocent-looking smile, she is quick to pass on the blame for the catastrophes she sparks, even accusing the innocent baby! The *Pulsatilla* child can be cunning and prankish: she taps her younger brother on his head (out of sight of the parents of course) when he takes a toy away from her or even when he gets attention from the parents (*fear of being neglected*). Jealousy towards siblings is rather overt. Here are some examples I saw in my practice:

When Dad comes home and a *Pulsatilla* child's younger brother, beating her to the door to greet him, is scooped up first, she lets out a high-pitched scream. When Mom talks on the phone, she screams again and grabs the phone. Once, her mother had to be in the hospital with the younger child for a week, and it terrorized her so much that whenever the phone would ring, she would start crying—making the connection with her mom's leaving her to visit the hospital. And now, every five minutes she asks for a hug from Mom: her CD, *all alone in the world,* is putting her in a perpetual state of terror that she will be left forever! The *Pulsatilla* child always demands all the attention for himself, no matter how many children are in the family. If he is the only child, then his parents are supposed to be there all the time just for him. You think one hour of playing after a hard day's work is enough? No! He demands that his parents play with him all day long, incessantly, never taking a break. And when the parent cannot entertain him, he wants to go shopping. Receiving a gift means to him that his parents love him. But of course they are buying things all the time! That's why Granddad, who buys a toy every time he sees little Miss *Pulsatilla,* is considered a good God-like person; parents of course fall into the enemy camp if they don't follow the same pattern. If the *Pulsatilla* child has only older siblings, she will gravitate to the one who spoils her, who becomes the *ersatz* father or mother.

Other Causalities

Other emotional triggers are *disappointment* (when not receiving the desired attention); *fright,* as the ego of a *Pulsatilla* person remains rather primitive, stunted by the lack of emotional support; *jealousy,* as others are always seen as competing with her for her source of love and support (husband, family); and stress (*emotional excitement*), as a *Pulsatilla* person does not have what Chinese medicine calls a good gall bladder—meaning the strength to make decisions. She is very *capricious, changeable and indecisive,* whether she is contemplating choosing a meal in a restaurant, clothing, an occupation, a game, or a career move. *Pulsatilla* is *full of desires, this and that,* reflecting her difficulty to make choices and stand by her plans (*irresolute; full of indefinite desires*). Often another person has to decide for her! *Pulsatilla's* sensitive nature invites situations of *mortification,* which often lead to *delusions, after mortification.* A *Pulsatilla* person is quickly overwhelmed by *mental labor.* It is also the remedy for any *ailment since puberty.*

Compensations

Regressive Infantile Behavior

Pulsatilla has made an art of the most effective method of making her nonnegotiable wishes known: regressive infantile behavior and screaming like a baby. In many cases, her screams bring about the unconditional surrender to her commands. As can be also the case in *Lycopodium*, this capitulation is the first one of the battles won, and the sweet taste of victory will never go away: it is sustained for the rest of *Pulsatilla*'s life! If not screaming for attention, regressive infantile behavior takes the form of bedwetting, misbehavior, or finger-sucking (*childish behavior*). In cases in which the child continues with or returns to such infantile acts, **we should find out what the child is retreating from instead of taking coercive measures** to stop the act of thumb-sucking itself. I have known parents to try punishment, reward, or tying up the thumbs in an attempt to cure this isolated symptom. But it is a fear of growing up that holds *Pulsatilla* in temporary paralysis: even though a part of the child wants to grow up, another part wants to remain in the safe shelter of the mother's womb. The outbreak of seemingly incomprehensible childish and unreasonable acts is, in fact, a return to some outgrown childish habit that gives a sense of security and protection.

Instability of Emotions

Pulsatilla laughs and cries at the same time or changes the mood from laughing to crying within minutes, resembling *hysterical behavior*. Changing moods (*weeping or laughing on all occasions*) is her M.O.: it does attract attention, and it also gets her out of situations that she does not like (such as testing at school or being rightly reprimanded at home). Shrieking in this case is only done to get attention; this is different from other remedies, in which the shrieking can come from frustration of not being understood. Often, when a younger sibling needs more attention because of sickness, *Pulsatilla* will resort to acting like a baby, sucking her thumb and wanting to sleep with the parents. When Mom goes on a trip for a few days, you can be sure that during these two days *Pulsatilla* will have potty accidents, though she is otherwise already dry (this equates to revenge and manipulation). Other regressive infantile behavior may include feigning disease or mistreating the family dog. Now we understand why the *Pulsatilla* child does not want to grow up! Being a baby assures her, in her mind, of the much-needed attention to which she feels entitled. The *Pulsatilla* child truly has two personas (*delusion of being double*; *delusion divided in two parts*), always using the one that best suits the situation, and always with the goal of receiving all the attention of adults. On one hand, she can start playing the adult, the parent, when a newborn has arrived by telling Mom: "I am worried when you leave him alone in bed," and "Feed him now, don't make him cry," "Let me hold the baby," "It makes me nervous that he will bump his head," etc. In fact, when *Pulsatilla* grows up, she looks forward to marriage and having children. On the other hand, though, the other persona is never far away: jealousy about the newborn leads to regressive infantile behavior, as mentioned before, and even if she is twelve or older, she suddenly needs help brushing her teeth. She is either an adult or a baby, never her own age, and the picture can change within hours. She will be either helpless or sassy, but nothing in between.

Sometimes, with a *Pulsatilla* parent, the child will become like a pet. A *Pulsatilla* mother will caress and fondle her child with overemotional physical demonstration when in the mood, but she pushes him off with indifference, impatience, or unconcealed annoyance and irritability when the child becomes tiresome or when her own mood has changed. This is baffling to her child, destroying his sense of security and the continuity of his emotional nourishment. A mother with an inflated anima can be overprotective towards a boy, and as a result he will completely fail in his masculine adaptation. Whenever a situation is too hard for him, the *Pulsatilla* mother, driven by her own CD and her own anxieties, believes that her child is ill or determines that he should do something more pleasant—because this suits her own temperament. Obviously, her child will learn to take advantage of every slight cold; when homework comes his way, or any annoying obligation, he will recall his need of support and lack of strength.

Self-Aggrandizement

No one can weave better fairy stories than *Pulsatilla*: she spins tales of lovely princesses to whom all things come as if by magic. Of course, such stories, in which she also creates imaginary companions (*delusions, of fancy illusions*), are nothing but an unconscious wish to obtain everything without effort, to secure friendships without ever being rejected because of her clinginess (*carried, desires to be carried and fondled*), an attempt to cover up a feeling of intense neediness that leads to the imprisonment of her life's desire: to be surrounded by many friends. In her stories, she can project lies (*liar*) and boasts, though in real life this would only cause others to laugh and mock her. Such stories are an attempt to cover up a feeling of inferiority (*want of confidence*). They are part of a person who is not willing to grow up like an ordinary little girl. But *Pulsatilla* tries to go one step further to make this dream world filled with grateful friends come true: she resorts to stealing (*kleptomania, steals money*) in order to acquire things for her intended friends and thus tie them to herself. I had one four-year-old patient who had stolen a purse from a classmate to give as a present to her mom on her birthday. She had wanted to please her mom, make her happy, and show her love. Unfortunately, it did not work, as she got into trouble—to her great surprise.

Another *Pulsatilla* girl, acting out destructively (the syphilitic part of this tubercular character) because she thought she was not loved, shoplifted cheap jewelry and gave it to her classmates to win them over as friends—until she was caught and her mother, calling her a thief, said that she never would be trusted again. This experience transformed her into the so-called perfect child (*anxiety conscience, as if guilty of a crime*; *remorse*); she became a straight-A student and added cleaning the house to her list of duties to please her mom (*yielding*). Coming home from school, she would clean for more than two hours, help her mom with dinner and dishes, and somehow still squeeze in her homework. In this case, the desire to attain perfection led to ritual and even obsessive behavior as *Pulsatilla* is *fastidious, and conscientious about trifles*. She felt she would be loved for it (*delusion, is forsaken*). Together with her amative behavior (*children are caressing and kissing everyone*), *Pulsatilla*, in her fantasy identification, makes an attempt at surrounding herself with friends to dissolve her CD, all alone in the world, and to save herself from having to face a realistic assessment of her own individual worth.

Pleasing Others to Assure Attention

While many children with autism show more interest in toys and objects than in persons, the *Pulsatilla* child is the opposite: she is people-oriented. Why? To escape her Cyber delusion, *she is all alone in the world* (which can come from either perceived or real aloneness), there is only one solution, and that is to express her great need for attention. Attractive and seductive-looking (like the *Phosphorus* child) as well as *servile and submissive*, she has no difficulty charming others to satisfy her excessive need for attention. Her looks are helpful: *effeminate, too coquettish*, always dressed and looking like a little princess or sailor. Following the dictum "you catch more flies with honey than with vinegar," *Pulsatilla craves affection but also kisses everyone, bordering on adulterous behavior*! Pulsatilla children are extremely *affectionate, which they manifest by kissing and caressing*. Invariably, this is the six-year-old coming back from school, giggling that there are at least three boys in love with her; if her parents praise her for being so attractive and popular, it can be enough to encourage the development of a lifelong image of herself as a princess. This is the naïve adult who, when Mr. Perfect puts his arms around her and kisses her gently on the lips, thinks that she is floating with the angels in heaven—this is not a fleeting moment, mind you, but a permanent state of bliss. She feels worthy of being kissed, and that provides enough self-esteem to propel her into a life of constant daydreaming. This is also the girl who, still at puberty, dreams that all men are in love with her and that she can choose whom to kiss: in other words, a little princess syndrome. Because of her *yielding* and *amorous* character, when she grows up, such *lasciviousness and nymphomania* often lead to *ailments from sexual excesses. They are cheerful and gay in bed,* and to fill the loneliness, even have the *delusion, that someone is always in bed with her. She dreams of men.* Because of the great need for attention, and just to be popular, *Pulsatilla will be submissive in her grief,* and when they are teenagers or older, *Pulsatilla* people can go so far as to agree to participate in sexual acts against their wishes (*submissive*), such as sadomasochism (another form of *ailments of sexual excesses* for *Pulsatilla*). She would starve herself to death (*anorexia nervosa; bulimia*) as she is convinced she looks ugly (*delusion body is odious).*

Pulsatilla children adore receiving kisses for the smallest reasons, including "medicinal" kisses to allay the pain when falling on their knees or scraping their elbows. Concerned mothers (the *Carbon* moms in the first place who detest any kind of pain) give extra affection to their two-year-olds in such "life or death" situations, but *Pulsatilla* is well aware, as she grows up, that injuries (no matter how small) are an opportunity to get attention.

The mother of one of my *Pulsatilla* patients could not understand why her child was the first one to welcome a friend, family member, or even a stranger with a smile and a hug, but then would refuse to even say goodbye when they left. It was because the *Pulsatilla* child was losing the attention of the person and pouting about it. Such a child wants to punish the person for leaving and not continuing to entertain her. She is so much a "people person" that she will invite everyone to come with her to show them how well she use the potty—and, of course, she expects a resounding "Bravo!" from the onlookers. She is the little princess everywhere. At home, she is the consummate little helper in the kitchen, where she wants to show how well she can cook (*amorous).* The *Pulsatilla* child at school prefers to be with the teacher rather than peers at recess time. She works hard at becoming the teacher's pet (and the pet of his aides) through her helpfulness, but of course it is all about seeking and getting attention. One *Pulsatilla* girl called her teacher and aides "my assistants."

Late Psychosexual Maturation

Whereas psychosexual maturation takes place with most children from age six on, the *Pulsatilla* child has a hard time growing up: the transition from the prenatal psyche into ego consciousness is a critical and a hard one for the *Pulsatilla* child; a child's psyche is not yet separated from the parents' unconscious, especially the mother's. It is exactly this transition that presents an obstruction to venturing away from the shelter of home and parents when she goes to school, begins to adjust to organized society, and starts to enter into relations with others. The difficulty for the *Pulsatilla* child becomes very clear now: she has a meltdown when entering school for the first time, pleading with her parents not to leave her. This close psychological identification is further revealed by the fact that little children often dream about the problems of their parents.

No matter how hard she tries, and no matter how much attention she receives, *Pulsatilla* is a bottomless vessel of craving for attention (*craving for affection in children*). Dissatisfaction is a permanent characteristic for *Pulsatilla*: *she is satisfied with nothing, extremely capricious and peevish about everything; well one hour, miserable the next. The child longs for this, now for that, even with good humor. He wishes now for this, now for that employment, but when given to him he will have nothing to do with it. Weeping, bursting into tears very easily* can initially be used as a weapon. *Pulsatilla weeps telling her symptoms; she weeps at everything whether joyful or sad or at answering a question.* This certainly can evoke sympathy and pity, but only for so long! Eventually it turns people off, as it stems from *envious and greedy behavior in which she wants everything for herself,* accentuating her lonely feeling and giving her real cause for weeping.

Clinginess

While the mother is the relatively fixed symbol of emotional nourishment and protection, she is not the only psychological umbilical cord attached to the *Pulsatilla* child. At school, *Pulsatilla* desperately looks for a good friend—and if he finds one, he clings to him quite literally: holding his hand firmly and hanging around his neck all the time, whether the friend wants it or not. At the same time, *Pulsatilla* can be nasty to everyone else because they might take this precious friend away, posing a threat to a relationship that is vital for the emotional survival of the *Pulsatilla* child. *Pulsatilla* submits to and identifies with the close friend, and through this symbolic participation in another person's life, *Pulsatilla* has the illusion of living

Golden Tips from the Masters

- On the physical plane, the syphilitic miasm is expressed on the bones with scoliosis, hallux valgus, etc., in other words, a "softness" of these bones and deformations.
- *Intolerance to heat* is remarkable and the *Pulsatilla* child's mood and her *confusion of mind* always improve when *walking slowly outside in fresh air* in spite of cold sensitivity.
- *Kali-sulph* is the mineral analogue
- If *Pulsatilla* does not hold, think about *Ipecac*
- Pathology on one side: the occurrence of symptoms on only one half of the body is very peculiar, including profuse sweating on one side of the face
- Pathology of the venous system, especially on right side of the heart. Prominent veins on dorsal surface of the hand
- Wandering pain in rheumatoid arthritis: rheumatism goes from joint to joint
- Extreme mother instinct: they adore children
- Cravings for ice cream, pastry, desire for butter, but aversion to fats which also aggravate, typical for a tubercular character (craving what aggravates them)
- #1 remedy for measles and German measles
- Loss of smell and taste (*Puls* is chronic of *Kali-bich*); also *Medorrhinum*
- Indicated in about half of the cases of pregnancy vomiting
- Convulsions from suppressed menses
- #1 remedy in leucorrhea (cream-like or bland or thick yellow or changeable) in young girls (#2 remedy *Sepia* or *Sulphur* according to the symptoms)
- Children talk frequently in their sleep
- #1 remedy for chalazia/styes
- Deafness after measles
- Asthma from suppressed eruptions in children
- *Pulsatilla* has a dry mouth and no thirst. *Mercury* has the opposite!
- If you start with *Pulsatilla*, be ready to follow with *Silica*, its chronic
- Good sequence of remedies: *Puls—Sil—Fluoric acid* (Kent)
- Indicated for the phlegmatic temperament, but little suited for persons who form their resolutions with rapidity and are quick in their movements (Hahnemann)
- Menses are suppressed from getting the feet wet

Sepia officinalis (Sep). Common Cuttlefish.

The Cyber Delusion

Sepia's Cyber delusion is ***her family will starve***. What does this mean or express for the *Sepia* person? Is her family lacking in necessities? Hungry? Does she need to provide for or protect family members? Does the CD express the dutiful feeling of this person? What is the true attitude of *Sepia* towards family? We must look at the additional fixed ideas in order to understand the nature of the *Sepia* child or adult. Other delusions that confirm the Cyber delusion's expression are *delusion, talking, persons as though near of* (*about midnight*) and *delusion, someone calls him, during sleep*. The latter fixed idea points to the appeal that is made from within on the *Sepia* person to take action, to get *busy* in order to avoid the family's doomsday or starvation. She has this fixed idea that rest is not possible, that she can't let her guard down; she fights inattention with every fiber of her being (*delusion, feels every fiber on* ***right*** *side* and *duty, too much sense of*)! The right side stands for the active side, the sword, the consciousness: it is here that *Sepia* wields her animus, her maleness, to get things done! But because of this relentless feeling of being needed, this delusion will change in the syphilitic phase to *duty, aversion to* and *aversion to domestic duty* as well as *escape from family*. The CD is also reflected in the *early responsibility* that is pushed on this *Sepia* person as a child. Perhaps, for instance, her mother died and she, as the oldest child, took over motherly duties (*maternal instinct exaggerated* and *too much sense of duty*).

The CD seems also to be supported by the *delusion, she is poor*, another important fixed idea also supported by the delusion, *is going to be robbed*. But how is she poor? *Sepia's* poverty can be expressed on any level: physical, emotional, or mental. On the physical level it has to do with her perceived poor health as expressed by some of the other delusions: *delusion,* ***three*** *doctors come; delusion. he is sick and for this reason will not work. She is filled with concern about her health and thinks she will have consumption and soon will die*. It is remarkable that this proving speaks of three doctors. In dreams, one of the connotations (there are other meanings too) of the number three as relatively fixed symbol is of some fateful point that has been reached, something unavoidable that will happen; something needs to be done to avoid the total abyss. How well this reflects *Sepia's* situation in the syphilitic stage of life that occurs later on!

Poverty on the physical level can also be reflected by stasis, stagnation, non-movement, and lack of progression. Physical poverty is created in *Sepia* by the repression of sexual functions, which now distorts the whole of the life activities of the body. It brings about conditions of stasis everywhere, leading to clotting of the menses, with a brown, dark discoloration; black spots or floaters in the eyes (*vision, colors, spots, floating*); *muscae volitantes* (according to TCM, blood is normally stored in the Liver, which is related to the eyes and can be reflected on the face with a redness of the left cheek only: a poverty of storage of blood); soreness and tiredness of the eyes with drooping eyelids; and a bearing-down feeling in the abdomen and uterus because of lax muscles. There is prolapse (sycotic weakness) of all organs, especially the rectum and the sexual organs, due to poor muscle tone (*worse standing, lifting, involuntary urination upon coughing, low back aches*)—which is another expression of hypoadrenalism. The latter will also cause urine incontinence especially after laughing but also after coughing. Sexual intercourse is intolerable because of tenderness of sexual parts to the touch: *genitalia, female, aversion to coition*; *enjoyment absent*; *coitus painful*. Even the menses can be replaced by profuse leucorrheal discharges for years. *Sepia*'s physical poverty is certainly expressed by her great exhaustion, often necessitating naps between 3 and 6 p.m. Also, *Sepia* can *faint all day long, from heat, cold, dampness, during menses, while kneeling in the church* and *from trifles*. She feels weary and trembles all over. The influence of the adrenal dysfunction on pigmentation and the aging process gives a typical external aspect to the *Sepia* patient: *rigid fiber, sallow complexion, yellow freckles, loss of hair, early graying,* and *premature aging*. The extreme tendency to *spasticity with globus and ball sensation* in various parts (felt in the prostate in men) is explained by the suppression of psychic and sexual impulses.

Regarding mental poverty, *Sepia*'s memory is especially affected in the exhausted syphilitic stage: *inability for mental activity*; *it is an exertion to think*. If the person needs to pursue additional studies, i.e. in order to advance her career, it becomes a chore: *I could not remember the things that I knew yesterday*; *it is hard work for me to study or think*; *I don't wish to study*; *I could not keep my mind on my books nor follow the lectures, my attention was wandering*; *when I study I cannot apply my mind to the subject but constantly think of something else*. In all these preceding provings we see poor concentration; *Sepia* can be a useful remedy for the overworked student or professional.

Other mental functions are affected: *when I am writing a letter, and I read it over, I found everything wrong; I had used wrong words and wrong expressions and so I gave it up in disgust. I cannot collect my thoughts and am unable to answer the simplest questions, which made me very unhappy.*

Poverty on the emotional plane does not mean a lack of emotions in general, but a lack of positive or anima emotions (warmth, love, etc.). The emotions go from violent anger (*ailments from emotional excitement*) to absolute *indifference, even to loved ones* and inability to bond with children and husband (*aversion to family members* and *aversion to husband*). These last emotions are linked to her drive for individuality and self-expression, which also explains her *aversion to sympathy, consolation and company*. All of these emotions are outgrowths of the repressed sexuality and of the eruption of the unconscious personality, a mixture of the animus and the shadow. Sadly, the kind of depression that may ensue leads those in its grip to isolate themselves socially. It is part of the pervasive perversity of depression that *Sepia* refuses the things that could make her feel better (*indifference to pleasure and to life*). Her spouse says, "Let's go to a movie or have a nice dinner out!" She replies, "I am too tired; I am too depressed." *Sepia's* depressed world becomes smaller and smaller until, failing to find opportunities for fun as well as for personal growth, the depression becomes the centerpiece of her life.

Sepia can come across as bossy because she says what she thinks and what is necessary and does not pad it with extra fluff. She can be sarcastic if people talk down to her (*mocking, sarcasm, with great intuition concerning other people's weaknesses*). She can become an overwhelmed mother who is prone to flipping out, running out of the house screaming that she is not coming back and that she will kill herself, leaving the rest of the family shattered and helpless. Many miles have been added on the family car by the exhausted *Sepia* mother on her escapes! Many rubrics reflect this exhaustive state: *nothing suits her, she finds fault with everything; she has the greatest irritability from the slightest cause; she is very indifferent towards everything, and has no proper sense of life; I have no more ambition and I simply don't want to do anything, either work or play; it is even an exercise to think; I feel like quarreling with everyone and become very much excited about a mere trifle and said some sharp things* (feeling ashamed of it at the same time). This *melancholic depression* and *adynamia* stem from hypoadrenalism. *Sepia* also has a high affinity for the thyroid and adrenal cortex.

What does *Sepia's* delusion *alone in the grave yard* point to? What is in the graveyard? It is the relatively fixed symbol of the resting place of the soul, when the body disintegrates, although the craters of the moon are the place where the soul rests in dreams. It can express a sense of isolation, but a desired one: no one visits her too often in the graveyard! At this point the body has fallen apart: "Leave my soul alone; I am done!" This reflects the sentiment: "Rest at last!" This delusion also stands for the unconscious, a deliberate retreat into the unconscious, confirmed by the *delusion, talking of water* and *the delusion, something comes from above which presses the chest*. Water is the relatively fixed symbol of the unconscious. The notion "from above" may manifest as the top story of a building, the peak of a pyramid, or an attic; all of these represent consciousness. In other words, *Sepia's* conscious life oppresses her chest (where the heart is), and she desires to withdraw—or has already withdrawn—into the unconscious (*graveyard, fancy illusions*)! It is also connected to the *delusion, of fancy illusions, when closing the eyes*. Closing the eyes is a symbol of her wish to avoid facing the reality of life, to escape into her dream world!

Sense of Duty

Among the "dutiful" remedies, *Sepia* takes a prominent place. Being dutiful can certainly be a positive characteristic if kept within reasonable limits. However, if *Sepia* were able to make healthy use of her dutiful nature, we would not use this characteristic to find the patient's simillimum. Of course, "reasonable" limits are different for different individuals. The personalities to be discussed here all think that their sense of duty is "reasonable," but those who live with them might beg to differ! Duty can be limited to family only, as it is in *Kali-c*, with the CD *an abyss behind her*, whose exercise of duty is more like a reign of dictatorship; duty can be focused mainly on one's own person and concerns (*Arsenicum*), in which case it is called selfishness—created by *Arsenicum's* CD, *she is being watched* and *her family will starve*—or a sense of duty can be felt toward the world as in the case of *Aurum*, driven by the CD *neglects his duty and deserves reproach*. While being dutiful to a reasonable degree is mainly a psoric trait, any of the above characters can express it with an intensity bordering on obsessive-compulsive behavior (sycosis).

The dutiful person is dependable, precise, and punctual. At the same time, such a person sets high standards for everyone and follows societal rules. The other side of the coin is that determination may give way to obstinacy, censorial behavior, and precision to the point of preoccupation with trifles and even OCD behavior. An overactive sense of duty can lead to lack of adaptability in new situations, rigidity in views, and inflexibility in approaching problems. It may lead in this situation to a life filled with burdens rather than joyful accomplishments—a life filled with guilt because of a perceived neglect of duty. Such individuals become sensitive to criticism because anticipated praise is not forthcoming; this leads to the creation of the delusion *he is not appreciated* (*Aur, Pall, Thuj*; to these, add *Calc-s* and *Lachesis*). This can result in smoldering, unexpressed feelings of rage, resentment, and depression in otherwise seemingly well-adjusted people.

For some people, "duty" means putting themselves on the "back burner," claiming that they want nothing for themselves. They live "only for others," and they are proud of it. This does not reflect unconditional love or unselfishness as they would like to think; neither is it a form of duty we want to emulate. It is, rather, an expression of selfish love. It enslaves the object of love to the lover's possessiveness. Two characters in our materia medica expressing this "selfish" love are *Ignatia* and *Hyoscyamus*; both have the proving *the pain and penalty of unrequited love*. And *Ignatia* only wants acknowledgement of her devotion as a reward!

Causalities

Sexual Excesses

Sepia's chief and most pronounced NWS is *ailments from sexual excesses*! How can that be? This would be surprising for any student of homeopathy. Features like clear skin, a symmetrical face and body, feminine facial features, and an hourglass figure are rarely hallmarks of a *Sepia* woman. *Sepia* is usually known as a rather asexual, manly woman with masculine propensities and appearance; she often has a narrow pelvis, deep voice, overgrowth of body hair with a tendency toward beard and mustache formation, and a lack of libido. In other words, the animus is in steady control! All this reflects *Sepia's* "masculine protest," a repression of her femininity and a rather anti-feminine attitude. At first, *ailments from sexual excesses* make us think of oversexed beings like *Fl-ac, Medorrhinum, Platina, Lachesis,* and *Lycopodium*, all of whose libidos in a certain stage tend towards hypersexuality. But when it comes to sexual intercourse, *Sepia* can say, "Not tonight, dear—or ever!" So if *Sepia* is not a sexual being, how did it land in this rubric? And who is she? As hard as *Sepia* tries to completely overthrow her expected feminine role, it is impossible for her to accomplish this in a short time span. We can use here an analogy with the cuttlefish that only is half successful in escaping from her enclosing shell. Even if *Sepia* tries to throw off her female temperamental and sexual/emotional tendencies, she can only slowly transform and disown women's primary expressions with the risk of creating pathology related to and symbolized by the mother vessel, the uterus.

Whence, then, this ailment from sexual excesses—and in black type, no less? It has everything to do with a sexually overworked body. And I don't refer here to masturbation, another reason for such NWS from sexual excesses (*Plat*, *Ph-ac*, *Origanum*, *Staph*, and *Hyosc*). But for *Sepia* I see *maternal instinct exaggerated* and *duty, too much sense of.* This will now clarify these sexual excesses: she loves to have a family (there is still anima in the beginning) and is a very responsible (although stern) mother who will not refuse sex with her husband (at least not in the initial stage) because it is part of her duty and it satisfies her maternal instinct.

The *Sepia* fish resembles the uterus, the place of human creation. The uterus, as with any vessel in alchemy and dreams, represents femininity, fertility, love, protection, and emotional nourishment; it is embodied in its purest form in the oyster or the soft, mushy, jellylike substance from which *Calc-c* is derived. *Sepia*, though, turns from introversion to extraversion, basically rebelling against the passive and protected femininity of *Calc-c* (the *Calc-c* or oyster has walled itself off from the environment with a thick, impenetrable shell). The oyster, producing for us the wonderful remedy *Calc-c*, has no limbs whatsoever and is always encased in its shell; its only visible expression consists in the slight opening and closing of the shell. It reflects the love of *Calc-c* for a protected world (its home and family) and the lack of desire to enter the outside world (it fears all the dangers to be found there; there is no need for legs as there is no wish to go outside of its protected world). Such a picture is even more pronounced in the *Bar-c* person, the undeveloped *Calc-c*, who has the delusion, *his legs are cut off* and *he walks on his knees*. The explicit difference between this and *Sepia* supplies us immediately with the idea of how different these two dutiful characters are. Just from the analogy with Nature's creatures, we can deduce that the *Calc-carb's* duty is very restricted, inwardly oriented or family oriented, with a great aversion to involvement in the outside world. She is the great mother, personal therapist, and cozy friend that will not disappoint you; she is warm, protective, has all the feminine curves in abundance, and is contemplative and passive; in other words, she is the absolute opposite of *Sepia*.

Duty for *Sepia* is also providing her children with ways to survive in the outside world; *Calc-carb's* duty is always to provide a safe haven for her "little" ones (even when they are grown up). Eventually, though, in the final phase, as the negation in the role of the woman extends itself to include the refusal of the mother's role, we find in *Sepia homosexuality* (*in love with her own sex*), *sexual frigidity* and *aversion to the opposite sex,* syphilitic expressions.

For *Sepia,* sex serves the purpose of creating a family (maternal instinct) and is not at all for pleasure, as reflected in the proving *after coition, anxious and restless the entire day.* But sexual satisfaction and any desire plummet often at the birth of the first child and reemerges, if at all, after the last child leaves home. *Sepia* often treats intercourse as a marital necessity demanded by the animus in man and treats sexuality with benign neglect until an affair sets off a crisis in which the sinning party will be exposed to *Sepia*'s wrath (*anger about former vexations; about past events; passionate; rage, fury*). Over time, as people settle into a typical pattern of sex, a drop in desire affects both men and women. But it is often the case in a woman like *Sepia* that the level of desire is lower to start with. Protection, duty, domesticity, and predictability are often the very things that stifle desire in the *Sepia* person. Her role as a wife, mother, and professional is not only overwhelming but also highly desexualizing; it is hard to shift into sexual mode from such roles. She is always worrying about the kids, whether the dog has been fed, and everything else on her to-do list. Ailments from sexual excesses, in this case, refer to multiple pregnancies and often multiple miscarriages (*disposition to miscarriages from fifth to seventh month*) for which progesterone shots will often be given preventively, though *Sepia* would do a much better job. Ailments from sexual excesses will refer also to a relationship with a hypersexual individual (*Lycopodium, Lachesis, Medorrhinum*), which can push any woman into this *Sepia* state. It also refers to the situation of many women in societies in which families with four or more children are still common or in places where boys are preferred, leading parents to keep trying until the desired son arrives (for example, in India).

Early and Excessive Responsibility

As mentioned before, the mother's Cyber delusion can make an early and dominant imprint on a *Sepia* child, an imprint that can even be made during intrauterine life if her mother suffers during pregnancy from emotional events and causalities that correspond to the *Sepia* proving. It is readily understandable that the pregnant mother, for whom the remedy *Sepia* is a wonderful remedy for many illnesses in and after pregnancy (morning sickness, herpes outbreaks, threatening miscarriage [especially between 5th and 7th month], leucorrhea, lower back pain, exhaustion, and postpartum depression among others), can easily transfer this intense feeling of being isolated and overwhelmed to the unborn fetus through mystical participation. As discussed above, the graveyard is the resting place of the soul. For the exhausted *Sepia* pregnant mother, it stands for a retreat into the unconscious which is undertaken because events in her conscious life threaten to overwhelm her. A *Sepia* child with such an inheritance (often in large families) is frequently saddled with the role of substitute/assistant mother, required to help out at a young age when she should still get to enjoy being a growing child. *Sepia* children who take on adult roles may appear mature and controlled, but they feel helpless and frightened. Their competence is achieved at the cost of youthful curiosity and exploration. Such a child rather focuses on required tasks than to deal with painful feelings like absence of the mother or father (because of drugs or alcohol), a kind of avoidance that often persists into adulthood and contributes to the formation of a workaholic.

As a child, *Sepia* demonstrates the extreme opposite of the passive immobility of the *Calcarea* child. *Sepia* is a *serious child* that is called to duty far too early in her individuation path because of a noble misfortune like the absence of the mother (due to death, alcoholism, sickness, drug addiction, etc.). Early on, the put-upon *Sepia* child becomes the sterner "mother" who rules the household with a practical, no-nonsense approach void of warmth. Initially, she is an extravert. In other words, everything is aimed at the object, not the subject, aimed at the goal to be reached—this is not done with much introversion, but with a plan of action, a plan of attack that secures the best result for everyone involved. Small wonder that someone whose anima (her female side) had to be suppressed from a young age in order to respond to the animus (her active male side) should have difficulty expressing her affection for others. Rather than kissing and hugging her younger siblings, she will be overprotective of them, a kind of displacement as this overprotection takes the place of expressing deeper feelings, which she is unable to do. Her emotional side has been stunted: if someone in the family dies, *Sepia* will not say or ask anything but will remain emotionless.

Emotional Excitement (Stress) and Fright

What is the stress about? Since *Sepia* takes on a traditionally masculine role, the stress she feels is related to business: home business and/or outside business, most often both. If this business fails in spite of her hard work, it becomes a disappointment (at home because the kids disappoint her, at work because of loss of position [*A/F loss of position* is italic for *Nux-v*, the acute of *Sepia*]). Such a loss can, of course, be viewed as a *humiliation* or *mortification and embarrassment* and can occur as a result of *mental work excess*. And when *Sepia* is criticized or *scorned* at work or at home, it forms part of the failure and *disappointment*. So another theme, besides the sexual excesses that are part of her duty and performance, is failure in business. In fact, the strongest theme that links these NWS together is precisely the enormous duty she puts on herself and her desire to succeed, the activity of her animus! This is a woman at the mercy of her animus! Instead of a relationship to her animus, she is possessed by it. Just as it would be for a man in his traditional role as the family breadwinner, embarrassment and humiliation for *Sepia* now become nearly synonymous; in fact, she *fears humiliation*.

What does the *NWS fright* relate to? At first we could say that she might be afraid that she will fail in her business, but she really does not have that fixed idea. We can't find *Sepia* in the rubric *delusion does not succeed* or in *she does everything wrong*, and we can't find *Sepia* in the lack of confidence rubric, not even in her final syphilitic state of exhaustion! The fright, then, mainly relates to her health. Her sense of duty creates the fear that she could become sick while so many depend on her: *cares, about domestic affairs*, at least in the initial psoric stage. But there is anxiety and *fear about health*, leading to fixed ideas of *being sick and three doctors needed*: there is pronounced *anxiety during fever, about her health, hypochondriacal, during flushes of heat*, while most of her other anxieties are less strong. Her fears are mainly *fear of apoplexy, of impending death, that she soon would die* and *fear for the physician*. In the provings, it is stated that *she is full of evil forebodings*. But in a way, all these NWS can be put together under one umbrella: that of a too-great sense of duty leading to her own demise.

What about the grief? It is mainly about the loss of business and possible disharmony in the family, where her rules are not followed and not everyone appreciates the great leadership she demonstrates or her strong animus which allows her to be decisive and get things done. She suffers from a defective primitive anima, and the grief is mainly expressed through weeping *when telling her symptoms* to her physician or *just uncontrollable and involuntary weeping* without giving any health information, overwhelmed as she is by sadness. Her thinking conscious function has now been forced into the background, and her inferior feeling function is in command. But, as one can see now, it looks more like hysterical, uncontrollable crying, as anything as archaic and primitive as her now-dominant feeling function—controlling both her body and mind—shows. But *Sepia* does not cry at movies; she is not a dweller or grudge-holder. She can talk about feelings, but she does not go through a box of Kleenex except at the physician's office!

Compensations

Action/Thinking rather than Feeling: A Stern Mother

Sepia, derived from the ink of the cuttlefish, is the extreme opposite of the passive immobility of *Calc-c*, both being members of the mollusk family (snails, clams, mussels, and oysters) and both considered dutiful remedies. It goes without saying that their dutiful behaviors will be quite different from each other. Looking at the cuttlefish, and drawing a parallel to describe our *Sepia* patients, the cuttlefish possesses some overdeveloped limbs (which evokes a picture of the *Sepia* person jogging) which cannot even be withdrawn into its shell. It has also a pair of fins which allow rapid locomotion. Clearly, *Sepia* stands for an externalization, evolving from the shell-enclosed, soft, and immobile quietness of *Calc-c* to an emancipating, fast-moving individual who takes tasks to heart and wants to resolve them with a speedy and no-nonsense approach. No mulling over, none of the hesitation, contemplation, or shyness of *Calc-c*: "What needs to be done must be done now," she says.

The *Sepia* person becomes the stern mother who rules the household with a practical approach, not a warm one, although initially she is an example of an extraverted person. *Sepia* can be a great companion: she is active, and practical; she is a go-getter, a mover and shaker, a person whose business is also outside of the family—and no male is safe from her competitive mind. *Sepia* is ready to fight for her own needs and rights, for cultural achievement and human dignity and causes. For the sake of her convictions and needs she is willing to neglect relationships and disregard old patterns that have outlived their usefulness like the old German adage of "Kinder, Küche, und Kirche" (children, kitchen, and church). She is the quintessential career and pioneer woman. She also has the capacity to structure and order her environment. She can be a wife and mother, but also a competent administrator and the creator of home and soul. She responds to practical and concrete rather than abstract situations and to the requirements of the moment. She listens, receives, carries, nests and nourishes, protects, and promotes growth. Rest and standing still are things *Sepia* hates in any situation, personal or otherwise.

Sepia's heavy reliance on Logos (thinking/animus) results in an imbalance between Logos and Eros (feeling/anima): *Sepia* is all about action, determination, business, and having opinions, hallmarks of the strong activity of the animus. Her resistance to the natural mother instinct causes unexpected difficulties in such a woman: she may experience sexual problems (*coition aversion to, coition, enjoyment absent*), failure of conception (*sterility*), miscarriage (*abortion, fifth to seventh month*), excessive *nausea and vomiting during pregnancy, cancer of the uterus, greenish leucorrhea,* and *amenorrhea.* Her shift to the Logos or conscious thinking function results in a development of intellect that suits *Sepia's* desire to fit in the working world; she may even dazzle her coworkers with a semblance of intellectual comradeship. But such intellectual development in *Sepia* is often accompanied by the emergence of masculine traits.

Restlessness and Industriousness

The *Sepia* person demonstrates extreme restlessness from a young age. There is *clenching and grinding of the teeth at night, kicking the feet during sleep,* and *making unusual movements with the hands with great perseverance.* Contrary to the placid, inert, motionless *Calcarea* person, *Sepia's* *industriousness* takes the form of *restlessness*: *she has no patience to remain long in one place*; she always wants to be busy (*occupation ameliorates her complaints*), and the more she runs around the better she feels (*ameliorations from vigorous movements*). Before she experiences the wonders of homeopathic *Sepia,* she tries to achieve a delicate détente with threatening depression by becoming a relentless road warrior, cycler or runner; this allows her to compete with really sporty people. There is great *internal restlessness for many days with hastiness*; *when she has scarcely begun work she would wish it was done.* It is only later, in her exhaustive state, that she will become indifferent: *she felt all day as if she did not care what happened*; *no desire to work. Inattentive and absent-minded.* We also find in the provings *sad about her health* and *domestic affairs, discontented with everything.* This *Sepia* person, child or adult, does not have to be told to clean up her room as she organizes her belongings and toys very properly and gets annoyed when someone disturbs this order (*rest, cannot rest, when things are not in the proper place*). Once *Sepia* has her menses, this cleaning becomes obsessive before the onset of menses (*industrious, mania for work, especially before menses*). Why this restlessness before menses? Her menses, in a pathological state, are clotted and brown, reflecting non-movement or stasis. It is as though *Sepia* tries to rectify this through exaggerated movement (cleaning) before the menses. It is an act of survival—an effort to store more blood in the liver. Other rubrics reflecting this restlessness include *generalities, motion of affected part ameliorates,* and *violent motion ameliorates,* but *Sepia* is **not** found under *slow motion ameliorates*!

Independence and Precocity

This compensation should not surprise us, as there is an accent on the animus and Logos or thinking function: *Sepia* can count on her intellect. In the beginning, in a healthy state, *Sepia* has an *unusual clearness of intellect and an ability to give close consecutive thought and greater quickness of memory*. In good health, *Sepia* has *an unusual quickness to recall well known facts, and answers quickly. And her answers are intelligent but curt* (opposite of the *Lachesis* person, intelligent but entering into long conversations, *jumping from one topic to another*). There is also another side to the coin: a woman or man (child or adult) who represses her or his anima or feminine side often turns into an opinionated, fidgety, nervous, even mean and narrow-minded individual. When the anima is suppressed as is the case in *Sepia*, and the animus is dominant, she may fall victim to unaccountable, surprising hysterical impulses (*tendency to hysterical spasticity with globus and sensation of a ball in inner parts*) when this repressed soul image takes its revenge. And the *Sepia* woman becomes obsessed with her animus-driven persona, someone who always knows better and reacts in a masculine way. Passion has very little to do with being passionate about relationships or showing affection. It will merely reflect her passion and drive about succeeding in personal goals, future, and work, leading to a tendency to lose control and turn into an angry individual (*the greatest irritability from slight causes; vexed and disposed to scold*). The over-protectiveness towards younger siblings and the drive to succeed are nothing but a hidden aspect of jealousy in the *Sepia* child (*jealousy between children*). As the *Sepia* person feels that she is unable to demonstrate real love and affection, she substitutes affection through excessive care and attention directed to younger siblings and to the tasks at hand. So her independence is more an expression of loneliness and displacement of affection with hyperactivity, often hiding bossiness.

Difficulty Socializing

Sepia children may remain isolated at school and need to be encouraged to participate in play. *Seriousness* has penetrated deeply into the *Sepia* child's psyche. Affection is not part of her makeup, which does not mean that she cannot be sweet, but she is rather passive in this domain. She can accept caresses and hugs but usually does not initiate affectionate behavior herself, not even with family members or babies: she neither rejects nor embraces overtures to affection (*affection stifled*). Therefore, this child, if not actively embraced by others at a play date or birthday party, feels rejected and is unable to take the initiative. Her emotional passivity contrasts strongly with her physical activity. In the consultation room, she looks too serious and indifferent to what is happening. No tears come out until the physician takes her aside and starts asking questions. At this point, she can weep uncontrollably (*weeping when narrating her symptoms*) as if she has been able to break the chains of her emotional isolation.

Weeping (in her case, a sign of an archaic rather than a dominant anima), although ameliorating her condition, is now nearly constant: *every few minutes inclined to cry, without knowing the cause; frequent attacks of weeping which she can scarcely suppress;* and *very melancholic during the menses.* And even her sensory senses are overtaxed as now *her nerves are very sensitive to the least noise and particularly to music and piano playing. She has also great sensitiveness to odor. Sepia* children also demonstrate an extreme aversion towards, and timidity in front of, strangers (*presence of strangers aggravates; averse to the sight of people*). Confrontation always aggravates her, especially when *contradicted,* which results in temper tantrums: anger is indeed easier for this child to express than fear or loving interaction with others. The *Sepia* child often suffers from *atopic eczema* (on bends of the joints of knees and elbows), possibly provoking more rejection and nasty comments from other children. *Sepia's* isolation stems from an utter vital exhaustion resulting from different causalities, requiring a deliberate withdrawal to nurse one's wounds and replenish the energy vessel.

Music and Nature's Expressions

Rather unusual positive compensations for the *Sepia* child are dancing and Nature's violent expressions such as thunderstorms and lightning (*generalities, thunderstorm, ameliorates*). *Sepia feels oppressed in sultry weather, but becomes more cheerful when it thunders and lightning:* these are symbols for forcefulness and power and motion, suitable for *Sepia's* animus and aversion to stasis! In contrast to *Phosphorus* and *Nat-c* persons, *Sepia* sleeps better when it thunders, and she loves walking in this weather as it gives her a stimulus and a kick which are needed to ameliorate the feeling of stasis. As a result, this improves her whole state of being, physically and emotionally. To improve the stasis of circulation and energy, which is at the basis of all her symptoms, *dancing ameliorates all her symptoms. Dancing ameliorates her mood,* as the *Sepia* person has a strong sense of rhythm—and, of course, as with any exercise, especially *violent motion,* dancing improves her stagnation in general. Therefore, running, walking, massage, yoga, and exercise and physical exertion in general ameliorate the *Sepia* person.

Withdrawal

The intelligent and quick-minded *Sepia* is overcome in her final, syphilitic phase by the heavy load of responsibilities related to her occupations at home and work. Her mind is often filled with sad memories: *busy with gloomy recollections. The recollection of past unpleasant circumstances puts her in extreme ill-humor* (this is < > *Nat-m, who rejoices in them*). Sepia *thinks of things she does not wish to think of...* we can see clearly many similarities with *Nat-m,* so don't go too fast from a *Sepia* layer to a *Nat-m* layer! In her exhausted state, *Sepia* becomes an asocial being, quite a contrast to her first phase. We even have in *Sepia* the proving *aversion to* ***social*** *intercourse, amounting to contempt.* Here, again, we make a differential diagnosis with *Nat-m*: *Nat-m* becomes asocial as a consequence of finding herself emotionally isolated by circumstances of deception, lack of emotional nourishment, and disappointed love, although she gives the appearance of being social by getting involved in volunteer work (a vocation). *Sepia* needs a **vacation, not a vocation** and couldn't care less about others at this point. Only a *Sepia* person in her end stage would welcome a life removed from the struggle for existence and living upon some solitary island where she would have nothing to do but lie in the sun. How she wants to run away and leave it all and have peace at last!

The *Sepia* woman will symbolically reflect the secretion of the ink sac of the *Sepia* fish, which is composed of melanin (found in the skin and in the back of the eyes in humans). In the patient requiring *Sepia* by the Law of Similars, this is the yellowish or brownish discoloration (including vitiligo) so often found, an endeavor perhaps to conceal or hide a particular emotion (for instance, the distress and shame that may follow a romantic breakup). Also, the patient's desire to get away, like the fish, may explain why the patient hides behind "a cloud of *Sepia*."

Golden Tips from the Masters

- A male *Sepia* has decreased sexual desire, back pain > lying on a hard surface, a history of fainting, and sensation of ball in prostate
- Great remedy for prolapse (sycosis underbuilt; rectum, uterus, vagina, bladder) and for a sensation of dragging or a heavy feeling of bearing down
- *Sepia* has the irritability of *Nux-v* (its acute) and the tearful dependency of *Pulsatilla*
- Has an affinity for the portal veins and liver (venous stasis)
- Insults more than any other remedy
- They don't care if they ever have sex again in the syphilitic exhausted phase; they may fake orgasms; they are disgusted at this point with anything having to do with sex
- Aloof, detached, with loss of motherly instinct in syphilitic phase
- #1 NWS birth control pills and progesterone treatment, hysterectomy, and menopause
- Marked tendency toward motion sickness
- Marked cravings for sour tastes, vinegar, sour pickles, chocolate when premenstrual
- Chloasma gravidarum and easy bruising
- Miscarriage in fifth to seventh month
- #1 remedy for postpartum blues
- #1 remedy for Addison disease
- #2 remedy for Raynaud's syndrome (#1 is *Agaricus*)
- Hypothyroid remedy (*Thuja, Nat-m*)
- For the nauseated, vomiting pregnant woman who has aggravation from the thought of food she craves or would like to have. Great morning sickness remedy
- Purple is a color that is quintessentially *Sepia*. Purple discoloration, particularly of the hands, due to venous stasis and associated with coldness of the extremities. The color is more of a violet shade and should not be confused with blueness
- Persistent empty eructations after eating
- Indicated in the obstinate vestiges of acute rheumatism
- Depression in male *Sepia* person following coitus and feeling of castration (autotomy)
- *Murex* is highly complementary to *Sepia*

- Headaches figure largely in *Sepia* picture
- Persisting leucorrhea (*Kreosotum*, *Graphites*) and *leucorrhea in young children* (*Puls*)
- #1 remedy for enuresis in first stage of sleep: the bed is wet as soon as the child is asleep
- Hands cold and feet warm or vice versa!
- *Sepia* can be used when menses fail to appear in mothers who do not nurse

Silicea (Sil).
Silica or Silicon dioxide or pure flint

The Cyber Delusion

The predominant fixed idea or CD of *Silicea* is that the ***left half of the body does not belong to her***. Symbolically, the left side of the body is the female side and everything that stands for it: protection (the shield), love for Nature and animals, creativity, intuition, and emotional nourishment. It is also associated with the moon, night, winter, death, and the underworld, as well as the subconscious. The lack of fusion of left and right (with right being responsible for action, will, planning, and decision-making) in this person is accountable for the fact that many of *Silica's* compensations serve as defense mechanisms. Without both sides being fused into a whole, it is psychologically much more difficult to become a confident person. The non-fusion also represents a child who, at age five, has not separated enough from the prenatal psyche—from the mother. All too often, this can result in the child becoming a terror at home (*defiant; abusive; intolerant of contradiction*), while his individuality and individuation have not yet progressed sufficiently to allow him to step confidently out of his home and explore the world. This confusion is present in *Silica's* sense of identity (*she becomes confused, and makes mistakes; she is unable to control herself; she is unsteady and confused in her actions and is always distracted as she imagines to be in two places at the same time*); her state is further confirmed by other delusions or fixed ideas: *delusion, head seems to be too large* and *her body is divided into two parts*. In other words, the fusion of the two halves of her body (left and right) has not taken place at the age when it should (from age five until puberty). It is the critical transition from the prenatal psyche into ego consciousness that the *Silica* child struggles with. When the child must learn to venture away from the safety of home and parents, when he goes to school and begins to adjust to organized society, starting to enter into relationships with the foreign object/subject world, *Silica* struggles to adapt like a moth coming out of its cocoon.

At age eight or nine, when a child typically frees himself from the closest ties in the family dynamic, *Silica's* delusions stop his transition toward ego consciousness. This is because one part of the child is firmly rooted in the family, *longing for home,* and *the child is obstinate and headstrong, and self-willed,* while the other part is timid about exploring the outside world (*he has timidity, about appearing in public and to talk in public and has the delusion, that he is about to receive an injury and that everything will fail*). *Silica*'s delusions reflect the struggle between the independence that this child seeks and the still-present dependence on his family. One half of *Silica* is autonomous, while the other half is still attached to the family. It is not uncommon for the child to have dreams reflecting the struggle between his desire for independence and his homesickness, or wish for continued protection. The Cyber delusion readily leads to secondary delusions about a dangerous world, explaining the timidity with which *Silica* approaches the outside world: *delusion, he is about to receive an injury*; *delusion, she is pursued by enemies* and *delusion, everything will fail.* Another delusion, *he has done wrong,* reflects his *lack of confidence,* making him feel insecure even about leaving the safety of his home; he is always looking for a secure, familiar person to accompany him (*delusion, someone walks besides him*). It is for this reason that *Silica* always has two fixed and opposite personas, the dichotomous good-bad or devil-angel child, and is unable to accommodate additional personae or to adapt his emotional clothing, as one must often do in order to deal with life's circumstances.

Causalities

Anticipation Anxiety about Expectations

Nash, in *Leaders in Homeopathic Therapeutics,* gives us a good physical description of the *Silica* child: *puny, delicate, with a nearly translucent skin, face pinched and an old-looking expression,* which prompted Elizabeth Hubbard, the well-known homeopath, to label *Silica* the "angel-child." To an inattentive observer, *Silica* might seem a spoiled little princess, the pride or trophy of the family who is totally unfit for household work. Some of her behaviors might certainly enhance that impression: *egotism*; *housekeeping, women, unable to do*; *duty, no sense of,* and *inability to manage finances,* as if she were destined for greater things, a more royal world (like *Phosphorus* and *Platina*). However, her timidity and lack of confidence do not allow her to reach the level of *nobility* (*delusion being noble*) of a *Phosphorus* (the queen) or a *Platina* (the empress), both of whom are much more established in the world than *Silica*. *Silica* feels that she needs to fulfill certain expectations that have been imposed on her by someone else in the family, an impression that provides another translation of the Cyber delusion, *left half does not belong to her.*

This fixed idea points to a control exerted by someone else; someone else possesses half of her body. She does not have the sense that she is being controlled, as does the *Alumina* child, who has the delusion of speaking with someone else's voice. Rather, the family's expectations for *Silica* to grow up to be that extraordinary person—proper, beautiful, smart, and perfect in everything she executes—exert inordinate pressure on the *Silica* child, and this may lead to an identity crisis. This child is told that everyone in the family is bright and that she should be too. She is exhorted not to dishonor this family of high achievers. Such demands create high anxiety, destroying the self-confidence of a *Silica* child, as she may easily become over stimulated and experience mental burnout (*over-susceptibility to nervous stimuli; ailments from mental work*). Having practiced for about a decade in Los Angeles/Hollywood, I encountered numerous *Silica* children who were expected to be the next Grace Kelly in spite of their inner shyness and performance anxiety, causing great *fright*. Their natural grace and beauty prompted many parents to expose these children to a world full of glitter, action, and competition, requiring more mental, emotional, and physical stamina than most of the children could muster.

The *Silica* child might be the oldest son or oldest daughter in the family and be expected to follow in the footsteps of a successful father or mother. Yet he does not want to be a career person, a CEO, a great sportsman or actor, or to continue the military tradition. Instead, *Silica* may want to be an artist or to dedicate his life to poor people, and he would be more likely to enjoy success in his chosen field. Conflict between a person's own nature and the demands of her family may create a *Silica* state. I have no doubt that this leads to the creation of additional *Silica* people, engendering a neurosis that is difficult to overcome. The *Silica* child is repeatedly told by his family (often an intellectual father) that if she behaves the way she is expected to, she will be accepted. She should go to a good university and not talk about enrolling in art school. Or, at least, if she simply must pursue art, she should go into the graphic design business—that's where the money is. "Just don't become another starving artist." *Silica* thus becomes totally *image-bound*, most likely in the family image which he needs to hold up.

Silica has to live up to a false ego, an ego created not by his own desires but by the expectations of others. His *delusion, everything will fail* becomes reality when he studies too hard and his mind becomes blank, which unfortunately leaves the mind quite unprotected and allows it to be penetrated by outside influences. *Silica's* timidity is so great that he feels he can't overcome this timorousness even when he is alone (*timidity when alone*). To live up to that false, strong image that is expected of him, the *Silica* child often dreams of becoming someone famous, even represented by a Superman or James Bond figure, to help him in pushing the door wide open to the threatening world. He needs that picture of an alter ego to bolster his confidence. *Silica* even has pronounced *dreams of humiliation*, and he has a *desire to be magnetized*. In other words, *Silica* is looking for the support, protection, and positive opinion of others because he is afraid he will fail or be injured (*delusions, will receive an injury* and *delusions, everything will fail*).

Silica is distinguished by a nature more refined than that of *Lycopodium*. *Lycopodium* children, especially, and to a lesser degree *Silica* personalities, consider family members to be inferiors whom they can address with selfish commands and control through irritability, inducing weak and apologetic answers. But the *Silica* child comes often from a cultivated background with high standards, and she always needs to give a worthy performance. *Lycopodium*, with its *love for power*, presents more arrogance and needs to feel superior to others (*dictatorial, talks with an air of command*), while *Silica* is easier to intimidate (*the slightest word brings tears; sensitive to and anxiety from noise*). Even a bad dream cannot be erased from her memory: *on waking at night from an anxious dream she remained very anxious and her heart beat audibly.*

Aggravation of Mental Work

Although *Silica* is an intellectual remedy (*it has great activity of the mind; great facility of thought and fluent expression*), mental work aggravates this child: *mental labor is very difficult; concentration is difficult when studying and reading; there is difficulty in fixing the attention; there is confusion while talking; comprehension is difficult, and distractedness is always present.* This is because she frets far too much over details (*she is conscientious about trifles* [details], and *she even has remorse about trifles and a sense of guilt about trifles*). *Silica's* perfectionism may express itself as follows: "I tend to get behind in my work because I repeat things over and over again." "Neatness is very important to me. Other people seem to accept lower standards from themselves than I do." In other words, this *Silica* child becomes very upset about the smallest mistake or imperfection in her homework, endlessly fretting over it and trying to correct it numerous times until perfection is reached. *Silica* does not just set very high standards for himself but places excessive importance on the self-evaluations that she bases on those standards. Mistakes are failures for *Silica*, and he believes he will lose the respect of others following failure: *forsaken, feels is not being beloved by his parents, wife and friends*. The performance aspect is intrinsic to his view of himself. Although *Silica gets confused and makes mistakes (she had almost put a watch into the saucepan to boil instead of an egg), and easily makes mistakes in talking,* it has nothing to do with the backwardness of a *Bar-c* but rather with the distraction of mind and the overactivity of the brain that result from paying attention to every tiny detail. Since *Silica* suffers from overexertion of the mind, any additional intellectual challenge can lead to a great fear of failure: *fear of failure, in business and in examinations; want of self-confidence, and undertakes nothing lest he fail.* Due to his sense of perfectionism, *Silica* can become a procrastinator. This child exhibits *fear of undertaking a new enterprise* and there is even a *delusion, that everything will fail. Silica*'s fixation on details can become so cumbersome that she *makes mistakes easily in talking,* may experience *constant vanishing of the senses,* and exhibits *prostration of the mind from reading* and *brain fag. Silica*'s lack of confidence becomes especially evident when she is forced to perform: *timidity when appearing in public* and *fear before an examination.*

Compare *Silica*, in her fear of examinations, with *Anac*, who often suffered the indignation of being criticized by the teacher and is now determined to prove himself by excelling in his studies, putting undue pressure on himself and ultimately suffering failure due to sudden memory loss. Compare *Silica*, also, with *Picric-ac*, who is ambitious, feels the need and duty to perform well and who as a consequence exerts himself and then *lacks will power to undertake anything*; and with *Arg-nit*, an overemotional, often irrational and impulsive individual with weakening mental faculties (*he feels very much affected bodily and mentally; he does not undertake anything lest he should not succeed*).

Fright

Ailments from fright are additional causalities; in view of his CD, these should not be surprising. One *Silica* child was terribly frightened when inadvertently left alone on the school bus by the driver. When discovered, he was crying, trembling, and even vomiting. After this incident, he announced that he did not want to go to school anymore. In spite of the growing desire to mature and to be independent, *Silica* has neither the communication, empathy, sensuality, and beauty of *Phosphorus* nor the arrogance and self-assuredness of the *Sulphur* personality, who is often ruled by delusions of grandeur and is fond of religious and philosophical debates. *Silica* is not the strongest of people either mentally or physically, as evidenced by *ailments from mental work* and *sexual excesses.* This commonly leads to obstruction in *Silica's* maturation and individuation process, leaving *Silica* with a rather infantile ego. Even someone with a well-functioning, self-confident ego, like *Sulphur,* cannot control everything that happens in his world; this is certainly true for *Silica,* who often drifts aimlessly and insecurely into his outside existence because of a lack *of firmness and spine,* also sometimes called *cowardice.*

Compensations

Intellect: A Gifted Child

Silica has a keen *intellect.* Just as with *Lycopodium,* a sense of physical weakness during *Silica's* early childhood years often results in feelings of *lack of confidence and timidity appearing in public.* The **law of compensation** is at work not only in the dream state but also during the conscious life of a human being: *Silica* has the tendency to compensate for her physical weakness by placing greater emphasis on her mental potential. A physically weak individual tends to lean more toward intellectual endeavors, even more when he is aware of a physical inferiority complex. *Silica* and *Lycopodium,* primarily, and at times *Sulphur, Lachesis,* and *China,* often carry this attitude to an extreme, developing into bookworms or brooding introverts, especially in their final syphilitic phases. Like *Sulphur,* they may also resort to philosophical, political, or religious ranting. *Silica* children impose perfection upon themselves (*Carcinosin*) and are often too serious. *Silica* wants to be number one in school (*Aurum, Nat-s, Sulphur,* and *Nat-m*) and often succeeds if she isn't thwarted by her detail-oriented mind, anticipation anxiety, and lack of stamina.

Silica is very affected by *admonition,* a sycotic trait: *even kindly admonition aggravates* (*Nat-m, Phosphorus,* and *Platina*). Of course, *Platina's* sensitivity has a different meaning: she is the empress, the perfect, spiritual, and passionate person who is aggravated and terribly insulted by the slightest criticism (*ailments from wounded honor*)! *Phosphorus* wants to become friends with the rest of the world, so admonition means disapproval and a chance to lose at least one friend. And who could disapprove of a person like *Phosphorus* who is always so sympathetic, full of care that something might happen to you, and truly interested in finding out who you are? *Nat-m,* the already mortally wounded soul in relationships, receives admonition like another nail in the coffin, as reflected in fixed ideas such as *she is persecuted* and *mother* (read: her nourishing vessel) *is dead. Silica's* fear of criticism in intellectual matters, though, has to do with the distraction of mind, the overactivity of the brain, and the undue attention he pays to minute detail; admonition will only destroy any vestiges of confidence that may remain. This is also very different from *Lachesis*' intellectual prowess: *Lachesis* is more competitive and aggressive, using her sharp tongue as a tool to make her point. *Silica* is an introverted thinking type, whereas *Lachesis* is an extraverted thinking type.

Their keen intellects lead *Silica* and *Lycopodium* to become lawyers, teachers, priests, or librarians—any profession with a maximum of sitting and a minimum of outdoor activity suits them (except accounting, as *Silica* has *an inaptitude for finances*). This avoidance of motion is another aspect of obstruction and stagnation, in this case on the physical plane. Not for nothing do we see in these remedies symptoms of stagnation, mainly in the GI tract (*Sil, Sulph, Lyc,* and *China* with constipation, flatulence, gas, borborygmata, etc.) but also in the cardio-vascular system (*Lachesis* with hemorrhoids, varicose veins, thrombosis, etc.). It is interesting to note that, in the above remedies, Nature compensates through modalities like *<from tight clothing, <from pressure of clothes and touch, >from motion and open air, >free secretions, >eructations, >from loosening clothing, >warm applications/food,* and for *Sil, >from profuse urination* (Gels).

Inflation/Deflation

Silica is a person (adult or child) with an excessive persona or mask: it is the contrast between the way the person really is and the way he appears! At home this child appears willful and outright hard towards those he loves (parents and siblings), but the true persona is one of extreme timidity when he appears in public. The behavior at home is in sharp contrast to the reality of the forces that motivate him (this is also true for the *Lycopodium* child, which makes a differential diagnosis difficult). The mask is worn for his own purposes, and he is afraid of being unmasked or of becoming the emperor with no clothes. *Silica* is deathly afraid that the public will find out that she is not precisely the person she presents herself to be, and that she will therefore be hurt: *delusion, about to receive an injury.* In reality, she is often an individual utterly lacking in self-confidence and self-assertion: *spineless; lack of character and want of grit, moral or physical* (similar to the *Lycopodium* child again). Therefore, *Silica* expends a great deal of effort in order to create and maintain a compensatory image. Shunning center stage—feeling shyness and social anxiety—is as natural as breathing, but *Silica* takes it to new heights! Social anxiety, the distress felt over being evaluated and observed by others, is especially painful for the person in a *Silica* state. This person is like a huge blown-up balloon that can be deflated with one needling remark (*she is easily offended, and takes everything in bad part; delusion about needles, about pins,* = symbolic!). Hence, there is a tremendous fear of failing in performances, especially when she is away from her home: *timidity appearing in public, and the delusion, everything will fail* as well as *anticipation about an engagement*. Even the stool of the *Silica* child is timid and bashful (*constipation from inactivity of the bowels* and *stool remains long in rectum*). The stool comes out, after severe straining, but it then slips back inside, as if it does not want to be seen in the outside world: *the stool when partly expelled recedes again; stool that has already protruded slips back again*!

Yielding/Unyielding Behaviors

When, as a stranger, you see a *Silica* child, you think of her as needing a remedy for the *yielding* character, a person who has *no grit or spine* as she shows a lack of **assertiveness**. This is only partially true: we may expect to find in this child some hardness and fixation comparable to the presence of silica in glass, quartz rocks, and amethyst: simultaneously fragile (breaks easily) and inflexible (cannot be bent). This hardness is also paralleled in silicon's electrically insulating and water-repellent properties. For some people, *biting and scratching* can be defensive maneuvers; notably, silica is a component of teeth and nails, providing their hardness. Often, alternative doctors give *Silica* as a supplement to strengthen the hair and nails. This, of course, is not homeopathy, but rather a crude way of providing for a nutritional lack of *Silica*. We do find homeopathic *Silica* indicated in some instances of fragile nails (*gray dirty nails, as if decayed, when cut scattering like powder and splitting into several layers* and *brittle nails, crumbling off of the nails and splitting*), but it is also indicated in case of *rough and yellow nails* and *thickened nails.*

Obsessive-Compulsive Behavior

Silica's preoccupation with trifles may lead to overt obsessive-compulsive behavior and fixed ideas. The *Silica* person checks and rechecks her work. She pays great attention to details because she fears that her work is not going to look good enough, leading to guilty feelings (*remorse about trifles*). Again, we see in this child the primary concern with image. *Silica* patients can also display superstitious behavior; they may feel that everything needs to be done in a certain obsessive-compulsive way—and perfectly. This behavior reflects the suspicious and doubting nature of *Silica*; she does not trust herself, and so must check and recheck everything she does. *Silica* thinks he is handicapped or weak: he is *unsteady and confused in his actions* and has the *delusion that everything will fail*; there is *want of self-confidence and lack of character, weakness,* and *neurasthenia*. *Silica*'s defense mechanism is trying to cover up this perceived weakness through fixed behaviors: she has the *most excessive scruples of conscience about trifles, as if he had done a great wrong,* and *she shows remorse about trifles*; there is even the fixed idea of *the patient thinking only of pins, fears them, searches for them, and counts them carefully*. The *Silica* child demonstrates fear of needles and injections (*oversensitive to steel points directed towards her*). *Silica* patients dwell on trifles and are very particular about order and cleanliness.

A *Silica* person will want to take survival courses and courses in herbology, botany, and the like so as to be prepared for anything. These courses become the crutch that *Silica* people lean on to strengthen their egos when in public. If they learn about homeopathy or medicine, it is not necessarily for the purpose of helping others; rather, it is primarily to help themselves overcome their shyness when faced with the outside world. These are all measures of compensating for a weak perceived ego with respect to the external world. The yielding character of *Silica* when separated from family stems from a lack of the energy and grit needed to impose her point of view on the rest of the world; this is quite different for *Lycopodium*, whose timidity is related to cowardice. Now the difference between these two remedies in the context of avoiding confrontation can be understood: *Silica* thinks she cannot win because of her mental and physical exhaustion, even if she has a personal opinion; *Lycopodium* does not want you to find out in this confrontation that he is just presenting a front, a mask, for a very insecure and cowardly person, and he will therefore speak with conviction (*dictatorial, speaking with a voice of command*).

For the *Silica* child, the fear of failure can be felt before beginning any task, whether it is a little one like cleaning up his room or a more demanding one like doing homework. *Silica* can be very fidgety during performances at school because she is too conscious of the impression that she is making: *overanxious about himself, ailments from anxiety and fear* and *restless and fidgety, starting (being startled) at the least thing, especially from noise*. In general, every task becomes a gigantic enterprise; there are no small tasks. It is not because *Silica* thinks that she is not capable of succeeding; like *Lycopodium*, rather, she is preoccupied with others' perceptions of her and her performance. She wonders what others think of her. No wonder *Silica postpones everything till next day* and has *ailments from anticipation*. Above all, the *Silica* child wants to protect her image, not only in the eyes of other people but also in her own. She does this by paying attention to detail, by maintaining excessive order, and by becoming overly fastidious. *Silica* is considered a perfectionist; for her, failure translates into humiliation, especially when she is *contradicted*. A *Silica* child's drawings display a great sense of detail and symmetry. This is because she feels she is being looked at and needs to keep up her image; a *Silica* child I presented in a live case for class drew with a crayon, one in each hand, perfect symmetric circles!

Fear of failure applies mostly to *Silica's* performance in public, where she feels less shielded than at home. A *Lycopodium* child immediately says, even at home, "I can't do this—I can't do my homework; please help me." He anticipates failure, which certainly conflicts with the tough, bossy, and intellectual attitude he usually projects. The *Silica* child, though, gets hopelessly lost in the minute details of the project, erasing and redoing every word she writes to perfection, which leads to mental exhaustion; however, she has no difficulty starting her work. If the pathology increases, though, and the *Silica* child or teenager is not helped, indecisiveness takes over, and she will not start a task or make a change of career unless she knows that she can do it with perfect success. Or, as one *Silica* expressed: "I am not going to start college and waste my time partying until I figure out what I want to do." But she wanted so much to live up to the picture of perfection that, years later, this person still had not made up her mind.

Outward Hardness/Induration and Obstinacy

Silica's defense mechanism is to project hardness in order to keep up her image: such a child has *irritability after consolation; has an irritable and peevish mood, easily getting out of humor; everything frets her and makes her peevish; she shows inquietude and ill-humor on the least provocation, and a disposition to fly into a rage; the child becomes obstinate and headstrong but she cries when gently spoken to*. *Silica* can even become violent when contradicted: there is *intolerance of contradiction; she has to be restrained from committing violence*. This contrasts sharply with the angelic behavior this child often demonstrates at school. *Silica's* obstinate defensiveness also gives way to another form of hardening: a local hardening, or induration. This focal hardening is found in *Silica's* proving symptoms: styes, hard cysts, glands, calcifications, and hardening of the breast muscle: *hardening of the left breast; the right breast is hard, painful and swollen at the nipple; and induration of the axillary glands.*

Another pathology related to *Silica*, the fistula (*fistula of the bones and joints*), reflects *Silica's* unyielding, stubborn, and tenacious character. A fistula penetrates tissue, creating a tunnel that brings the interior process to the outside. We can imagine it as something like the slow, arduous process of digging the underwater tunnel from Great Britain to France (*generalities, fistulae, caries of tibia and fibula*). *Silica* also appears in black type for *fistula of the bones* and *fistulae of the joints* (both *Sil* and *Phosphorus*). Do not underestimate the stubbornness of a *Silica* person! Lung fibrosis is another form of induration. When pneumonia evolves from its acute stage, requiring *Aconite*, to a subacute stage, requiring *Bryonia*, to a chronic situation, there will be a chance of fibrosis, especially in the presence of conditions that cause chronic irritation of the lungs (as with longtime smokers or patients with chronic emphysema). This chronic stage is a sycotic phase requiring remedies like *Silica*: *chest, inflammation, lungs, neglected*; and *chronic neglected pneumonia, passing over into suppuration*. Keloid formation is another local hardening that responds to *Silica*: *skin, keloid* (*Sil*, Graph); *multiple keloids which appeared after excision of a tumor.* While the above physical expressions are sycotic manifestations, it may be noted that *Silica* is a strong tri-miasmatic remedy. *Longing for home, sensitive to noise, great anxiety, disposed to weep, inclination to startle, itching on a hairy scalp, oppression of stomach after eating, very sleepy after eating, sour eructations, and bashful stool* are some of the psoric expressions.

The same hardness is seen on the emotional plane. While the timidity, yielding, *gentleness* and self-consciousness of *Silica* are well known, this other hard side is not as familiar: *defiant; consolation, kind words aggravate; egotism; when crossed has to restrain himself from doing violence.* This hard side is the compensated state of *Silica*, the behavior that *Silica* adopts to protect and shield herself from the world. Induration can occur on the mental level as well. *Silica* is well known for fixed ideas (*pins, counting; delusion, head is too large; delusion, body is divided*). As adults, *Silica* patients can compensate for these traits with their behavior, and they may therefore appear to be very outgoing, sociable people. They may make you think of *Phosphorus* or *Sulphur*. *Silica* might have the mildness of *Phosphorus*, but not its exuberance or independence (in TCM, *Silica* belongs to the Earth element, *Phosphorus* to Fire!).

To discover a person's uncompensated picture, we need to ask more questions about what he was like as a child. Was he timid and shy? If so, this is his true nature, for which he has now found ways of coping; therefore, we always pay great attention to the uncompensated symptoms of the child. It is interesting to know that *Pulsatilla*, with its soft, gentle, and yielding behavior, is the acute of *Silica*. It is as if, when the situation becomes chronic, the yielding behavior of *Pulsatilla*, initially uncompensated in *Silica*, needs to transform into the hard, fixed survival mode of the compensated *Silica*: *child becomes obstinate, headstrong*. At this point, we can see the persistence of the Cyber delusion: that one side of the body does not belong to her.

A compensated *Silica* person, acting in survival mode, will tempt an inattentive physician to assume the role of prosecutor during examination—just what the *Silica* person is afraid of. Although this is a natural reaction for the physician when confronted with a silent patient, examiners should ask themselves: why and for what purpose is this patient silent? In the case of *Silica*, the silence is due to timidity; in *Nat-m*, the patient hides out of fear of being hurt; in *Platina*, the silence is due to the person's haughtiness; in *Lycopodium*, there is a fear that her cowardice will be discovered; in *Sulphur*, the silence is due to his egotism and feeling of intellectual superiority, while *Calc-c* needs to be silent because he is mulling things over.

Dreams

Dreams often give us a way of discovering the patient's inner feelings, especially when he is taciturn. *Silica* is no exception to the dream rule of compensation. In spite of outwardly hard conscious behavior, there is a lot of fear in *Silica*'s dreams, well hidden to keep up that image of strength: *dreams, being pursued by wild animals, cats and dogs, ghosts* (only *Sil*); *dreams, animals, thieves, and ghosts*; *half-awake dream, as if innumerable spirits wanted to seize him*; *when he woke up, he could not move a limb, and lay in a sweat with great anguish and palpitation dream that he had to die*. A four-year-old *Silica* patient of mine had a nightmare in which a crab came out of the sea while he was playing at the beach. After one dose of Silica 30C, the dream theme changed to a fairy coming to his aid, chasing the crab away and saving him. It is not unusual for the simillimum to change the theme of dreams. If *Silica* feels she is being pursued by such dangers, it is no wonder that she feels timid on one hand and, on the other hand, feels the need to stand strong and rigid (*dreams, of being wrongfully accused of a crime*, only remedy in this rubric). *Silica* also has some pleasant dreams, *amorous, vivid and enthusiastic*, which reflect the amorous side of a person who is shy and yielding in public but can let go of the timidity in dreams. In fact, in the liberated unconscious world, *Silica* dreams of a great sexual and loathsome character showing up: *dreams of a loathsome, repulsive character; lewd dreams and strong sexual impulses; lewd dreams and emission of semen.* Here we see clearly the law of compensation at work: these dreams reflect the opposite of the conscious attitude.

Looking for Support (Desire to be Magnetized)

Silica really relies on the people in his family first: they are the safest ones to lean on, and they are always present and available (*delusion someone walks besides him*). It is the structure and the cohesiveness of the family that saves the *Silica* person; without a stable family, she *feels forsaken and not being beloved by her parents, wife or friends.* (This is interesting when we consider that houses and other durable structures are made of stone and cement, which contain a large proportion of silicon dioxide.) The *Silica* family can also extend beyond the parent-child nucleus. If there is neglect by parents, this can be overcome by the *Silica* patient's relationship to his grandparents. But the *Silica* child will *never* look for support from strangers because of his *timidity about appearing in public.* For *Silica*, the home and family are everything: this child *longs for home and for his relations at home.* Compare this to *Sulphur* and *Phosphorus* children, whose goals are to leave the home as soon as possible and conquer the world. The *Silica* person has one foot firmly planted in the family home and puts the other one hesitantly and very carefully out of the door: she exhibits a *yielding, faint-hearted, anxious mood.* During an interview with a physician, this child will always speak to the parent accompanying her, not directly to the doctor. *Silica* might also look for the support of a stronger child at school (often a bully!), a famous person, an athlete, guru, or band member (being a groupie), as he can associate himself with the other person's name and fame and ride on his coattails: *desire to be magnetized.* He does this to satisfy the ego or image and, at the same time, to resolve the problem of *timidity appearing in public.* The persons with whom *Silica* associates often become part of their extended family. Also, *Silica* could be the shy little sister or brother who follows a popular older brother, a high school football star—a relationship which may give the *Silica* person the delusion that he, too, is great.

All compensations and all forces influencing the *Silica* person contribute to unconsciously maintain her Cyber delusion: the contrary wishes of parents who force the child to follow their dominant conscious function instead of her own; the considerable compensations of hiding a shadow which is so vastly different from the mask; her yielding behavior in public versus her almost tyrannical attitude in the family; dreams of humiliation versus amorous ones; the great facility of thought and, nevertheless, the easy overpowering of her mental capacity. *Silica* seems to be the prototype of the person full of contradictions, which does not help solve her confusion regarding her real identity—it makes for an extremely obstructed personality with an excessive persona. One example from the practice:

> An 18-year-old girl was overanxious about the impression she made, what other people thought of her: Do I look good? Do I look perfect? She had a tendency to postpone everything. She plucked out all her eyebrows because she could not make them identical, drawing them on her face instead. It could take her two hours to decide on jewelry as it all had to match, so she liked to buy things in sets. It took her a long time (usually two hours) to leave the house because she was caught up in so many rituals. As a child, she had had imaginary friends and remembered them all. She could only wear one pair of socks, and if they were not on perfectly she would panic and rip them off. It would take time to calm her down until she tried again. In school, she had a terrible time with homework because she would have to recopy it many times until it was perfect. She applied lotion over her entire body daily and could not be without hand lotion during the day. When she had a horseback riding class when she was about 12, she had to leave the class to put emergency lotion on as she could not stand to touch the dry dusty leather of the reins. She liked the horse, but not the work; she did like dressing up in western outfits to show the horse. When her mom hung up her clothes she ripped them all down because they were not on matching hangers. When her room was remodeled, the tile in the bathroom was made to match the comforter in her bedroom.
>
> The slightest admonition brought tears. She would hide behind her mother's legs when meeting new people and refused even to say "please" and "thank you." In preschool, she had sneered at other kids, telling them that they were stupid and that she did not want to play with them. Of course, she changed her

attitude eventually when she made no friends. She was always playing dress-up, not doing her homework. She said she was not going to do anything until she decided what she wanted to do in life—and not let her parents decide for her. She resented any suggestion about a possible career, and she was not going to be a person who changed her mind. She had a disposition to fly into a rage when with her family, and she was obstinate and bossy with everyone at home. She had an inability to manage her finances. Pressure from family could lead to an identity crisis and the delusion that everything would fail. She maintained her privacy at all costs and was hard toward family and yielding toward the world. She thought of trifles and reproached herself about them. When older, she established a nice home where everything matched. She made lists of what she needed for her home and lists of ingredients for what she would try to cook. She had eight sets of dishes and replaced any piece that broke to maintain the set. When replacing one glass, there was a problem as they were sold in sets of four. She then would want her mother to take the extra three glasses and put them in storage. She would fight with her dad when he rearranged a few items in her perfect kitchen. She was an intellectual, with great activity of thoughts, and was fluent and great with words. Every job was big—there was no small job. But as she paid too much attention to detail, mental work aggravated her and caused headaches as she got stuck in the details. Unsurprisingly, she responded well to homeopathic *Silica*, overcoming the allopathic OCD label!

Golden Tips from the Masters

- Sea sand (Silicea marina), mainly composed of *Silica*, *is a great remedy for constipation and suppuration of glands*. J. H. Clarke prepared it from sand from the beach, "just as it was left by the tide." Unlike *Silicea terra*, he advised us to use it *where Nat-mur symptoms are present in a Silica case*, especially in cases of constipation since both remedies are of great value in such a condition
- Compton Burnett ("Dr. Gout") recorded a case in which a boy was eating sand at the beach in spite of his parents having forbidden it. Burnett told the parents to let him do it. The boy kept eating the sand for 14 days, during which time his health vastly improved. After 14 days, he neither craved nor ate sand any longer
- *Silica* is the homeopathic surgeon: it can open ripe abscesses and to remove splinters; used in abscesses after *Hepar-s*, which helps and expedites suppuration, to open the abscess without causing scars
- *Silica* hates wind and always covers ears and head with a hat
- Great indication for sweaty feet and hands: sweat drips from their fingers; #1 remedy for suppression of perspiration from the feet
- #1 remedy for seizures after DPT and #2 after *Thuja* for ailments from vaccinations
- Craving for cold food although they are chilly (lack of vital heat)
- *Mercury* and *Silica* are inimical! Always use *Hep-s* as an intermediate! (*Merc—Hep—Sil*)
- *Kali-s—Puls—Sil* is a good sequence
- *Silica* is excellent for unresolved pneumonia, for a chest with prolonged coughing and catarrh that does not clear up
- Acne in face with nodules under the skin or with small scarred holes
- Children with big head, thin legs and small, full, and round abdomen
- Delayed development in children
- One of the main remedies in asthma for children because of lack of stamina
- *Silica* represents image, refined nature, firmness in family, timidity towards strangers, magnetization by family, local hardness, and struggle between yielding and firmness
- Constipation <when traveling (*Nux-v*, *Lycopodium*)
- Heat makes her sick, yet she wants it; suffocation in a warm room, >in open air
- Very useful in diseases of the bone with fistula, caries, and necrosis
- The child always wets the bed during the first sleep (Nash)-also *Sepia*

Staphysagria (Staph).
Stavesacre

The Cyber Delusion

Staphysagria's Cyber delusion is ***someone walks behind him*** (*Staph, Sil, Anac, Med and Calc*). For the remedies belonging in this rubric, "walking behind him" has different meanings and can be negative or positive. *Silica* needs a stronger positive force in the outside world to boost his confidence and has also the *delusion someone walks besides him*. *Calc*-c needs the same protection to boost his immature and fearful ego (*he talks about nothing but murder, fire and rats*); he needs a family member or friend to hold his hand as he is *anxious that people will observe his confusion* and to keep him from falling victim to his Cyber delusion, *he is about to sink into annihilation*. The person behind him is an assurance that he is supported ("I have your back!") and protected from everything that can happen on the outside; the person behind him gently nudges him forward from his inert, hesitant attitude. *Calc*-c needs a little push to spring into action as he mulls things over. *Medorrhinum*, as he projects his own shadow, is suspicious of everyone (as he is the one hiding certain aspects of his life—the sexual one, for instance) and therefore looks constantly over his shoulder to see if anyone wants to harm him, projecting the darkness and evil of his unconscious onto others. For him, the person behind him is always a threat, someone suspect. In *Anacardium's* case, it is an oppressive negative force, a controlling and dominating father figure that brings *Anac* to the brink of dissociation and schizophrenia. For *Lachesis*, this delusion is a mixed bag. On one hand, it is negative, as he is often overcome by the CD *he is about to receive an injury and he is wronged*; he is indeed fearful of bodily harm, like *Nat-m*, but the accompanying person can also be positive: *Lachesis* can *be under the influence of a powerful being*, often one who supplies him with nighttime inspiration for his fertile, active mind. A rather negative aspect of this delusion is that *Lachesis* gives his power away, projecting it onto a mana personality (for Polynesians, a mana personality is he who is full of power and wisdom) who acts as his guru and life force. Giving his power away will always hinder him on his path to individuation; his individuality is stifled when he subjects himself to the judgments of a more enlightened person. *Mag-m*, suffering from ailments from deceived friendship and anger, is always anxious and hurried as the peacemaker and caretaker with a strong sense of responsibility; her delusion *she is friendless and neglected* makes this person walking behind her a rather negative influence. *Sanicula*, a very touchy and low-energy person who *cannot bear to be touched* and has a great *fear of the darkness*, constantly looks behind her like *Medorrhinum* and feels rather threatened by the dark figure that follows.

What does *Staphysagria's* CD mean? Is the shadowy figure a benevolent presence or a threatening one? It looks as if there is always a person walking behind *Staphysagria*, navigating and controlling her slightest movement. She cannot be herself! In other words, she is constantly letting someone else invade her boundaries, submitting her ego to someone else. The latter is also the essence of the *Carcinosin* victim, and *Staphysagria* is the number one associated remedy of *Carcinosin*. In practice, this means that when a patient is stuck in a *Staphysagria* situation, he is betraying his own soul and on his way to creating cancer in his body; cancer serves as a final warning for him to change the direction in his life. It is interesting that we find *Silica* and *Calc-c* also in the rubric *someone walks besides him*, indicating in their cases the benevolent character of the shadow person. But we don't see *Staphysagria, Medorrhinum*, or *Anac* in this rubric. *Staphysagria's* CD reflects a lack of freedom of choice and of decision-making; someone is shadowing her, but not necessarily in a benevolent and protective way. This is confirmed by other delusions that express how she feels about this guidance: *delusion she is pursued; she is persecuted; she is unfortunate; she is criticized; of insults; and she will be murdered.*

The fixed ideas of being criticized and belittled and of receiving insults indicate the real character of *Staphysagria's* relationship with that shadow figure. There is no talk of *being under the influence of a powerful being* as there is with the mesmerized *Lachesis*, who actually derives support and inspiration to follow her chosen path from this delusion. *Staphysagria* feels persecuted, unfortunate, and that she will be murdered—all expressions of her loss of control over her life. What *is* already being killed, murdered, and obstructed is her personality and individuality, her freedom of choice. In other words, she is totally dominated, leading to much anxiety and even anguish. *Staphysagria* never achieves authenticity, as authenticity entails honoring one's own emotional needs and desires. This control by a person on whom one is dependent on an ongoing condition, not a question of episodes as it is with *Lyssin*, who intermittently loses support from the one he depends upon. The *Staphysagria* person has received so many black eyes in her relationships that it has become part of her persona. The abuse prevalent in *Staphysagria* has created a permanent state of anxiety, worse even after escaping her cruel reality in a short sleep (*anguish after a nap*), a state that *Staphysagria* eventually considers normal. It has become part of her luggage, of her personality, expressed by the delusion *past anxious thoughts and things are present.* Nothing is forgotten! This fixed idea has become part of her identity! The truth is, though, that some unbearable deeds are too painful to acknowledge, too heartbreaking to face. For this reasons, investigating and understanding recurrent dreams can be a wake-up call for the patient. The *Staphysagria* person often dreams of being driven in a car with someone else at the wheel of the car, a symbol of her life being directed by others and of her not being in control of her own destiny. Dreams only recur when the patient neglects to listen to the message, just as a bill collector comes back for unpaid bills. Hopefully, through intake of homeopathic *Staphysagria*, her inner voices will begin issuing stentorian commands.

But what happens initially? How does *Staphysagria* deal with the shadow figure? *Staphysagria* is almost like a split personality. On one hand, she endures all this cruelty, control, and criticism; on the other hand, her pride forbids her from reacting to the perpetrator directly and immediately. There is a little voice in her saying: "Don't react; don't show your anger." The *delusions, as to the greatness of her body; things appear small and humility of others while she is great* (a delusion she has in common with *Platina*, who really is convinced that *she does not belong to this world*) tell us that *Staphysagria* does not want to stoop to the level of the perpetrator. She is above all this, and the little voice in her reminds her that she is a much better person than her antagonist. She chooses the mighty high road, but is this beneficial for her? Only her story will tell! What can be foreseen is that a continuous barrage of insults chips away piece by piece at *Staphysagria*'s exterior armor.

One of the least known aspects of *Staphysagria* is haughtiness. The idea that *Staph* shares the delusion *humility of others while she is great* with a character like *Platina* may raise some eyebrows—but, as usual, things are not as they might appear on the surface. This fixed idea must lead to different compensations and probably has an altogether different meaning and causality for each of the two personalities. The roads of these two remedies may share a starting point, but they diverge quickly when *Platina* and *Staphysagria* are compared. The delusion *humility of others while he is great* is a problem of perception for these two as they are both sensation types. They both have this delusion of grandeur and can be *haughty*, yet the interior distortion behind the delusion could not be more different!

Platina covers her feelings of isolation with a true superiority complex, and the delusion of grandeur comes from a basic belief that she has no equal: *delusion, being noble, he is a great person, as if exalted.* She can find no one who is her sexual or spiritual equal, and has the delusion, *she is alone in the world; delusion, is deserted;* and *she has no place in the world.* Her Achilles heel is her egotism, and the compensation for *Platina* is that she has developed a very inflated view of herself, leading to the delusion *people seem mentally and physically inferior; a delusion, as to greatness of her body;* while *everything in the room is diminished, while she is tall and elevated;* Platina feels *enlarged, is very tall; her head is enlarged; is swollen; things appear small, he himself seems too large* and *on entering the house after walking; everything seems too narrow.* These delusions are the mental equivalent of a loss of sense of proportion in ocular vision. In her mental vision, objects seem small, and this makes *Platina* look down on everyone with pride. She lives to gratify herself as if only she mattered, as if only she were in the world. Her world is truly small, as she seeks to satisfy her passions with no concern for others. The irony in considering herself to have spiritual superiority is that her greed is largely for temporal things: *delusion, of wealth.* Hers is an egoistic hedonism compounded by narcissism. She can be *pompous; feels important, and squanders money; she is a boaster; braggart* and ultimately *discontented with everything.* And so, like a self-fulfilling prophecy, *Platina* ends up alone in the world. She becomes depressed and tires of the world. As the saying goes, it's lonely at the top. So it is for this ice witch whose goal is self-glory. This is quite different from *Staphysagria's* story as shown before!

Causalities

Indignation and Lost Honor

There are many ailments from (A/F) for *Staphysagria*; however, though many are black type, they are not equally weighted. The primary NWS is *ailments from indignation* on every level: emotional, mental, and physical; it is for this reason that *Staph* is known as the rape remedy. A rape can occur on any of these levels and be perpetrated by different people: at home, at work, in different relationships, and even during recreation—we are all familiar with obnoxious coaches! Though being berated at work or benched at a game doesn't seem life-threatening at first glance, it must be considered that one's identity is very closely tied to those groups; strong criticism threatens one's sense of membership as does the fear of exclusion, abandonment, and ostracism. Criticism makes a person feel attacked and unloved, and can be so damaging to a person's sense of self that it has an effect similar to abuse. One common manifestation of indignation and rudeness, especially in the workplace, is the behavior of the bully boss. Such a boss misuses power and humiliates people in front of others. She can be verbally abusive and overly controlling as she micromanages. He quarrels with his victim and, as he does so, contemptuously and unfairly lobs criticism at his subordinate. At home, a spouse may belittle his mate in front of others—and then insist it is all in good fun, though the victim is seething with rage, heartbreak and mortification. A variant of indignation and hostility is passive aggression, which is demonstrated in such behaviors as dragging one's heels on a project, remaining silent for a whole day as if the other person is a ghost, failing to respond to a meaningful request, or failing to disclose useful and necessary information to a colleague. As can be seen, instances of rape are more common on the mental/emotional levels than on the physical level, the one most often associated with this hideous crime. There is even the unjust *loss of position* (meaning losing one's job to suit the financial interests of the stockholders and CEO of the company, common in today's corporate environment), which can be considered an *ailment from indignation* that turns *Staphysagria* into an individual who *cannot support injustice*, into a remedy picture of *Causticum*, bent on vengeance to even the score.

The perpetrator's control of *Staphysagria* can be so extreme that the victim loses all self-esteem, loses touch with reality, and lives in a daze with the *delusion, everything looks strange* and *familiar things look strange*. The controlling person, who always possesses a syphilitic streak to bolster his own fragile ego, seeks out his victim and exerts his power through rudeness, insensitivity, and cold-blooded control, even under the banner and persona of professionalism (*ailments from rudeness of others*; *from mortification with indignation*; *from reproaches*; *from honor wounded*; *from embarrassment*). The perpetrator's goal is always the same: to damage the self-esteem and self-worth of his victim, to make her feel ashamed of herself as a member of society and to reassure that the animus in the victim is nothing but a silent, obedient and subservient dwarf, an entity "happy" to live a voiceless life! It is sheer manipulation and signals insensitivity and, often, cruelty in an individual. Sometimes, a perpetrator uses her own disease to control and tie her victim to her, appealing to an exaggerated and misplaced sense of duty on the part of the victim. Unless *Staphysagria* can escape from her situation, these negative events remain with her: *she suffers grief from long past offenses and dwells on past disagreeable events* (Nat-m). For *Nat-m*, dwelling on these sad thoughts can serve as the motivation for her career as a crusader or a reason to live. For *Staphysagria*—and here is the difference between *Staph* and *Nat-m*—dwelling on past injustices only creates yielding, submissive, and resigned behavior in later stages, building up inner pressure (*ailments from suppressed anger*, even resulting in *headaches from grief* (also *Ign, Aur, Calc, Puls*) and making her, because of the weight of psychogenic causes, the most likely remedy to become a cancer victim in the future. As Jung often asserted, Nature will visit you with a disease if you suppress your emotions!

There is also a kind of physical rape unknown to allopathy and the public in general. Often, a patient who has undergone surgery complains of pain at the site of the incision for months or even years afterwards. The body, psychologically, is rejecting the assault—just like the assault of frequent catheterization is expressed by recurrent bladder infections. You can imagine what is done allopathically to alleviate pain in the scar: doctors open it in precisely the same place, adding a second rape incident. Don't use remedies such as *Bell-p, Arnica*, or *Calendula* in this case as they do not reflect the emotional NWS of the "crime." They do not take the totality of the patient into account. *Staphysagria* is indicated!

Disappointment and Silent Grief

An example from my practice shows how such a NWS has lifelong consequences—not only for the victim, but also for other family members, imprinting the crime of indignation on others and perpetuating the emotional state—leading in turn to its trans-generational continuation. For women, a negative experience with the father leads to a malformation of the animus (corresponding to the paternal Logos and dominant thinking function) and can be responsible for a *Staphysagria* state:

> I had a patient who experienced extreme discord with, and even hatred for, her father because he cheated on her mother who did not stand up for herself; the strife was so serious that, from a young age, she developed a hatred towards men in general (due to a negative experience on the formation of her animus). Unbeknownst to her, she became just like her hated father. This patient was successful in business (showing the strength of her animus) and married for the

> first time at age 40; she soon divorced and then married a younger person, whom she dominated in the same way that she and her mother had been dominated by her father. Obviously she got tired of this relationship too. She told me that an inner voice was telling her that all men were alike and that she could trust no man. If she married she would only repeat the tragic experience of her mother. Her hatred of men, first aroused by her experience with her father, dominated her feelings so strongly that her idea about her father became her impression of all men. Whenever a real man came into her life, she projected this father image onto him. She was estranged from her father, but his image still ruled her mind, as could be seen in her behavior toward the second man she married. She had pretended to take on the role of a woman while unconsciously adopting the attitudes of a man. In some cultures, it would be said of such a woman that she was possessed by the ghost of a man. In one sense, she became a man; in another, she tried to assert her superiority over men, which undermined her feeling function. It made it impossible for her really to be a woman, especially in any relationship with a man. In marriage, she always struggled for supremacy, just as she was doing in business. She refused to listen to the woman's voice within herself, which could have told her that her hatred and bitterness toward her father had permeated her attitude toward all men, squashing her feeling function. By some strange law of the antipathy of similars, she loathed her father not because she was so different from him, but because in some ways she was so much like him.

Not unexpectedly, her disgust for men might have been lurking in her unconscious, which can only be revealed by a dream, the messenger of her unconscious; her chief complaint, though, severe pain and bladder infection after each sexual encounter (*bladder, cystitis, in newlywed women*), revealed the hidden disdain and repulsion she felt towards men, experienced as physical violation or rape. In the case of a negative father complex leading to a distorted animus, as was the case with this patient, there often are various disturbances of the sexual function/genitourinary tract: for instance, menstrual disorders, aversion to sex, lack of libido, painful coition or vaginismus, and honeymoon cystitis because the anima has been injured. In this patient, a typical *Staphysagria* situation was created through the *disappointment, the suppressed anger with silent grief* and *anger with indignation.*

Compensations

How does *Staphysagria* cope with this cruelty in her life? Does she react vehemently? Does she find anything positive in her bleak life as does *Nat-m*, a remedy often confused with *Staphysagria*? Can she find a balance between her pride and healthy reactions, helping her to stand up for herself in front of her abuser?

Escape into a Dream World: Delusion, of Fancy Illusions

It is not unusual for a *Staphysagria* person to be abused, dominated, and even prevented from communication with the outside world. *Staph* feels more and more incapable of connecting to people (because of shyness, shame, embarrassment, brainwashing, self-reproach, secrets, etc.) and, consequently, flees into a dream world to create imaginary friends and lovers. *Nat-c*, *Nat-mur*, and *Staphysagria* are all examples of this tendency. Each of them has fixed ideas on the same theme of *fancy illusions*. Note that these personalities all bear the hallmark of loneliness and isolation. *Staphysagria is absent-minded in a dreamy state*; additionally, all three personalities are often estranged to some degree from their family, which creates great *grief*. *Staphysagria* dreams or daydreams—not only about a different world, but also about an ideal lover (*amorous*). She may concoct a platonic love for someone she admires—her neighbor, a coworker, or her homeopath; however, she may also fantasize about someone whom she has never met, such as a singer with a beautiful voice. Kind words from her treating homeopath can easily catalyze the process of transference, in which he will now replace her father, lover, or friend—sometimes a hindrance to true healing.

Rather than reaching out to others, *Staphysagria* isolates herself so much in her dream world that, in spite of being a lonely person, she *has aversion to the presence of other people*; *she desires solitude, and even has aversions to all persons*, preferring to indulge in her created escape world although she follows such indulgences with self-reproach (*reproaching herself from indulging to sexual fantasies*—only remedy, referring also to her *masturbation tendency*). Lingering in her reveries allows her to *dream about a different future*. As the real world has no authentic meaning for her, the escape into the fabricated artificial world creates a ray of hope; it is for this reason that we often see a changeable behavior in *Staphysagria*: she is *discouraged alternating with courage and hope*. Her escape is so complete that she can neglect her family to indulge in her fancies (another reason for estrangement from her family): *escape from her family and children on waking*;

thinks she had fancies happened, even preventing sleep. And to artificially inflate her subdued ego, *when in company, she always speaks about herself.* All these exaggerated mental efforts lead to another secondary NWS: *ailments from mental exertion.*

Religion and Sex

Religion is another possible positive tool for *Staph*; she does not use it to the extent that characters like *Aurum, Lachesis, Platina, Hyoscyamus* or *Verat-a* do, but she does experience *anxiety about salvation*—like *Lachesis*, praying to God to relieve her from this hellish life, and experiencing *anxiety, scrupulous as to her religious practices.* Tested so harshly in daily life, she also *fears to lose her religious faith.*

Where religion is used as a positive tool, sex is never far away. Look at remedies like *Platina, Lachesis, Lil-t,* and *Kali-br,* characters that fluctuate between these two compensation states before falling into one or the other. *Staphysagria* is no exception. But *Staphysagria's* timidity, lack of confidence, low self-worth, damaged ego, and especially his aversion to all persons and *to the opposite sex,* can turn the sexual libido inwards and results in *excessive masturbation.* Only *Platina* and *Origanum* masturbate more than *Staphysagria.* It creates a secondary NWS, *ailments from sexual excesses, creating dullness of the mind after masturbation,* a NWS loss of fluids creating a significant weakening of her Vital Force. Masturbation is another escape route for *Staphysagria,* one that allows her to fantasize about the ideal person (*persistent sexual thoughts intrude leading to libertinism and lascivious behavior*), but, as mentioned above, these thoughts do not lead to overt sexual behavior as with *Hyosc, Plat, Phos, Sel, Orig,* and *Fl-ac.* While *Platina* will actively pursue the search for the ideal soul mate, *Staphysagria* will create him in her dream world, since she is *highly excitable* and easily aroused by these sexual thoughts. This is a set-up for inevitable failure; *Staphysagria* often suffers *from disappointed love* as she always becomes very timid whenever she meets someone she is romantically interested in and cannot make any overtures! In TCM, this indicates that she has a deficient Gall Bladder (the organ that provides the courage to make decisions).

It is important to note that masturbation is not one-dimensional and does not always carry the same motivations and consequences; likewise, one must investigate the motivations for masturbation, both in the conscious and the unconscious. The motive of *Staphysagria* is clear: unable to access—or afraid of—the natural act (because of rape, indignity, or platonic love), she resorts often to masturbation. The greatest danger of masturbation (besides the loss of fluids leading to asthenia) is that it tends to isolate. It provides the person with a means of short-circuiting his emotions without experiencing any partnership at all; she remains in isolation with her sex instinct, and the expression of this isolation is masturbation. And then there is the psychological impact: the hangover which generally follows the act of masturbation is an expression of the guilt that arises when one flees from the normal directional experience to the non-directional experience (*reproaches herself, from indulging to sexual fantasies, only remedy*). With each return to masturbation, the sense of guilt is deepened, and so a vicious cycle is formed with constantly increasing isolation and guilt.

Staph's conscientiousness about trifles refers to the exaggerated importance she places on small things: even when someone says hello to her to be nice, she believes that he loves her. Small gestures such as opening the door for *Staph* are blown out of proportion, and the other party has no inkling of *Staphysagria's* thoughts and interpretations. (This also makes us think of *Ignatia*.) These disappointments, persistent sexual thoughts, and fantasies, along with excitability about trifles, lead to excessive masturbation. Masturbation, in turn, can quickly degenerate into lasciviousness and enjoyment beyond what is normal, therefore creating dis-ease as well as ailments from sexual excesses and confusion. *Staphysagria becomes a hypochondriac from masturbation, even driving her to suicide while she can become indifferent in general and indisposed to talk*!

Avoidance of Direct Confrontation

Staphysagria relentlessly looks for outlets such as masturbation, religion, and escape into a dream world to relieve his built-up pressure and pent-up anger. *Staphysagria* has a moral superiority complex, a delusion of grandeur that comes from her pathological suppression of emotions. This moral superiority complex serves to cover feelings of deep guilt, humiliation, or shame: *delusion, she has committed a crime*. On the other hand, she feels that she can and must always remain dignified, and to *Staphysagria* this means refraining from showing anger. She is a person with a Victorian manner, a vestige of a time when anger and contradiction were considered evil and when their existence was not acknowledged in outstanding people. But the suppression of such feelings threatens to invade and poison her conscious life. *Staphysagria* has the delusion, *she is criticized*; she becomes indignant and yet believes it is beneath her to express any anger: *delusion, everything beneath him seems too low down*. The egoistic pride of a *Staphysagria* does not permit her to stoop to expressing negative feelings! She does not become angry in the presence of the perpetrator (*yielding*). The *Staphysagria* person, who is excitable and easily aroused to anger, seldom manifests this openly and does not fight back; rather, she wilts and wishes to avoid confrontation if at all possible (*Lyc*). Confrontation is too painful, and it hurts her pride, so she quickly learns to submit rather than fight. She throws out no harsh words like *Nat-m* or *Lachesis*; unlike *Causticum*, she controls her thoughts of correcting injustices through active deeds. *Staph* will do anything to please; she does not react in the presence of the perpetrator and indulges in self-reproach (*delusion, she is unfortunate*). When she *reproaches others* and shows *hatred to those who have offended,* it is done in silence as her sense of moral superiority dictates. *Staphysagria* must realize that there is a right way to rock the boat, to be assertive, determined, courageous and rational, to express "spirit and breath" and to stop worrying about the approval of others—regardless of her social position.

The problem is that this timid, quiet person develops a judgmental and self-righteous attitude (*delusion, himself seems too large*). She judges others just as she rigidly as she does herself: she *reproaches others,* is overly *sensitive to rudeness,* and is *sensitive to moral impressions*. Superficially, she is initially *yielding* because she really fears anger and confrontation. But this compensation, that she is too dignified to fight, backfires when she erupts at times and may even *throw things in anger,* usually when alone at home—and so begins the cycle, once again, of shame and self-loathing (usually from past psychological or sexual abuse). She keeps what she feels to herself, and her overdeveloped sense of righteousness is enough to destroy her life. In the end, she may stay in an abusive relationship like a martyr or, at any rate, subjugate her desires. *Staphysagria* is trapped in her own pride. While *Platina* has a pathological desire for spirituality, sex, and pleasure, *Staphysagria* has a pathological desire to please others.

Staphysagria's life is a struggle for survival; it is a life of hiding. The reality is that she cannot stand up for herself or move forward (*delusion, someone is behind her; she is falling backward; his legs would go out from under him*—only *Staph!*). Legs are a symbol, in dreams, for moving forward on the path of individuation; legs are the support system that allows a person to follow life's libido. *Staphysagria,* obviously, often lacks the legs to move forward and be her own person; she is afraid for anyone to see her weakness and exert power over her, and it is for that reason that she exhibits a moral superiority toward others. Thus, she compensates with the *delusion, as to greatness of body* and with *humility and lowness of others while she is great*. She fears losing self-control and therefore keeps herself tightly in check and in line with what she considers proper; in this way, she convinces herself that she transcends those who, to her, are base: *Staphysagria's* delusion of grandeur is that she is above those abusers who are small and vexatious as well as those she perceives to be rude and non-virtuous, as they are beneath her moral level. *Staphysagria* has been wounded so thoroughly in life that she is not able to be indifferent, to refuse to show disapproval, or to let go of her attachment to feeling superior to the non-virtuous. Unfortunately, *Staphysagria* does not realize that her judgments of others are often as brutal (*abusive, insulting; critical*) as those to which she has been subjected all too often in her life (*ailments from mortification*).

Whether the *Staph* patient is right or wrong, she swallows her pride and goes on with her daily activities. She does not allow her indignation to be expressed naturally—they are too dignified to fight (*delusion humility of others while she is great*—this is her form of haughtiness). Instead, he goes home sick or goes to bed *trembling* with a *pale and livid face* and exhausted, *suffering from pride, envy* or *chagrin*. Once at home, out of sight and safely away from the scene of the crime, *she might throw things*, but she still gets sick from the conflicts around her (*rudeness, ailments from*). Hering captures the essence of Staphysagria: *there is great indignation about things done by others and grieving about the consequences*. This leads easily to *fear of losing control*, and even *fear of losing her reason*.

It becomes very clear that *Staphysagria* is indicated in those states in which anger is not fully expressed. I wish to emphasize "not fully expressed" because *Staphysagria* is useful not only where anger has been totally suppressed but also when it is seldom or partially expressed. Kent says it differently: "One who is in good health can easily put aside a controversy, knowing that he has done what is right, but a *Staph* patient when he has to control himself goes all to pieces, trembles from head to foot, loses his voice, his ability to work, cannot sleep and a headache follows."[33]

Resignation in Final Stage

In resignation, one admits the facts of a situation but claims an inability to do anything about it owing to what one perceives as constraining or overwhelming circumstances. The intent

33. Kent, *Lectures*, 895.

is to escape into a dream world or to give up. As mentioned before, the *Staphysagria* person will never confront her abuser about his undignified actions. The question, then, is how to awaken the resigned, suppressed person, be it your patient or family member, so that her moral superiority can be converted and transformed into a self-preserving action: only judiciously applied homeopathic *Staphysagria* can do so! Note that homeopathic *Staphysagria* can bring a person into a *Causticum* state; she may now do more than stand up to the abuser: she may become an active fighter for others in similar circumstances. The sequence of remedies *Staphysagria—Colocynthis—Causticum* can bring the victim into a normal balance before the extreme violence of *Causticum* takes over. Well-adjusted doses of *Staphysagria* have a remarkable tendency to evoke *dreams about battles and murder and dreams full of bitterness*. Even more commonly, dreams appear in which the patient finds herself now at the wheel of her car instead of sitting in the back seat, symbolizing her decision to finally determine the course of her life. Such dreams offer *Staph* encouragement to stand up for herself, and this encouragement can change the victim into a fighter who no longer takes abuse. The intake of homeopathic *Staphysagria* often leads to many badly needed divorces, helping the victim to find the courage to act. Without effective homeopathic treatment, the *Staphysagria* person does not speak out; rather, she suppresses her emotions and then suffers for it. She accepts inconvenience and injustice, but she cannot escape their influence: *horrible things and sad stories influence her greatly*. If no help is available, *resignation often replaces resentment* as the dominant emotion, especially given that she also suffers from *weakness of memory for places, for what she is about to say, often a result of these unmerited insults*. There is none of the bitterness and hatred we find in *Nat-m* or *Nit-ac*—only acceptance of her fate.

At the end of life, people who have not had the courage and strength to express their feelings regret it deeply. Sartre said, "An essential freedom is the ability to say no." Certainly *Staphysagria* does not say no as often as she should. It is hard for her to demand and assume the role of an equal partner in a relationship, but subjecting oneself to the constraints of constant acquiescence can be incredibly depleting. *Staphysagria* never honestly articulates her feelings, which in the end results in festering resentment, a corrosive bitterness (*anger, throws things away*), or complete resignation. None of these provides the real sense of lightness for which we strive in life: the knowledge that one does not need to suppress feelings, that the receiver will accept our expressions with love and consideration. This brings *Staphysagria* back to her Cyber delusion that someone is always right behind her, a permanent controlling shadow—and unfortunately, her suppressed anger and resignation will lead to many strong physical expressions such as *chorea,* with *uncontrollable shaking of the head* and *trembling of the extremities, "tic nerveux" in children, chattering of the teeth, impotence* (as well as *Lycopodium*, the most indicated remedy), *prostate suffering, spasmodic pains in vulva and vagina, stitching headaches and stitching heart pains* (like *Kali-c*), and *griping twisting pain in the abdomen and extremities.* These illnesses are often the sole reason for consulting the physician, and they indicate the intensity of suppressed emotions that are finding their only outlet on the physical plane. In addition to homeopathic doses of *Staphysagria*, dreams (as discussed above) often offer encouragement to *Staphysagria* to stand up for herself.

Cases from the practice:

Example 1:

I remember the case of an elderly woman I treated for an angry, itching, torturous eczema. It was a clear-cut case of the silent suffering of Staphysagria. When I asked how she acts when angry, she said with a sweet, convincing smile, "I never get angry." Through further questioning though I discovered that her husband had had an affair with a younger woman at the office, gone on vacation with her, and had even offered to get a divorce from his wife (but his mistress wanted no commitment). By accident, my elderly patient had found all this out, but she never even told her husband that she knew. From that point in time, she had developed an intensely angry-looking, red, and inflamed psoriasis that covered her torso, front and back! In her delusion, she believed she was morally above her husband, his lover, and the affair, so she did not even mention it. But emotions that can't be consciously expressed have to find a place in the dark unconscious, torturing and keeping the unfortunate patient captive, resulting into the expression of excruciating skin problems.

Example 2:

In a very graphic *Staphysagria* case, a man took his son to a baseball game and was utterly disgusted by the drunken, loud fans sitting behind them. He could not confront them, because, as he expressed it, that would be beneath him, and he wanted to set an example for his son. Then insult upon insult came when they spilled beer and even vomited on him. That night, while sleeping on the couch (his wife and he were not getting along), he felt as if hot oil were being poured over his head (such burning indignation!), and the hair all over his body fell out (alopecia universalis). There is nothing grand about the inability to voice anger when it is called for; it simply leads to the silent suffering of the morally haughty *Staphysagria*.

Example 3:

The direct consequences of lack of grit can be seen in the case of a patient who retired and was taking care of his wife, who was suffering from manic depression. His only hobby was dancing in a club once a week, but his wife was very critical of him whenever he took another partner although she herself was too tired to dance. If he went somewhere without her, she always made him feel guilty and isolated herself from him. Whatever he did for her at home was never good enough. She said, “You do everything for others but nothing for me,” which of course was not the truth. But she stayed in bed and demanded that everything be done for her. Because of her continuous criticism and rudeness, he stopped attending the weekly dance, which caused him great grief and disappointment. Shortly after this, tics appeared around his mouth; he was plagued by the twitching, as well as by chattering of the teeth—to the extent that food would come out of his mouth while he was eating. This led to further social isolation, as it caused him great embarrassment. Finding no healthy outlet for the suppressed anger, Nature had punished him with the deepest pathology of the central nervous system: tics and twitching.

Golden Tips from the Masters

- Closest remedy to *Staph* is *Carcinosin*, with *ailments from domination*. *Staphysagria* is the #1 concordant remedy of *Carcinosin*
- Easily offended by the slightest word or action which she feels is directed to her (*admonition aggravates*)
- Peculiar symptom: swallowing while speaking (only *Staph*)
- Bulimia because of low self-worth
- Because of the sweetness and yielding, it can be confused with *Pulsatilla*, but there is much more suppressed anger in *Staph*
- *Staphysagria* women can lose their libido because of too many cystoscopies, catheterizations, or gynecological investigations
- #1 for honeymoon cystitis
- #1 for styes on eyelids after suppressed anger
- #1 for prevention of mosquito bites
- *Staphysagria* gets physical symptoms from vexation: headaches, stomach pain, trembling lips, chronic cough, and abdominal pain. Children hit themselves after vexation/ indignation
- Is a marvelous remedy for injuries to sexual organs
- Pain in the coccyx after a fall (*Hyper*)
- Loss of hair because of indignation and suppressed anger (compare to loss of hair in *Ignatia* after shock or hearing bad news, and in *Ph-ac* after grief)
- Smarting sore pain in the inner canthi of the eye in a patient who has never had anything wrong with her eye
- Lice in hair (also *Psorinum*)

Stramonium (Stram). Thorn apple. Jimsonweed

The Cyber Delusion

Stramonium's Cyber delusion is that ***he imagines he is quite alone in a wilderness and abandoned***. *Stramonium* experiences a sense of isolation and total abandonment in a world full of perceived dangers—a world of natural disasters populated with all kinds of wild animals and rival clans. The Cyber delusion is supported by the *delusion, of being devoured by animals, of dogs attacking him* and the *delusion, that he was killed, roasted and being eaten. He imagines he is alone and is frightened in a dangerous world. Frightful figures, such as cats, rabbits, dogs* (especially huge black dogs), *rats and mice approach him from every side*. The *Stramonium* child has a constant vision of *an executioner standing before him; he endeavors to escape, and he imagines he is alone all the time and is afraid.* One can only imagine how terrifying it is for the *Stramonium* child's mind to be inundated by such gruesome visions. The wilderness in *Stramonium* is literally linked to many fixed ideas about animals; *delusion, dogs attack him; bugs, cockroaches, mice, rats, rabbits* are all animals figuring in the fixed ideas and nightmares of these children. Human beings are also part of the animal world, and human behavior is more often unpredictable than that of animals. For the *Stramonium* child, therefore, human beings are among the animals they most fear (*the executioner standing in front of them*).

The wilderness theme encompasses even more than animals and humans. Fear and fright are indeed the first reactions (sycosis). Fear for *water* (*hydrophobia*) and *the noise of rushing water* are predominant. Water is the relatively fixed symbol for the unconscious; just as with the *Magnesium* remedies, *Stram* also has many dreams about water; these dreams represent repression of emotions such as fear and abandonment, relegating them to the unconscious in order to allow the person to deal with life's everyday challenges. Repression is indeed deeper than suppression: suppressed contents are always recoverable, but repressed material resists recovery and leads to forgetting. It is not surprising that the intensity of the conscious feelings matches the intensity of the messenger of the unconscious: his dreams, or, rather, nightmares.

Stramonium, the acute of *Calc-c* (and therefore just as much in need of a safe home to survive as *Mag-c*, the skilled orphan), is overwhelmed by nightmares when the control mechanisms of the conscious are not at work. The frightened child indeed has awful nightmares (*he seemed to be in a condition of frightful excitement, appearing to be occupied with the most vivid fancies, at times, frightful images; does not recognize his friends and family, calling bystanders as if absent*) and delirious attacks. *Stramonium's* violent reactions and apparently dull mind are inexplicable to bystanders and to the child himself. It is when *Stram* is in this state that the homeopath possesses a tool to penetrate the child's unconscious, coming to understand what the patient feels when his conscious mind is unable to clarify.

In order to restore *Stramonium's* sense of security, he must implement a fast and vigorous alert-response system. The *Stramonium* child exhibits extraordinarily volatile, wild, changeable behaviors which seem inexplicable. Perplexed parents wonder how their child could hug them one moment and, without provocation, bite them the next. It seems impossible to reconcile this child's need to be with a trusted companion (such as the mother or another family member) with wanton lashing out and behaving like a wild animal towards that very same caretaker.

To understand what triggers such erratic behavior and the child's need to resort to the dichotomous compensations of amativeness and extreme violence, we must first recognize that the mind of a child in the *Stramonium* state is more than unruly. He is plagued by horrible nightmares. Allopathy has assigned him a variety of diagnostic labels, from ASD to OCD to ADHD. Such young, neurotic, delusional persons—untrained and inexperienced—are afraid of life. Their delusions (fixed ideas) will reflect these ruling emotions; the delusional themes are—among others—insecurity, confusion, danger, anxiety, simple and crude egotism, and fear of bodily harm.

Causalities

Fright and Abandonment

Fright and fear are among the major emotions during pregnancy: fear of the delivery in first-time pregnancy, fear of losing the baby (especially if the woman has suffered miscarriages before), fear of bleeding, fear of bad results after tests (for instance, genetic testing for older women), fear of having a child with special needs, fear of being alone when there is a crisis, and so many more in times of economic uncertainty. The real issue, or NWS, is abandonment by a parent or trusted person, perceived or actual (*Lyssin*). *Lyssin* and *Stramonium* are the main remedies for *hydrophobia* in which patients react to water with high-pitched screams, shudders of fear, and paroxysms. *Stramonium* does not feel up to defending himself against all of the horrifying, threatening things in the world, especially animals such as insects, beetles, or dogs (*delirium of fear, as though a dog were attacking; he suddenly turned to the wall, exclaiming, "there are those bugs, help me to catch them, and after them a procession of beetles;" he began to grow worse, biting a man's hand, sometimes crying out that she saw cats, dogs and rabbits; fear of wild animals and black dogs; woke suddenly in night and said there were snakes under and about him; looked wild, screamed and pointed to them*).

Remember that this feeling of abandonment coupled with fright is easily transferred during pregnancy from mother to child when the mother feels forsaken by her partner. Pregnancy can change even the most independent and confident woman into a very vulnerable individual; this is especially true during first pregnancies or those involving medical difficulties. The feeling of fright is easily replaced by the emotion of anger, which is less threatening to the ego of the individual. Even postpartum, such fear can be a trigger and can transform a normally developing child into an overly dependent child—one whose behaviors may be assigned a range of labels from OCD to ADHD and even autism or ASD.

A typical example of a *Stramonium* situation is provided by the case of a six-year-old child:

> The child, after many practice trials, was deemed fit by his parents to find his way by himself to a friend's home close to his school. However, on his first time walking alone, he got lost and was terrified and crying! An adult asked him if he was OK, but he wiped away his tears and said "yes" as he never showed his feelings to strangers (*presence of strangers aggravates*)—which is also typical of the *Lycopodium* and the *Sepia* child. Later, he did find his friend's home, but after that he would not let his mother out of his sight and cried every time she left him at school. He now needed to be reassured up to fifteen times a day that his mother was going to pick him up and that she still loved him (*delusion, forsaken*). (A *Nat-m* child would have a similar reaction.) And when, the following week, his beloved dog was attacked by another dog, the combination of the

two unfortunate events within a short period imprinted him with the feeling of being all alone in the wilderness.

The classic allopathic diagnosis linked to *Stramonium* is *separation anxiety*. The crux of the *Stramonium* child's suffering is the terrible fear of being left behind in a wilderness full of animals and having to fend for himself. Especially when twilight and darkness come, the *Stramonium* child demonstrates a separation anxiety which will continue until day breaks again. Another causality can be a fright such as a death in the family (*hearing bad news*), which rocks the delicate stability of the *Stramonium* child's immature ego: *after a dreadful shock, occasioned by the death of his brother who fell dead in his arms, talked incoherently, struck at all around him with his foot and hands.* I have seen many three-year-old *Calcarea* children sink into a *Stramonium* state after hearing of one or more deaths in the family: the immature ego cannot process such events. Fright and lack of protection against death, especially one's own death, propels these children to incomprehensible reactions. Although *Stram* is only a normal type remedy in the rubrics for *ailments from hearing bad news, Stramonium* is the acute of *Calc-c* (which is a black type remedy for it), also demonstrating extreme dread of physical suffering and dying.

A *Stramonium* state is often produced when a *Calc-c* child gets caught in the middle of the divorce of his parents, especially when the two parties continue to fight. A *Calc-c* child is unable to choose between the two parents, and the ongoing turmoil between them can obstruct the child's cure! When parents fight, the *Stramonium* child feels forsaken and unprotected. Pathology such as Tourette's syndrome is one of the consequences.

Anger

Where there is fright, there is anger. Fright is the mother of anger; in Traditional Chinese Medicine, the water element linked to the emotion of fright is the mother of the Wood element, the seat of anger. There is much anger in the *Stramonium* child, but it has to do with *abandonment by a parent or trusted person* (abandonment either real or perceived). There is *violent anger*, and *being besides himself*; *Stram* also demonstrates *anger from contradiction, anger with a red face* as well as *anger at trifles* and *anger on waking. Admonition* (*A/F reproaches*) plays quite an important role in the life of a *Stramonium* child. This is understandable given that, for *Stramonium*, being reproached by a parent leads immediately to the idea that he will be abandoned in the wilderness and left on his own.

Compensations and Consequences

Need for Protection (Desire for Company)

We can see that, for the rather primitive and immature *Stramonium*, escaping from the wilderness will require use of all the tools he can muster. The first reaction to these delusions is separation anxiety (the main allopathic diagnosis) because of fear of the dark with fear of being alone at night; therefore, a *desire for company at night* is a first positive compensation (*from the darkness, being alone, and in the morning, her state is aggravated*). *She wants sunshine and light*—a second positive compensation—the fear of being in the dark and to a lesser extent of being alone, *in the evening after sunset*. In fact, it does not have to be dark yet. The uneasiness in the child sets in when the light of the day starts deepening (*twilight aggravates, Pulsatilla, Calc-p*). Although we don't find *Stramonium* under the rubric *twilight aggravates*, it should be added to it. Even when the *Stramonium* child is out with his parents, he wants for them all to return home quickly before full darkness sets in. *Stramonium*, the acute of *Calcarea carbonicum*, needs protection in his quest for a formation of the ego; absence of parental support will lead to extreme separation anxiety. The first reaction is *looking for support* (psora): *she wants light and company*. *Stram* is *startled from fright from his sleep*, and his fear factor is one of sheer panic (*much excited and rather delirious, under the impression of some immediate danger, clinging to the person who had him in her lap; this child awakens terrified, knows no one, screams with fright, clings to those near, startled with great forces and alarm, crying out that she is going to fall, clings to her mother with as much desperation, as if she were going to be thrown from a precipice; wants to be kissed; mania for light and company, cannot bear to be alone*). No wonder these children are anxious at night, with *weeping and whimpering*. Once the *Stramonium* child wakes up from a nightmare, she looks for a familiar face: *when his father got him to recognize him, the boy said: "Why, papa, is that you?" and commenced stroking with his fingers his father's face.*

Overcome by fixed ideas about the world as a wilderness, his fears get the best of him. A sensitive *Stramonium* child is especially afraid of being alone and in the dark. Darkness creates panic in this child (*desire for light*). He will not sleep alone (a night light is not enough), and he is plagued by nightmares during which he wakes up, thrashing and screaming and not even recognizing his parents around him (*frightful images; he does not recognize his friends and family, calling bystanders as if absent*). In other words, the *Stramonium* child will wake up in terror, calling out for his parents or a familiar face, but because he is in a semi-comatose frightened state, he does not even recognize them until after much verbal and physical reassurance. This need for protection is so great that one *Stramonium* child said to his mother, "If you die, I will swallow a coin so I will die with you" (*attached strongly to others; clinging in children to the mother*). While it may be tempting to try to soothe the patient with allopathic drugs, this will result in the suppression of emotions that need to be processed, delaying the individuation process and meanwhile saddling the patient with harsh side effects.

Many children view the world as a dangerous place that cannot be entered without the unrelenting and continual support of close family or friends. Some individuals therefore remain obstructed personalities (failing to complete the maturation process) as their fear hinders them on the path of individuation, the process by which a person becomes an individual in a psychological sense—that is, a separate unity or a whole apart from the masses. In the case of the *Stramonium* personality, there will be an intense search for that supportive person or entity. The success or failure of this enterprise will make all the difference in the *Stramonium* person's future. For those successful in connecting to others, the added protection gives them a sense of some normalcy and belonging as well as the security they look for. (If they remain in their delusions, though, that protection will hinder their spiritual growth to an extent determined by their level of dependency.) For those not able to connect, the compensations will be limited strictly to dealing with daily battles: every tool available will be used for the sole purpose of survival. We must not forget the tremendous influence of traumatic intrauterine events during which an increased wish for protection is a normal reaction of the pregnant mother. Depending upon the intensity of these emotions of perceived or real abandonment and fright, many children's personalities will already be obstructed at birth unless the mother is properly treated during pregnancy.

Need for Light

During the daytime, the *Stramonium* child does everything possible to avoid natural factors that represent the relatively fixed symbols of the unconscious: for example, running water, fading light, or flickering lights from ambulances, which often elicit strong unexpected reactions and even convulsions. *Stramonium* needs the strong and steady (not flickering) light of the conscious world and is afraid of the dark unconscious, where he feels helpless. The longing for light is the longing for consciousness and understanding (for instance, a small light in a dream is an allusion to deficiency of understanding). The color black is another symbol of the unconscious and much feared: *he is deadly afraid of black dogs, black figures, black objects and people,* and visual hallucinations are predominant in his pathology. This continuous switch from light or conscious to darkness or unconscious is also expressed by the delusions that *he is double, that he is God* (light), *then the devil* (*darkness*); this dichotomy will indeed be expressed in the schizoid behavior of the *Stramonium* child, who can be an angel and then a violent devil. The desire for company is aroused especially at night (*from the darkness, being alone, and in the morning, her state is aggravated; she wants sunshine and light; fear of being in the dark and to a less extent of being alone, in the evening after sunset*).

Primitive and Foolish Reactions

Stramonium exhibits foolish behavior to hide her deep suffering. The *Stramonium* child, overcome by extreme fears, will resort to primitive and foolish reactions to obtain the much-needed support of the person or people he wants to protect him, usually his parents. The most primitive reaction is a sexual one. To draw attention, the child might resort to obscene behavior: *full of wit, but indecent behavior sometimes; his thoughts ran upon obscene things, and he frequently put his hands to his erected penis. He says many foolish things, and shows constant senseless chatting. He is talking to himself and finds pleasure in his own talking. He talks of nothing but one subject. His foolish behavior can be outspoken as expressed in delirious laughing, making faces and behaving generally like an intoxicated person, or like a fool, pulling his clothes, making laughing grimaces, with a staring look; making all kinds of faces and imitations of motions, gestures and voices of different animals. There is loquacious delirium, with desire to escape out of bed; he runs about; stammering and muttering before a word comes out; convulsive attacks and mouth full of rattling phlegm. He is sitting up and talking incessantly, and always wants to go away. He exhibits the wildest restlessness and hurries off too fast, with all his might, if he wants to go to another place.*

Jealousy is always present in this child: anyone competing for the attention of his parents presents a danger in that the child may not have their support when needed (which is all the time, especially when it gets dark). Jealousy is an emotion easily aroused in the pregnant woman, who can feel insecure about her looks and may fear that her husband will turn his attention to other women (*she had many strange fantasies, such as imagining that lovers are concealed behind the stove; wife complaining of husband neglecting her*). Such strong emotions carry over to the unborn fetus all too easily. Such delusion and suspicion creates a child who wants his parents all to himself and complains that they do not pay enough attention to him. This child *could only be pacified by holding his chest pressed close to his mother's breast.* In such cases, a differential diagnosis with the *Hyoscyamus* and with the *Pulsatilla* child will be necessary.

Religion

Overly concerned about his mom's welfare (as she was his protector), one of my young *Stramonium* patients prayed every night that his mom would live for 130 years (*wants to read the Bible all day; religious affections in children*). This child generally read to his dog every night, but when they visited his grandma and his mom told him that he could not read to his dog at grandma's house, he cried out, "Why is God doing this to me? Why does he hate me?" (*narrow-minded in religious questions*). Because sex is not yet available as a compensation, religion is the displacement that children seek. And indeed, in their quest for protection and to be saved from imminent danger, *Stramonium* people often resort to religion in a maniacal way (*religious mania; pious looks,* and *praying, despairs of her salvation*).

Violence and Anger

Stramonium is a remedy indicated in many children with behavioral problems stemming from *ailments from anger with fright.* These children are very *passionate* and *easily provoked into a rage.* The Cyber delusion explains some of these violent reactions; for a child who views the world as a very dangerous place in which he can rely solely on himself (*delusion, he is all alone in the wilderness and abandoned*), there is a perceived choice between killing first and being killed. Fear is always the mother of the angry and violent reactions in such children—one of many important reasons to provide them with a safe and emotionally nourishing environment.

One patient told me that she tried to stop the unruly behavior of her *Stramonium* son by threatening him: "If you don't behave properly, I will put you out there with the wild animals!" This reaction was the worst one possible for this child in particular—because it fueled his Cyber delusion! The child's terrifying delusions commonly force him into a state of high alert because of his feeling that he needs to defend himself; he is thrust into the intensity of a life-or-death situation, resulting in an archaic and automatic resolve. This often leads to violent behaviors in children which are incomprehensible to their concerned parents. So strong is this force of terror, so alien to the conscious experience of a normal human being, that the child appears possessed. It is instinctive fear, though, that unleashes these astounding abilities, unlocking reserves of strength that are otherwise concealed. There is a desire to attack, to *break things, tearing things, biting,* all of which are accompanied by increased physical strength during delirium (*delirium, of furious mania, requiring several persons to hold her; wildness of manners; she would, while held in her mother's lap, suddenly start as if in error, with outstretched arms and glaring eyes, and with such an effort that it required much exertion to hold her, in his rage, he wants to kill people; when her mother took her up, she became furious and began to scratch and bite; the child wanted to bite and strike at those around her; constant staring about, then a fixed gaze, with sudden starts of the arms and lower extremities, then sudden and furious screaming, biting and scratching and tearing with the hands, and kicking; threatens to use a knife on those about him; he breaks chairs with incredible quickness and destroys things*). In this stage, he even wants to be left alone (not at night though): *when spoken to, he appeared peevish and irritable. He is not disposed to do any real work.* For the child in school, the mental destructive phase (*confusion; insanity, behaves like a crazy person; malicious, spiteful and vindictive; runs about*) will bring him the label of a dangerous, uncorrectable, and dull child with ADHD.

Dullness of the Mind

The *Stramonium* child faces many problems in school: *he uses wrong words in talking. He desires to relate a story, but cannot connect a sentence and he cannot find the right word and becomes displeased at this interruption.* There is an *inability to give a proper answer;* there is a rapid change of ideas *so that he seldom completes a sentence. Stammering and stuttering* are often present. *There is dull, difficult thinking; he cannot think clearly about anything and loses thoughts before he can give their utterance. He feels stupid in the head, and is unable to articulate and becomes indifferent to everyone and everything.* He also suffers from a morbid sensitivity from offenses (*A/F, ailments from reproaches*): *crying, with indignation to give offense and to feel offended.*

Differential Diagnosis with *Hyoscyamus*

Normal type is a 1 in the provings, *italics a 2 in the provings,* and **bold type a 3 in the provings.**

Stram	Hyosc
CD: ***all alone in wilderness***	**CD:** ***is going to be sold***
NWS: **fright—forsaken** by trusted person—*from reproaches*	NWS: *forsaken*—**jealousy**—*grief*—**disappointed love**—*fright*
Separation anxiety results in:	Separation anxiety results in:
Clinging, **frightened**, restlessness, stammering; sometimes indecent; *religious mania* (speaks of devils—*praying*—reading Bible)	*Cunning,* outspoken **sexual behavior, lewd talk, jealousy with killing**; entire loss of modesty—**religious affections—restlessness**
Foolish behavior shown in:	**Foolish behavior** shown in:
Laughing; making faces; imitating voices of animals—**gestures**—*naked*	**Laughter**, **gestures**, *dancing;* **lewd** behavior (**nakedness**)—catching at air
FEARS: **alone—dark—twilight—anything black—of being injured—water—tunnel**	FEARS: **alone—water**—*being sold (betrayal)—men—being poisoned*
VIOLENCE: rage with **increased strength—tearing**—*breaking*—**biting—striking—destructive**—*kill*	VIOLENCE**: rage with increased strength**—*breaking—biting*—**striking—killing with knife—destructive**
Accuses partner of faithlessness	**Accuses partner of faithlessness**
Nymphomania	**Nymphomania—shameless**
MENTAL: *wrong words*—dull—loses thoughts—*cannot answer*	MENTAL: weak memory for what he has **heard and read**; *improper words*
More fear than apathy	Alternation of delirium and apathy
Aversion to answer	**Aversion to answer**
Desire for company, <alone **at night**	**Desire for company, <alone day/night**
Delirious from fright	**Delirious from jealousy**
	Refuses to eat
Stammering	**Muttering**—*talks to himself*

Golden Tips from the Masters

- Remedy for active mania and explosive dementia (mania and violence), close to *Lachesis*, which is more often induced by alcohol
- Lesser known etiologies: stroke, heat stroke, high fever, and head injury
- Fear of pain and something wild is about to happen
- *Stram—Hyosc—Bell*: highest fevers + mania + delirium; *Stramonium* works more deeply than *Belladonna*
- Remedy for Huntington's chorea
- Remedy for rabies (*Bell, Lyssin*)
- Pupils dilate immediately upon reprimand
- Affects cerebral nerves, then skin, then sexual organs
- Holds a position between *Belladonna* and *Hyoscyamus*: more mania than *Belladonna*; lacks the inflammatory intensity of *Belladonna* and has more congestion than *Hyoscyamus* but not *Hyoscyamus's* weakness. *Stram* is the most loquacious of the three; he also throws himself about and jerks the head. *Hyos* is the most insensibly dull and twitches. *Bell* starts or jumps, waking from sleep
- Painlessness (pain not felt as a normal person would) with complaints of pain (*Opium*)
- Fever highest at noon + dry hot skin + suppressed urine: *Stramonium*!

Sulphur (Sulph).
Brimstone

The Cyber Delusion

From childhood to adulthood, the *Sulphur* personality is propelled by the Cyber delusion that ***his old rags are as fine as silk***. This refers not only to his appearance—which is not necessarily beautiful, as this person is often *tasteless in dressing*—but, for *Sulphur*, *eccentricity* is equal to beauty (*too much coquettish*). Both polarities—indifference and excellent grooming—exist side by side when it comes to neatness in *Sulphur's* appearance. This person can be *indifferent to his personal appearance*, which one translates here as standing out by wearing clothes from a thrift store or throwing together whatever he can find on a given morning regardless of color, style, or size. His retro style of dressing is indeed noticeable. Plaid jackets and saddle shoes make him look as if he is always sneaking a quick break from a low-budget comedy act.

An individual's choice of garments is an effective way to display rejection and cynicism of society, and clothing is often an incredibly accurate indicator of what a person thinks of himself and his life course. It is a way of making a statement. Dressers like *Sulphur* flaunt their creativity and express their defiance, and they welcome the attention that results from it; it helps to reinforce the identity of a person who wants to be more than just another pretty face in the crowd. *Sulphur* wants to be himself, and also to be seen as a unique individual. *Sulphur*'s style reflects his real Self, his character and personality; anything less would be just a costume. Sometimes, completely accidentally, he may wear a perfectly appropriate outfit that matches the color of his eyes, deluding a *Phosphorus* person that he has stepped straight out of *GQ* magazine. But the next day, the same *Sulphur* man might wear that light blue pullover with orange flowery pants. *Sulphur* may also display a bumper sticker on his refrigerator claiming that the only domestic quality he has is that he lives in a house. *Sulphur's* desire to be unique trumps his wish to belong. While most persons are groomed from early childhood to conform to social norms, *Sulphur* belongs to a select group of people who seem uniquely resistant and immune to such grooming. The norm and the wisdom of the crowd repel him like charged magnets, so he is likely to be active and well-versed in the world of alternative medical treatments.

One sees equally the *Sulphur* person who is tidy, polished, and up to date with the latest mode. There is one thing he is sure of: all of the things he possesses are extraordinarily wonderful. He is in love with them, so they can't be discarded! All these possessions (including wife and children) are so beautiful and valuable not, of course, on the basis of an objective value judgment, but simply because they are his. I even remember an adult *Sulphur* patient who needed new shoes but did not know his shoe size as his shoes were borrowed.

This Cyber delusion that *his old rags are as fine as silk* reflects the essence of the *Sulphur* person as a whole: he considers himself the most intelligent and most interesting personality, with the brightest future ahead, as everyone will rightfully recognize his extraordinary talents. Oscar Wilde comes to mind! At all stages in his life, *Sulphur* thinks that the world is going to come out and greet him. In other words, we are referring to a benign form of narcissism: benign in that he is often someone who achieves things rather than just having things. He is unscripted, unedited, and wholly authentic (*eccentricity*). Who cannot recognize this inspirational belief in his greatness and creative genius? His judgment is not entirely wrong. His drive to be an individual does set him apart from the ordinary, and due to his intelligence, he is indeed capable of producing interesting ideas and concepts (*desire for literary work*). He is someone who calls himself *nulli secundus*, Latin for "second to none," from a young age. There is a certain haughtiness to this *Sulphur* person. He would fully agree with Voltaire's statement that "*La terre est couverte de gens qui ne méritent pas qu'on leur parle,*" loosely translated as "The world is crawling with people who aren't worth talking to." Why discuss and defend his highly developed maverick philosophies with people who have nothing in their heads but mundane thoughts such as a 9 to 5 job, raising children, and pursuing a life of fictitious happiness, the script of life of a *Calc*-c? His kind of unforgiving judgment (*censorious, critical*) is often justified because he has all the evidence on his side, which is why a cynic like *Sulphur* arouses much interest and often provokes much hilarity. His CD, a delusion of grandeur and inflation, is reflected in everything he possesses: his mind, his character, his company, his achievements, his children, house, car, wife, and pets. Because they are his, they are necessarily more beautiful, grand, extraordinary, and intelligent than anyone else's.

If *Sulphur* happens to be the CEO of a desirable company, he sees himself not as a mere individual but as the personification of the company he leads—all because of his grandiose self-regard. He aims to produce work that goes beyond the successful; he wants it to change the world. One who has been bestowed with many gifts, brilliance, intellectual daring, and often a high social position, can draw the attention and ire of the devil. The possessiveness of *Sulphur's* character, therefore, can lead to dark consequences when the ugly dragon of jealousy rears its head, for his wife (cultured and moneyed) is just another glorious property: *brutal jealousy from gentle husband, driving him to strike his wife.* Men and women (see *Lachesis*) experience jealousy differently, and it is the threat of sexual infidelity that most stirs jealousy in men like *Sulphur* and *Lycopodium*. Jealousy can cause men, especially, to explode violently, and it is such jealousy that motivates the majority of spousal murders. It is not jealousy that is to be blamed per se; it is the delusion that a loved one has committed an infidelity when none has occurred. *Sulphur* feels he has to defend his good name by acting violently against a wife who has "dishonored" him (*ailments from wounded honor*).

Sulphur's CD and his focus on establishing a unique identity are supported by other grandiose delusions: that *he is a great person*; *his clothes are beautiful*; *he has delusion of fancy illusions, delusion that he is very tall, delusion as if he is rich as well as grotesque delusions,* and *delusion of wealth.* In Hering, we read: *a coat looks like a beautiful jacket, a cap like a beautiful hat; a foolish happiness and pride, thinks himself in possession of beautiful things.* Certainly, many fixed ideas of this *Sulphur* person point to a feeling of superiority; this is a human being who is destined to see his name in big letters on a big building, as one of my patients exclaimed. Wealth and beauty are in the eye of the beholder, but the *Sulphur* person has his own criteria. Though it might appear foolish to others, the *Sulphur* person takes pride in the most common possessions, however old and useless they might be (*a foolish happiness and pride, thinks himself in possession of beautiful things*).

Sulphur often resembles, at some later sycotic or syphilitic stage, a manic depressive person in whom the contrast between the two phases of mania and depression is markedly apparent. Because of his grandiose delusions, his avarice and his hoarding tendencies (even of useless old things) can be matched by foolish spending. In fact, he thinks he is so rich that *he destroys his things, throws them away thinking he has an abundance of everything, reflecting a megalomaniacal madness.* And yet the opposite can be seen when he thinks he needs to hoard for safety: he can exhibit the *delusion he comes to want* and *delusion he is getting thin,* reflecting the worry he feels for his family (*cares and worries about family*—most important remedy in this rubric). He loves a bargain; if he buys gas and then two blocks later passes a gas station where the price is two cents less per gallon, he will obsess about it for an hour and berate himself for not having known there would be a less expensive gas station up ahead. He feels pain upon opening his wallet to pay for something that he has spent too much on. He is, however, very intelligent. Well versed in medical literature (*reading, passion to read medical books*), he invests in items in certain categories. He will splurge on healthy food, vitamins or other functional items as well as interesting books. As for the rest, he exercises a rigid self-control: he will not buy it unless it is on sale! When he finds something in store that is organic *and* less expensive, he has hit the proverbial jackpot, stretching his dollar! He can be cheap, but he is certainly never dumb in his search for good value.

Obviously, such behavior leads to a certain degree of disorganization, but *Sulphur* is not aware of it. *Sulphur* has no objection to putting things away, but he can't ever figure out where they should go, and there is no overall design as to where things ought to be. Books and papers in his office are spread on the floor, desk and anything that can hold something. Don't call him disorganized: he knows exactly where everything is. It feels as though there is safety and comfort in accumulation. It doesn't even matter what the things are. Even old envelopes seem to have a meaning or value that one could almost call preciousness. He certainly gets upset if someone moves them or, God forbid, throws them away. There is some kind of security in having all this stuff lying around all over the place for the *times that he will get thin*!

Sulphur is passionate in body and spirit, and he often displays *vanity*. All of the delusions we see refer to *Sulphur's* need for recognition or appreciation, his need to be validated for the tremendous effort he is making (at least in his mind), his need to earn the respect of his peers as an outstanding individual, as a person who truly is the bride at every wedding and the corpse at every funeral. In other words, it is fame and acknowledgement he strives for ("Did you notice me? How could you miss me?"). *Sulphur* (like *Verat-a*) represents *the need for an ego*, a name (*despair of social position*), an image, the need to be somebody important, to be recognized, to be counted in, the need to be proud of oneself. Imperial heights are the aspiration and central theme in this state of megalomania, which in realty is quite foolish given that even the most casual observation of lives of kings and emperors reveals loneliness and misfortune.

Causalities

Success and Failure: Embarrassment

Driven by his CD, the *Sulphur* person experiences a constant struggle between the buildup of his ego and the possible humiliation which could follow were he to fail in his undertakings. He has a big ego (*egotism, self-esteem*), which does not necessarily mean that he is egotistical; rather, it indicates a libidinous drive for individuation, a striving to become an independent individual. It is not selfishness that aims at creating around it an absolute uniformity of type. *Sulphur* leaves other people's lives alone and recognizes an infinite variety of types; he accepts it all and knows he is the "alpha dog." *Sulphur*, with his perceived greatness of mind and body, is apt to experience many moments in life in which that greatness is not recognized; he may even be ridiculed, or things might not work according to his plans. It is easy to understand that the greatest ailments from (A/F) for the proud *Sulphur* person are moments in which his fancies and great plans are failing, or simply moments at which he loses a coveted position as the leader of a gang: *ailments from embarrassment and loss of position* are among the most distressing A/F that he must endure. Thwarted ambition, the feeling of dishonor, and embarrassment or shame—or, plainly, what he thinks of other people's opinions of him—are most difficult for *Sulphur*. He must, at all costs, avoid embarrassing situations or situations in which he might be scorned (*ailments from being scorned*). For *Sulphur*, creating a legacy is an indisputable dimension of life.

Failure in business, not being elected class president, bankruptcy as a result from his grandiose can't-go-wrong enterprise, losing a card game, or not having a perfect score on an exam—all of which equate in his mind to *ailments from literary and scientific failure* and *ailments from shame*—will bring him nothing but loss of face and loss of self-esteem. When his status falls, *Sulphur's* sense of shame rises. The above A/F are also incidents of *hearing bad news* for him, a ripping off of his excessive mask. So he becomes very sensitive to criticism as this is directly perceived as being *insulted and disgraced*. He can become irritable and angry; alternating with his feeling of hurt pride, these are followed by *mortification* and indignation. There is *lamenting, because he is not appreciated* and *hatred of persons who do not agree with him*. However, a *Sulphur* person does not stay irritated and can move on quickly (*irritable with easy and quick remorse*). But there is nothing that shakes the *Sulphur* person to his core like being humiliated and embarrassed. He is so sensitive to this crime that *Sulphur* withdraws (*aversion to the company of others, desire for solitude* and *aversion to being approached*) to lick his wounds and ponder how to make a comeback. This might take quite a while as *he can feel himself a failure,* which gnaws at his usual self-confidence for some time.

Most of his causalities have nothing to do with family matters but are related to the ways in which humiliating events affect him personally; they relate almost exclusively to occurrences that seem to decrease (at least in his mind) his standing in society. *Sulphur* cloaks his true self for fear of embarrassment and shame, working hard to create a grand façade. If he does not measure up to any of his self-identified attributes and standards, then he feels sure that he is falling from his throne (*ailments from egotism*).

A person cannot possess two opposite functions of consciousness in equal amounts and strength; when a situation asks for the feeling function, *Sulphur's* untrained and primitive function exposes his weakness as he is *sentimental and horrible things affect him profoundly.* He approaches the world with his intellect instead of with his archaic feeling function. And rather than using intuition as his subordinate conscious function, he resorts more to sensation, as we see the proving: *impelled to touch everything; does not know if objects are real until he has touched them.* This also refers to the genuine pleasure *Sulphur* derives from counting his money or logging into his online bank accounts: "Am I really this rich?" he asks himself.

Compensations

Collecting/Hoarding

For the *Sulphur* person, there are two reasons for becoming a hoarder. One is to bolster his ego and appearance, a rather benign form of narcissism; he might, for instance, portray himself as a much richer person than he is (*delusions of wealth*). But the second reason is an opposing one: he is always afraid that he will not have enough to survive (*anxiety about the future* and *full of worries*), that he needs to take care of himself or he will end up on the street (*delusion, he is thin; delusion he will come to want,* and *fear of poverty*). Material things are usually high on his list: this is the child who knows the value of things from a young age. He is an antique collector, and he always makes sure he ends up with the prized possessions of other children (*bargaining*). Sharing with other children is not always on his list (*frugal*) unless his peers recognize and accept him as the leader and flatter him (*he gives everything when flattered*). The *Sulphur* child can be a study in contradiction in several ways: he can be very fastidious (everything needs to be in the right order and he is very tidy in the way he dresses), or he shuns bathing, recognizing that water is the most desired commodity on earth and also is unimpressed with advertisements for fruity-smelling shampoos (in reality, he does not like to be washed as it often aggravates an itching eruption). Once a *Sulphur* person told me, while sweating profusely (*perspiration, exertion aggravates*; *perspiration while walking*) during our tennis game, "To perspire is a gift from Providence. It saves me the trouble of urinating." And the weekly tennis game, he told me, was the only time he allowed himself to shower in the club house (saving water at home, of course!). However, appearance is important to *Sulphur*. He can be extra clean (*he loves cats*, the groomers among animals), but can also be the opposite, with old rags and a *dirty appearance* because beautiful clothes don't resonate with his inner soul. Being himself and original in his appearance is therefore another trait of *Sulphur's* appearance; there are times that he really does not care how he looks, considering himself above any criticism about the way he presents himself. And he *does not know if objects are real until he touched them*. We often see the *Sulphur* child getting his savings account booklet out, just touching it, or counting the coins in the piggy bank, getting pleasure from gazing at them fondly, showing them to friends, assuming that everyone is as interested as he is, and then putting them away without feeling the need to use them at that point (*frugal*; *delusion he might come to want*; *delusion he is thin*, reflecting the fear of poverty in the future). Of course, people who lived through the Great Depression that followed the 1929 stock market crash have remained very affected by it, often throughout life.

Before one calls *Sulphur* a true materialist in the sense of *Nux-v*, one must remember that this is a person who has a deep sense of true values; these values include a de-emphasis on show. A house, for *Sulphur*, is intended as a small improvement on a cave, and a car is simply a means of transportation from point A to point B which functions safely, economically, and with a reasonable degree of comfort. A *Sulphur* person can be wired to be frugal; a *Sulphur* lawyer making $500,000 a year is just as likely to be a tightwad as a *Sulphur* waiter making $20,000 a year: in cheap he trusts!

Intellect

Sulphur can signal his brain power in a variety of ways: with wit, wisdom, breathtaking conversations or withering criticism (*censorious, critical*). Objective cues as to a person's intelligence include the speed of reaction time, fluency of speech, and spontaneous humor. A *Sulphur* person is very capable in each of these realms. Oscar Wilde, an example of a great *Sulphur* wit, informed the customs official upon arriving in the United States in 1882: "I have nothing to declare but my genius." "Genius," said Jean-Paul Sartre, "is the brilliant invention of someone looking for a way out." *Sulphur* considers himself a genius, as defined by having an unusually powerful intellect—and others are prone to agree. He routinely explodes conventional methods, always taking a fresh, unexpected approach. *Sulphur* looks unconventional and relaxed, but the sparkle in his eyes is that of someone vigilant, incisive, and capable of mischief. Give him a small chance and a never-ending flood of eloquence, poetry, metaphor, and hyperbole will begin. Listening to *Sulphur* when he speaks is like drinking from a fire hydrant. Sometimes it is invigorating and restorative; at other times, it is a shock to the system.

The life of *Sulphur* is a constant struggle: not merely a metaphorical one against want or boredom, but also an actual struggle against other people. He is rather intolerant of anyone whom he considers mediocre, and he does little to hide his contempt. He does not hesitate to interrupt another speaker and finish the sentence for him. *Sulphur* is in love with the sound of his own voice, another expression of his benign narcissism. Often blessed with a dazzling intellect, he does not ask questions about others, but he talks about himself in a way that sweeps everyone up with his exuberance and confidence; others don't even notice that they are being addressed rather than included in a conversation among equals. There is flamboyance in the way he talks, but one can also discern flashes of sarcasm and irreverence. *Sulphur* never hesitates to inject a contrary viewpoint, whether at a department meeting, a lecture, or Grandma's Thanksgiving dinner. He uses conversation to stave off boredom and to keep himself constantly stimulated; he usually prefers to do this by finding a topic he can dominate and use to show off his knowledge. As a teacher, he is eloquent and garrulous, brimming with ebullience and energy, often known by his students as a raging extravert. His narcissism is identified with a partial aspect of himself: his intelligence, his wit, his fame. This behavior is intended to spur others to ask who on earth this outstanding person might be. No wonder, when and if he is in the mood, everyone around him feels he is the wittiest and most fascinating person in the room; he is a virtuoso when it comes to commanding a group's attention. He is so quick to make new friends—from ne'er-do-wells and rednecks to doctors and execs—that his network often results in multiple marriages among his contacts. Happily, this also provides him with an endless supply of uproarious stories.

Of course, all this does not mean that this somewhat benign narcissist is not an interesting person; he is, indeed, well versed in religious, political, and metaphysical subjects (*dwelling on religious and philosophic speculations*), and he is able to produce interesting (and somewhat eccentric) ideas that shake the core of the conformist person and even of the scientist. *Sulphur* tends to have an unusually strong sense of certainty that emboldens him to air unpopular opinions. *Sulphur* can lecture with an authority and in a manner that can easily change people's views. Knowing that he is the standard by which all others are judged and come up short, *Sulphur* is well aware that he knows more about every subject—and if he doesn't, it is only because the subject is boring and not worth knowing about!

People tend to admire Mr. *Sulphur* but, on the other hand, they often feel inferior and intimidated. No one wants to play the fool in the presence of those who don't suffer fools gladly; and when feeling like deer in the headlights of his dazzling intelligence, they are afraid that they will be toyed with or not taken seriously. Often known as an *enfant terrible*, *Sulphur* (as well as *Lachesis*) can use the power of his intellect like a sword. Both personalities exploit their ability in the same way that Marilyn Monroe exploited her beauty. *Sulphur* is an outspoken, *critical person* but is very forgiving of those who recognize his genius (*flattery, gives everything when flattered*). Of course, he is *censorial* of others who, by his standards, do not make sufficient effort to reach their potential. When he hears an opinion on a topic he is not familiar with (which is rare!), he feels the need to form an opinion too. Call him Mr. Opinionated (*censorial*). *Sulphur* gives his life meaning by attempting to change the status quo and transform things into what he believes they ought to be; he is not in the least concerned with scoring high on a personality test or on the social popularity index. As his audience tunes in to the pitch of his voice and the steeliness in his eyes, he knows he is a righteous defender of the truth, a leader, and so he will never be insulted if called a weirdo or a quack. *Sulphur* is proud to be among the weirdos! *Sulphur* men and women stand alone, cut off from the world by a sense of distance from other people that is not an illness and cannot be cured (and, in any case, they do not want to be cured).

The *Sulphur* child is a person with great ambitions, which leads to *aversion to play in a child*, and *inability to play*. From a young age, helped by his intelligence, he is already scheming to get ahead of everyone, to possess the most, to always win in games, and to be the leader of the pack (this child loves to be the center of adulation and approval). A *Sulphur* young person is often a seething and belligerent pupil who will not submit to the stultifying practices that surround him, so as a student, he is quite isolated by his defiance. Complaints about his monopolizing the class discussion dog him all through school; boredom and simmering adolescent aggression often may lead such a youth to play pranks. *Sulphur* can grow up without making many close friends, but he armors himself against rejection and mockery by adopting a hard shell of indifference and using his intelligence to strike back. *Sulphur's* standoffishness and sense of superiority are ways of coping with loneliness. If he cannot believe himself to be lovable, he takes feeling powerful as a substitute. *Sulphur* is convinced that it is his birthright to be famous (*intelligent but naïve*), as his dominant conscious function is always thinking to the point of *theorizing and boasting* coupled with either intuition or sensation. He is often the editor of the high school paper or president of his class, and he has a droll, somewhat earthy sense of humor which is often shocking to people who don't know him well.

Fond of philosophy and politics, *Sulphur* is a man of letters with an extensive library; he appears to alternate between choleric and melancholic temperaments. His kind of fleeting depression is not so much the hopeless despair of a *Calc-c* or an *Aurum*; for *Sulphur*, it is caused by the ignorant people in this world who refuse to see his genius and by the perpetual injustice of a life in which lazy and stupid people obstruct him in his lofty goals. He is convinced that most human beings are deserving only of contempt.

With single-minded determination, he excels in his capacity for enjoying intellectual pleasures (when healthy and balanced; *easy comprehension and active concentration*; *ability for philosophy*), which are available to him on many levels, from the simplest jesting and conversation to the highest achievements of the mind. His witty conversations signal intelligence and creativity. Independence of spirit is a hallmark of the *Sulphur* person as he writes and speaks with little respect for authority, detesting the hollow conformism which he finds in society in general. Being notoriously disdainful of authority, during his studies *Sulphur* conspicuously avoids attaching himself to any single mentor just to preserve his independence. He knows he is smart, though he really is not haughty, and, in fact, he does not hesitate to work on cultivating his humility. Although often blessed with all the powers of genius and understanding in a degree far beyond the ordinary, he can be at the same time visited with an afflictive disorder like hypochondria (*reading, passion to read medical books*; *hypochondriasis, driven to suicide*).

Sulphur can be a charismatic person in his psoric phase; he is *cheerful and gay, and gives everything when flattered*. He *is full of reverence for those around him*. Of course, this reflects how much he needs adoration of his genius even more than he needs money or possessions. The eternal butterfly *Phosphorus*, with her dominant feeling and primitive thinking functions, is attracted to him like a moth to the light. *Sulphur's* charisma bends the light waves in a room with his incredible confidence and self-esteem. It certainly does help that once *Sulphur* falls in love (the word "falls" is especially appropriate here as love allows his primitive feeling function to emerge and be projected), he shows a generosity towards the beautiful *Phosphorus* (who now becomes one of his most beautiful possessions) that seems to utterly belie the hoarding instinct discussed above. No wish of the beloved should go unfulfilled, and gifts, after all, are things that he will be remembered by. He becomes a supremely generous, passionate, inspirational, and caring hero for whom nothing seems impossible!

Alcohol, to which *Sulphur* turns so readily in times of stress (*dipsomania, drinking on the sly*), is initially a benefit for his mental activities; surprisingly, it affects his faculties advantageously while brightening and intensifying his consciousness: *mental strength increases, more intelligent during drunkenness*. There is no better profession for *Sulphur* than that of a journalist or writer. Often with an outsized appetite for cigarettes, scotch, and company with long and winding conversations, *Sulphur* even gets the benefit from alcohol when it comes to mental prowess. This is the journalist who takes a quick bite for lunch, washes it down with a few glasses of wine and scotch and a similar quantity of post-prandial cognac, and then proceeds to haul himself around the desk and produce the needed article to perfection—no need for a second draft. This is the journalist who can subject himself to any humiliation and discomfort in order to obtain material for his column. He does not shy away from the truth, offending even venerated members of society as he sticks to his guns. He could be called an alcoholic, but he never becomes the falling-down-drunk sort.

In a counterweight to intellectual pleasures, on the side of suffering stands *boredom*, which for *Sulphur* is a veritable scourge. Want and boredom are indeed the twin poles of human life. When not stimulated in class, he checks out (*absorbed and buried in thought and building air castles*) and escapes into a creative dream world (*delusions of fancy illusions*), *leading to dullness in this child and only understanding questions after repetition*. It is when he suffers from boredom that this child is labeled with ADHD and ASD, as he is also *displeased with everything and his confusion of mind is greatest throughout the morning*. He has no lack of true intelligence; he has *abundant ideas and great clearness of mind, with an active memory, and vivacious speech*, but he is *impatient,* especially when things are not going according to plan. While this can be very positive, it also turns easily into a negative trait involving *theorizing, building air castles.* This causes *thoughts intruding and crowding around each other, leading to stagnation of thoughts. Sulphur* might be the king of *theorizing,* but air castles sometimes have to be torn down; this is always a source of grief and *loss of honor,* a particularly painful A/F for a *Sulphur* person. He is often *busy fruitless, with an obsession about trifles or details, leading to prostration of the mind and brain fag,* which leads teachers and parents to believe that he has many problems *concentrating while studying.* And as he is focused on his own world (*where he is longing for repose and tranquility*), he has a *weak memory for names of his peers* and people in general.

Insensitive and Critical

As mentioned before, due to his archaic feeling conscious function, *Sulphur* prefers to approach the world with his strong intellect rather than his Achilles heel, the weak feeling function. *Sulphur* needs a rational explanation for everything. There are no situations in his mind that cannot not be resolved with strict factual and rational thinking, which usually makes for a very *critical and censorious person who can be averse to amusement and refuses to answer* when an appeal is made upon his feeling function or emotions.

Insensitivity (not in his own eyes, but in others') can be a hallmark: *Sulphur* never hesitates to pursue his creative passions and recognition for fame, justice, and other mind-boggling pursuits while his partner will be left to deal with the colorless practical necessities of life: children, house-related obligations, taxes, etc. Gandhi gave up his legal practice to begin his mission, leaving his family destitute. Would a family-oriented *Calc-c* do this? Never! But for *Sulphur* Gandhi, there was no return. His higher mission of peaceful resistance superseded any fleeting concern that may have crossed his mind. He saw it as his duty to stimulate the fire of justice in the belly of the British Empire. He risked going against the tide of popular opinion to defend causes he believed in. Inspired by the greatness of his goal, this self-absorbed person used stubbornness and selfishness for the greatest good for all: justice for people who needed an inspirational leader to help them crawl out of the darkness of their existences. Being a morally motivated nonconformist, Gandhi helped fight wrongdoing in society and became a hero by pulling himself away from the group to take solitary action. There is also another kind of *Sulphur*: the one who likes taking care of his family (*Sulphur* is the most outspoken remedy for *cares about his family*) and the one who wishes he had been a cave man so that he could whack the saber-toothed tiger on the head and taken him home to eat for dinner.

Sulphur can be a male chauvinist, which until recently was relatively unproblematic in Western society; often, he thinks that women should be educated not for work, but just in order to be interesting to men and to have something to fall back on if her husband should die young or turn out to be unreliable. Another area of insensitivity for *Sulphur* is sexuality: his selfishness and self-centeredness are at their height when he claims that the sex in his relationship is great, having no clue that his partner is climbing the walls. Having a tendency to hypoglycemic headaches with annoying irritability in the morning, he usually shovels his food into his wide-open mouth. When his wife makes pancakes for both of them, he has wolfed down his half before she finishes cooking them; as his wife is about to sit down and join him, he gets up to leave because he has finished eating. This is a typical display of *Sulphur* insensitivity; his wife hopes that sharing a meal might be a little more of a social event, but he does not notice; he has other things on his mind. As intelligent as *Sulphur* is, he could increase his love for humankind if he would consider that the highest form of human intelligence is the ability to observe without judging others (*censorial*).

Competitiveness and Suspicion

If this child wants to be a leader, a sense of competition is inherent in him. He shows *courage* to start things and *obstinacy* in finishing them, but this can also be the source of much negative behavior towards himself and others. When things are going wrong, he *gets angry with himself about his mistakes, is easily discontented with himself and feels himself a failure*. Besides *reproaching himself*, he can show *envy at qualities of others* and *hatred and revengeful behavior* toward competitors. *Sulphur* is often *suspicious and mistrustful* toward others, as his competitive streak can easily yield secondary delusions: *delusion that he is about to receive an injury* (everyone wants to take his leadership position); *that he is being injured* (everyone is out to undermine him) and *the delusion that he is persecuted* (paranoia). *Sulphur* also tends to suffer from suspicion, which takes the form of fixed ideas that others are always out to rob him from his prized possessions, his favorite things, and his money. This equates to a kind of depression that causes him to see and look for dangers where none exist: *delusion about criminals*; *delusion of emaciation* (losing property/money/toys/books), *delusion he will come to want,* and *he is getting thin* and *being doomed,* all secondary delusions expressing his need to look out for himself. In order to ensure that he remains competitive, *Sulphur* is industrious; he can belong to the vast number of people who work hard all week long and who, on Sundays, suffer weekend neurosis—that is to say, when confronted with days of idleness, *Sulphur* is overwhelmed by the emptiness of his life and suffers from weekend headaches (*Ars, Nux-v*). This isolates him further from his peers. Paradoxically, his ego and his critical behavior contribute to his ability to serve as a leader while causing him to be shunned by others who may only see the bully in him. No wonder his sleep is never peaceful (*restless at night*): *he kicks, mutters and moans* and *whines in his sleep* and, being a hot person, *wants to sleep naked.* A distinction between the *Sulphur* child and the *Lachesis* child can be difficult.

Religion

Frequently, homeopathy students make the mistake of emphasizing one facet of a certain characteristic; in a remedy's proving, though, we often see two opposites. As has been established, *Sulphur* is always a person of extremes: very tidy or very untidy (*dirtiness, children urinating and defecating everywhere*; *dread of being washed in children*); he can also be very generous, propelled by his delusion that he is rich, and on the other hand, sometimes he is tightfisted and selfish. We see a similar dichotomy in the context of *Sulphur's* religious beliefs. We can find the strongest atheists (*Lachesis*) among *Sulphur* people, as expressed in the rubric *godless and want of religious feeling.* As the individualist he is, even in the face of death, *Sulphur* will renounce God. However, a *Sulphur* personality also *dwells on religious and philosophical speculations*; *he can be very religious and has anxiety about his soul's salvation, and fears to lose his religious faith*; *he has anxiety about salvation with excessive religious scruples.* Constant, fanatical praying provides comfort in hard times (*a little girl with religious insanity takes passages of Scripture literally and acts upon them*). The religious ranting (*religious mania*) goes hand in hand with philosophical brainstorming, as seen above (*racks his brains about metaphysical subtleties* [Calc-c]).

Isolation: The *Sulphur* Hermit

At the end of his life, *Sulphur* becomes a hermit, often a man of great intellect and insight, who will elect to live in solitude. The quality of intellectual company cannot be substituted with quantity of company: for *Sulphur*, a hundred fools will never equal one wise man (him!). What accompanies him in his self-imposed solitude is what a man is by himself. Having become an introvert, he easily reaps secret joy from his solitary life. He simply prefers traveling through his own interior universe. He has become the ultimate individualist, so his wish for solitude evolves naturally and inevitably. When entirely alone, he is entertained by his own thoughts, no longer having to rely on the diversity of various people, boring conversations, or fleeting amusements. While young, obtaining fame was an exquisite and highly desired goal, but *Sulphur* now flees renown like the pest. Most of the pleasures generally sought after have become entirely superfluous for him. *Sulphur* will look for quiet, leisure, and a tranquil and modest life that is as undisturbed as possible. He will seek seclusion, even solitude. As his life comes to a close, it becomes clear that this last stage will not be constructed around close relationships with others. His individuality, so strongly honed during his life, accompanies him always and everywhere; everything he experiences now is touched and painted by it. He begins to think of company as a fire at which the prudent man warms himself at a distance; he resolves, even when with others, to remain aloof for fear of losing his own integrity. A life of retirement and solitude for *Sulphur* has a beneficial influence on his peace of mind, for he escapes living in the sight of others; he is no longer forced to politely heed the annoying casual opinions and conversations which were so unbearable to him during his productive life. As this is the time in life when man is deserted by love, looks, desire to travel, delight in sports, and aptitude for social and sexual intercourse, the hermit *Sulphur* becomes well aware that what he has in himself will outlast any of those. For *Sulphur*, genuine and profound peace of mind is reached only in complete retirement. He welcomes isolation and the opportunity to occupy himself, undisturbed, with his own thoughts and works; everything else becomes not only unnecessary, but even burdensome. He becomes like Robinson Crusoe, content on his deserted island. Love of solitude, for *Sulphur*, is the result of experience and reflection, both of which have increased with the years. And even if his life's work goes virtually unnoticed during his lifetime, he is one not to think that the world is right and that he has been wrong. He is convinced until his dying day of the supreme value of his work; he is certain that will it have an everlasting and beneficial effect on mankind. Even at the end of his life, when the curtain falls, he gladly looks back on what he has done and bows for the last time, undaunted by what others may say.

An Example of a Sulphur Personality

St. John Philby lived in the first part of the 20th century. The father of Kim Philby (the British master spy for the KGB), St. John was one of those English men who had a lifelong attraction to the Far East. He became a Muslim and took a Saudi slave girl as his second wife. He lived in Mecca, dressed as an Arab, could hold his own on a desert ride with any tribesman, ate camel meat, and spoke French, German, Urdu, Persian, Arabic, Pushtu, and Punjabi. He spent most of his life short of money, and on the rare occasions that his writings were successful, things were already going well financially. However, he was rarely depressed or discouraged. Showing immense energy, he led a rich and varied life. His outspokenness caused many to dislike him; his utter conviction that he was right and everyone else wrong made him some powerful enemies. (The fact that he frequently *was* right did not ease matters.) His married life was strange, to say the least—he always discussed his new mistresses with his wife, yet she remained loyal to him. His children and grandchildren adored him. He once wrote, "My ambition is fame, whatever that may mean and for what it is worth. I have fought for it hard."[34] This he achieved. One sees in this *Sulphur* the imperfections we all contain; above all, though, this man is an individual, which is more than can be said of most people in this world!

34. Quoted in Philip Knightley, *The Master Spy: The Story of Kim Philby* (New York: Vintage, 1990), 21.

Golden Tips from the Masters

- *Sulphur* is a fire remedy, a volcano ready to erupt, and its acute is *Nux-v*
- *Sulphur* can be lazy unless he wants something; then, he will do it 150%
- Excellent remedy if remnant (fatigue, cough) of an acute disease remains as it triggered the growth of the psoric miasm (allopathy calls them sequelae of the disease; homeopathy calls them flare-ups of the hydra-headed psoric monster)
- Can't tolerate wool clothing and is allergic to feathers
- "Homeless" remedy: bad odor; unclean; untidy, broken skin
- Early morning diarrhea (5 a.m.) driving him out of bed, and weakness and empty feeling in stomach around 11 a.m.
- People who are NWS vaccinations in spite of the right remedy (better than *Thuja*)
- Asthma from suppressed itch; asthma alternating with psoriasis; asthma in the summer
- Postpartum fever: *Sulph* CM—one dose always cures
- Every time she urinates she jumps from a sharp pain
- The similarity with *Tuberculinum* is so great that every *Sulphur* case which fails to respond to *Sulphur* should be considered a *Tuberculinum* case (E. Whitmont)
- Good sequences of remedies: *Sulph—Calc-c—Lyc* and *Sulph—Sarsaparilla—Sepia* (Kent)
- Asthma alternating with skin symptoms: *Sulphur*. Asthma coexisting with skin symptoms: *Ipecac*. Asthma alternating with rheumatism: *Nat-s*

Tarentula hispanica (Tarent). Tarantula spider

The Cyber Delusion

Tarentula has the CD ***she believes she is insulted.*** Looking at the whole picture of *Tarentula* to understand the essence of this remedy, it will become clear to the reader that *Tarentula* feels insulted when her love is not acknowledged (*ailments from unrequited love*). Here, we see the parallel with *Ignatia,* who wants only recognition and acknowledgment for what she so "selflessly" (we know better in *Ignatia's* case!) does for the person to whom she is dedicated. *Tarentula's* Cyber delusion is supported by the delusion *she is going to be assaulted* (rejection of love is an assault on the psychological plane and *she will receive an injury*) and the *delusion, strangers are in the room,* which refers to the lack of connection with the people in her immediate environment and life. In the case of *Tarentula,* the "stranger" refers to the lover/husband whom she loves and to whom she so desperately wants to attach—but his reactions are those of a stranger: non-compliant, indifferent, uninterested in responsibilities, and sending out feelings of estrangement! *Tarentula's* disconnection is also expressed by *aversion to company to the presence of other people* and *desires solitude but yet has fear of being alone.* One sees the desire to connect for safety and intimacy, but the fear of rejection, the coldness of the desired person, and the ensuing disappointed love lead her to various contradictory compensations; which of them she unconsciously employs depends on her prevalent miasmatic state.

Insults and abandonment can come in different forms. In one case, the husband of a pregnant woman started gambling, lying, and squandering money; he assaulted his wife daily with fights and physical abuse, even throwing her to the floor. Her mother, however, inanely advised her to ignore him, hoping he would become less aggressive. By giving such advice, the woman's parents became "strangers" too as the pregnant mom felt totally isolated and lonely at the hands of an abuser. In another case, a husband reacted to the news that his wife was pregnant again by exclaiming, "No, not another screamer!" This led to the birth of a child in an ASD state who needed *Tarentula*.

Inevitably, the CD leads to secondary delusions reflecting isolation, dependency, low self-worth and a feeling of vulnerability: *delusion legs are cut off* (Bar-c) and *delusion of being smaller*, being thrown into a scary world. Taking into account the passion with which *Tarentula* approaches her goal (just like *Lachesis*), the risk is great that dark elements of her repressed unconscious will crash into her consciousness and upset the ego's balance: *delusion, she will become insane*. *Tarentula* has been indicated in many cases of true insanity (dissociation)! There is a *loss of will power*, but not always to the extent that the ego loses total control over the conscious life, which would result in a psychosis: *consciousness of the unnatural state of mind, hence despondency, moral depression and disgust for everything*.

Causalities

Unrequited Love

This NWS is well described in T. F. Allen's *Encyclopedia of Pure Materia Medica* as *insanity on account of an unfortunate love, causing profound grief and anxiety*. Of course, we have here the creation of a potentially large group of delusions related to love (unrequited, disappointed, deceived, and so on), especially in women. Insanity is the most extreme outcome, but many struggle for years before falling into the depths of psychosis, suffering from various neuroses of which hysteria is one of the most dramatic: *hysteria, severe attacks, increased by moaning and relieved by sighing; hysteria with bitter belching; ludicrous and lascivious hysteria in a woman*. The unrequited love refers to the hopeless longing of *Tarentula* for the subject of her love and desire (similar to that of *Ignatia*), but with very little or no return. When it comes to real love, the person reaches at least the infatuation stage and connects with his partner on the psychological level rather than just on the physical level. Having invested so much in her partner with no return, it is clear why *grief, disappointed love and unhappy love* would feature prominently in *Tarentula's* story; in this, *Tarentula* does bear a resemblance to *Ignatia* as both feel betrayed by the object of their love. *Tarentula* is prone to *anorexia nervosa; eat, refuses to eat,* (black type remedy) *anguish about the future* and even *dementia with the sadness*.

Anger and Vexation

The perceived insult coupled with the feeling of isolation in a scary world leads to *Tarentula's* numerous ailments *from anger and vexation*—understandable given her feeling of being misunderstood or rejected. Fear is often replaced with anger, which is safer in terms of the preservation of the ego; the anger may come *from emotional excitement,* caused by the event and *from hearing bad news.* For the *Tarentula* child (still in a rather primitive mode and having no dominant function of conscious until reaching the age of about 18), every word, action, and situation is perceived through the lens of that fixed idea that he will be assaulted (*ailments from reproaches and punishment*). In this context, we can understand *Tarentula's* violent, impulsive, and initially incomprehensible reactions towards others, including *biting and convulsions, even biting himself, abusive behavior, cursing and swearing, contrary, and refusing to answer.* Such a child appears **asocial** at home as well as at school. His *disobedience* and *restlessness* make it difficult for him to follow strict rules or comply with the organized structures of a child's life in the family and at school.

Compensations

The needs stemming from these fixed emotions, resulting from her perceived idea of being rejected and insulted or simply not getting the attention of the object of her love, are met by an array of compensations, initially positive ones. They serve the patient, at least initially, in that they help to dull the pain of this CD; eventually, though, they turn into negative, syphilitic counteractions. *Tarentula* seems not to be particularly psoric, and is rather obsessive; he also demonstrates destructive egotism, especially in the form of hysterical manifestations (sycosis) about "me," leading to destruction (syphilis) when results are not forthcoming.

Cunning and Mischievous

Tarentula is a very cunning individual and will initially take purportedly positive steps to resolve the only worry he has: getting the attention of his "lover." In case of a child, this inevitably means having his needs met by the opposite-sex parent, most often the mother, who has transferred a strong emotion to the unborn fetus through the psychic umbilical cord intra-utero: that of a perceived insult which has been inflicted on the pregnant mother by husband, family, or friends. This can take many forms: it may be a literal insult in words, but it can also be that she perceives herself as not having received enough attention from her lover (or husband, family, friend, teacher, guru, etc.)—whether false or true. If it is false, perhaps her partner simply has to go on a trip and will be absent for some time, If it is true, it may be that he has no interest in the child, for which he should take responsibility; after all, this child is the fruit of their love. And if the future father insists on giving the child up for adoption, the situation is more intense—especially if the cunning female hoped to tie her lover to her in a marriage of which he wants no part.

A *Tarentula* child is cunning enough to *incite others* in class, so he is sure to derive pleasure from such incidents without taking the blame. He takes additional delight in seeing others punished. And if sly misbehavior does not work, she might get the attention of others by feigning illness: *feigned paroxysms, a girl simulating fainting and insensibility, looks sideways to watch the effect produced on those around her* (*delusion, of being sick*); this is very different from the CD of *Sepia*, who is truly exhausted and wants reprieve from a hectic life. *Tarentula* shows *suddenly fox-like destructive efforts, requiring utmost vigilance to prevent damage, followed by laughter and apologies; she is very destructive and mischievous, amusing and cheerful.*

Contrasting Moods

Tarentula has a vast array of superimpositions of contrasting moods: a palliative, not a curative compensation for *Tarentula*. These moods are frequently seen in people who have to banish some chronic worry. Among these people we often find the best wits, the finest stand-up comedians who use aspects of their misery in life as material and whose jokes are often spiced with a grain of bitterness and irony. Others will hide their pain under a forced cheerfulness, which, because of its artificiality, makes everyone uncomfortable: they feel the pressure behind the expression of these false sentiments.

Tarentula's contrasting moods could well fool anyone, homeopath and lover included. They are, however, cunning inventions of *Tarentula* stemming from her chronic worry that she will not be loved. We already know that such a fixed idea can be the trigger for dissociation and real insanity (*paroxysms of insanity; no sleep for five days, sings loud and suddenly springs from bed destroying everything she could get hold of*). But *Tarentula* certainly tries hard through these moods to tie the lover to herself, and often she succeeds: the prey falls into the trap of the cunning spider, the real *Tarentula*. Who would not be deceived by her extreme *desire to joke, to play and laugh; extreme gayety*? This sounds like a person anyone would want to get to know. But there is a dead giveaway in the exaggerations that reveals her sycotic nature: *she laughs at the slightest cause and her disposition to joke and laugh is extreme. There is ludicrous hysteria, and the making of ridiculous gestures.* But that this is a contrasting mood is well expressed by the following proving: *happy mood and gayety in the street, disappearing on coming indoors and replaced by deep sadness and laughter is followed by crying.*

Music

In trying to attract others, *Tarentula* uses *music* as a tool to express her neurotic and desperate attempts to get attention, although it also serves to relieve her anxious state: *great excitement caused by music; she sings till she becomes hoarse and exhausted; the musical aria, called, "Tarantella" charms and pleases the person; he keeps time with his head, trunk and limbs; music cheers up, amuses and relieves; the good effect of music continues.* But make no mistake: it is not classical music (*Aurum* and *Natrum*) she listens to; rather, it is chaotic, fast music which resonates with her frantic inner mental state. The child *Tarentula* displays extremely foolish behavior: *the patient laughs, dances, runs and gesticulates, without noticing he is an object of astonishment.* It is very easy, as one can see, to label this victim with ADHD or even autism as he seems to be living in his own world, unaware of others' wonderment at his foolish behavior. In any case, though, music seems to be one of the great tools (*excitement from music; music ameliorates the restlessness of extremities*) capable of liberating *Tarentula* from the chains of her inner restlessness (*music ameliorates the restlessness of extremities*).

Activity and Restlessness

Tarentula spares no effort to succeed: *restlessness of hands and legs, constant motion and cannot remain in one place* and *mania for work* are just a few more of her exaggerated sycotic expressions. It is, in fact, *fruitless activity*: nothing real is achieved and no goal seems to be pursued. In addition, guidance from the young *Tarentula's* parents is unsuccessful due to her total *disobedience* and *impulsive behavior. She is restless busy with involuntary motions of the hand as if knitting.* Her *restlessness of the legs takes on an insane character.* All this behavior is bound to shift over to the syphilitic miasm as a loss of control begins to occur: *mania, abuses everybody, with singing, tearing clothes and her own hair, destruction followed by laughter.* She *always is in a hurry, in movements and while walking and always implies others to hurry.*

> I had a five-year-old patient, diagnosed with ASD, who would run all around my office, destroying everything he could get his hands on. At the same time, he would exhibit sexual behavior (the other great sycotic tool of *Tarentula*) by humping his older sister while they were playing on the floor or smelling and stroking his mother's hair while sitting on her lap. This sexual behavior is one of the greatest tools that *Tarentula* possesses to attract the "lover," and it is another form of the restless activity.

As an adult, *Tarentula* often succeeds in avoiding progression to a more destructive/harmful phase, due in large part to her ability to use *sex* as the ultimate tool to turn her lover into the desired possession: there is *extreme sexual excitement; violent nymphomania in which she cannot suppress her lascivious inclination; lasciviousness, almost to insanity; excitement of the sexual appetite, which nothing can control; and shamelessness, exposing the person*. As soon as the *Tarentula* person is aware of her sexual prowess, she will use it and make it difficult for her partner to leave: "We fight all the time but the sex is great!" exclaims the other party. What this victim does not know is that sex for *Tarentula* is just a restless exercise; it makes her feel better only because she controls the situation. But she feels worse *from coition*. However, *under the influence of sexual excitement, she shows a better disposition and mood*. We might not see it in very young children (*Tarentula* is not in the rubric *masturbation in young children*), but as soon as her sexuality blossoms after puberty begins, sex will become a major weapon (*sexual desire increased*). Before puberty, as discussed above, this "sexuality" will be mainly expressed as amativeness and affection; she will hug and kiss anyone who shows friendliness towards her, somewhat like *Pulsatilla*. It does not have to be her mother or father—anyone will do, as *Tarentula* is not codependent in the way *Hyoscyamus* is.

Overcome by Emotions and Destruction

Sycosis, and fruitless efforts in general, are bound to turn people off and lead the unfortunate *Tarentula* patient subsequently to syphilitic reactions of violence and destruction (*threatens to kill and to destroy*) alternating with withdrawal and indifference. *Tarentula*, with its *short patience* and *impulsive* character, follows the same path from sycosis to syphilis. If love, foolish behavior, and sex (*change of temper, in a good-natured man, to the point of becoming intolerable; under the influence of sexual excitement, he showed a better disposition and mood*) don't help him get attention, then *cross, angry behavior and abrupt speech* are tried (*mood, alternating*). Then *destruction of everything that she can lie her hands on, mocking old people with their age and if restrained becomes even more violent* (*anger, violent; anger when touched*). This *anger when touched* can also be translated on the emotional plane: a child can become violent from apparently innocent remarks directed towards him: *striking his friends from anger*. A suggestion from a schoolmate like "Tie your shoes!" can be met with rage; *Tarentula* may hit the other child in the face. The *Tarentula* child *does not answer when questioned, refuses to answer* and *has aversion to answer*—making social interaction difficult and, at times, almost impossible. *Concentration during conversation is difficult* and *he is very contrary and obstinate. And presence of other people aggravates his symptoms, he has desire for solitude*. These further provings suggest behaviors seen in children labeled as ADHD or ASD!

Secondary delusions appear if no positive intervention has been accomplished, reflecting her loneliness and despondency without love: *lamentation, with suppressive pain in the heart, as if a misfortune had befallen her. There are crying spells without a cause*. Sadness, grief, melancholy, and moral depression are not only almost constant symptoms of the sting of *Tarentula*; they have also been present in a striking manner during the different provings of this medicine: *excessive grief, accompanied by thoughts of death*. As her exaggerated efforts have been fruitless, it is no wonder that she *becomes indifferent and has disgust for everything. There is desire to lie down* (the opposite of the sycotic restless phase) *without any light and without being spoken to*. The unfounded fears come up, becoming fixed ideas that he will be harmed: *fear, which could not be stopped, in a young woman; questioned about it, she tried to find a cause, and leaves others to think there is one but really there was none. Fear and shaking, the patient cannot find a suitable place where to hide himself: thinks he is going to be assaulted. There is great fear of impending calamity* and *great desire to be alone with fear of being alone. No attention is paid to conversation, not even the most interesting one. Then there comes dullness of the mind where the patient does not wish to answer the questions asked. Little intelligence and poor memory are exhibited*, and *she does not understand the questions posed to her*. The patient might stay in these secondary delusions, or she might fall back into the Cyber delusion that she is unloved and insulted by everyone, since no one seems to understand the depth of her grief or her desire for love.

Examples of Tarentula Cases from the Practice:

Example 1:

Beginning in the fourth month of pregnancy, a patient of mine suffered from ecclampsia and was told that it could be fatal. Her mother had promised to be there at the delivery, but was not. Her absence was an act of unrequited love and rejection. The expectant mother had to undergo an urgent C-section because of highly dangerous BP; her survival was uncertain, and now her own mother informed her by phone that she was not going to come since "the Lord had his plans already set up for [her]; no need for Mom to come." This rejection and insult ensured that the baby was born in a *Tarentula* state.

Example 2:

Another case, this one more difficult to decipher, involved an adopted child; though some facts about the birth mother were known, the adoptive mother of the patient was absolutely unaware of the NWS. I saw the patient in my office when he was six years old; below, I have included rubrics in the text of his story, and have also included descriptions provided by his adoptive mother in quotes. One can recognize many important features of *Tarentula*, to which the child responded beautifully:

The child shows reckless and *foolish behavior*. He dances like a monkey to music (*foolish behavior; sensitive and ameliorates to music*); he is impulsive and cannot sit still unless he is watching TV (*restlessness*). He does not like contradiction (*intolerant of contradiction*) and he annoys people to the point of being malicious (*maliciousness*). "He never obeys me. When he plays outside, I have to go get him and literally pull him into the house (*disobedience*). What worries me, though, is that he talks to any stranger, like workers in the street (*amativeness*). He often *refuses to answer* or answers totally unrelated to the question. He acts the same way at school. He is cruel (*malicious—cruelty*) to the dog (which is blind), hits him or jumps on him. He tells lies about his older sister, that she is mean and teaches him bad words and offends him. Of course he does this when he is caught saying bad words" (*cunning*).

All this fixed behavior could be traced back to his birth mother (when I asked about it): she had become pregnant with her second child "so that her boyfriend would marry her"! The birth mother's first child (a girl) had been adopted by the same family. Both children had the same sets of birth parents *and* adoptive parents, but the outcome was one hundred percent different: the first-born child, the girl, was a normally developing and affectionate child! Why? Early in the pregnancy of the first child, the parents had agreed to give the child up for adoption, so there were no negative feelings attached to the situation, and therefore, also not to the child. However, the birth mother became pregnant the second time with the intention of forcing her boyfriend to marry her, and she only decided to give the second child up for adoption two weeks before his birth—because her boyfriend still refused to marry her! These circumstances qualify as *ailments from unrequited love,* a feeling that was transferred to the unfortunate child intra-utero. When he came to me for an examination, he still showed all the symptoms of *Tarentula* (triad of *cunning, restless,* and *mischievous*), which was his simillimum.

Example 3:

Another patient, a young woman pregnant for the first time, experienced early contractions in her second month of pregnancy. She phoned her husband, who refused to come home and told her to phone again if things got worse. This was an "insult" which stayed with her until the delivery. As she was wheeled into the delivery room, her husband fainted by her side, and all of the nurses ran to help him—leaving his pregnant wife undergoing contractions all by herself. She thought, "He always gets away with taking all the attention!" She felt insulted once again by the nurses' actions. Not surprisingly, the baby boy was born in a typical *Tarentula* state.

Example 4:

Another case of mine involved a 15-year-old girl. When I met her she would do anything to draw attention, especially cutting things with scissors and laughing about it (*destructiveness, cunning*). She would tear her clothes (*destructiveness of clothes; tears things; mania, tears clothes*) and become aggressive if she was not getting attention (*obstinate; violent anger*). At school, she would slap the teacher if she was forbidden something (*contrary, obstinate; intolerant to contradiction*). She was easily bored and did not like doing things for longer than a certain amount of time, always doing things without much purpose (*fruitless busy*). She was physically strong and would jump on the trampoline with her sisters. She was fearless and did not seem to understand the concept of danger. She was tied down in her chair when eating; otherwise, she would not stay at the table (*restlessness, anxious, compelling to rapid walking*). As a seven-year-old, she had refused to eat for 14 days (*refuses to eat, anorexia nervosa*). There were still days she would not eat or would eat just one meal. She had excessive hair on her extremities (*hirsutism*). Although her normal speech was limited to one word, she could sing a song fast (*singing*). When younger she had cried frequently, and often tried to run away (*wants to escape*) by jumping out of the window. She was easily startled in sleep and destroyed her mattress (*destructive*). She was generally *disobedient* except when her mom showed sadness, and then she would obey (*looking at others in distress aggravates*). When she saw a lady crying, she went to her and kissed her (*sympathy, compassion*). Every little noise woke her up (*sensitive to noise*). When I saw her, she was constantly moving in her chair. Her hands were restless (*hands, gestures, grasping at things; hands, motion, involuntarily*), and suddenly she got up and started dancing violently as if in a trance, not caring if others paid attention (*dancing wild; music ameliorates restlessness of extremities; shamelessness*). She was moving constantly from one place in the room to another (*runs about; hurry in movements*). She loved to paint her nails and always was looking for coloring crayons to use (*colors, charmed by blue, green, and red*). As there were crayons in the room where I saw her, she looked at them while watching her mom from the corner of her eye (*cunning, mischievous; deceitful*) before quickly taking one. The intrauterine story was revealing: the mother had been very happy to be pregnant (she already had two children), but her husband's first reaction to the news, as noted in the previous section, had been to say, "Not another screamer!" (Their first child had been a difficult one.) The mother said that she had been "offended" by his reaction (*delusion, is insulted; A/F disappointed love; A/F unhappy love; from unrequited love*).

Example 5:

Another case of mine involved an 11-year-old girl who, showed many *Tarentula* characteristics. She was considered a high-functioning child with ASD. Her mother had died in a car accident when the girl was four, but her problems had started before that time. Even now, her stepmother remembered that when she had met the girl at age five, she was someone who "hardly needed sleep;" she woke up at different hours (*restlessness, tossing in bed; goes from one bed to another*). She had an unusual craving for dairy (milk, cheese, cottage cheese, sour cream). She loved rigid schedules and was always concerned about planning and making sure nothing unusual would happen. But she only had a five-minute attention span (*concentration difficult* and *tries to escape*): she would not listen at all (*contrary; disobedient*). She was impatient and loved touching everything, but did not like to be touched herself (*touched, aversion to be*). She was easily distracted and wandered back and forth like a caged animal (*restlessness compelling to rapid walking*). She was very restless, and even during the interview, she asked at least five times: "Are we done yet?" She walked freely around in the big examining room, and often approached the mother and even the homeopath (me), kissing us, embracing us (*amorous, amative*), and saying things through the microphone like "I can be good, and then I can be bad" (*playful, laughs immoderately and with stupid expression*), then cruising around again. She never played with toys and never engaged in pretend play. The only thing she enjoyed was going shopping at the mall with her stepmom—but first, she had to be trained to stay close to her stepmom. Otherwise, she would not be allowed to come along, since she always wandered off and tried to escape (*runs about*). (In my office, though, she stuck close as she felt insecure in this new situation.) She was very *destructive* in general, ripping pages out of books, cutting sheets, and so on (*tears things*). She did this early in the morning, getting up early before anyone else in order to be able to rip and tear things without interference (*cunning*). She could be mean to her little brother and to other children (*malicious, spiteful*); she would do things like put her brother in hot water or push children out of the car (when it was not moving) and then laugh about it (*sardonic laughing*). She was intelligent but also *cunning*. In school, she never talked about what other children were talking about; she did not participate (*unobserving*). During the interview, too, she went behind the homeopathic students, lay down, pulled up her shirt, and caressed her abdomen (*naked, wants to be; obscene, lewd; shamelessness, exposing the person*). But when she saw that some of the students were looking, she quickly pulled her shirt back down and stood up. There were many instances of talking to herself; when her mom told her to clean up her room and checked back five minutes later to remind her, she heard her talking to herself: "OK, [citing her name], start doing this." She loved to go to bed with the lights out. She loved *dancing wildly* to the exciting music of Hilary Duff. She really always knew what she was doing (*cunning*). She loved to massage her own body (*lascivious, lustful*) and seemed to be in her own world (*delusions, of fancy illusions*). She could be very *disobedient*, and her mom had to repeat some directions very often. She disliked ceiling fans: the noise and movement disturbed her (*sensitive to noise*).

Her birth mom had had three miscarriages before becoming pregnant with her. She was happy to be pregnant, but she never felt the baby moving. It was reported by the stepmom that her husband had also been happy about the pregnancy. But in reality, I didn't know anything first hand since the father was not at the interview. The birth mom had worked for an advertising agency and loved it; she had been funny and close to the family. Both the patient and her brother suffered from arthrogryposis, a debilitating condition causing stiffness, deformity of hand joints, and muscle weakness. Her younger brother, also diagnosed with ASD, was more severely affected than she was. The only thing missing here was the secret story of the mom. We can clearly see, though, that the behavior of this girl was mainly sycotic. On the father's side, there was indeed mainly sycosis; looking at the pregnancy history of her mom, the sycotic miasm might well have been transferred to her intra-utero (we must note the three previous miscarriages, which indicate the strength of the sycotic miasm). The girl's restlessness, short attention span, and foolish behavior were very pronounced. Together with the amativeness, kissing, disobedience, destructiveness, and cunning and malicious behavior, the picture of *Tarentula* showed through very well. We can also see that a differential diagnosis with *Hyoscyamus* is necessary. *Hyoscyamus* is not as restless, but she is much more shameless and sexual than *Tarentula*. Notably, this girl did not lie down to stroke her abdomen in front of everyone, but out of sight, and she stopped immediately when she saw that some of the homeopathic students had observed it. This confirms the "foxy" nature of *Tarentula*: when no one looking, she tears things and exposes herself.

The remedy (*Tarentula* 6C, 2 drops from RSB in a 4-oz cup and 2 drops from the cup, very infrequently given with increased succussions) improved her level of concentration and restlessness considerably: she was able to sit down for long periods of time, which she did voluntarily. She interacted much more with her brother than she ever had before, and she even completed her homework while riding in the car.

Golden Tips from the Masters

- Physical and mental agitation
- Aversion to self-control (for instance, in cigarette smokers)
- One of the best remedies for boils
- Remedy for spider bites (*Hypericum*)
- Intense headaches as if hundreds of hot needles were being thrust into the brain (*Bell*), relieved by rubbing the head against a pillow
- Important remedy for anorexia nervosa
- Nymphomania due to extreme hyperesthesia of the genitals (*Plat*)
- Great sequence of remedies: *Ars—Thuja—Tarentula*

Thuja occidentalis (Thuja). Arbor Vitae

Thuja, taken from the twigs of the tree, was introduced and proven by Hahnemann himself. Called the "anti-sycotic king," *Thuja* played an enormous role in Hahnemann's time but gained even more importance during both World Wars and when the spread of sexually transmitted diseases peaked in the sexual revolution of the 1960s. Subsequent suppression of these illnesses (as seen with use of antibiotics) has forever soiled the next generations even before they are born and has sped up every pathological process in humankind. *Thuja* obtained its early fame when von Boenninghausen, ahead of any allopathic intervention, used it to cure and prevent smallpox epidemics in the 19th century.[35]

The Cyber Delusion

Thuja's Cyber delusion is ***body is delicate***. This sense of oneself as fragile (*frail, sensation of being*) and vulnerable is confirmed by other fixed ideas: *body is brittle*; *body is lighter than air*; *body is thin and could not resist the least attack*; *body is in danger of coming into pieces and being made of glass*. The lack of protection and strength is also expressed in such delusions as *he is diminished and too thin* and *delusion, of emaciation*. This spirit of weakness leads to secondary delusions; one theme of these is fear of one's demise: *delusion, he was about to die, his time has come to die,* and he *was pursued by enemies*. It goes so far that the patient will refuse to shake hands because of the pain it would cause: *he will not be touched, sensation of being frail, and has fear of others approaching him as it will give her sudden twitches* and *she will not see her physician as he seems to terrify her*. Thuja's fragility is also observed in difficulties adjusting to weather changes, especially when exposed

35. C. M. F. von Boenninghausen, *Lesser Writings of von Boenninghausen* (New Delhi: B. Jain, 1991), Concerning the Curative Effects of Thuja in Small-pox, 3.

to damp weather: *wet weather aggravates, foggy weather aggravates, approach of a storm aggravates,* as well as *storm aggravates* and *windy and stormy weather aggravates.*

Another theme is a compensation for *Thuja's* CD of vulnerability; consciously or unconsciously, he gives his power away to others in his search for protection: *delusion, head belongs to another; errors of personal identity;* and *he is under super human control.* Just like *Silica* and *Calc-c,* who fear the outside world, *Thuja* needs a companion—not so much to protect him from feared confrontations with the outside world, but mainly to hold his hand as he is utterly confused (*sees people besides him; someone walks besides him*). Confusion, in itself, is a third delusion theme: he is *divided in two parts; he is cut in two parts and does not know upon awaking which part he has possession of; mind and body are separated; he is separated from the soul and familiar things seem strange.* This aggravation upon awaking (*can scarcely collect his senses for half an hour in morning on waking; unable to go on with her dressing and constantly needs reminding*) is a strong sycotic expression in general, not just for *Thuja.* Experiences of extrasensory perception (ESP) are usually not welcomed by *Thuja;* they are, rather, feared. Unlike *Lachesis, Phosphorus, Calc-c,* and *Silica,* who feel at home with ESP (under the rubric *desires to be magnetized*), *Thuja* derives no benefit from such experiences. I had a 50-year-old patient who suffered from multiple expressions of sycosis: hypertension for years, not improved with meds; diarrhea, hemorrhoids, and polyposis in the rectum; rheumatic pains in the hands; and blocked nostrils when going to bed. But what clinched the remedy was that he delayed going to bed because he had the unpleasant experience of waking throughout the night with a feeling that people were in his room and touching his head, which created the feeling he was going insane (*fear of insanity; delusion, he is insane*). A dose of *Medorrhinum* first addressed the strong family and personal sycotic background; then, *Thuja* brought a remarkable improvement in all symptoms with blood pressure 120/80, good sleep, no rheumatic pains, disappearance of hemorrhoids, and smaller-feeling polyps. *Medorrhinum* and *Thuja* both have symptoms such as *foreboding, delusions sees faces and head is caressed on by someone.* The confusion seen in the case above can be so strong that, if not corrected by the remedy, the patient can succumb to dissociation and insanity: *commences every sentence anew without ability to finish in spite of every effort of memory; insane woman will not be touched or approached.*

Thuja is in danger of dissociation, or at least of becoming a split personality and creating an alter ego (supported by the delusion, *he is too weak to survive as a whole* and alluded to above with regard to the separation of soul and body). This is also seen in the delusions about a living being in his abdomen: *delusion, voices are in his abdomen; hears voices in his abdomen; animals are in his abdomen as well as in the fear, of insanity, of losing his reason.* This is a rather threatening entity, not a supportive one, contributing to *Thuja's* sense of vulnerability!

Yet another, fourth theme of delusions emerges as a result of the CD and feelings of weakness and perceived threats: an escape from the adult world into a dream world, dangerous when one feels like glass. We see this in the *delusion, of fancy illusions,* in a wonderful world where he has the delusion *of hearing music. Thuja* feels out of place among his peers, something he has in common with *Nat-m,* as he is always pushed and pulled between the dream world and the human world. This might well be due to the fact that *Thuja,* even when abused, or a *Thuja* child caught in the middle of a family dispute, has a strong sense of guilt (*anxiety, as if guilty of a crime*) and always feels responsible for having brought this calamity on himself. Slowly but surely, because left unexpressed, this guilt will build up and these thoughts will return (*dwells on past disagreeable events*) until the pressure cooker blows its lid, especially when *things don't go their way* (*violent anger*).

All of these delusions are part of the extensive shadow side of *Thuja,* for which compensation through an excessive persona is required to achieve any kind of control and balance in *Thuja's* life. When such a vast shadow side is present, offering protection and serving as a defense mechanism, an excessive persona or mask has to be present—similar to *Lycopodium,* with which *Thuja* shares similar psychological problems of identity and alienation (a process of a sycotically overbuilt persona to hide the sycotically underbuilt shadow side). Indeed, *Thuja* demonstrates his overbuilt characteristics through the fixed ideas of *appearance of building stones, he is heavy* and *delusion of a higher power;* he is a person who needs to strengthen himself for public appearance, like *Silica* and *Lycopodium.* This is not the only time that we will find *Thuja* in the same bed as *Lyc* and *Sil*! However, compared with *Lyc* and *Sil* (who are afraid to be discovered for who they are and are very image-oriented), *Thuja* is much more calculating. He finds out that showing his emotions freely does not pay off in society. Strong, one-sided attitudes in the conscious mind often furnish opposite dreams, called compensating dreams; in *Thuja's* case, dreams unmask him and try to steer him in the direction of true individuation: *dreams of falling* are yet another reflection of the vulnerability of *Thuja,* who cannot maintain the mask in his sleep.

Dreams of falling can refer to fears of loss of security or coming down to earth from an overly lofty attitude (which would be more typical of a *Nux-v* than a *Thuja* person). In addition, if one uses fantasy to try to get away from reality—as *Thuja* does—dreams of falling may occur when this escape is taken away and reality breaks through. If *Thuja* has a dream of falling into an abyss or pit, it might represent the fear of meeting the hidden side of oneself. *Thuja* also has dreams of death: his own or others'. Death in a dream seldom refers to the actual death of the dreamer; rather, it points to the profound archetypal process of transformation that can take place if only *Thuja* finds the courage to listen to his dreams. The same theme is found in patients who, in their dreams, enter a house familiar to them in which the rooms begin to multiply in a disorderly way. The dreamer then stops wandering through the house and becomes afraid to investigate further. The house is the relatively fixed symbol of the self—of the dreamer himself—, representing his body, attitudes, and personality. Different parts of the house refer to different parts of the dreamer; for instance, the attic represents consciousness or light, while the cellar or basement depicts the unconscious. Such a dream in a *Thuja* person reveals several feelings: fear of investigating the unknown (unconscious), incapability, and confusion about the integration of the dark unconscious element into the conscious in order to further the individuation process. In Kent, *Thuja* is also under dreams of *calling out*, the opposite of the persona or compensation of fortified building stones (exaggerated mask versus the opposite shadow). This fortified mask is also seen in the introverted attitude of *Thuja*: *remarkably earnest mood in a young girl*; *very earnest frame of mind in spite of the cheerfulness of those around him*, certainly a strong contrast to his close family member, *Medorrhinum*.

Causalities

Why is such an extreme form of protection needed, and where does *Thuja's* fragility came from? *Thuja's* ailments from (A/F) hold some initial surprises; as always, though, upon deeper investigation, the secrets of the A/F show themselves to match the CD and its accompanying delusions.

Sexual Excesses

Thuja is the king of sycosis, and sex rules in this miasm! It is important, first of all, to distinguish between truly lascivious behavior and the more fragile state from sexual excesses seen in *Sepia*, in which the genital system is exhausted and burnt-out. *Thuja's* sexual excesses are more akin to those of *Medorrhinum* in that sex is not considered as the means for procreation but, rather, as a constant source of pleasure, especially when sex is experienced too early or emerges as a sudden hurricane at puberty. *Thuja* is linked to, and interlocked with, *Medorrhinum*—to the point that both remedies are needed to cure a case of strong sycosis such as asthma (for one); *Thuja* also acts vigorously on the genitourinary tract relieving inflammation, ulcers, fig-like tumors (from the Greek *sycon*, or "fig"), and other symptoms allied to the sequelae of gonorrhea.

The main sexual outlet for *Thuja* is masturbation, done secretly and beginning at a young age (*Bufo*). Parents ought to be careful not to scold such children as they will later vividly recall the sense of shame and anger connected with the experience, which then had to be denied and repressed. These children have an early fixation on sex and grow up with feelings of attraction to the same gender *with indifference to the opposite sex* and promiscuous sex. So *Thuja* certainly figures in homosexual persons suffering from socially induced guilt; as they are quite introverted, *Thuja* people tend to hide their passions as they also feel unloved and unattractive and are disgusted with their genitalia.

Quarrels

Looking at the provings, we ascertain that *Thuja* quarrels with family members rather than with outsiders: *abusive to husband*; *abusive to mother and aversion to husband and mother*; *irritability to her family*. That her quarrels occur with the two most important sources of emotional support for any human being—the mother and the partner—is strange; however, these quarrels have their origin in contradiction. The conflict is fueled by *Thuja*'s anxiety, thoughtlessness, and depression: *anger from contradiction*; *violent anger when things don't go after his will and easily angered about trifles*. The provings tell us that such a child can become quite *ugly in his behavior*. This last characteristic is often seen in children afflicted with autism: angry when they lose a game, angry when they don't get complete attention from a parent, angry when they ask for a present and are refused, and so on. T. F. Allen expresses it thus: "The child is excessively obstinate and on the slightest contradiction it throws itself to the ground in rage and loses its breath and passionate in unexpected attacks."[36] One sees similar behavior in *Tuberculinum* and *Lycopodium*, complementary remedies to *Thuja*. This ugliness of temperament and hardness on the emotional level manifest themselves also on the physical level with the formation of tumors.

36. T. F. Allen, *The Encyclopedia of Pure Materia Medica* (New Delhi: B. Jain, 2000), 601.

Thuja's ugly behavior is quite similar to *Lycopodium's* anger, in which lust for power predominates; with *Thuja,* though, it comes from a position of weakness rather than one of power. *Thuja's* hostile behavior comes from forgetfulness and dissatisfaction with life (*low spirited and morose; passionate and dissatisfied; feels as if she cannot exist any longer*). Thuja's ire does not target strangers (just like *Lyc*) due to her *cowardice and aversion to presence of strangers.* Unfortunately, *Thuja* can be very *obstinate and headstrong, with fixed ideas and hysterical behavior,* all sycotic expressions.

In terms of emotional triggers, the number one stress factor is a father who is cruel to the mother during pregnancy. Any quarrels (*A/F discords between chief and subordinates*) lead to a high stress level in the expectant mother, resulting in the release of a flood of stress hormones (adrenaline, noradrenaline, serotonin) which come into contact with the unborn fetus via the amniotic fluid. We can only imagine that, if such a situation has already been created intrauterine, a blossoming sycotic state will worsen upon receiving that first hepatitis vaccination at birth: *anxiety after vaccination.*

Vaccinations

With the present worldwide epidemic of autism spectrum disorders, the issue of vaccinations as a causality has become all-important and has engendered heated controversy. But when the impassioned rhetoric is dismissed and when the proving symptoms of *Thuja* and its indication in many human conditions are examined, the link between vaccination and ASD indeed reveals itself to be a strong causal relationship. Kent, writing in the late 1800s in his *Lectures on Materia Medica,* asserts: "Thuja is a pre-eminently strong medicine when you have a trace of animal poisoning in the history, as snake bite, small-pox and vaccination."[37] Let's investigate the various rubrics in which we can see the correlation between ASD and vaccinations:

Important rubrics of *Thuja* linked to autism

- *Generalities, history of repeated vaccination*: Thuja, Carcinosin, Malandrinum
- *Forgetfulness*: *would scarcely collect his senses for half an hour in morning on waking; unable to go on with her dressing, constantly requiring reminding.* This we often see in children with

37. Kent, *Lectures,* 945.

ASD who need much help in dressing, whereas before vaccination they could dress themselves.

- *Makes mistakes in talking, writing and looking. Commences every sentence anew without ability to finish in spite of every effort of memory. Cannot think, talks slowly as if hunting for words; uses wrong words. Speaks in monosyllables and very slowly.* Thuja is in the rubric for *talking, slow learning to talk*!
- *Imbecility of mind and loss of speech after vaccination*! It is this proving that draws our attention; it expresses exactly what we are looking for. Unless we find this disappearance of speech in other remedies, this can become a cardinal specific remedy for ASD!
- *Restless sleep, cries all day, occasional flow of saliva from mouth, looks like an idiot. Nervousness to such a degree that approach of a stranger gave her sudden twitches.* If this appears after vaccinations and was not present before, we can exclude *Bar-c*, as the *Bar-c* state is an innate one that is present from birth.
- *Thoughts vanish so that he does not know what to say; inability to fix the attention and to think.* Focusing is known to be another difficulty for children suffering from autism, contributing to the inability to learn language
- *The child is exceedingly obstinate; on the slightest contradiction throws himself to the ground in rage and loses his breath.* This proving is often seen in behaviors of children with ASD.
- *Imbecility and restless after vaccination*
- *Head pain from vaccination*: only *Thuja*!
- *Eye pain, post orbital, after vaccinations*: only *Thuja*!
- *Eye inflammation, after vaccination*: only *Thuja*!
- *Face, eruptions, acne, from vaccination*: only *Thuja*!
- *Stomach, pain, from vaccination*: *Thuj* black type and only remedy
- *Rectum, diarrhea after vaccination*: *Thuj, Sil*
- *Respiration, asthmatic, after vaccination*: *Thuj*, Carc
- *Cough, after vaccination*: *Thuj*, Carc, *Sil*
- *Extremities, emaciation, upper limbs, after vaccination*: *Thuj* only remedy
- *Extremities, paralysis, lower limbs, after vaccination*: *Thuj italic* and only remedy
- *Extremities, suppuration, fingers, nails, after vaccination*, *Thuj*, black type and only remedy
- *Extremities, swelling, shoulders, after vaccinations*: *Thuj*, only remedy
- *Extremities, swelling, upper arm, after vaccinations*: *Thuj, Sil*

- *Extremities, felon, root of nail, from vaccinations*: only *Thuja*
- *Sleeplessness, after vaccination*: *Thuj, Mez, Carc*, almost constant symptom in ASD
- *Sleep, restless, after vaccinations*: *Thuj*, only remedy!
- *Skin, eruptions, boils, from vaccinations*: *Thuj* and *Sil*!
- *Skin, eruptions, eczema, discharging, after vaccination*: *Thuj, Sil*
- *Skin, eruptions, eczema, after vaccinations*: *Thuj, Mez*
- *Skin, eruptions, after vaccinations*: *Thuj, Mez*
- *Skin, after vaccinations*: *Thuj*, only remedy
- *Generals, development arrested, from vaccinations*: *Thuja*, only remedy
- *Generals, convulsions, after vaccinations*: *Thuj, Sil, Carc, Variol, Cic*
- *Generals, repeated family history of vaccinations*: *Thuj, Sil, Bar-c, Graph, Med*
- *Generals, history, personal, of repeated vaccinations*: *Thuj, Carc, Maland*
- *Anxiety after vaccination*: only *Thuja*!
- *Rage, from contradiction*: *Thuj, Ign*
- *Anger, violent, things, when things don't go as he wishes*: only *Thuja*
- *Anger from contradiction*: *Thuj* (*he is irritable, especially if anyone says anything of which he does not exactly approve*, T.F. Allen)
- *Jealousy in children*: *Thuja*
- *Cannot endure soft tender music without tensive spasms of the heart* (*Thuja*): I remember a child with autism demonstrating anger and throwing things at her mother when her mother sang a little song for her; this behavior stopped the moment her mom stopped singing
- *Peevishness; cries all day; eyes stare vaguely* and *occasional flow of saliva from the mouth; he looks like an idiot: Thuja*

Compensations

Hiding

Given that fragility is *Thuja's* main issue, one would think that many common psoric compensations such as companionship, religion, industriousness, and an eye for detail would be eagerly demonstrated; however, this is not the case. Being the king of sycosis, secrecy is always prominent in *Thuja*; he treats his family with abuse at the slightest contradiction, is feverishly impatient, and is hard to communicate with: he is *contrary, haughty and violent when things are not going his way*. These are not characteristics that endear *Thuja* to those who must interact with this individual. *Thuja avoids the sight of people, has desire for solitude* and has *aversion to presence of strangers*. There is a feeling of not belonging to his family, something that the injured *Thuja* has in common with *Sepia*, as he prefers to be alone in his misery (*shuns people*). Looking for support from others is not in *Thuja*'s book; instead, he hides and flees (*nervousness to such a degree that approach of a stranger gave her sudden twitches*). Driven by his CD of fragility, *Thuja* insists on *not being touched* and yet *is impelled to touch everything*, a characteristic often found in children with ASD. Even when syphilis is the true background of ASD, many sycotic traits are commonly found in what the famous nineteenth-century homeopath Compton Burnett called the creation of **vaccinosis**; he found the worst cases of vaccinosis to afflict those in whom the vaccination did not take. Often there are other *Thuja* rubrics present in ASD, for example: *cannot tell what is wrong, ugly in behavior, sensitive to music, walks in circles*, and *speech monosyllable*.

Hiding in *Thuja* also takes the form of deception, lying, and cheating, something that Kent in his *Lectures on Homeopathic Materia Medica* describes thus: "Irritability is likely to be shown toward individuals about the house, toward the husband and the mother; yet she is able to control herself among strangers and the doctor may not be able to find out about it, because she has in her nature a disposition to cheat."[38] The deceitfulness that Kent attributed to *Thuja* is not like the conniving, manipulating behavior intended to build up *Nux vomica*'s heap of gold, nor is it analogous to the cunning behavior of *Tarentula*, which is intended to tie a person to her sexually. As expressed by Kent, *Thuja* practices deceit in order to guard herself in her vulnerability (*delusion, made of glass* compensated by the *delusion, appearance of building stones*), to prevent others from seeing through her mask and discovering her frightened and injured soul.

Religion and Industriousness

Religion, a typical sycotic expression (*his whole existence consists of extremes*), takes the *form of pious fanaticism* in *Thuja*, who is *too occupied with religion coupled to despair about religious salvation*. Rather

38. Kent, *Lectures*, 946.

than balance, religion brings imbalance to the fragile *Thuja* and is part of the formation of the excessive persona and the delusion of appearance of building stones. Driven by guilt (*anxiety as if guilty of a crime*; *reproaching himself*), he imposes on himself a strict moral/religious mask to subdue the dark delusions hidden in his subconscious.

T. F. Allen states that *Thuja* "herself desires with anxiety and despair to be taken to an insane asylum, and there to be treated very harshly and strictly, so that her fixed ideas may be subdued and banished. She desires the strict restraint of the asylum as she cannot take the trouble to banish all sorts of bad thoughts. She fancies she has committed a sin and is now punished by real insanity."[39]

It is no wonder that *Thuja*, when sexual escapades have failed and she is overwhelmed by her delusions, seeks further help in the church: *she constantly longs for the offices of the church in order to banish her sinful thoughts of suicide*. In the proving, industriousness is ruled out: *mental dullness with pious fanaticism* and *no desire to work* and *indisposition to any kind of intellectual labor. There is want of disposition to do anything*, and she is *unfitted for every work on account of confused whirling of thoughts in the head*.

Conscientiousness about Trifles

Thuja has a great eye for detail: this remedy is black type for *conscientious about trifles*, and *occupied with trifles*, or, as T. F. Allen says, *excessively thoughtful about a trifle*; however, this is a consequence of, or leads to, confusion. It also reflects an obsessive self-interest and rigidity and a fanaticism about health, diet, and image. Where obstinacy might be helpful in others, in *Thuja* it takes a more sycotic and obsessive tone: *the child is excessively obstinate*.

Hurry and Confusion

Psoric tools for *Thuja* are virtually non-existent; sycosis and syphilis are the main expressions. There is always *hurry in everything*: *in mental work, in movements, in occupation* and *while walking*. Hurry and confusion do not mix well, so this leads to many *mistakes in speaking*, in which *Thuja* uses *wrong words*, and *mistakes in writing*, in which *Thuja omits words and syllables*. *Restlessness* is present throughout *day and night, with tossing in bed and walking in her room in circles and inability to*

39. Allen, *Encyclopedia*, 600.

accomplish the simplest task. There is a tendency to *talking hastily with ill humor and swallowing words.* Other strong sycotic characteristics like *deceit* and *jealousy* **are less** strongly present than might be expected, probably because of confusion and withdrawal from the real world.

Mistakes and Dipsomania

As much as *Thuja* tries to build a strong fixed persona, the mask often shows up as a broken mirror when *Thuja* is confronted with finding her way back to reality, holding a conversation, or writing. This broken mirror continuously challenges *Thuja* as she attempts to successfully complete the simplest of tasks, contributing to an ever-increasing confusion and melancholy and feeding her various delusions. *Thuja* is the king of sycosis, but excessive sycosis always leads eventually to syphilis, or lack of control, as excessive Yang ultimately turns into excessive Yin. True to its speedy nature, *Thuja* pushes quickly through the sycotic cycles, which leads to further isolation with loss of essential tools. The patient first starts finding that *thoughts are vanishing while speaking, speech becomes slow; he starts answering slowly* and experiences *confusion* in many forms, and then he suffers from secondary delusions such as *familiar things seem strange; errors of personal identity appear* ("Who am I?"). He acts like he is *intoxicated and starts losing his way in well-known streets. Everything looks like in a dream, with absent mindedness.*

Thuja starts every sequence anew without ability to finish it in spite of every effort of memory. He makes mistakes in writing very frequently; with the greatest attention he changed or omitted at one time letters, at another syllables, at another time whole words. As Thuja sinks into a fog (*could scarcely collect his senses for half an hour, in the morning on waking*), we see increasingly the dependency of *the very despondent* Thuja on others.

Thuja is easily frightened and easily offended; she therefore takes everything in bad part and becomes quarrelsome, especially when intoxicated. She is *weak in character* (Lyc), so *dipsomania* becomes an outlet. For *Lycopodium*, alcohol use is a result of a wish to assume a business persona (*employs every possible means to increase his ambition*) and remove any inhibitions that might otherwise weaken his power position (*dictatorial, speak with a voice of command and power of love*). *Thuja*, prone to extreme swings from anxiety to exhilaration (sycosis) and with delusions reflecting the inner weakness, finds comfort in alcohol use too. In her case, though, the main goal is to fall in a state of happy oblivion (*his whole existence consists only of extremes, wherewith he is always irresistibly inclined to agreeable excitement; these happy and exalted reveries constantly increase from day to day, overstepping all bounds...spirits are excited, lively and loquacious, the effect of alcohol*). *Thuja's* *disposition to slander* and *weakness of will* lead to a downward spiral: there is *loathing at work, indifference to pleasure, discouragement.* But *Thuja's* worst fear is borne out as his memory weakens to the point that he is *forgetful on which side of the street his house was.* Helplessness is expressed as a constant *fear of evil, a strong irresolution,* and *an inconsolable anxiety about his family while on a short journey. Thuja* turns into an *imbecile, who does not seem to understand a question, does not answer and cannot count. She does not care for her children or relatives* (*Sepia*) *and stares into space. Thuja's* relationship with *Sepia* is also expressed in the *mental depression after childbirth, as she thinks she must die from a slight rupture of the perineum.* Anxiety and fears turn into a syphilitic *anguish which does not allow Thuja to sleep.* The disintegration of his personality (*loss of will; feels as if she cannot exist any longer*) brings *Thuja* back to his CD as his vulnerability peaks.

Golden Tips from the Masters

- *Thuja* is the great antidote to tea and vaccination (Clarke)
- Disgust and ugliness is a key idea (fishy odor, discharges, warts, naevi, and growths). Disgust alternates sometimes with desire for what disgusts them
- *Thuja* is the chronic of *Arsenicum*: in sycotic diseases like asthma will follow the acute use of *Arsenicum* to cure as *Arsenicum*, a great acute for asthma will not be able to cure the disease itself. An anti-sycotic like *Thuja*, *Nat-s*, *Medorrhinum* or *Nit-ac* is always needed for a true cure of asthma.
- Emotionally close to *Nat-m*
- Called "the great masquerader" and "the king of the urinary system" (uremia, prostatic trouble, nephritis, chronic urethral discharges)
- Tendency to birthmarks, warts and naevi
- Stunted growth in a child
- Keynote: aggravation from cold damp
- Sweats on uncovered parts while covered parts are dry. Never sweats with clothes on, only when uncovered
- Intolerance to onions and garlic
- Leading remedy for condylomata. Not indicated in non-specific urethritis (NSU)
- Constipation improves when nose starts running, and nose can run with each defecation
- #1 remedy for rectal and colonic polyps
- Most prescribed remedy for vaginitis (for instance, yeast infections after antibiotics)
- Great wart remedy, except for plantar warts, which respond better to *Nat-m* or *Causticum*
- Left-sided headache like a nail being pounded into the head
- Great affinity for the thyroid (with *Nat-m* and *Sepia*)
- A dose of *Thuja* routinely given after a vaccination minimizes the bad effects
- For women with mustache growth and coarse black hair on legs (hirsutism)
- Complementary remedies: *Aur*, *Nit-ac*, *Medorrh*, *Lyc*, *Sulph*, *Puls*, *Ign*, *Kali- bich*, and *Colocynthis* are acutes of *Thuja*

Veratrum album (Verat-a). White Hellebore

The Cyber Delusion

Verat-a is a person who tries to hide his insecurity, and particularly his great desire for social status, behind a façade that belies his struggle. This is a child who exhibits disruptive and destructive ADHD behavior just to fit in, to be accepted as a "somebody." As an adult, *Verat-a* lies, steals, feigns, and belittles—and she does not shy away from violence. As we will see, *Verat-a* leaves no stone unturned—most of the time, unfortunately, with negative compensations. Just like *Lycopodium*, *Verat-a* struggles with the disparity between who he really is (shadow side) and how he wants appear to others: strong and important (*Lycopodium* = excessive persona). He is essentially the extravert feeling type: his emotions easily lead to an array of delusions.

The motivation and drive behind *Verat-a's* compensatory behavior is his Cyber delusion: ***delusion he is a prince***. The differences between *Verat-a* and *Lycopodium* are immediately evident: *Lycopodium* wants power, respect, and acceptance from his peers and co-workers and uses his conscious thinking function and gift of intelligence to achieve it. *Lycopodium* has an excessive persona, whereas *Verat-a*, as expressed by his CD, identifies with his persona of "being a prince," a pseudo-ego with which it is impossible for him to see himself as part of common humanity. He feels with his whole heart that he is a prince and desires to be treated as such. It is a form of malignant narcissism, as it is not supported by any mental acumen, performances, or deeds. He has no special character traits to show off: his ego has become identified with the royal persona simply because, for instance, he has come into riches through an inheritance; this allows him to play the kind, noble prince (*delusion of wealth*; *gestures, makes ridiculous gestures*; *insanity after gaining fortune*; *squanders money*). His prince persona smiles and is courteous and gently condescending, while his ruthlessness, his volatile emotions and *find faulting attitude* are invisibly harbored in his shadow side. In some of his revealing dreams, symbolic for his rigid persona, his clothes will stick to his skin, as if his skin cannot breathe, simply because his persona is an iron mask—it creates a lopsided false personality, which does not allow for emotional growth! *Verat-a* has more serious doubts than *Lycopodium* about his place on the social ladder (*despair about social position*) and compensates even more by taking on the airs of someone with an elevated status (*delusions of grandeur*). The Cyber delusion is also expressed by the following delusions:

Delusion, he himself is Christ
Delusion, he is distinguished
Delusion, he is in communication with God
Delusion, he is a great person
Delusion, he is in heaven talking with God (only remedy!)
Delusion, he is a person of rank
Delusion, as if he is rich
Delusion, he is a messenger of God (only remedy!)

In the above delusions, we see immediately that *Veratrum* has religious overtones which *Lycopodium* does not share. In fact, *Veratrum* has more marked religious delusions than delusions of grandeur; many of his compensations have a religious overtone, especially as the pathology becomes deeper. For example, if *Veratrum* can't succeed in the business world, he will try to rise in the ranks of obscure religious groups or will make sure he is photographed in the company of religious or world leaders. *Veratrum* especially appreciates the power of the church, with its many seemingly docile followers. *Veratrum* will do anything to receive an audience with leaders in society, and he will go to great lengths to be photographed with a president, a religious leader, an actor, or a sportsman to increase his social value—in his own eyes and in the eyes of others. In the process of identifying himself with Christ and God, he develops an extraordinary degree of narcissism.

The delusion that *he himself is Christ* reveals the hidden agenda of the *Veratrum* person especially clearly; this fixed idea is the basis of his actions and thoughts. The true symbol of Christ is the symbol of the savior, the hero of love: a hero who does not want power or try to rule others, who does not want to possess worldly goods. The real Christ is a hero of giving and sharing who appeals to the hearts of people. *Veratrum* believes himself—erroneously, blinded by delusions of grandeur and desperate longing to be someone—to be a savior of the poor and of the underdog. In reality, his aim is to conquer, as he seeks fulfillment through social standing, fame, pride, and power. His kind of religion does not help *Veratrum* to transcend his narcissism and egoism or to flee his inner isolation. *Veratrum* wants to be able to say that he has done something interesting in life and made a difference. His skill lies in his prowess to hold on to power and prestige, so instead of giving, sharing, and being, he is an individual more interested in having, exploiting, and forcing. There is a blatant division between the persona he projects in society and the real being, the man without clothes behind the mask. Such a stark discrepancy leads to extraordinary compensations that are, unfortunately, mostly destructive for the *Veratrum* personality and his associates.

Causalities

Honor Wounded

Above all, *Veratrum* has a fervent desire to be recognized, to be somebody. This strong need for social status certainly stems from a mistaken perception. In contrast to *Lycopodium*, *Verat-a* is not an intellectual, an outstanding student, or an exceptional professional; he is a rather unsophisticated soul, and this fact leads to the NWS *deceived ambition*. *Nux-v* has this NWS as a black type remedy; the difference is that the materialistic *Nux-v* has the drive and tools to reach his goals, and so he often does become a leader. *Veratrum* has the ambition, but not the tools, as we can see from the delusions and provings. Young *Verat-album's* goal, in spite of his limitations, is to be accepted and respected by his parents and peers; often, since he does not have the needed skills (*imbecility*), he discovers that there are other ways to achieve special status. Unfortunately, as noted in the compensations, these other ways are mostly negative. *Verat-a* may wheel and deal his way into becoming class president rather than winning the election based on merit or popularity. As an untreated *Veratrum* ages, this state will deepen in the adult with *pecuniary loss* or *business failure*, which in this case is equal to *ailments from* (*A/F*) *wounded honor* (*consequences of injured pride or honor*). Failing to be elected class president is also considered a business loss and an ailment from wounded honor. As an adult, *Veratrum* may put on a surgical gown while on vacation (when in reality he is an electrician) in order to be perceived as important. Or if thirsty to be accepted, she may fake pregnancy: *fancies herself pregnant or that she will be delivered soon* (*delusion she is pregnant*). These examples show the extremes *Veratrum* uses to attract attention, to be noticed.

Compensations

Search for Fame

In order to heighten his pleasure, *Veratrum* supplements his basic human needs with luxury, delicacies, alcohol, pomp, mania, boasting, lascivious sex, and display. His desires are unlimited, and each gives birth to a new one (*boaster, rich, wishes to be considered rich*; *dipsomania*; *gourmand*). Nothing could suffice to still his cravings and fill the bottomless pit of his heart. He wants to keep up with the Joneses—a nagging preoccupation known as status anxiety. *Veratrum* is foolish enough to exchange the bulk of his life for splendor, rank, pomp, honors, and titles (*despair about social position*; *pompous*). But all the pleasures experienced by the dull consciousness of this simpleton are very poor in comparison with the fullness of life of *Phosphorus* or the true intellect of *Sulphur*. What *Veratrum* wants is fame, but he will never have a claim to fame based on achievement of extraordinary actions or works; this is something about which he can only fantasize. *Veratrum* is a person who engages in extensive image creation or image protection, but there is little connection between his self-promotion and true achievements.

Busy Fruitless Behavior

Although he will deny it vehemently in view of his tasks, which he perceives as noble, *Veratrum* really is *busy fruitless*. There is restlessness in his activities, and this restlessness, alternating with inertia and scheming, keeps him from the possibility of finding meaning in life. Of course, he always speaks more than he says, and he darts from place to place in search of a person or place to confirm for him that there is, in fact, a great need for him and his work in the world. "Go, go!" is his mantra: he finds sitting still, patience, and meditation to be a waste of time.

There is no person in the materia medica more concerned with the way others regard him (*despair about social position*). But *Verat-a*, endlessly seeking esteem and honor, is imprisoned by the limits of his own consciousness, and cannot go beyond these limitations despite his attempts. His excessive persona can change like a chameleon—but it has only one purpose: to increase his value in the eyes of his fellow men. Unfortunately, wealth and rank are no guarantees of inner happiness; this is especially true for *Veratrum*, who feels the need to masquerade indefinitely. He works to maintain his disguise until either he is found out for who he is (and even then, he wages a foolish campaign to reinstate himself) or he runs out of money (which has usually been obtained through an inheritance).

Veratrum gives the impression of being very busy, but his actions are mainly fruitless: *busy restlessness, attempts a great many things, but becomes always tired of them and accomplishes nothing.* Another essential component of his nature is reflected in *an unreasonable hyperactivity* (ADHD). This unreasonable hyperactivity also fits children who can't sit still and or exhibit monomania (such as tapping their fingers or feet for hours on end). This is compulsive behavior, but it often has no specific goal. I once had a patient who, for days at a time, would rip a telephone book into very fine, narrow strips (*tears things; Stram*).

Lying and Cunning

Veratrum is also an expert liar. "One can lie with the mouth," Nietzsche writes, "but with the accompanying grimace one nevertheless tells the truth."[40] *Veratrum's* facial expressions, along with a certain falseness or impropriety in bodily appearance and posture, give away his dishonesty (*attacks of rage with swearing; restless wild look with cold sweat on the face*). Veratrum exploits others as he takes things away from them by force or cunning (*deceitful, sly*); this includes stealing things (like personal notes) to use them against his victims (*inclination to talk about faults of others*). Often feeling insecure about himself, he builds himself up at the expense of others. One can see what a false Christ this person is, in spite of the power of his religious expressions and preaching abilities. *Veratrum* is always ready to make biting remarks about anyone he considers easy prey, anyone who may be momentarily weak. *Veratrum* is a package of lies, anxiety (especially about salvation and social position), and competitiveness all rolled up into one scheming and insolent individual.

If loquacity and religion don't help him achieve his ambitions, *Verat-a* resorts to lying about his achievements (*boaster, wishes to be considered rich*), bullying, or discrediting others to make himself look better. We see in the provings: *never speaks the truth, does not know herself what she is saying.* He will lie, even unconsciously, about his performances, goals, and wealth—just to feel elevated, even temporarily, to the higher social status he so desperately desires. As

40. Friedrich Wilhelm Nietzsche, *Beyond Good and Evil*, trans. Helen Zimmern (Aeterna, 2011, Kindle edition), 53.

mentioned above, *Veratrum* also feigns disease (*he asserts that he is deaf and blind; she asserts she has labor pains; she boasts she is pregnant; she announces her imminent confinement*). In fact, if he has any money (usually, as we have established, it comes from an inheritance), he hands it out to the less fortunate (homeless people, prostitutes) or uses it to bribe his classmates into supporting his leadership. As is true of so many who unexpectedly come into unearned money, *Veratrum* spends it with gusto and throws it away with great élan. His motivation, again, is not generosity; he is no philanthropist like *Aurum*—he only wants to be looked upon as a rescuer and hero for the underdog. Although unearned wealth exempts him of want, it delivers him now to a boredom that must be ameliorated with daily outward fruitless activity as he never finds peace within himself. He also lacks the tools to even contemplate this idleness.

Verat-a may buy expensive presents for his friends or accumulate expensive clothes for himself, even if doing so maxes out his credit card! This irresistible impulse to buy expensive things for others (or self) is very characteristic of *Veratrum*. There is no better audience to preach to than the one you have just bribed (*squandering his money, proud of his position*)! And if that does not help him achieve the desired status, he does not hesitate to get the goods, so to speak, on his opponent (which could be anyone who is more successful or has a higher social status) by snooping in his past or in his private documents in order to discredit him: *disposed to talk about faults of others; if irritated scolding and calling names*. All of this leads him back to the steadfast idea that he is someone special and that he has really reached a special position in society: that of a prince!

Religion

Veratrum has the delusions he comes close to sainthood, or a messiah, or the greatest of anything. This impression of sovereignty, which fills him with such pride, cannot be kept inside; because of his CD, he is virtually compelled to act on it. He wants to be recognized by all and loved by all—nothing less. This is enough to create many of his delusions of megalomania. He has an urgent mission to fulfill, and an emergency message that only he can deliver—a message that will affect the world (*pompous, important; insanity, megalomania; delirium, religious*). The importance of this message is continuously growing in him, and now he has become a prophet and declares himself a warrior for God. His mind becomes feverishly obsessed with points of religious doctrine. Everything he reads and sees reveals to him that the world is in

References

Allen, T.F. *The Encyclopedia of Pure Materia Medica.* New Delhi: B. Jain, 2000.

Artemidorus. *The Interpretation of Dreams (Oneirocritica).* Translated by Robert J. White. Torrance, California: Original Books, 1975.

De Schepper, Luc. *Advanced Guide for Professional Homeopaths.* Santa Fe, NM: Full of Life Publishing, 2008.

Hahnemann, Samuel. *The Chronic Diseases, Volume 1.* New Delhi: B. Jain, 1997.

Jung, Carl G. *Analytical Psychology: Its Theory and Practice: The Tavistock Lectures.* Translated by R.F.C. Hull. New York: Vintage Books, 1968.

---. *The Development of Personality: The Collected Works of C. G. Jung, Volume 17.* Translated by R.F.C. Hull. Princeton University Press, 1991.

---. *Dreams.* Translated by R.F.C. Hull. Princeton University Press, 1974.

---. *The Portable Jung.* Edited by Joseph Campbell. New York: Penguin Books, 1976.

---. *The Practice of Psychotherapy: The Collected Works of C. G. Jung, Volume 16.* Translated by R.F.C. Hull. Princeton University Press, 1933.

---. *The Psychogenesis of Mental Disease: The Collected Works of C. G. Jung, Volume 3.* Translated by R.F.C. Hull. Princeton University Press, 1960.

---. *Psychology of Dementia Praecox.* Translated by R.F.C. Hull. Princeton University Press, 1960.

---. *The Psychology of the Transference.* Princeton University Press, 1966.

Kent, J.T. *Lectures on Homeopathic Materia Medica.* New Delhi: Aggarwal Book Centre, 1990.

Knightley, Philip. *The Master Spy: The Story of Kim Philby.* New York: Vintage, 1990.

Maoshing, Ni. *The Yellow Emperor's Classic of Medicine: A New Translation of the Neijing Suwen with Commentary.* Translated by Maoshing Ni. Boston: Shambhala, 1995.

Nash, E.B. *Leaders in Homeopathic Therapeutics.* New Delhi: Jain Publishers, 1989.

Nietzsche, Friedrich Wilhelm. *Beyond Good and Evil.* Translated by Helen Zimmern. Aeterna, 2011. Kindle Edition.

Schopenhauer, Arthur. *Essays and Aphorisms.* Translated by R.J. Hollingdale. London: Penguin, 1976.

Schroyens, Frederik. *The Essential Synthesis.* London: Homeopathic Book Publishers, and Archibel S.A., 2007.

Sechehaye, Marguerite. *Autobiography of a Schizophrenic Girl: The True Story of "Renee."* Translated by Grace Rubin-Rabson. New York: Penguin, 1994.

Tyler, Margaret. *Homeopathic Drug Pictures.* New Delhi: B. Jain, 1996.

von Boenninghausen, Clemens Maria Franz. *The Lesser Writings.* New Delhi: B. Jain, 1991.

Whitmont, Edward. *Psyche and Substance.* Berkeley: North Atlantic Books, 1991.

Wilde, Oscar. *De Profundis, Complete Works of Oscar Wilde.* New York: Harper Collins Publishers, 1958.

Other Books by Dr. Luc

Advanced Guide for Professional Homeopaths

This book follows *Hahnemann Revisited* and *Achieving and Maintaining the Simillimum.* The latest findings about potencies, miasms and observations of Hering are fine-tuned for clinicians. Eleven intrauterine questions and eleven questions for the homeopath to see if the clinician has the right remedy are explained in detail with clinical examples. In addition, the Cyber delusion is defined and ways of finding it in the clinic. This is an invaluable guide for any professional in practice.

Achieving and Maintaining the Simillimum:
Strategic Case Management for Successful Homeopathic Prescribing

A companion book to *Hahnemann Revisited*; this unique book teaches the reader the most difficult aspect of homeopathy—how to stay on the right course in the challenging path to cure for a chronic patient. "Dr Luc—Homeopath, Hahnemannian scholar, and lecturer—has written a monumental work that will unite all homeopaths. This book documents and teaches Hahnemann's advanced methods, unknown to 90% of practitioners in the world. This long awaited companion book to *Hahnemann Revisited* is a must for every homeopath. This book will help homeopaths become better prescribers and better case managers. More importantly, studying this book will help you restore health to your clients in the most rapid, gentle and permanent way—our highest ideal of therapy (Aph.2)"

Homeopathy and the Periodic Table Braving the Elements—Bridging the Gap
Between Homeopathy and the Elements of the Periodic Table

"Exploring and using only the provings from renowned and reliable sources such as Hahnemann's *Chronic Diseases*, and *Materia Medica Pura*, from Hering's *Guiding Symptoms*, T.F. Allen's *Encyclopedia of Pure Materia Medica*, and von Boenninghausen's *Materia Medica*, Dr. Luc has created a fascinating book about the relationship between homeopathy and the periodic table. A chapter on dream interpretation in homeopathy, used to clarify the proven elements in the periodic table, introduces the serious student of homeopathy to yet another way of finding the simillimum. A MUST for every sincere and serious practitioner."

Hahnemann Revisited A Textbook of Classical Homeopathy for the Professional

A complete and comprehensive guide to the discovery, diagnosis and healing of chronic and acute conditions through homeopathy has served as a guiding light for homeopaths around the world since publication in 1999, and has become the authoritative textbook for homeopathic education. It has been translated into seven languages and is a magnificent treatise covering Homeopathy's foundations, healing process, and the true hereditary factors in medicine—the chronic miasms. Written in an engaging style by a world renowned homeopath who has successfully practiced his art of medicine throughout both the industrialized and less developed countries of the world, this is the first complete, comprehensive modern homeopathic textbook. Some topics covered include: miasmatic prescribing, LM potencies, prioritizing symptoms, using the timeline, the "Never Well Since," case management, adjusting for hypersensitives, nosodes, constitutions, as well as an explanation of Homeopathy and Traditional Chinese Medicine. It is organized into: 25 chapters, 5 appendices (including forms for the practice, sample cases and an extensive chart of symptoms and their miasms), and includes 44 diagrams. *Hahnemann Revisited* provides its readers insights in the mind, body, and soul of the individual; detailing the true basis of health and dysfunction in the spirit Hahnemann intended. This textbook is timeless and will be groundbreaking for generations to come.

The People's Repertory

A guide to acute prescribing for laypeople, including a mini-repertory and materia medica of over 100 remedies commonly used for acute complaints. It also includes an explanation of how to put acute remedies in water for better results, and a description of the half-dozen most common constitutional types.

Human Condition Critical

An explanation of chronic prescribing in homeopathy from the patient's perspective. Includes an explanation of LM potencies and how they work and basic guidance for patients on improving the Vital Force with good nutrition and a healthy lifestyle.

TO ORDER BOOKS BY DR. LUC:

Please visit Dr. Luc's bookstore at his website at drluc.com